# Internationales Symposion der Deutschen Ophthalmologischen Gesellschaft vom 12. bis 14. April 1980 in Freiburg

# Herpetische Augenerkrankungen

## *Herpetic Eye Diseases*

Herausgegeben von
Rainer Sundmacher

Mit 175 Abbildungen und 127 Tabellen

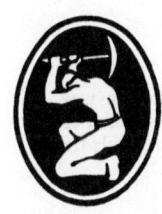

J.F. Bergmann Verlag München 1981

Dozent Dr. Rainer Sundmacher
Augenklinik der Universität Freiburg
Killianstr. 5, D-7800 Freiburg i.Br.

ISBN-13:978-3-8070-0324-5     e-ISBN-13:978-3-642-80499-1
DOI:  10.1007/978-3-642-80499-1

CIP-Kurztitelaufnahme der Deutschen Bibliothek
Herpetische Augenerkrankungen : Internat. Symposium d. Dt. Ophthalmolog. Ges. vom
12. - 14. April 1980 in Freiburg im Breisgau = Herpetic eye diseases / hrsg. von Rainer
Sundmacher. - München : J. F. Bergmann, 1981.
ISBN-13:978-3-8070-0324-5
NE: Sundmacher, Rainer [Hrsg.]; Deutsche Ophthalmologische Gesellschaft; PT

Satz: Fotosatz Service Weihrauch, Würzburg

2119/3321-543210

# Inhaltsverzeichnis — Contents

## Virologic Aspects

## Latency

---

\* Papers which were presented as posters are signified by *P*

## Clinical Virology

## Antivirals

## Different Clinical Experiences

## Interferon

## Keratoplasty

## Zoster Ophthalmicus

## Cytomegalovirus Diseases

# Teilnehmerliste — List of Participants

Abels, E., Dr.med., Schillerstr. 3, 7858 Weil a.Rh.

Arrata, M., Prof. Dr.med., 84 Rue de Rivoli, 75004 Paris, France

Bahmann, D., Dr.med., Seestr. 17, 6460 Gelnhausen

Baringer, R., Prof., M.D., Dept. of Neurology, Univ. of California, San Francisco, Cal. 94121, U.S.A.

Barth, J., Dr.med., Ottostr. 4, 7000 Chur, Schweiz

Behrens-Baumann, W., Dr.med., Univ.-Augenklinik, Robert-Kochstr. 40, 34 Göttingen

van den Bergh, D., Dr.med., Universitaire Instelling Antwerpen, Universiteitsplein 1, 2610 Wilrijk, Belgium

Bettge, F., Dr.med., Rietstr. 3, 7730 VS-Villingen

Bialasiewicz, A., Dr.med., Kurt-Schuhmacher-Str. 38/40, 3000 Hannover

Bigar, F., Dr.med., Univ.-Augenklinik, Rämistr. 100, 8091 Zürich, Schweiz

van Bijsterveld, O.P., Dr.med., Koninklijk Nederlands Gasthuis voor Ooglijders, F.C. Dondersstraat 65, Utrecht, The Netherlands

Blaul, Gudrun, Dr.med., im Klostergarten 2, 6701 Gönnheim

Bloch-Michel, E., Dr.med., 3 Rue Péguy, 75006 Paris, France

Blochinger, A., Dr., Fa. Dr. Winzer, Mainaustr. 146, 7750 Konstanz

Blyth, W.A., Dr., Bacteriology Dept., Medical School, University Walk, Bristol BS8 1TD, England

Böke, W., Prof. Dr.med., Direktor, Univ.-Augenklinik, Hegewischstr. 2, 2300 Kiel 1

Bourne, W.M., M.D., Mayo Clinic, Rochester, Minnesota 55901, U.S.A.

Brenner, J., Dr., Dispersa AG, Postfach 1086, 8401 Winterthur, Schweiz

Brewitt, H., Doz. Dr.med., Augenklinik der Med. Hochschule, Karl-Wiechert-Allee 9, 3000 Hannover

O'Brien, J., Ph.D., Dept. of Ophthalmol. Med. College of Wisconsin, 8700 West Wisconsin Ave, Milwaukee, Wis. 53226, U.S.A.

Bunaes, Unn Benum, Dr.med., Pilestredet 15, Oslo 1, Norway

Burfitt-Williams, G.C.T., M.D. 175 Macquarie St, Sydney, Australia

Cantell, K., Prof. Dr.med., Central Public Health Laboratory, Mannerheimintie 166, 00280 Helsinki 28, Finland

Carreras Matas, B., Prof. Dr.med., Recogidas 39, Granada, Spain

Carter, Clare, B.Sc., Bristol University, Dept. of Surgery, Bristol Royal Infirmary, Bristol BS8 1TD, England

Centifanto, Ysolina M., M.D., L.S.U. Eye Center, 136 South Roman St, New Orleans, Lousiana 70112, U.S.A.

Chastel, C., Prof. Dr.med., Dépt. de Bactériologie Virologie, Faculté de Médecine, B.P. 815, 29279 Brest Cedex, France

Cheng, Y.C., Prof., M.D., Dept. of Pharmacology, School of Medicine, Univ. of North Carolina, Chapel Hill, N.C. 27514, U.S.A.

Chromek, W., Dr.med., Herkomerstr. 111, 8910 Landsberg am Lech

Cioli, S., Dr.med., Clinica Oculistica S. Orsola, Universitá Bologna, Via Massarenti 9, 40138 Bologna, Italia

de Clercq, E., Prof. Dr.med., Rega Institute, 10 Minderbroedersstr., 3000 Leuven, Belgium

Cobo, M., M.D., Duke University Medical Center, Durham, North Carolina 27710, U.S.A.

Colin, J., Dr.med., Centre Hospitalier Régional, Service Daviel, 29279 Brest Cedex, France

Collum, L.M.T., F.R.C.S., 9 Fitzwilliam Place, Dublin 2, Eire

Corydon, L., Dr.med., Hovmarksvej 73, 8700 Horsens, Denmark

Dann, D.F., M.D., Lutwyche Rd, Lutwyche 4030, Brisbane, Australia

Darougar, S., Dr., Institute of Ophthalmology, Judd Street, London WC1H 9QS, England

Delgadillo, R.A., Dr., Department of Medicine, University of Antwerp, U.I.A., 2610 Wilrijk, Belgium

Denis, J., Dr.med., Clinique Ophtalmologique de l'Hôtel-Dieu, 1 Pl. du Parvis Notre Dame, 75181 Paris Cedex 04, France

Dieckhues, B., Prof. Dr.med., Univ.-Augenklinik, Westring 15, 4400 Münster

Drew, C.D.M., Dr., The Wellcome Foundation Ltd, 183 Euston Rd, London NW1 2BP, England

Dünzen, R., Dr.med., Bahnwegle 1, 7813 Staufen

Dunnick, June K., Ph.D., National Institutes of Health, Westwood Bldg, Room 750, Bethesda, Maryland 20205, U.S.A.

Easty, D., F.R.C.S., Bristol Eye Hospital, Lower Maudlin Street Bristol BSI 2LX, England

Egerer, I., Doz. Dr.med., I. Univ.-Augenklinik, Spitalgasse 2, 1090 Wien, Österreich

Epstein, D., M.D., Dept. of Ophthalmology, Karolinska Hospital, 10401 Stockholm 60, Sweden

Erbe, M., Dr.med., Univ.-Augenklinik, Robert-Koch-Str. 4, 3550 Marburg

Falcon, M.G., F.R.C.S., Moorfields Eye Hospital, City-Road, London EC1V 2PD, England

Faulborn, J., Prof. Dr.med., Univ.-Augenklinik, Mittlere Str. 91, 4056 Basel, Schweiz

Felgenhauer, W.-R., Dr.med., 1 Promenade Noire, 2001 Neuchâtel, Schweiz

Feuerhake, C., Dr. med., Augenklinik der Med. Hochschule, Karl-Wiechert-Allee 9, 3000 Hannover

Field, H.J., Dr., Div. Virology, Dept. Pathology, Addenbrookes Hospital, Cambridge CB2 2QQ, England

Foster, C.S., M.D., Mass. Eye and Ear Infirmary, Department of Ophthal., 243 Charles Street, Boston, Mass. 02114, U.S.A.

Franke, Ida, Dr.med., Uferstr. 12, 5600 Wuppertal-Barmen

Gerhard, H., Dr.med., Wasserhohl 15, 6702 Bad Dürkheim

Görtz, Gisela, Dr.med., Oskar-Kühlen-Str. 41. 4050 Mönchen-Gladbach

Gomahr, H., Dr., Gödecke AG, Mooswaldallee 1–9, 7800 Freiburg

Grabner, G., Dr.med., II. Univ.-Augenklinik, Alserstr. 4, 1090 Wien, Österreich

Granzow, Viola, Dr.med., Augusta-Anlage 30, 6800 Mannheim 1

Grimm, J., Dr., Behringwerke AG, Jägerstr. 14–18, 7000 Stuttgart 1

Guimaraes, R., Dr.med., Av. Alfonso Pena 3112, 30.000 Belo Horizonte-MG, Brazil

Gywat, L., Dr.med., Rauracherstr. 33, 4125 Riehen, Schweiz

Härting, F., Dr.med., Univ.-Augenklinik, Hufelandstr. 55, 4300 Essen

Hagenau, W. und G., Drs.med., Univ.-Augenklinik, Röntgenring 12, 8700 Würzburg

Hahr, S., Dr.med., Univ.-Augenklinik, Robert-Koch-Str. 4, 3550 Marburg

Hardt, B., Dr.med., Univ.-Augenklinik, Schleichstr., 7400 Tübingen

Hartmann, Chr., Dr.med., Univ.-Augenklinik, Joseph-Stelzmann-Str. 9, 5000 Köln 41

v. Haugwitz, M., Dr.med., Neckarstr. 55, 7300 Esslingen

zur Hausen, H., Prof. Dr.med., Direktor, Institut für Virologie am Zentrum für Hygiene der Univ., Hermann-Herder-Str. 11, 7800 Freiburg

Heimann, J., Dr.med., Grabenstr. 4, 7770 Überlingen

Hellenthal, J., Dr.med., Univ-Augenklinik, Prittwitzstr. 43, 7900 Ulm

Hetland, R., M.D., 420 Pine Lane, Los Altos, California 94022, U.S.A.

Hill, T.J., Dr., Bacteriology Dept., Med. School, University Walk, Bristol BS8 1TD, England

Hilsdorf, C., Dr.med., Chefarzt der Augenklinik, 9053 Teufen, Schweiz

Hoffmann, F., Doz. Dr.med., Augenklinik im Klinikum Steglitz der FU, Hindenburgdamm 30, 1 Berlin 45

Holmgren, T., M.D., Dept. of Ophthalmology, Central Hospital, 63188 Eskiltuna, Sweden

Holtmann, H.W., Prof. Dr.med., Univ.-Augenklinik, Venusberg, 5300 Bonn

Holtmann,    ., Dr.med., Univ.-Augenklinik, Venusberg, 5300 Bonn

Horchler, W., Alcon Pharma GmbH, Habsburger Str. 134, 7800 Freiburg

van Husen, H., Dr.med., Hauptstr. 1, 7822 St. Blasien

Jaeger, W., Prof. Dr.med., Direktor, Univ.-Augenklinik Bergheimerstr., 6900 Heidelberg

Jeker, J., Dr.med., Mittelsdorfstr. 59, 5033 Buchs, Schweiz

Jones, B.R., Prof., F.R.C.S., Institute of Ophthalmology and Moorfields Eye Hospital, City Road, London EC1V 2PD, England

Junker, C., Dr.med., Moorgärten 16, 2848 Vechta

Jungwirth, C., Prof. Dr., Institut für Virologie und Immunbiologie der Univ., Versbacher Landstr. 7, 8700 Würzburg

Karobath-Baum, E., Dr. med., Krankenanstalten der Rudolfstiftung der Stadt Wien, Boerhaavegasse 8, 1030 Wien, Österreich

Kaufman, H.E., M.D. Prof. and Chairman, L.S.U. Eye Center, 136 S Roman Street, New Orleans, Lousiana 70112, U.S.A.

Klauber, Anne, Dr.med., Eye Department, Rigshospitalet, Blegdamsvej, 2100 Copenhagen, Denmark

Kneer, M., Dr.med., Beyerstr. 18, 7900 Ulm

Knöbel, H., Dr.med., Augenklinik Univ.-Krankenhaus Eppendorf, Martinistr. 52, 2000 Hamburg 20

Kok-van Alphen, Clare, M.D., Dept. of Ophthalmology, Academisch Ziekenhuis-Leiden, Rijnsburgerweg 10, Leiden, The Netherlands

Kollmar, F., Deutsche Wellcome GmbH, Postfach 109, 3006 Burgwedel 1

Kommerell, G., Prof. Dr.med., Univ.-Augenklinik, Killianstr., 7800 Freiburg

Korra, A., Prof. Dr.med., Univ. Eye Clinic, 17 Raml Station Square, Alexandria, Egypt

Kortüm, G.F., Dr.med., Univ.-Augenklinik, Schleichstr. 12, 7400 Tübingen

Kosik, Doris, Dr.med., Klinik für Augenkrankheiten, Kantonsspital, 9000 St. Gallen, Schweiz

Koskenoja, M., Dr., Hannikaisenk. 11–13 B. 36, Jyváskylá, Finland

Kraus-Mackiw, Ellen, Prof. Dr.med., Univ.-Augenklinik, Bergheimerstr., 6900 Heidelberg

Kritzinger, Erna E., F.R.C.S., Birmingham and Midland Eye Hospital, Church Street, Birmingham B3 2NS, England

Lalau, C., Dr.med., Dept. Ophthalmology, Academisch Ziekenhuis-Leiden, Rijnsburgerweg 10, Leiden, The Netherlands

Leaford, Tricia, The Wellcome Foundation Ltd, 183 Euston Road, London NW1 2BP, England

Lenhard, V., Dr.med., Institut für Immunologie und Serologie der Univ., Im Neuenheimer Feld 305, 6900 Heidelberg

Lichtwer, H., Dr. Gerhard Mann GmbH, Brunsbütteler Damm 165–173, 1000 Berlin 20

Lienert, F., Dr.med., Gustav-Vorsteher-Str. 5, 5802 Wetter 1

Linden, T., Dr.med., Univ.-Augenklinik, Westring 15, 4400 Münster

Löbering, H.G., Dr., Dr. Thilo u. Co GmbH, Rudolf-Diesel-Ring 21, 8021 Sauerlach

Lopes Cardozo, O., Dr.med., Hospital Free Univ., Dept. Ophthalmology, de Boelelaan 1117, 1081 HV Amsterdam, The Netherlands

Lorenz, Birgit, Dr.med., Univ.-Augenklinik, Mathildenstr. 8, 8000 München

Luther, Eva, Instituto Barraquer, Calle Laforja 88, Barcelona-21, Spain

Maas, G., Prof. Dr.med., Direktor, Hyg.-bakt. Landesuntersuchungsamt, Postfach 3809, 4400 Münster

Mackensen, G., Prof. Dr.med., Direktor, Univ.-Augenklinik, Killianstr., 7800 Freiburg

MacLachlan, J.E. and Anne, Drs., 124 Kent Rd, Pascoevale 3044, Victoria, Australia

Mahoney, K., The Wellcome Foundation Ltd, 183 Euston Road, London NW1 2BP, England

Marsh, R., F.R.C.S., Moorfields Eye Hospital, City Road, London EC1V 2PD, England

Masuyama, Y., M.D., Dept. of Ophthalmology, Miyazaki Med. College, Kiyotake, Miyazaki 889–16, Japan

Maudgal, P.C., Dr.med., Academisch Ziekenhuis St. Rafael, Kapucijnenvoer 7, 3000 Leuven, Belgium

Mayer, H., Dr.med., Augenklinik des Katharinenhospitals, Kriegsbergstr. 60, 7000 Stuttgart 1

McGill, J.I., F.R.C.S., Southampton Eye Hospital, Wilton Avenue, Southampton SO9 4XW, England

Mellin, Fr. Dr., Univ.-Augenklinik, Hufelandstr. 55, 4300 Essen 1

Merk, W., Dr., Dr. Karl Thomae GmbH, 7950 Biberach an der Riss

Mertz, M., Doz. Dr.med., Augenklinik rechts der Isar, Ismaninger Str. 22, 8000 München 80

Miestereck, H., Dr.med., Dr. Thilo und Co GmbH, Rudolf-Diesel-Ring 21, 8021 Sauerlach

Moser, H., Dr., Behringwerke AG, Postfach 11 40, 3550 Marburg 1

Müller, O., Dr.med., Konradstr. 7, 5000 Aarau, Schweiz

Murray, K.S., Dr., 24 Collins Street, Melbourne 3000, Australia

Mustakallio, Anja, Dr., Solnantie 9.A.6., Helsinki 33, Finland

Naumann, G.O.H., Prof. Dr.med., Direktor, Univ.-Augenklinik, 8520 Erlangen

Nesser, Ulrike, Dr.med., Getreidegasse 27, 5020 Salzburg, Österreich

Neubauer, H., Prof. Dr.med., Direktor, Univ.-Augenklinik, Joseph-Stelzmannstr. 9, 5000 Köln 41

Neubauer, L., Dr.med., Univ.-Augenklinik, Mathildenstr. 8, 8000 München

Neumann-Haefelin, D., Doz.Dr.med., Institut für Virologie am Zentrum für Hygiene der Univ., Hermann-Herder-Str. 11, 7800 Freiburg

Noeske, D., Dr.med., Augenabteilung des Johanniter-Krankenhauses, 5300 Bonn

Nordmann, G., Dr.med., Augenklinik am St. Josefs-Hospital, Dreieckstr. 17, 5800 Hagen

Öberg, B., Doz. Dr., Astra Läkemedel AB, Research and Development Lab., 15185 Södertälje, Sweden

Oh, J.O., M.D., Ph.D., Proctor Foundation, Univ. of California Med. Ctr., San Francisco, Cal. 94143, U.S.A.

Ohrloff, C., Dr.med., Univ.-Augenklinik, Venusberg, 5300 Bonn

Orsoni, Jelka G., Dr.med., Clinica Oculistica dell'Università, 43100 Parma, Italia

Ossendorff, I., Dr.med., Eichenhofstr. 21, 5231 Lindlar

Ottovay, Eva, Dr.med., Eye Department, Rigshospitalet, Blegdamsvej, 2100 Copenhagen, Denmark

Pape, R., Prof. Dr.med., Brucknerstr. 37, 7600 Offenburg

Papendick, U., Dr., Birkendorfer Str. 65, 7950 Biberach an der Riss

Papst, W., Prof.Dr.med., Chefarzt, Augenklinik AK-Barmbek, Rübenkamp 148, 2000 Hamburg 60

Polack, F.M., Prof., M.D. Dept. of Ophthalmol., Univ. of Florida, College of Medicine, Box J-248, Gainesville, FL 32610, U.S.A.

Pollard, R.B., M.D., Dept. of Medicine, Infectious Diseases, Univ. of Texas Medical Branch, Galveston, TX 77550, U.S.A.

Prusoff, W.H., M.D., Prof. and Chairman, Dept. of Pharmacology, Yale Univ. School of Med., 333 Cedar Street, New Haven, Conn. 06510, U.S.A.

Raptis, N., Dr.med., Schützengraben 5, 7880 Bad Säckingen

Ravenscroft, T., Wellcome Research Laboratories, Langley Court Beckenham, Kent BR3 3BS, England

Raydt, G., Dr.med., Univ.-Augenklinik, Mathildenstr. 8, 8000 München 2

Reich, M.E., Dr., Univ.-Augenklinik, Auenbruggerplatz 4, 8036 Graz, Österreich

Renard, G., Dr.med., Service d'Ophthalmologie, Centre Hospitalier Régional, 29279 Brest Cedex, France

Rentsch, F., Doz. Dr.med., Univ.-Augenklinik, Postfach 23, 6800 Mannheim 1

Rippel, W., Dr.med., Obere Landstr. 3, 3500 Krems, Österreich

Röhr, W.D., Dr.med., Uhlandstr. 17, 8400 Regensburg

Roesen, U., Dr.med., Lt. Arzt d. Augenabteilung des St. Josefskrankenhauses, Hermann-Herder-Str. 1, 7800 Freiburg

Romano, Amalia, Dr.med., 86 Gordon Street, Tel Aviv, Israel

Rossignol, A., Dr.med., Clinique Ophthalmologique de l'Hôtel-Dieu, 1 Pl. du Parvis Notre Dame, 75181 Paris Cedex 04, France

Roussos, J., Dr.med. (see Dr. Rossignol)

Royer, J., Prof., Université Besançon 25000, France

Runge, J., Dr.med., Dr. Thilo und Co GmbH, Rudolf-Diesel-Ring 21, 8029 Sauerlach

Rutllan, J., Dr.med., Instituto Barraquer, Calle Laforja 88, Barcelona-21, Spain

Sawada, A., M.D., Prof. and Head, Dept. of Ophthalmology, Miyazaki Med. College, Kiyotake, Miyazaki 889-16, Japan

Scriba, Marianne, Dr., Sandoz Forschungsinstitut GmbH, Brunnerstr. 59, 1235 Wien, Österreich

Seydewitz, F., Dr.med., Fritz-Geiges-Str. 22, 7800 Freiburg

Shiota, H.M., M.D., Ph.D., Dept. of Ophthalmology, Tokushima Univ. School of Med., Kuramoto-Machi, Tokushima, Japan

Singh, M., M.D., 57 Joshi Colony, The Mall, Amritsar, India

Smolin, G., M.D., Proctor Foundation, Univ. of California Med. Ctr., San Francisco, Cal. 94143, U.S.A.

Söser, Margarete, Dr.med., Univ.-Augenklinik, Anichstr. 35, 6020 Innsbruck, Österreich

van de Sompel, W., Dr.med., Universitaire Instelling Antwerpen, Universiteitsplan 1, 2610 Wilrijk, Belgium

Soyer, Patrice, Laboratoires Luneau, 3 rue d'Edinbourg, Paris VIII, France

Spaleck, C., Dr.med., Holbeingasse 2, 8078 Eichstätt

Sundmacher, R., Doz. Dr.med., Univ.-Augenklinik, Killianstr., 7800 Freiburg

Schenk, D., Dipl.-Biol., Asta-Werke AG, Kaiserstr., 4802 Halle i. W.

Scherz, W., Dr.med., Wesselswerth 34, 43 Essen 16

Schildberg, P., Dr.med., Allmendenweg 8, 4660 Gelsenkirchen-Buer

Schmack, E.N., Dr.med., Wermingser Str. 47, 5860 Iserlohn

Schmidt, D., Doz. Dr.med., Univ.-Augenklinik, Killianstr. 7800 Freiburg

Schmitter-Westerman, Grünewaldstr. 7, 2880 Brake

Schmitz-Valckenberg, P., Dr.med., Löhrstr. 139, 5400 Koblenz

Schultz, R.O., M.D., Prof. and Head, Dept. of Ophthalmol., Med. College of Wisconsin, 8700 West Wisconsin Ave, Milwaukee, WI 53226, U.S.A.

Schwartz, F., Dipl.-Biol., Selecta-Verlag, Passinger Str. 8, 8033 Planegg

Stärk-Zamboch, Gudrun, Dr.med., Lüpertzender Str. 29, 4050 Mönchengladbach 1

Stolze, H., Dr.med., Augenklinik im Klinikum der RWTH, Goethestr. 5100 Aachen

Streissle, G., Dr., Institut f. Immunologie und Onkologie der BAYER AG, Aprather Weg, 5600 Wuppertal 1

Sturrock, G.D., F.R.C.S., Univ.-Augenklinik, Mittlere Str. 91, 4056 Basel, Schweiz

Tams, G., Dr.med., Augenklinik im ZKH, St. Jürgen-Straße, 2800 Bremen

Tapasztó, I., Dr.med., Villám I. u. 8, Kecskemét, Hungary

Tenner, A., Prof. Dr.med., Kneippweg 11, 7988 Wangen/Allgäu

Thiel, H.J., Prof. Dr.med., Univ.-Augenklinik, Hegewischstr. 2, 2300 Kiel

Thompson, P., M.D., Clinique Ophthalmologique de l'Hôtel-Dieu, 1 Pl. du Parvis Notre Dame, 75181 Paris Cedex 04, France

Thon, B., Dr.med., Augenklinik, Krankenanstalten der Rudolfstiftung der Stadt Wien, Boerhaavegasse 8, 1030 Wien, Österreich

Tjoa, S.T., Dr.med., Hospital Free University, Dept. Ophthalmol. B 445, de Boelelaan 1117, 1081 HV Amsterdam, The Netherlands

Townsend, Jeannette J., M.D., Dept. of Pathology, 595 HSW, Univ. of California Med. Ctr., 3rd and Parnassus Avenues, San Francisco, California 94143, U.S.A.

Trauzettel-Klosinski, Susanne, Dr.med., Univ.-Augenklinik, Schleichstr., 7400 Tübingen

Treffers, W.F., Dr., Kerkstraat 18, Mook, The Netherlands

Trousdale, M.D., Ph.D., Estelle Doheny Eye Foundation, 1355 San Pablo, Los Angeles, California 90033, U.S.A.

Tullo, A.B., F.R.C.S., Bristol Eye Hospital, Lower Maudlin Street, Bristol BS1 2LX, England

Uchida, Y., M.D., Prof., Dept. of Ophthalmology, Tokyo Women's Med. Coll., 10 Kawada-cho, Shinjuku-ku, Tokyo 162, Japan

Unger, H.H., Prof. Dr.med., Günterstalstr. 9, 7800 Freiburg

Varnell, Emily, Prof., L.S.U. Eye Center, 136 S. Roman St, New Orleans, Lousiana 70112, U.S.A.

Victoria-Troncoso, V., Dr.med., Dept. of Ophthalmology, Rijksuniversiteit-Gent, de Pintelaan 135, 9000 Gent, Belgium

Völker, Dr.med., Univ.-Augenklinik, Venusberg, 5300 Bonn 1

Völker-Dieben, H.J.M., Dr.med., Diaconessenhuis, Houtlaan 55, Leiden, The Netherlands

Voigt, G.J., Dr.med., Evang. Krankenanstalten, Du-Nord, Augenklinik, 4100 Duisburg 11

Waller, W., Doz. Dr.med., Univ.-Augenklinik, Josef-Schneider-Str. 11, 8700 Würzburg

Waring, G.O., III, M.D., Prof., Dept. of Ophthalmol, Emory Univ. Clinic, 1365 Clifton Road, N.E., Atlanta, Georgia 30322, U.S.A.

Waubke, Th.N., Prof. Dr.med., Direktor, Univ.-Augenklinik, Hufelandstr. 55, 4300 Essen 1

Weber, U., Dr.med., Univ.-Augenklinik, Robert-Koch-Str. 40, 3400 Göttingen

Wendel, Elke, Dr.med., Danzigerplatz 4, 6700 Ludwigshafen

Westkott, H.G., Dr.med., Wickeder Hellweg 81, 4600 Dortmund 13

Wilcke, R., Dr.med., Augenklinik, Kantonsspital, 6004 Luzern, Schweiz

Wilhelmus, K.R., M.D., Moorfields Eye Hospital, City Road, London EC1V 2PD, England

Winter, R., Dr.med., Augenklinik im ZKH, St. Jürgen-Strasse, 2800 Bremen

Witmer, R., Prof. Dr.med., Direktor, Univ.-Augenklinik, Rämistr., 8006 Zürich, Schweiz

Witschel, H., Doz. Dr.med., Univ.-Augenklinik, Killianstr., 7800 Freiburg

Wollensak, J., Prof.Dr.med., Direktor, Univ.-Augenklinik im Klinikum Charlottenburg, Spandauer Damm 130, 1000 Berlin 19

Wright, P., F.R.C.S., Moorfields Eye Hospital, City Road, London EC1V 2PD, England

Yamane, S., M.D., Dept. of Ophthalmology, Tokushima Univ. Med. School, Kuramoto-Machi, Tokushima, Japan

Yates, W., Dr., 2A Mylne St., Toowoomba 4350, Australia

Zirm, M., Doz. Dr.med., Univ.-Augenklinik, Anichstr. 35, 6020 Innsbruck, Österreich

Zotti, Anneliese, Dr.med., Augenklinik, Krankenanstalten der Rudolfstiftung der Stadt Wien, Boerhaavegasse 8, 1030 Wien, Österreich

# Danksagung

An erster Stelle sei meinem Lehrer Prof. Mackensen und den DOG-Vorstandsmitgliedern der Jahre 1978–80 mit ihren Vorsitzenden Prof. Küchle, Prof. Neubauer und Prof. Böke sowie dem Schriftführer Prof. Jaeger dafür gedankt, daß sie mir die Organisation dieses Symposiums anvertrauten und mir bei der Durchführung alle Unterstützung gewährten.

Daß das Symposium dann in einer freundlichen und effizienten Weise stattfinden konnte, ist das Verdienst sehr vieler Mitarbeiter der Universitätsaugenklinik Freiburg und anderer Universitätsstellen, die unbürokratisch und mit Begeisterung geholfen haben. Als Beispiel für viele nenne ich nur Frl. Kukula, Fr. Mattes, H. Bernhard, H. Gruber, H. Preuninger, H. Walzer, H. Welz und Dr. Haug. Auch die Stadt Freiburg mit ihrem Oberbürgermeister Dr. Keidel erwies sich als liebenswürdige Gastgeberin.

Bei der anschließenden redaktionellen Arbeit waren die Mitarbeiter des J.F. Bergmann Verlages, München, eine große Hilfe.

Meiner Frau und meinen Kindern danke ich sehr dafür, daß sie Verständnis für die erforderliche Arbeit aufbrachten und mich trotz zu häufiger Abwesenheit dennoch weiter zur Familie rechneten.

R. Sundmacher

Den nachstehenden Firmen danken wir für ihre Unterstützung.
We would like to thank the following companies for their support: Gödecke, Freiburg – Dr. Thilo, Sauerlach – Dr. Winzer, Konstanz – Titmus-Eurocon, Aschaffenburg – Alcon Pharma, Freiburg – Dr. Mann, Berlin – The Wellcome Foundation, London – Basotherm, Biberach – Dispersa Baeschlin, Winterthur – Astra Läkemedel, Södertälje – Bayer, Wuppertal-Elberfeld – Behring, Marburg – Thomae, Biberach – Spingler-Tritt, Jestetten

Sundmacher, R. (Hrsg.):
Herpetische Augenerkrankungen
© J.F. Bergmann Verlag, München 1981

# Ansprache des Ersten Vorsitzenden der Deutschen Ophthalmologischen Gesellschaft

W. Böke, Kiel

Ladies and Gentlemen,

I would like to welcome all of you on behalf of the "Deutsche Ophthalmologische Gesellschaft" – the German Ophthalmological Society. We are particularly glad that this meeting has attracted so many participants and such a large number of experts from all over the world. Thank you very much for coming.

Indeed, our topic is not only a very important one, but a very exciting one, too. Much progress has been made in the field of herpetic ocular disease during the last ten years. However, many problems must still be solved. I think that this meeting will be a further step forward in improving both the scientific understanding of the host-virus interaction within the ocular structures as well as our knowledge of the best treatment of its clinical manifestations.

However, before we begin, let us take a look back to the time when nobody knew that corneal disorders can actually be caused by herpes viruses.

Seventy years ago, the dendritic keratitis was considered to be a degenerative lesion. From *1912–1914, Wilhelm Grüter*, later Professor of Ophthalmology at the University of Marburg (Germany), studied this experimentally. He demonstrated its infectious nature by transferring human herpes material onto the rabbit cornea. Grüter was the first to successfully reproduce the dendritic keratitis experimentally in rabbits and he postulated its viral origin.

Unfortunately, World War I stopped further studies and postponed the publication of the results obtained so far by Grüter. It was not until 1920 that Wilhelm Grüter reported his revolutionary findings to the "Deutsche Ophthalmologische Gesellschaft" in Heidelberg.

I think there is no better way to start our meeting than to remind ourselves of his discovery, which certainly belongs to the major events in ophthalmological history of the early 20th century.

I hope that this meeting will be a successful and pleasent one for all of you.

Thank you very much.

Wilhelm Grüter (1882–1963)[1]

---

[1] Für die Überlassung der Fotografie von W. Grüter danken wir H. Neubauer, Köln.

Sundmacher, R. (Hrsg.):
Herpetische Augenerkrankungen
© J.F. Bergmann Verlag, München 1981

## Begrüßung

D. Sasse, Freiburg, Dekan der Medizinischen Fakultät der Albert-Ludwigs-Universität

Meine sehr verehrten Damen und Herren, sehr geehrter Herr Vorsitzender,

zum internationalen Symposium der DOG über herpetische Augenerkrankungen darf ich Sie im Namen der Medizinischen Fakultät unserer Universität Freiburg ganz herzlich begrüßen. Wie Sie alle wissen, ist es ein besonderer Vorzug solcher Symposien, daß sie sich ganz speziellen Themen zuwenden können, um durch die Kombination von theoretischer und klinischer Forschung den aktuellen Stand einer Problematik von allen Seiten zu beleuchten.

Nun, daß dieser Überblick über ein solches Spezialgebiet sehr gründlich geschieht und alles andere ist und natürlich auch sein will als irgend eine „Fortbildungsschnellbleiche", dafür bürgen nicht nur die Namen der Veranstalter hier, denen ich ganz herzlich meinen Dank sage, sondern auch die große Zahl der Referenten. Nicht zuletzt läßt auch der noch verhältnismäßig große Zeitraum von insgesamt zweieinhalb Tagen mit recht frühem Beginn und spätem Ende Sorgfalt erkennen. Dieses alles spricht für eine Gründlichkeit, die eigentlich allen Medizinern eigen sein sollte, zu der aber die Augenärzte in besonderer Art historisch verpflichtet sind. Vielleicht ist es Ihnen allen bekannt – mir war es bis vor kurzem, dies muß ich zugeben, neu –, daß der Hippokratische Eid, der, wie Sie wissen, durch die Mittlerrolle der arabischen Medizin zu uns ins Abendland gekommen ist, in antiken Lehrbüchern mit einem Zusatz versehen wurde. Zusätzlich zu dem allgemeinen Satz: „ich werde niemandem ein tödliches Gift verabreichen" steht hier als ein fachärztlicher Appendix: „oder eine Salbe, welche die Sehkraft zu vernichten oder zu schwächen in der Lage ist". Hier haben wir also sozusagen eine schon recht frühe fachärztliche Anerkennung mit einem allerdings etwas drohenden Hinweis.

Mögen Sie also von hier wissenschaftlichen und ärztlichen Gewinn mitnehmen und lassen Sie sich in den wohl doch noch verbleibenden Zwischenzeiten auch etwas anrühren von der Stadt und von der Umgebung Freiburgs, auf die wir hier – allerdings ganz ohne eigenes Verdienst – immer sehr stolz sind.

Sundmacher, R. (Hrsg.):
Herpetische Augenerkrankungen
© J.F. Bergmann Verlag, München 1981

# Begrüßung

G. Mackensen, Freiburg, Direktor der Universitäts-Augenklinik

Sehr verehrte Kolleginnen und Kollegen, liebe Gäste aus vieler Herren Länder, Spektabilität,

die Freiburger Augenklinik, selbst in einem länderverbindenden Grenzgebiet Deutschlands gelegen, freut sich, in diesen Tagen Gastgeber sein zu dürfen für eine stattliche Zahl von Wissenschaftlern, die sich mit dem speziellen aber wichtigen Problem der Herpesviruserkrankungen des Auges in den verschiedensten Gegenden der Welt befassen. Sie alle sind herzlich willkommen und wir danken Ihnen für Ihre Teilnahme. Viele werden nach London weiterreisen, um dort die 100-Jahresfeier der Englischen Ophthalmologischen Gesellschaft miterleben zu können und im Anschluß daran wird Sie der VI. Europäische Kongreß in Brighton angezogen haben. Wir sind glücklich, daß uns diese weitaus glanzvolleren Kongreßereignisse die Möglichkeit gaben, Sie über Freiburg zu leiten und zu einem Arbeits-Symposium zu vereinen.

Bitte verstehen Sie, wenn sich aus dieser Grundauffassung einige Konsequenzen ergeben. Es wird intensiv zu arbeiten sein. Auch der Rahmen unseres Symposiums ist einem Arbeitstreffen angepaßt. Statt gesellschaftlich repräsentativer Umrahmung wollen wir Ihnen und den begleitenden Damen schlichte landesübliche Unterhaltung zur Entspannung bieten. Wir hoffen, daß dies Ihre Zustimmung findet, ja wir erwarten sogar, daß Sie auf diese Weise mehr von den Eigentümlichkeiten dieses Landes zwischen den Vogesen und dem Schwarzwald und von der Art, in ihm zu leben, erfahren. Es ging uns auch darum, die Kosten gering zu halten, um den Assistenten die Teilnahme zu ermöglichen.

Wichtig ist es mir, daß hier ein Symposium abgehalten wird, das von einem Wissenschaftler unserer jüngeren Generation geplant, vorbereitet und gestaltet wurde. Ich freue mich darüber, daß die Deutsche Ophthalmologische Gesellschaft Rainer Sundmacher diese Gelegenheit gab, nachdem seine Arbeiten auf dem Gebiet der Viruserkrankungen des Auges Interesse gefunden haben, und ich danke unserer Fachgesellschaft dafür, daß sie in dieser Weise unseren wissenschaftlichen Nachwuchs fördert. Mich werden Sie dementsprechend in der Rolle dessen sehen, der mit Interesse beobachtet, wie sich einer seiner aktiven Mitarbeiter nun auch in einer solchen Aufgabe bewähren wird. Allein die Liste der Symposiumsteilnehmer spannt meine Erwartungen hoch.

Dr. Sundmacher hat viele seiner klinischen Studien zusammen mit dem von Professor zur Hausen geleiteten Institut für Virologie ausgeführt. Sein Partner ist dort Dr. Neumann-Haefelin. Dies Symposium gibt mir Veranlassung, für diese mustergültige und kontinuierliche Zusammenarbeit zwischen einem Institut und einer Klinik zu danken und sie zu empfehlen. Sie lernen Herrn zur Hausen als Präsidenten der ersten Sitzung kennen.

Ich hoffe, Sie werden sich in Freiburg wohlfühlen, unsere Augenklinik als einen Platz empfinden, an dem man sich bemüht, unsere Wissenschaft voranzutreiben und an dem man weltoffen ist.

Das sind meine Gedanken, die ich dem Symposium voranstellen möchte.

Sundmacher, R. (Hrsg.):
Herpetische Augenerkrankungen
© J.F. Bergmann Verlag, München 1981

## Eröffnungsansprache

R. Sundmacher, Freiburg

Meine sehr verehrten Damen und Herren, Spektabilität,

auch ich möchte Sie hier in Freiburg ganz herzlich willkommen heißen und Ihnen wünschen, daß alle Ihre Erwartungen an dieses Symposium erfüllt werden. Eine meiner Erwartungen zumindest ist schon eingetroffen: Das Auditorium ist reichlich gefüllt mit Herpes-Spezialisten und Herpes-Enthusiasten vieler Fachrichtungen und Länder, die sich auch nicht davon haben abschrecken lassen, daß wir uns weitgehend in Englisch werden unterhalten müssen. So viel Interesse ist, glaube ich, ein gutes Omen.

Ladies and Gentlemen,

I think I need not stress how glad I am to welcome you all to Freiburg. Many of you have traveled quite a few miles and I would like to say how much I appreciate your efforts.

Before we start with the program, I have to make some announcements.

I would like the English-speaking community to keep in mind that the majority of us are not native speakers and that you, therefore, should speak up as clearly as possible.

I have been asking the chairmen to be very strict with the time schedule. When you start with your presentation, you will get a green light; one minute before the end of your time, the light will change yellow and then red. Red means that you must stop immediately unless you want the chairman and the audiance to kick you out.

We should try to make the discussions as effective as possible. We have four portable microphones down here and two stationary upstairs. Before you start talking, get yourself a microphone, wait for a sign from the chairman, then say your name – we need this for identification of the tapes – and only then start with your question; preferably only one at a time. The speaker should answer immediately. It would certainly be helpful if you wouldn't forget that other people may also have some questions. Please, do not present "prepared discussion remarks together with some slides" unless you have obtained permission from the chairman before the session.

If, up to the end of the discussion time, "vital" questions could not be placed or answered, I would suggest that you give me your question on a sheet of paper, and we will see whether we can include it together with the answer in the report.

To make posters more attractive, we have integrated them in the program with a normal discussion time. The author will be down here to briefly summarize his poster, and a slide of the poster will help you remember details of it and any questions you may have. To make this a meaningful arrangement, it is mandatory that you study the posters before the sessions.

If you have already clarified a problem in a private discussion with the author but feel that this problem may be of general interest, we would welcome your comment in the audience.

And now let's start: It is a real pleasure to ask Professor zur Hausen, virologist and herpes and tumor viruses specialist, to chair the first session.

# Virologic Aspects

Sundmacher, R. (Hrsg.):
Herpetische Augenerkrankungen
© J.F. Bergmann Verlag, München 1981

# Herpesviruses — Common Properties and Heterogeneity

D. Neumann-Haefelin, R. Sundmacher, Freiburg

**Key words.** Herpes viruses – physical and biological properties, HSV-1 strain specificity and heterogeneity, dendritic keratitis

**Schlüsselwörter.** Herpesviren – physikalische und biologische Eigenschaften, HSV-Stammeigenschaften und Heterogenität, Keratitis dendritica

**Summary.** The natural occurrence of herpes viruses has been demonstrated within a broad range of animal species. All herpes viruses share typical properties of the group, such as common morphology and the ability to establish persistent infections. Nevertheless, the different herpes viruses of man (HSV 1 and 2, VZV, CMV and EBV) as well as those of animals are quite distinct from each other. Immunological cross-reactivity and molecular DNA studies have shown that there is more affinity between biologically similar herpes viruses of different host species than between different herpes viruses of one individual species (except HSV 1 and HSV 2). All members of the herpes virus group studied so far display an extensive heterogeneity of strains. Sixty-three corneal HSV 1 isolates were compared for intratypic strain differences. Studies of biological properties (neurovirulence in mice) and biochemical analysis (DNA cleavage with restriction endonucleases) revealed considerable differences between individual strains. Attempts to correlate biological and biochemical strain characteristics with clinical features failed. One explanation for this outcome may be that many other pathophysiological factors are involved in the pathogenesis of herpetic diseases. Nevertheless, further studies on the heterogeneity of viral strains are considered necessary for elucidation of the pathogenesis of herpetic diseases.

**Zusammenfassung.** Herpesviren kommen im gesamten Bereich der Wirbeltiere vor und besitzen ohne Unterschied die Strukturmerkmale der Herpesvirusgruppe:

Das komplette Virus besteht aus dem von einer lipidhaltigen Membran umschlossenen Ikosaederförmigen Nucleocapsid (ca. 100 nm Durchmesser;

162 Capsomere) und enthält als Virus-Genom einen DNS-Doppelstrang mit einem Molekulargewicht von ca. 100 Millionen. Die allen Herpesviren gemeinsame wichtigste biologische Eigenschaft ist ihre Fähigkeit, persistierende Infektionen hervorzurufen. Abgesehen von diesen Gemeinsamkeiten sind die menschlichen Herpesviren, Herpes simplex Virus Typ 1 und Typ 2 (HSV 1 und 2), Varizellen-Zoster Virus (VZV), Zytomegalievirus (CMV), Epstein-Barr Virus (EBV) ebenso wie die tierischen Herpesviren sehr verschieden.

Immunologische Untersuchungen und molekulare DNS-Analysen haben gezeigt, daß zwischen den biologisch ähnlichen Herpesviren verschiedener Wirtsspezies engere Verwandtschaft besteht als zwischen den verschiedenen Herpesviren einer bestimmten Spezies. Die einzige bisher bekannte Ausnahme, die sich wahrscheinlich aus der Evolution erklärt, stellt die sehr nahe Verwandtschaft zwischen den menschlichen HSV-Typen 1 und 2 dar. Bei allen Mitgliedern der Herpesvirusgruppe läßt sich eine sehr starke Heterogenität einzelner Stämme feststellen. Dies mag an der Größe und dem besonderen Aufbau des Herpesvirus-Genoms liegen, wodurch wahrscheinlich eine besonders häufige genetische Rekombination ermöglicht wird. In den vorliegenden Untersuchungen wird über Stammunterschiede bei 63 kornealen HSV 1-Isolaten als Beispiel für intratypische Heterogenität berichtet. Untersuchungen biologischer Eigenschaften (Neurovirulenz bei Mäusen) und biochemische Analysen (DNA-Spaltmuster mittels Restriktionsendonukleasen) zeigten erhebliche Unterschiede zwischen den einzelnen Stämmen. Versuche, diese Unterschiede der biologischen und biochemischen Marker mit den klinischen Verläufen zu korrelieren, schlugen allerdings fehl. Eine Erklärungsmöglichkeit hierfür liegt vielleicht darin, daß außer den Stammeigenschaften der Herpesviren noch viele andere pathophysiologische Einflüsse bei der Genese herpetischer Erkrankungen beteiligt sind. Dennoch sind weitere Untersuchungen der Heterogenität der einzelnen Herpesstämme mit verschiedenen Methoden wünschenswert und notwendig, um den Einfluß der

Virus-Stammspezifität auf die Pathogenese herpetischer Erkrankungen zu klären.

Herpesviruses are enveloped, spherical particles composed of a core containing double stranded DNA, and of 162 capsomeres. The symmetric architecture of the capsid gives the particle the shape of an ikosahedron, which is common to some other virus groups, too.

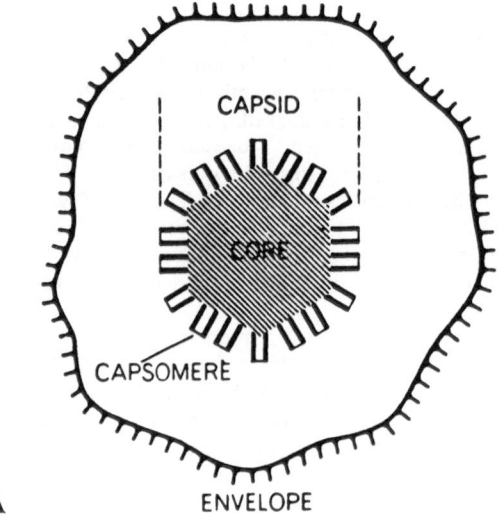

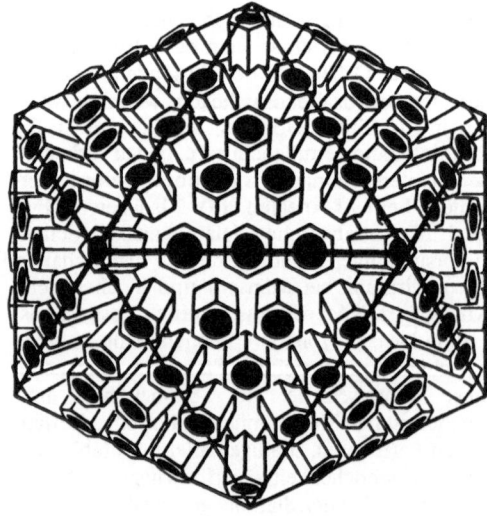

**Fig. 1A and B.** Structures of the herpes virus particle. **A** Architecture of the complete virion. **B** Model of the nucleocapsid. (From: Horne RW. The structure of viruses. Copyright 1963 by Scientific American, Inc. All rights reserved)

However, the diameter of the nucleocapsid, about 100 nm, is characteristic, as is the appearance of the capsomeres with deep 4 nm wide holes in them. Therefore identification in the electron microscope is quite easy and reliable as far as the *group* is concerned, whereas within the herpes group different members are morphologically indistinguishable [18]. The complete herpes virus particle is wrapped into a lipoprotein envelope, which is obtained from host cell membranes during generation of mature virions. As it bears the receptors for adsorption to the host cell, the envelope is a prerequisite for viral infectivity (Fig. 1).

Table 1 lists a number of viruses that share the structural characteristics just mentioned, and thus are classified as herpes viruses. This list, being still far from complete, was compiled mainly to indicate that herpes viruses occur over the whole range of vertebrates: from man and monkeys through other mammalian animals down to avian, fish, amphibian and reptilian species. Another property, common to all herpes viruses beside morphology, is their ability to induce persistent infections. In man as well as in animals this may result either in various disease conditions, or in a silent carrier state. In addition, there are infections with certain herpes viruses that lead to the formation of tumors, either in the natural host – like Marek's disease of chickens or the Lucké tumor of frogs – or in experimental hosts – like herpes virus saimiri or herpes virus ateles in monkeys. It is not the task of this short review to go into the problem of oncogenesis by herpes viruses. However, the breadth of expression of different herpes *infections* that is observed despite many common properties of herpes *viruses*, should be emphasized.

Older comparative studies [19] suggested multiple connexions between different herpes viruses. They were mainly based on serological investigations. Today we know that many of these data resulted from unspecific cross reactions. Recently introduced novel methods of peptide analysis by immunoprecipitation [6, 9] are going to revise the picture of antigenic relationship, and have so far revealed that some of these herpes viruses are more distantly related.

In the last few years another approach for determining the nature of herpes viruses was very successful, and shed light on fundamen-

**Table 1.** Examples of herpesviruses harboured by different vertebrate hosts

| Human herpesviruses | Other mammalian herpesviruses | Avian herpesviruses |
|---|---|---|
| Herpes simplex virus 1 and 2 | Equine abortion virus | Marek's disease virus |
| Human cytomegalovirus | Equine herpesvirus 2 and 3 | Turkey herpesvirus |
| Varicella-zoster virus | Equine cytomegalovirus | Duck plaque virus |
| Epstein-Barr virus | Pseudorabies virus | Avian laryngotracheitis virus |
| | Bovine rhinotracheitis virus | Owl herpesvirus |
| *Simian herpesviruses* | Bovine cytomegalovirus | Lake Victoria comorant virus |
| Herpes B virus | Bovine mamillitis virus | Pigeon virus |
| Herpesvirus saimiri | Feline rhinotracheitis virus | |
| Herpesvirus ateles | Canine herpesvirus | *Fish, amphibian and reptiliano herpesviruses* |
| Herpesvirus aotus | Herpesvirus cuniculi | |
| Patas monkey herpesvirus | Herpesvirus sylvilagus | Channel catfish virus |
| Baboon herpesvirus | Guinea pig herpesvirus 1 and 2 | Frog virus 4 |
| Simian EB-like viruses | Rat cytomegalovirus | Lucké virus |
| Simian varicella-like viruses | Murine cytomegalovirus | Snake herpesvirus |
| Simian cytomegaloviruses | | |

tal features of the group: the analysis of herpes virus DNAs.

Some of the principles and methods [1] in this work are illustrated in Figs. 2 and 3, mainly focusing on herpes simplex virus type 1 (HSV 1) as an example. As already mentioned above, the herpes virus genomes consist of double stranded DNA. Its general structure in the virion is a single linear molecule of about 100 million Daltons molecular weight (Table 2). DNA double strands will separate into the complementary single strands upon treatment with heat or alkali. This process is reversible, which means that the single strands will renaturate (reanneal) under appropriate conditions.

If there exist any repeated and simultaneously inverted sequences in the double strand, parts of the single strands will be complementary to each other and selfanneal, forming one or several loops (Fig. 2, left). These can be visualized in the electron microscope. In the search for genome homology of *different* viruses, denatured DNAs of

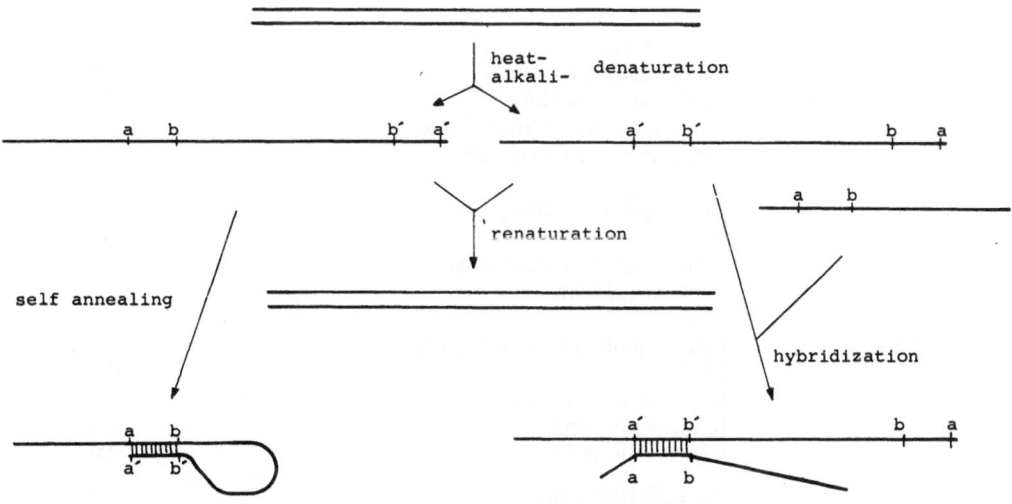

**Fig. 2.** Principles of the detection of intra- and intermolecular DNA homologies

5

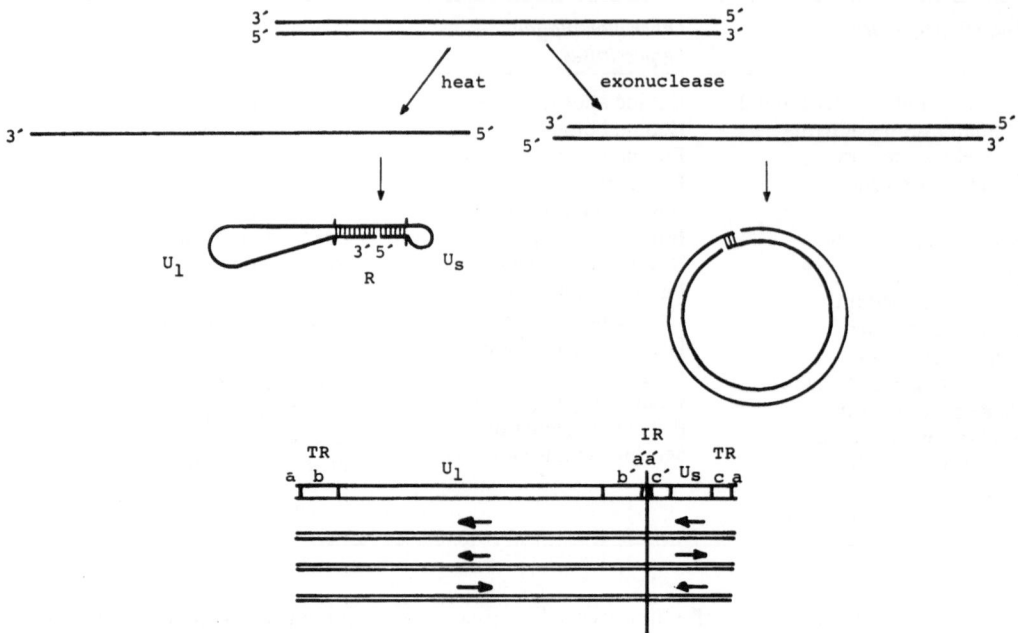

**Fig. 3.** Analysis of the basic structure and arrangement of HSV 1 DNA. $U_1$ = unique long region; $U_s$ = unique short region; R = repeated regions; IR = internal repeats; TR = terminal repeats

**Table 2.** Current nomenclature of herpesviruses

| Family: | Herpesvirus group | |
|---|---|---|
| | | DNA Mol. weight/$10^6$ |
| Subfamily Alpha: | Herpes simplex virus group | |
| | HSV 1 | 98 |
| | HSV 2 | |
| | Herpes B virus | |
| | Bovine mamillitis virus | 88 |
| | Equine abortion virus | 92 |
| |    probably other equine, feline, | |
| |    canine etc. herpesviruses | |
| Subfamily Beta: | Cytomegalovirus group | |
| | Human CMV | 142 |
| |    probably other mammalian | 132 |
| |    cytomegaloviruses | |
| Subfamily Gamma: | Lymphoproliferative virus group | |
| | EBV | 105 |
| | EBV-like simian viruses | |
| | Herpesvirus saimiri | 103 |
| | Herpesvirus ateles | 90 |
| ("Orphan" | Varizella-zoster virus | 80 |
|   perhaps Delta) |    probably related simian viruses | |

these viruses are mixed and incubated under annealing conditions. The complementary regions of otherwise heterologous single strands will hybridize (Fig. 2, right). By the use of radioactively labeled DNA those hybrid double strands may easily be detected.

Fig. 3 shows what happens, when annealing and hybridization techniques are applied to herpes simplex virus type 1 DNA. Heat denatured DNA of intact single strands will form two loops which are linked by a double stranded "handle" of annealed DNA regions [13]. In the right hand experiment of Fig. 3 an intact HSV 1 DNA double strand is treated with an exonuclease digesting only the nucleotides of the 3' ends of each strand. If there is homology of the terminal sequences, the resulting single stranded 5' ends are complementary, forming so-called sticky ends, and the DNA molecule will circularize upon annealing. This phenomenon is found with DNA of herpes simplex virus as well as all other herpes viruses investigated so far.

The interpretation of these findings is given by the arrangement of the herpes simplex type 1 DNA in Fig. 3. Two unique regions ($U_1$ and $U_S$) are bounded by the repetitious sequences. These are inverted at the internal site of the genome (IR), relative to the terminal sequences (TR). Further experiments revealed that this arrangement is present in four isomeric forms in any population of herpes simplex particles [5], as at the joint between the internal repeats of the long and those of the short region, switching back and forth may occur as indicated by the arrows.

Figure 4 shows the arrangement of herpes simplex DNA together with some other herpes virus DNAs in the circular form. It turned out that several herpes viruses display a certain limited similarity to the herpes simplex arrangement, like human cytomegalovirus (CMV) and pseudorabiesvirus (PRV), whereas others are quite different, such as Epstein-Barr virus (EBV), herpes

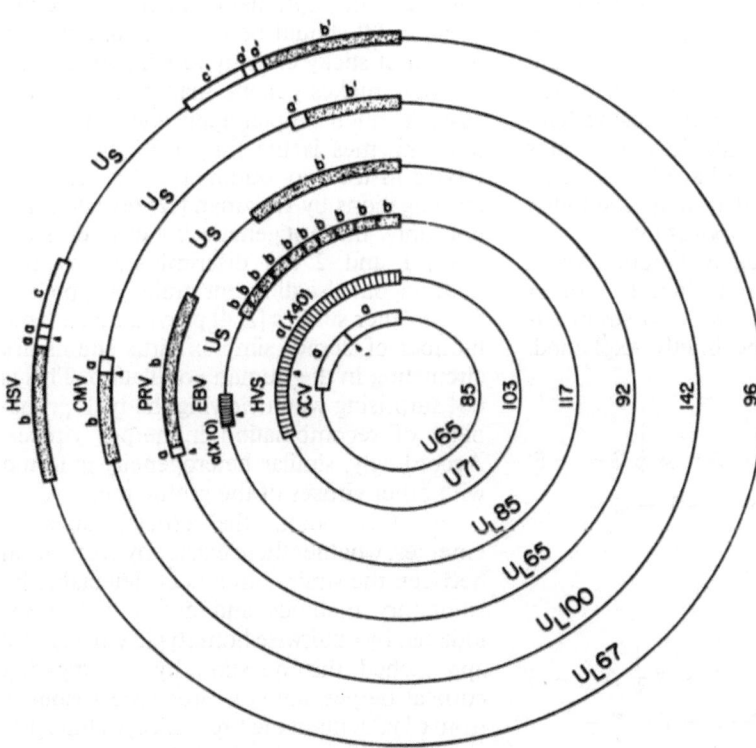

**Fig. 4.** Sequence arrangement of different herpes virus DNAs. Figures indicate the molecular length ($1/10^6$ Daltons) of the unique regions (U), the unique long regions ($U_l$), the unique short regions ($U_s$) and the whole genomes, respectively. (Cold Spring Harbour, 1979; Fourth Meeting on Herpesviruses)

virus saimiri (HVS), or the channel catfish virus (CCV). In studies on DNA sequence homology, cross hybridization could be demonstrated only in biologically similar viruses of *different* hosts. Human Epstein-Barr virus and Epstein-Barr-like simian viruses, human and monkey cytomegalo-viruses, herpes simplex virus and the simian B virus, and perhaps bovine mamillitis virus reveal homologies at least to a limited extent. This may be a consequence of evolutionary affinities. Negative hybridization results were obtained with different herpes viruses of the *same* host. The only exception is the 50% homology between the herpes simplex virus types 1 and 2.

On the basis of molecular data like sequence homology, or genome arrangement and length (Fig. 4), and of biological properties, a new subgrouping of herpes viruses was recently adopted [7]. Viruses of roughly similar DNA size and arrangement seem to fit well into subfamilies called alpha, beta, and gamma (Table 2). Varicella-zoster virus is still an orphan in the scheme, because its purification and analysis at the molecular level is largely restricted by culturing difficulties. The provisional state of this nomenclature should be noted, as for instance Marek's disease virus and turkey herpes virus, both causing lymphoproliferative disease, and thus candidates for gamma, turned out to have DNA structures rather more similar to herpes simplex virus than to Epstein-Barr virus [3].

Another fundamental technique, which has become important in the investigation of general DNA structures *and* viral strain differences as well, will be briefly explained.

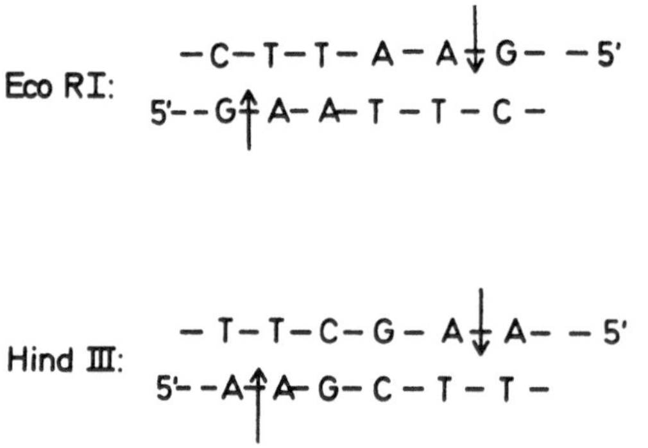

Eco RI:

$$-C-T-T-A-A \downarrow G- \ -5'$$
$$5'--G \uparrow A-A-T-T-C-$$

Hind III:

$$-T-T-C-G-A \downarrow A- \ -5'$$
$$5'--A \uparrow A-G-C-T-T-$$

**Fig. 5.** Recognition sequences of Eco RI and Hind III restriction endonucleases

This is the use of the so-called restriction enzymes, bacterial endonucleases, whose action is restricted to a certain sequence within a DNA double strand. Two examples are given in Fig. 5: Eco RI derived from E. coli and Hind III from Haemophilus influenzae. By those enzymes, DNAs are cleaved into well defined fragments dependent on the occurrence of the recognition sequence (Fig. 6). The fragments are designated A, B, C, D, a. s. on. according to their length. For separation and size determination the fragments are usually run by electrophoresis through an agarose gel, where they form bands in positions due to their particular size (Fig. 6).

Several techniques based on restriction enzyme cleavage have become most valuable tools in the process of characterizing DNA viruses. In the past few years they have facilitated a variety of new approaches towards functional maps of viral genomes, which cannot be described in detail in this short overview. Anyway, the sequence identification of DNA fragments by the so-called blot hybridization technique [14] and the large complex of optionally directed recombination [8] should be mentioned. The formation of sticky ends by restriction enzyme cleavage makes genetic manipulations very easy. A much simpler application of restriction enzymes is the fingerprinting of viral DNAs in the way outlined in Fig. 6. Early investigations by Roizman [12] revealed that not only the antigenetically distinct HSV types 1 and 2 are discriminated by this method, but also different strains of type 1. In fact, further studies [2, 4] proved that a large number of herpes simplex virus strains are circulating in the human population. This is not surprising when viewing the high probability of recombination in herpes viruses. Accordingly, similar heterogeneity is found with other viruses of the group, too.

At this point, the crucial question emerges, whether there exists any correlation between the strain differences detectable by laboratory methods and different diseases induced by otherwise homotypic viruses. We approached this question by investigating corneal herpes simplex virus type 1 isolates from 63 patients of the Freiburg eye clinic [10], using methods which have been previously described in detail [11]. Simultaneously, these patients were included in therapeutic studies [15–17] and thoroughly scored for differences

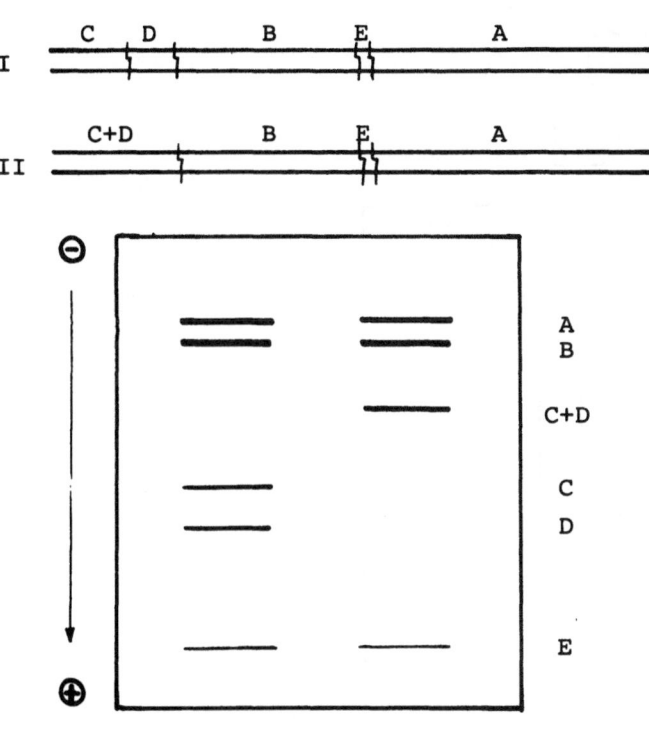

**Fig. 6.** Map of restriction enzyme cleavage sites on two DNA double strands (I and II) discriminated by the missing cleavage site, with II, between fragments C and D. Different patterns resulting from agarose gel electrophoresis of the fragments

in clinical features. Restriction enzyme cleavage of the viral DNAs revealed heterogenous patterns, as was expected. Figure 7 shows pairs of electrophoresis patterns of DNA fragments generated by Eco RI and by Hind III. The seven different herpes simplex type 1 DNAs discriminated by these enzymes are representative for 38 viral DNAs obtained from different patients. Rather disappointing was the outcome of attempts to correlate the clustering of DNA markers with clinical findings: Neither by subtle analyses of disease his-

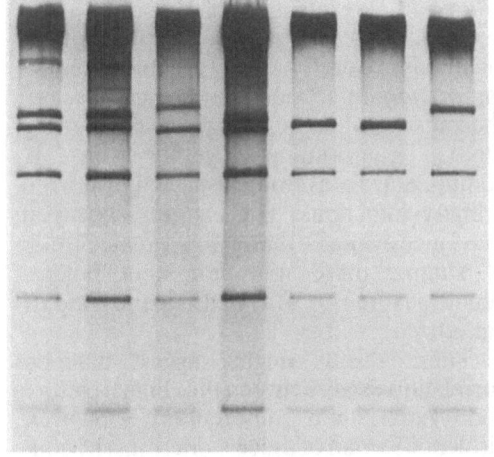

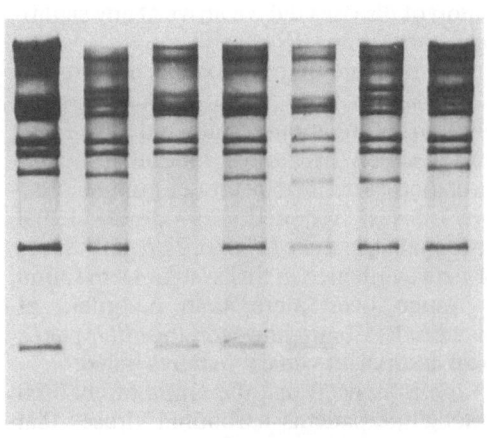

A                                                                                                                                    B

**Fig. 7A and B.** Agarose gel electrophoresis patterns of Eco RI (**A**) and Hind III (**B**) digests of corneal HSV 1 isolates

9

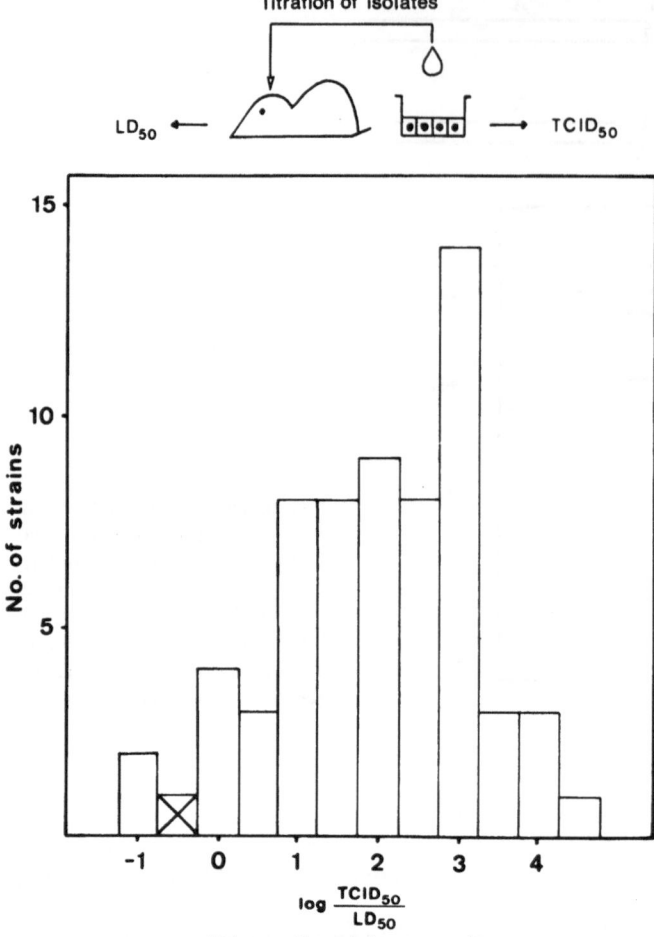

**Fig. 8.** Range of neurovirulence of 63 corneal HSV 1 isolates and the MacIntyre laboratory strain (X)

tories and courses, nor by an overall classification of diseases did we arrive at any significant correlation [11].

At the same time we extended biological examinations onto these isolates. Parallel titrations in the mouse brain and in cell culture resulted in figures indicating neurovirulence, as defined by the cell culture infective doses required to cause lethal encephalitis in mice (Fig. 8). The differences of neurovirulence in this system were found to range over more than 5 orders of magnitude. Again, however, the attempt at a correlation with clinical features failed.

It was noticed that the group of children among the patients harboured viruses that were mainly found to belong to the most virulent ones in the mouse assay. We suspected that at least in some of these cases primary

herpes simplex infections had occurred at the ocular site. In order to prove whether particular strains are preferentially capable of inducing *primary* infections with clinical disease, the most virulent isolates were retested by DNA fingerprinting together with 12 additional isolates from suspected or proven primary infections. The patterns shown in Fig. 9 give evidence that, as in the major group of strains, there was prominent heterogeneity, in the Eco RI as well as in the Hind III pattern.

These results might suggest that no correlation exists between the clinical picture and viral strain differences. However, virulence in man of a given virus must be considered as a result of a variety of viral *and* host factors. Particularly in the case of recurrent herpetic disease, the function of host control

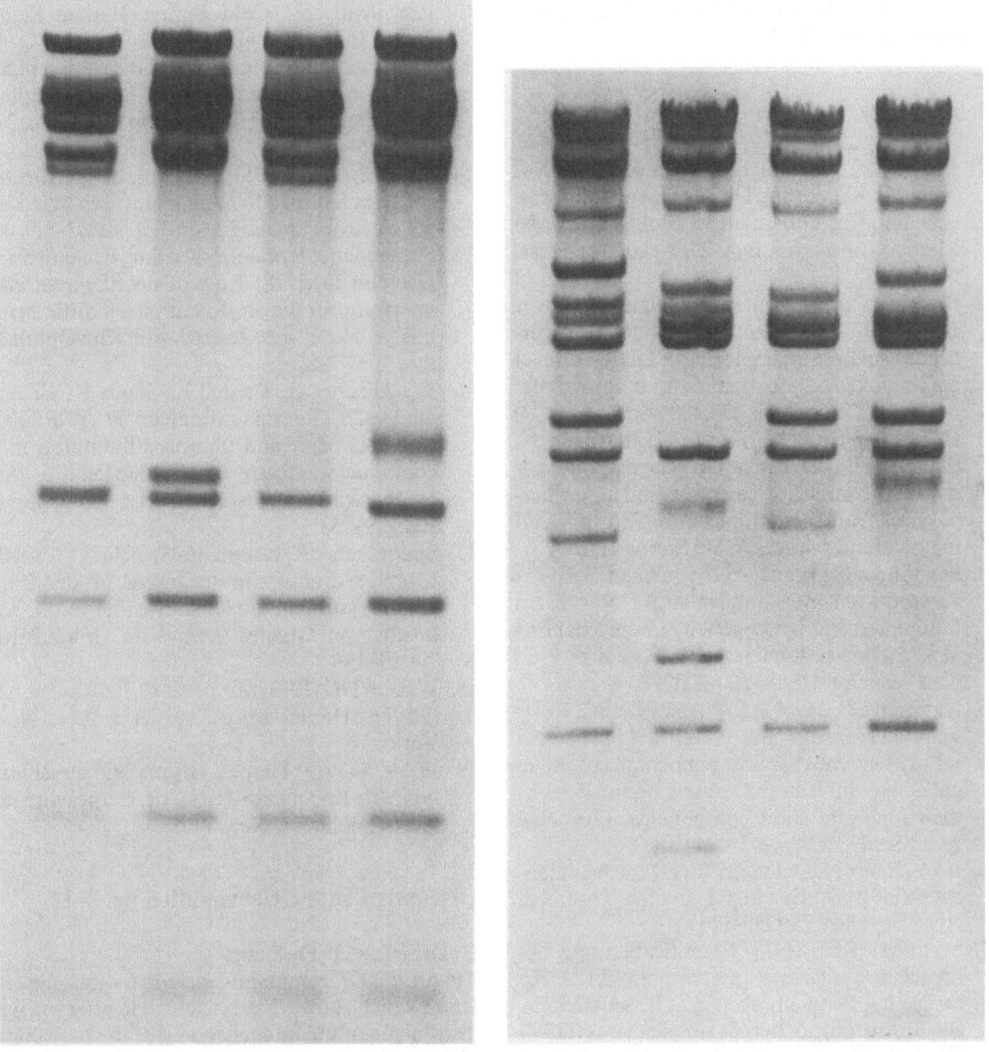

A

B

**Fig. 9A and B.** Agarose gel electrophoresis patterns of Eco RI (**A**) and Hind III (**B**) digests of corneal HSV 1 isolates derived from patients suspected for primary ocular herpes

mechanisms may play a major role in pathogenesis. The variability of viral properties implicated in this complex may be considerable, too. This is likely with herpes viruses in particular because of their extremely large genome and the probability of recombination. On the other hand, many sites in the genome and several gene products may be involved in the processes determining virulence. Thus, one viral strain may become more virulent by means different from another strain; and both again may display quite dissimilar properties in the laboratory animal as compared to man.

In conclusion, we feel that the lack of correlation as yet between laboratory markers and clinical features of ocular herpes simplex virus infections is not surprising from the virological point of view. From the ophthalmological standpoint it is neither if one considers the broad spectrum of herpetic ocular diseases.

Further investigations of viral structural and functional differences will be the only way towards understanding the implication of viral properties in pathophysiological mechanisms.

**Acknowledgment.** The experimental part of this work was supported by the Deutsche Forschungsgemeinschaft (Ne 213/1).

## References

1. Britten RJ, Graham DE, Neufeld BR (1974) Analysis of repeating DNA sequences by reassociation. In: Grossman L, Moldave K (eds) Methods of enzymology 29. Academic Press, New York
2. Buchman TG, Roizman B, Adams G, Stover BH (1978) Restriction endonuclease fingerprinting of herpes simplex virus DNA: A novel epidemiological tool applied to a nosocomial outbreak. J Infect Dis 138:488–498
3. Cébrian J, Kaschka-Dierich C, Berthelot N, Sheldrick P (1979) Inverted repeats in the genomes of Marek's disease virus and turkey herpesvirus. Pers. communication. Fourth Meeting on Herpesviruses, Cold Spring Harbor
4. Hayward GS, Frenkel N, Roizman B (1975) Anatomy of herpes simplex virus DNA: Strain differences and heterogeneity in the locations of restriction endonuclease cleavage sites. Proc Natl Acad Sci USA 72:1768–1772
5. Hayward GS, Jacob RJ, Wadsworth SC, Roizman B (1975) Anatomy of herpes simplex virus DNA: Evidence for four populations of molecules that differ in the relative orientations of their long and short components. Proc Natl Acad Sci USA 72:4243–4247
6. Ito Y, Spurr N, Dulbecco R (1977) Characterization of polyoma virus T antigen. Proc Natl Acad Sci USA 74:1259–1263
7. Matthews REF (1979) Classification and nomenclature of viruses. Intervirology 12:129–296
8. Morse LS, Pereira L, Roizman B, Schaffer PA (1978) Anatomy of herpes simplex virus (HSV) DNA. X. Mapping of viral genes by analysis of polypeptides and functions specified by HSV-1 × HSV-2 recombinants. J Virol 26:389–410
9. Mueller-Lantzsch N, Yamamoto N, Hausen H zur (1979) Analysis of early and late Epstein-Barr virus associated polypeptides by immunoprecipitation. Virology 97:378–387
10. Neumann-Haefelin D, Sundmacher R, Wochnik G, Bablok G (1978) Herpes simplex virus types 1 and 2 in ocular disease. Arch Ophthalmol 96:64–69
11. Neumann-Haefelin D, Lenz T, Sundmacher R (1979) Strain characteristics and features of ocular infection of herpes simplex virus type 1 isolates. Med Microbiol Immunol (Berl) 167: 239–250
12. Roizman B, Kozak M, Honess RW, Hayward G (1974) Regulation of herpesvirus macromolecular synthesis: Evidence for multilevel regulation of herpes simplex 1 RNA and protein synthesis. Cold Spring Harbor Symp Quant Biol 39:687–701
13. Sheldrick O, Berthelot N (1974) Inverted repetitions in the chromosome of herpes simplex virus. Cold Spring Harbor Symp Quant Biol 39: 667–678
14. Southern EM (1975) Detection of specific sequences among DNA fragments separated by gel electrophoresis. J Mol Biol 98:503–517
15. Sundmacher R, Cantell K, Haug P, Neumann-Haefelin D (1978) Role of debridement and interferon in the treatment of dendritic keratitis. Albrecht von Graefes Arch Klin Ophthalmol 207:77–82
16. Sundmacher R, Cantell K, Skoda R, Hallermann Ch, Neumann-Haefelin D (1978) Human leukocyte and fibroblast interferon in a combination therapy of dendritic keratitis. Albrecht von Graefes Arch Klin Ophthalmol 208:229–233
17. Sundmacher R, Neumann-Haefelin D, Cantell K (1976) Successful treatment of dendritic keratitis with human leukocyte interferon. Albrecht von Graefes Arch Klin Ophthalmol 201:39–45
18. Watson DH (1973) Morphology. In: Kaplan AS (ed) The Herpesviruses. Academic Press, New York
19. Wildy P (1973) Herpes: History and classification. In: Kaplan AS (ed) The Herpesviruses. Academic Press, New York

## Discussion on the Contribution pp. 3–12

H. zur Hausen (Freiburg)
Thank you Dr. Neumann-Haefelin for this presentation which shows that considerable progress has been made in the understanding of the molecular biology of herpes viruses; but as we will learn from subsequent contributions, a number of biological phenomena and virus-host interactions are still very poorly understood. Are there questions?

J. Wollensak (Berlin)
Did you find any correlation between the therapy with antimetabolic substances and different strains?

D. Neumann-Haefelin (Freiburg)
No, we didn't find any differences in this respect.

R. Baringer (San Francisco)
Did you look at any of the coat glycoproteins of your HSV isolates, and did you attempt to make any correlation? I ask this because it may be the glycoproteins which are primarily responsible for the virus-host interaction.

D. Neumann-Haefelin (Freiburg)
No, we didn't do any protein analysis in this work.


J.O. Oh (San Francisco)
Have you done comparative study between type 1 and type 2 Herpes simplex virus on biologic and biochemical characteristics?

D. Neumann-Haefelin (Freiburg)
All HSV strains investigated in this study were type 1 isolates.

Sundmacher, R. (Hrsg.):
Herpetische Augenerkrankungen
© J.F. Bergmann Verlag, München 1981

# Herpes Simplex Virus Strain Specificity: Virulence Correlates

H.E. Kaufman, New Orleans

**Key words.** HSV-1 strain specificity and heterogeneity, stromal keratitis, glycoproteins

**Schlüsselwörter.** HSV-Stammeigenschaften und Heterogenität, Stromaherpes, Glycoproteine

**Summary.** We know very little about why some people get recurrences of herpesvirus infections and others do not, and why some herpes infections are particularly severe and others are not. Considerable work has been done on host immune responses, but there is relatively little information available concerning the differences among strains within a given type of herpesvirus.

In examining strains of herpesvirus type 1, we find that the avirulent strains are inherently different from the virulent strains in terms of the ocular disease they produce. The avirulent strains colonize the ganglion and are shed into the tear film, yet these strains do not cause disease and prevent ganglionic colonization with the more virulent strains. It has been shown that a large proportion of the adult population carries antibodies to herpesvirus, indicating that previous infection occurred, even in the absence of overt disease. A large proportion also have herpesvirus in the ganglia, and enzymatic cleavage mapping indicated that all ganglia are infected with the same herpesvirus strain. It may be that, in most of us, the clinically-evident herpesvirus disease is related more closely to the particular strain of herpesvirus with which the patient was infected than to the state of the host immune system, although, if the immune system is totally suppressed, even benign organisms can cause disease.

We have attempted to correlate observed differences in the biochemical structures and metabolic processes of the various virus strains with the different types of disease produced by these strains, and it appears, for example, that those strains producing necrotizing stromal disease produce highly immunogenic glycoproteins unlike the strains that produce only epithelial disease.

**Zusammenfassung.** Warum manche Menschen an Herpes-Rezidiven leiden und andere nicht, und warum einige Infektionen ausgesprochen schwer verlaufen und andere nicht, darüber wissen wir eigentlich nichts. Über Immunreaktionen des Wirtes ist sehr viel gearbeitet worden, nur verhältnismäßig wenig aber über die „intratypischen" Stammunterschiede beim Herpes simplex-Virus. Nach unseren Untersuchungen gibt es virulente und avirulente Herpes simplex-Virus-Typ 1-Stämme. Die avirulenten scheinen sich im Ganglion auszubreiten, werden in den Tränenfilm ausgeschieden, führen aber zu keiner Erkrankung und können vielleicht sogar einen gewissen Schutz gegenüber den virulenteren Stämmen bieten. Wenn wir uns überlegen, daß die meisten Patienten ohne erkennbare Immunsuppression an Herpes erkranken, dann kann man sich vorstellen, daß hauptsächlich die Stammunterschiede der Herpesstämme und weniger der Zustand des Immunsystems für die Art der resultierenden Erkrankung verantwortlich ist. Obwohl das Immunsystem natürlich auch eine Rolle spielt und bei völliger Unterdrückung des Immunsystems auch sonst avirulente Erreger eine Erkrankung erzeugen können.

Wir haben versucht, biochemische Unterschiede bei den verschiedenen Isolaten mit dem klinischen Verlauf bei den Patienten zu korrelieren, von denen sie isoliert wurden, und fanden dabei, daß z.B. Stämme, die eine nekrotisierende Stromaentzündung hervorrufen, auch gleichzeitig hochgradig immunogene Glykoproteine induzieren, während Virusstämme, die nur einen epithelialen Herpes hervorrufen, dies nicht tun.

Fewer than 25% of the population infected with herpesvirus show clinical signs of herpetic ocular disease, and of those who do, some have only superficial, transient infections and others suffer severe, sometimes blinding disease. As the immunological aspects of herpesvirus infection have been elucidated, it has been suggested that the victims of severe and disabling herpetic infections are in some way immunodeficient, which allows the virus to do more damage than would be possible in a normal, immunocompetent host. However, because I find it difficult to accept the idea of so many immunodeficient individuals, I believe that other factors must be involved.

The differences between type 1 and type 2 herpesvirus have been delineated [5]. Within these types, however, there is tremendous diversity among the various strains, as work with herpesvirus in laboratory animals has shown. Some isolates of herpesvirus type 1 cause trivial disease and minimal infection relatively independent of titer. Others produce death in a high proportion of animals, and still others produce moderate disease, stromal necrosis and other manifestations that seem peculiar to the isolate but relatively independent of the amount of the virus in the inoculum [12]. That is, there are virulent strains and relatively avirulent strains, and there are strains that produce stromal disease in a high proportion of animals and strains that do not. If we stipulate that immunodeficiency cannot be a primary factor in randomly selected rabbits, it seems to follow that herpesvirus isolates vary considerably in their disease-causing potential.

Stevens and Cook [11] and Baringer and Swoveland [2] have established that herpesvirus can colonize the sensory ganglia, and Nesburn et al. [9] and others have shown that both sensory and sympathetic ganglia can be colonized by herpesvirus. Studies of trigeminal neurectomy indicate that the ganglion can serve as a source of reinfection for cutaneous herpesvirus in patients who never had previous clinical disease; irradiation of the trigeminal ganglion can cause bursts of virus shedding and recurrent herpetic infection in animals [10].

Virus shedding has been observed both in the saliva and in the tears [6]. In general, virus does not seem to persist in the cornea or in the skin after infection. Virus shedding into the tears frequently precedes corneal involvement in the rabbit. It is not clear whether shedding into the tears is the source of corneal infection in all cases, or whether virus can infect the cornea directly from the nerves. Infection of the central cornea has been seen in patients having corneal transplants with no effective innervation. This suggests that some, if not all, recurrences may develop through tear shedding. At this time, however, the interrelationship of virus in the tears, virus in the ganglia, and corneal recurrence is not clearly understood, and will require further examination for complete clarification. The work of Subak-Sharpe has shown by enzymatic cleavage mapping of DNA that ganglia from any one cadaver all have the same herpesvirus type 1 virus (although herpesvirus type 2 may infect the sacral areas in the same body), suggesting that one virus colonizes our ganglia and that later colonization by other viruses does not occur [7].

We can show that isolates from some patients produce mild disease in animals and isolates from others produce severe disease. We know that the relatively avirulent viruses infect the corneal epithelium, can colonize the trigeminal ganglion, and can be shed in tears in the absence of overt disease. In other words, the avirulent virus strains carry out the same infective processes that the virulent strains do, and there is no apparent defect in the infective process of the avirulent strains that can account for their non-disease producing character.

We have found that rabbits and also presumably patients infected with relatively avirulent herpesvirus strains appear to be protected from more virulent virus. These benign strains infect and colonize the ganglion, but they do not produce disease unless the host is massively immunosuppressed, and they prevent colonization by more virulent strains. These strain differences within a type are easily demonstrated in normal immunocompetent rabbits, as is the fact that some strains tend to cause clinically apparent recurrences and others do not. Of course, if the immune system is totally depressed, even a very mild virus strain might be capable of producing disease, just as cytomegalovirus, *Toxoplasma gondii* and *Candida albicans* do in renal transplant recipients who are chemically immunosuppressed to prevent graft rejection.

Although stromal disease almost certainly involves both virus multiplication in the stroma and host immune response to the virus, studies by Centifanto indicate that some viruses are more likely to cause stromal disease than others. Although these studies are still in the early stages, they suggest that these virus strains that cause stromal disease may produce common, highly antigenic glycoproteins. It is tempting to speculate that these glycoproteins enhance the host response, and perhaps even tissue tropism, and that host response to the virus is determined not only by the host immunological status, but also by the specific antigenic composition and biologic properties of the infecting virus strain. This suggests that, within a herpesvirus type, we may find the specific biological correlates that will explain variation in recurrence rate and the tendency to specific kinds of disease seen in some individuals.

It appears that most of us are infected with relatively avirulent herpesvirus, and that nature has vaccinated us with symbiotic "non-disease producing" strains in a kind of herpesvirus infection roulette. Immunization with non-DNA-containing components early in life may not be able to completely prevent infection throughout life, but immunity to the most damaging viral components might select against the virulent strains and favor colonization by less damaging virus. We would like to suggest that a primary factor in whether overt herpetic disease develops and recurs in a particular patient may depend on whether he was infected initially by an avirulent virus and perhaps thereafter protected, or by a "bad" virulent virus with the potential to cause severe disease whenever reactivation occurs. We also do not know why so large a proportion of herpetic disease patients, with signs of previous herpes infection and possibly virus in the trigeminal ganglion, *do not* get recurrent epithelial disease [1]. A statistically significant increase in HLA-B5 tissue types has been seen among patients having frequent corneal epithelial herpetic recurrences [4, 13] although the proportion is small. It may be that the D locus will correlate more closely with epithelial corneal recurrences, but this has not yet been investigated. No such correlation between tissue type and recurrence rate has been observed in patients with stromal disease [8].

Although much attention has been focused on the immune status of the host as the determining factor in the kind of and severity of herpetic disease that develops after infection, it may be that the virus strains themselves deserve a closer look. Our study of herpesvirus type 1 strains and their specificity in the production of particular kinds of ocular disease in varying degrees of severity is just beginning, but already, we have evidence that this approach may prove to have both theoretical and clinical implications.

**Acknowledgment.** Supported in part by USPHS grants EY02672 and EY02377 from the National Eye Institute, National Institutes of Health, Bethesda, Maryland.

## References

1. Baringer JR (1974) Recovery of herpes simplex virus from human sacral ganglia. N Eng J Med 291:828–830
2. Baringer JR, Swoveland P (1974) Persistent herpes simplex infection in rabbit trigeminal ganglia. Lab Invest 30:230–240
3. Carroll JM, Martola EL, Laibson PR, Dohlman CH (1967) The recurrence of herpetic keratitis following idoxuridine therapy. Am J Ophthalmol 63:103–107
4. Colin J, Chastel C, Saleun JP, Morin JF, Renard G (1979) Herpes oculaire recidivant et antigenes HLA; etude preliminaire. J Fr Ophthalmol 2:263–266
5. Dowdle WR, Nahmias AJ, Harwell RW, Pauls FP (1967) Association of antigenic type of Herpesvirus hominis with site of viral recovery. J Immunol 99:974–980
6. Kaufman HE, Brown DC, Ellison EM (1967) Recurrent herpes in the rabbit and man. Science 156:1628–1629
7. Lonsdale DM, Moira Brown S, Subak-Sharpe JH, Warren, KG, Koprowski H (1979) The polypeptide and the DNA restriction enzyme profiles of spontaneous isolates of herpes simplex virus type 1 from explants of human trigeminal, superior cervical and vagus ganglia. J Gen Virol 43:151–171
8. Meyers-Elliott RH, Elliott JH, Maxwell WA, Pettit TH, O'Day DM, Terasaki PI, Bernoco D (1980) HLA antigens in herpes stromal keratitis. Am J Ophthalmol 89:54–57
9. Nesburn AB, Cook ML, Stevens JG (1972) Latent herpes simplex virus. Isolation from rabbit trigeminal ganglia between episodes of recurrent ocular infection. Arch Ophthalmol 88:412–417
10. Nesburn AB, Green MT, Radnot M, Walker B (1977) Reliable in vivo model for latent herpes simplex virus reactivation with peripheral virus shedding. Infect Immun 15:772–775
11. Stevens JG, Cook ML (1971) Latent herpes simplex virus in spinal ganglia of mice. Science 173:843–845
12. Wander AH, Centifanto YM, Kaufman HE (1980) Strain specificity of clinical isolates of herpes simplex virus. Arch Ophthalmol 98:1458–1461
13. Zimmerman TJ, McNeill JI, Richman A, Kaufman HE, Waltman SR (1977) HLA types and recurrent corneal herpes simplex infection. Invest Ophthalmol Vis Sci 16:756–757

Sundmacher, R. (Hrsg.):
Herpetische Augenerkrankungen
© J.F. Bergmann Verlag, München 1981

# Herpes Simplex Virus Strain Specificity and Ocular Disease

Y.M. Centifanto-Fitzgerald, New Orleans

**Key words.** Herpetic keratitis – strain virulence, stromal keratitis, glycoproteins, dendritic keratitis

**Schlüsselwörter.** Herpeskeratitis – Virulenzunterschiede, Stromaherpes, Glycoproteine, Keratitis dendritica

**Summary.** The disease pattern of herpesvirus (HSV) strains in herpetic ocular infections seems to be an inherent property of the strain. The avirulent strains replicate in the corneal tissue, colonize the ganglia and shed virus just as the virulent strains do, but these avirulent strains do not produce overt ocular disease. In the five reference strains, differences in viral polypeptide composition were found mainly in the region of ICP 5 to ICP 20. The glycoprotein profiles showed differences in the number of glycosylated bands present and in the presence or absence of glycoprotein $C_2$ and its precursor. In an initial survey of the viruses producing severe stromal disease, we found several strains lacking expression of glycoprotein $C_2$. This polypeptide marker may be useful for epidemiological studies of the relationship between viral polypeptides and ocular disease.

**Zusammenfassung.** Der spezifische Krankheitsverlauf nach Herpes simplex-Virus-(HSV)Infektion scheint stark von den jeweiligen Eigenschaften des infizierenden Stammes abzuhängen. Avirulente Stämme vermehren sich genauso wie die virulenten im Hornhautgewebe und besiedeln die Ganglien, erzeugen aber im Unterschied zu den virulenten Stämmen keine manifeste klinische Erkrankung. Bei den fünf von uns untersuchten Referenz-Stämmen fanden wir Unterschiede im viralen Glykoprotein-Muster hauptsächlich in den Bereichen ICP 5–ICP 20. Die Glykoprotein-Profile unterschieden sich in der Anzahl der glykosylierten Banden und auch durch das Vorhandensein oder das Fehlen des Glykoproteins C2 oder seiner Vorstufe. In einer Pilot-Studie an Herpes-Stämmen, die einen schweren nekrotisierenden Stromaherpes erzeugt hatten, fanden wir mehrere Stämme, die kein Glykoprotein 2 bildeten. Hiermit ist vielleicht ein Polypeptid-„Marker" gefunden, mit dessen Hilfe man epidemiologische Studien zur Korrelation zwischen Virus-Polypeptiden und Augenerkrankungen durchführen kann.

## Introduction

Herpes simplex virus type 1 is associated with ocular infections and, in this capacity, produces a spectrum of disease that ranges from very mild conjunctivitis to invasive necrotizing stromal disease. It is not clear what determines the outcome of the infection, and, in most cases, the host immune response has been assigned a primary role in the determination of this outcome. Although we recognize the importance of the host immune response, it is evident that differences within strains exist and that part of the disease pattern process may be due to the virulence of the infecting strain.

To this end, we studied the biological and biochemical characteristics of herpes simplex strains to determine whether differences among strains could be correlated with the type of disease produced in the host. Variation in the antigenic type and polypeptide composition among strains has been established [3, 6, 7]; also it is known that virus strains that differ significantly in their immunological specificity also show differences in their membrane proteins [4, 11].

With this in mind, we sought to analyze the infected cell polypeptides (ICP) and the membrane proteins of a group of fresh clinical isolates and several laboratory reference strains of herpesvirus type 1. This work, which included five reference strains and 20 clinical isolates, encompassed disease patterns and infective processes in the rabbit cornea, and virus-specified proteins. The herpesvirus strains were divided into those causing epithelial disease, those producing deep stromal involvement, and those producing minimal disease (avirulent strains).

## Methods and Results

The herpesvirus reference strains used were RE, Shealy, F, McKrae and CGA-3. These strains, as well as all the clinical isolates, were grown in HEp-2 cells on Medium 199 supplemented with 1% fetal calf serum, 1% glutamine and antibiotics. The reference strains have high passage history and the clinical isolates were studied at passage 1 or 2.

### Avirulent Strains

Studies with the avirulent herpesvirus strains sought to determine whether inherent deficiencies in the infective process of avirulent strains may account for their non-disease-producing pattern. The avirulent strains produced minimal disease, primarily punctate staining of the cornea; only 8–12% of eyes infected with these strains were involved by day 8. In comparison, infection with the more virulent strains produced dendritic corneal ulcers and involved a majority of eyes by day 6.

The herpesvirus strains were able to replicate in the corneal tissue in the absence of disease; virus shedding was seen as early as 2 days post infection, continuing to day 9. Cultures of the trigeminal ganglia were positive in 70 to 75% of the animals, which is consistent with recovery rates seen in virulent strains. Thus, there appears to be no deficiency in the infective process of avirulent herpesvirus strains that could account for their non-disease-producing character.

### Ocular Disease

New Zealand white rabbits were infected with each virus strain and examined for the development of degree and kind of ocular disease, virus shedding, viral replication in the cornea, and colonization of the trigeminal ganglia. Our studies of the ocular disease of the reference strains [13] revealed that the kind of disease produced seemed to be an inherent property of the virus strain. Those strains producing stromal disease (Shealy and RE) did so consistently, with very low inoculum, as compared to the strictly epithelial disease producing strains, which did not cause stromal disease even at high doses.

RE and Shealy strains produced severe epithelial and stromal disease (Table 1); the $ID_{50}$ values obtained show these strains to be highly virulent. The McKrae and F strains produced moderate epithelial disease with less stromal involvement. CGA-3 strain produced dendritic ulcers with no stromal involvement. In vitro sensitivity to antiviral drugs such as idoxuridine correlated with the severity of the disease, i.e., the more virulent viruses required a higher concentration of antiviral agents to inhibit 50% of the viral growth in vitro.

### Virus-Specified Proteins

The clinical isolates and reference strains were grown in HEp-2 cells in the presence of $^{35}$S-methionine or $^{14}$C-glucosamine for the

**Table 1.** Herpesvirus-produced ocular disease

| Virus | Disease Pattern | $ID_{50}$ | Severity of disease | Sensitivity to IDU ($ED_{50}$) |
|---|---|---|---|---|
| RE | Epithelial, stromal geopraphic defect | 2.75 | Severe | 1.65 |
| Shealy | epithelial, stromal geographic defect | < 3 | Severe | 1.4 |
| McKrae | Epithelial, geographic defect | 4.5 | Moderate | 1.35 |
| F | Classic dendritic ulcers | 3.78 | Moderate | ND |
| CGA-3 | Classic dendritic ulcers | 5.18 | Mild | 1.15 |

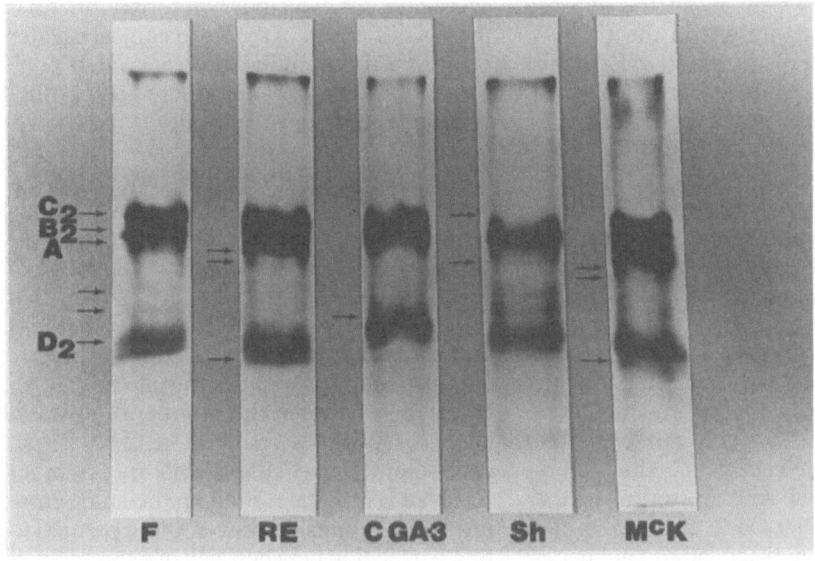

**Fig. 1.** Autoradiogram of an SDS-polyacrylamide gel slab showing the electrophoretic separation of the $^{14}$C-glucosamine-labeled glycoproteins of the five herpesvirus reference strains. Arrows indicate the differences seen in the numbers and kinds of glycosylated polypeptides resolved in the various herpesvirus strains

analysis of viral polypeptides and glycoproteins, respectively. Infected cell pellets were solubilized in NP-40 and immune precipitated with the homologous antiserum prior to electrophoretic separation in 8.6 or 9% polyacrylamide gels cross-linked with DATD. Polypeptide bands were resolved by staining with Coomassie brilliant blue and by fluorography.

## Reference Strains

Analysis of the infected cell polypeptides of the five reference strains showed some differences, mainly in the region between ICP 5 and ICP 20. Since this region contains the broad glycoprotein bands [5], it seemed necessary to study the membrane proteins that are the predominant immunogen in an infected cell [12]. The analysis of the glycoproteins by the metabolic incorporation of $^{14}$C-glucosamine showed differences in not only the number but also the kind of glycosylated polypeptides resolved (Fig. 1, Table 2).

Regarding the major groups of glycoproteins, we can see that $C_2B_2A$ complex was present in all strains except the Shealy strain, in which a lack of $C_2$ was observed. The $D_2$

**Table 2.** Membrane proteins of herpesvirus type 1 reference strains

| Glycoproteins | CGA–3 | F | Shealy | McKrae | RE |
|---|---|---|---|---|---|
| $C_2$ | + | + | | + | + |
| $B_2$ | + | + | + | + | + |
| A | + | + | + | + | + |
| pC | | | + | | + |
| 97K | | | | + | + |
| 89K | | | | + | |
| 83K | | | + | + | | + |
| 73K | | | + | + | + | + |
| E | + | | | | |
| $D_2$ | + | | + | + | + | + |
| pD | | | + | + | |
| 53K | | | | + | + |
| Total number of Bands | 5 | 7 | 7 | 8 | 9 |

A comparison of the glycoprotein profile of the five reference strains shows differences in the number and relative amounts of glycosylated bands and also differences in the presence or absence of individual polypeptides. Glycoproteins that are the predominant viral immunogen are more abundant in the RE (stromal-disease-producing) strain than they are in the CGA–3 (mild-epithelial-disease-producing) strain

21

glycoprotein was present in all the strains. Glycoprotein E was present in the CGA-3 strain. The presence of glycoprotein $E_2$ in this syncytium-forming strain is consistent with the findings of Baucke and others [1], in which the Fc-binding protein is reported to be present in larger amounts in syncytium-forming strains. In general, aside from the major group of glycoproteins, several glycosylated polypeptides and precursors were resolved, such as pC, which was resolved in the RE and Shealy strains.

Because of our interest in the apparent absence of glycoprotein $C_2$ in the Shealy strain, which produces the most severe stromal disease, $^{14}C$-glucosamine-labeled infected cells of each reference strain were immune precipitated with antiserum to the KOS strain and subjected to electrophoretic separation on SDS-polyacrylamide gel using the same experimental conditions. It was found that $C_2$ was present in these profiles, confirming our earlier suggestion that the apparent absence of $C_2$ was due to the particular antiserum used, rather than to an inherent defect in glycoprotein production. Subsequent work in our laboratory has indicated that the failure of this antiserum to resolve glycoprotein $C_2$ in the HEp-2 cells infected with the Shealy strain of herpesvirus was related to the immunogen used to raise the antisera [2]. In essence, we found that rabbit kidney cells, when infected with the Shealy strain, do not express glycoprotein $C_2$ and exhibit the classic cytopathogenic effect of polykaryocyte formation, indicative of a lack of glycoprotein $C_2$. It is important to note that the Shealy strain is not defective in the production of glycoprotein $C_2$ in HEp-2 cells, and that such protein is definitely resolved by using antisera prepared with a different immunogen. However, it appears that the virus strains that do not express glycoprotein $C_2$ in the rabbit kidney cells are found to be stromal-disease-producing strains in the rabbit eye.

Glycoproteins that are the chief viral immunogen are more abundant in the RE strain, which produces stromal disease, than they are in the CGA-3 strain, which produces mild epithelial disease.

Clinical isolates

With this in mind, we analyzed the fresh clini-cal isolates for two kinds of information: (a) is there a difference in the fresh clinical isolates regarding the number of glycosylated polypeptides, and (b) are there any other variations in the glycoprotein $C_2$ and its precursors.

Because stromal disease is not an "all-or-none" phenomenon (that is to say, virulent virus injected into the rabbit eye can cause stromal disease in varying degrees of severity), we compared the virus strains that produce severe stromal disease with those that produce minimal or no stromal disease.

Our initial survey showed no direct correlation between the number of glycosylated polypeptides resolved in the stromal-disease-producing strains and the number resolved in the mild-epithelial-disease-producing strains. However, there seemed to be a correlation between lack of expression of glycoprotein $C_2$ and stromal disease, i.e., four out of five strains that produce stromal disease showed an impaired expression of glycoprotein $C_2$ in the rabbit cells. Of these four virus strains, two are clinical isolates and two are reference strains genetically defective in the production of glycoprotein $C_2$.

**Discussion**

$C_2$ glycoprotein, which is present in the herpesvirus-infected cell membrane, plays a role in the fusion of these membranes [8] and in the production of polykaryocytes. It has been shown that glycoprotein $B_2$ promotes the fusion of membranes and that glycoprotein $C_2$ acts to suppress this fusion. The wild type herpesvirus strains, with a full complement of glycoproteins, cause the infected cells to round up and form aggregates, but rarely to form syncytia. However, herpesvirus mutants that lack glycoprotein $C_2$ and thus lack the fusion suppressor produce polykaryocytes upon infection of cells. This phenomenon of fusion, or tight adhesiveness, is of interest to us for two reasons. First, it provides a mechanism by which a virus could travel from cell to cell without entering the extracellular fluid. Second, it provides new viral antigenic determinants to the adjacent cell. Both the fusion and the provision of new antigenic determinants are of significance in the stromal disease process and must be examined in the evaluation of the postulate that the chief cause of stromal disease may be the stimulation of the host immune system by viral antigens present in the stromal cells [9, 10].

Because the number and class of glycoproteins expressed in a herpesvirus infected cell are determined not only by the virus genome but also by the host cell genetics, a generalized statement pertaining to glycoproteins and stromal disease-producing viruses cannot be made unless the methodology (cells used to grow the virus, preparation of antiserum, and animal model employed) is strictly and clearly defined. In the rabbit system, we have shown a correlation between expression of glycoprotein $C_2$ and the occurrence of stromal disease.

We feel that, although this constitutes only an initial survey, such a polypeptide marker will be useful for epidemiological studies on the relationship between viral polypeptides and ocular disease.

**Acknowledgment.** Supported in part by USPHS grants EY02389 and EY02377 from the National Eye Institute, National Institutes of Health, Bethesda, Maryland.

# References

1. Baucke RB, Spear PG (1979) Membrane proteins specified by herpes simplex viruses. V. Identification of an Fc-binding glycoprotein. J Virol 32:779–789
2. Centifanto YM, Kaufman HE HSV strain specificity and ocular disease. III. Stromal disease.
3. Halliburton IW, Randall RE, Killington RA, Watson DH (1977) Some properties of recombinants between type 1 and type 2 herpes simplex viruses. J Gen Virol 36:471–484
4. Hampar B, Mujamato K, Martos L (1971) Serologic classification of herpes simplex viruses. J Immunol 106:580–582
5. Heine JW, Spear PG, Roizman B (1972) Proteins specified by herpes simplex virus. VI. Viral proteins in the plasma membrane. J Virol 9:431–439
6. Honess RW, Watson DH (1977) Unity and diversity in the herpesvirus. J Gen Virol 37:15–37
7. Killington RA, Yeo J, Honess RW, Watson DH, Duncan BE, Halliburton IW, Mumford J (1977) Comparative analysis of the proteins and antigens of five herpesviruses. J Gen Virol 37:297–310
8. Manservigi R, Spear PG, Buchan A (1977) Cell fusion induced by herpes simplex virus is promoted and suppressed by different viral glycoproteins. Proc Natl Acad Sci USA 74: 3913–3917
9. Metcalf JF, Kaufman HE (1976) Herpetic stromal keratitis. Evidence for cell-mediated immunopathogenesis. Am J Ophthalmol 82: 827–834
10. Metcalf JF, McNeill JI, Kaufman HE (1976) Experimental disciform edema and necrotizing keratitis in the rabbit. Invest Ophthalmol 15:979–985
11. Roizman B, Keller JM, Spear PG, Terni M, Nahmias A, Dowdle W (1970) Variability, structural glycoproteins, and classification of herpes simplex viruses. Nature 227:1253
12. Spear PG (1976) Membrane proteins specified by herpes simplex viruses. I. Identification of four glycoprotein precursors and their products in type 1-infected cells. J Virol 17: 991–1008
13. Wander AH, Centifanto YM, Kaufman HE (1980) Strain specificity of clinical isolates of herpes simplex virus. Arch Ophthalmol 98: 1458–1461

## Discussion on the Contributions pp. 15–23

H. zur Hausen (Freiburg)
Thank you, Dr. Centifanto. Before we start with the discussion, let me make one brief comment. The analysis of individual strains of HSV by DNA analysis after cleavage with restriction enzymes has, without doubt, shown that there exist strain specific differences − irrespective of the type studied. These differences have turned out to be useful epidemiological markers. Right now, however, it would be meaningful to focus the discussion on markers which are correlated specifically with HSV pathogenicity, and I think that your contribution on glycoprotein patterns and changes in these patterns between individual strains does provide a good basis for this discussion.

W.H. Prusoff (New Haven)
In view of the fact that deoxyglucose has such a profound effect on the synthesis of glycoproteins, is it possible through the use of deoxyglucose alone, or perhaps in combination with another more potent viral agent, to either decrease the virulence of those viruses which might escape inhibition if the glycoproteins are critically involved in virulence or to achieve a synergistic or additive inhibitory effect?

H.E. Kaufman (New Orleans)
That is a fascinating question. As an isolated therapeutic agent in animal systems, deoxyglucose is a very weak antiviral. The question is, can it be

selective, so that, even if it does not kill all of the virus, some of the deleterious effects of virus infection are prevented. This has not, to my knowledge, been looked at, and certainly should be.

Another possibility may be to find markers of the viruses that do "bad" things. For example, there may be glycoproteins common to the most harmful virus strains. If we could use, perhaps, a non-DNA-containing immunogen to select for infection by a less harmful, or "good" virus strain instead of a "bad" one, some of these effects might be preventable. But this is also an idea for the future.

**H.J. Field (Cambridge)**
I just wondered, if you superinfect the contralateral eye with your virulent strain, does the opposite ganglion become colonised with the new virus?

**H.E. Kaufman (New Orleans)**
Most of the time, the ganglia on both sides have been infected in our primary infections. We have not tried infecting only one eye. However, the work of Subak-Sharpe and his group has shown that, in man, there is only one virus found in all ganglia, at least above the waist.

**Y.C. Cheng (Chapel Hill)**
I would like to make one brief comment. HSV type 1 and type 2 can induce many biochemical changes as you all know, and among them, there are three enzyme activities. Those are thymidinekinase, DNA-polymerase, and the DNAse. The enzymes induced by type 1 and type 2 are different, not only in terms of their kinetic properties but also in terms of their immuno-specificity. Therefore, using enzymes as a marker for differentiating between type 1 and type 2 viruses is a possible, viable way. In general − no matter which strain you are talking about − all HSV 1 strains induce a similar type of thymidinekinase, and the same applies to HSV type 2. Therefore, chemotherapeutic agents developed against a virus-specific enzyme derived from one strain are likely to work on all HSV strains, at least of the same HSV type.

Then I would like to adress Dr. Kaufman: Have you tried to correlate the severity of the diseases caused by various strains of HSV 1 with the inductivity of thymidinekinase, since you probably heard there is a big debate whether or not the TK strain could exist in a latent form.

**H.E. Kaufman (New Orleans)**
It has been shown that the thymidine kinase of HSV type 1 is different from that of type 2, and that inhibitory drugs can be used to separate type 1 and type 2 viruses. This is beautiful work. However, the thymidine kinase within type 1 tends to be similar, so similar drug effects would be expected. In our laboratory, we haven't looked at thymidine kinase as a marker; this is a very sophisticated technique.

**Y.C. Cheng (Chapel Hill)**
It's a very simple technique. We have it.

**H. zur Hausen (Freiburg)**
Dr. Kaufman, would you like to comment on some experimental and molecular epidemiological observations which appear to indicate clearly that reinfections by different strains of HSV are possible? How does this fit with your opinion that a prior infection with an avirulent strain could prevent subsequent infection by a virulent one?

**H.E. Kaufman (New Orleans)**
There are two papers that I know of. One was from the National Dental Institute, many years ago, on some patients with a couple of different infections with herpes labialis. Using neutralization kinetics, the investigators determined that the reinfections may have been different strains. This technique seems to me to be less than wholly reliable in this determination, however.

The other paper, by Andre Nahmias and his co-workers, also suggests the possibility of reinfection by different strains.

At this time, we do not have the data to state positively that colonization by one strain prevents reinfection by another strain. We don't know why the virus goes from the ganglia to the skin and back, and we don't really know whether reinfection is possible. It may be that reinfection by a different strain is only superficial and does not colonize the ganglion, which may be protected by the original infection. All of these questions need further study, and we are only at the beginning of the search for answers.

**H. zur Hausen (Freiburg)**
Thank you. We should also mention the older study by Blank and Haines who showed that reinfection at a different site with an isolate derived from the same patient led to recurrent herpes at the new inoculation site.

**H.E. Kaufman (New Orleans)**
This also seems to occur clinically. For example, in the past, virus from a patient with herpes labialis would be injected into the arm. The arm would develop a second site of infection, although the virus presumably was already in the ganglion. All this needs further explanation.

# Latency

Sundmacher, R. (Hrsg.):
Herpetische Augenerkrankungen
© J.F. Bergmann Verlag, München 1981

# Latency in Neuronal Tissues of Herpes Simplex and Varicella Zoster Virus*

R. Baringer, San Francisco

**Key words.** HSV – ganglionic colonization and latency, sensory ganglia, varicella-zoster virus

**Schlüsselwörter.** HSV – ganglionäre Infektion und Latenz, sensible Ganglien, Varizellen-Zoster Virus

**Summary.** Latent Herpes simplex virus in sensory ganglia of animals has now been repeatedly demonstrated after peripheral inoculation, and with a lesser frequency after intravenous injection. Persistence of virus in the central nervous system can also be demonstrated after peripheral inoculation. HSV type 1 has been recovered from trigeminal, superior cervical and vagus ganglia of humans and HSV type 2 has been recovered from human sacral ganglia. It is probable that these ganglionic sites serve as reservoirs for the recurrent oral or genital eruptions commonly encountered in clinical practice. Despite efforts by a number of investigators to determine how HSV persists in ganglia, this question has not been answered with certainty. Whether the common persistence of HSV 1 in trigeminal ganglia is related to HSV 1 encephalitis is also uncertain. Numerous attempts to recover latent HSV from olfactory bulbs at routine autopsy have been unrewarding, suggesting that the virus may not reside there in latent fashion. Restriction enzyme analysis of HSV 1 strains isolated from trigeminal ganglia and the brain of a patient with encephalitis revealed virtually identical patterns. However, virus was grown from the trigeminal ganglia 5 days after explantation, suggesting an acute infection at that site. Thus, the role of latent virus in the trigeminal or other sites in humans in the production of the encephalitic illness remains obscure.

Evidence for latency of varicella-zoster virus in cranial and spinal ganglia is lacking despite an abundance of clinical data suggesting the dorsal root ganglia as the likely site for residence of the virus. While the virus has been demonstrated in spinal ganglia of patients recently affected by cutaneous zoster, we have been unable to demonstrate it in explants of thoracic or cranial ganglia obtained at routine postmortem examination.

**Zusammenfassung.** Herpes simplex-Virus-Latenz in sensiblen Ganglien ist bei Tieren wiederholt nach peripherer Virusinokulation und etwas weniger häufig auch nach intravenöser Virusinjektion nachgewiesen worden. Darüber hinaus kann man auch eine Viruspersistenz im zentralen Nervensystem nach peripherer Inokulation nachweisen. HSV Typ 1 konnte beim Menschen aus dem Ganglion trigeminale, dem Ganglion cervicale superius und aus Vagus-Ganglien isoliert werden; HSV Typ 2 hat man in menschlichen Sakralganglien gefunden. Wahrscheinlich dienen alle diese Ganglien als Ausgangsort für rezidivierende Herpes-Erkrankungen im Gesichts- und Genitalbereich, wie sie klinisch so häufig vorkommen. Wie die Viren allerdings in den Ganglien persistieren, kann trotz erheblicher wissenschaftlicher Bemühungen bis jetzt noch nicht mit Sicherheit gesagt werden. Auch ist noch völlig unklar, ob die häufige HSV 1-Persistenz im Trigeminalganglion etwas mit einer HSV 1-Enzephalitis zu tun haben kann. Zahlreiche Versuche, latentes HSV aus den Bulbi olfactorii anläßlich von Routine-Autopsien zu gewinnen, sind fehlgeschlagen und deuten eher dahin, daß es latente Herpesviren in dieser Hirnregion nicht gibt. Wenn man HSV 1-Stämme von Patienten mit Enzephalitis aus dem Gehirn und aus dem Trigeminalganglion mit Hilfe von Restriktionsenzymen analysiert, zeigen sich praktisch identische Spaltmuster. Bei uns vermehrte sich ein aus dem Trigeminalganglion gewonnenes Virus aber bereits 5 Tage nach der Explantation, was eher für eine akute als für eine latente Infektion des Ganglions spricht. Damit bleibt die Bedeutung von latentem Herpesvirus im Trigeminalganglion oder anderen Orten für die Entstehung einer Herpes-Enzephalitis weiterhin unklar.

Eindeutige Beweise für eine Latenz des Varicella Zoster-Virus in kranialen und spinalen Ganglien fehlen, obwohl alle klinischen Befunde eindeutig auf die sensiblen Rückenmarkganglien als wahrscheinlichen Ort der Viruslatenz hinweisen. Während man das Virus in Spinalganglien von Patienten, die erst kürzlich an einem kutanen Zo-

---

* The written version of Dr. Baringer's presentation is a reprint from Nahmias AJ, Dowdle WR, Schinazi RF (eds) (1981) The human herpesviruses. An interdisciplinary perspective. Elsevier, The Netherlands

ster litten, nachweisen konnte, fanden wir es bislang nie in torakalen oder kranialen sensiblen Ganglien, die anläßlich von Routine-Autopsien gewonnen wurden.

Over a half century ago Goodpasture [1], who first demonstrated that herpes simplex virus (HSV) travelled along neural routes, suggested that the virus might have the potential for remaining in a persistent state within nervous system tissue. However, it was not until 1970 that Plummer and associates [2] were able to demonstrate this. In a series of rabbits inoculated intramuscularly with HSV 6 to 11 months earlier, they were able to recover HSV from "ganglion and cord cells" when these were co-cultivated with primary rabbit kidney cells for periods from 8–43 days in vitro. It is not clear whether the virus was present in the cells of the dorsal root ganglion or the spinal cord, but it was clear that virus which was not present in the free state was recoverable using these techniques. Stevens and his associates performed similar studies in mice inoculated in the footpad with HSV [3]. Animals that recovered from paralysis were killed and the spinal ganglia associated with the sciatic nerves were explanted and maintained as organ cultures. One to 2 weeks after explantation supernatant fluids from such explanted ganglia contained HSV. At the same time spinal ganglia taken from such mice and examined by histology, electron microscopy and by fluorescent antibody techniques did not reveal intranuclear inclusions, viral particles or viral antigen. Portions of other nervous system tissue which were treated in the same way as the latently infected ganglia did not yield virus. This constituted the first demonstration that the latent virus was present in spinal ganglion cells after peripheral inoculation.

Subsequent work by Stevens [4] indicated that the speed of travel of HSV in nerve trunks approximated the speed of retrograde transport of proteins within nerves and was far too rapid to be accounted for by sequential infection of Schwann or endoneural cells. Utilizing autoradiographic techniques, these same workers demonstrated that when latently infected ganglia were maintained in the presence of tritiated thymidine, viral DNA synthesis took place in isolated neurons. In pulse-chase experiments it was possible to demonstrate that subsequent viral DNA synthesis took place in satellite cells. Nucleic acid cytohybridization experiments demonstrated only rare neurons to contain viral DNA; after transplantation of ganglia additional neurons were found to contain viral DNA suggesting that the virus might be maintained in many neurons in a latent or static state. The same group [5] demonstrated in rabbit and mouse models that the latent virus could be detected after peripheral inoculation, not only within the appropriate segmental sensory ganglia but also within appropriate segments of central nervous system tissue. Finally, Cook and Stevens [6] demonstrated that after intravenous inoculation latent HSV could be demonstrated in cervical and thoracic dorsal root ganglia with great frequency and with lesser frequency in the anterior and posterior portions of brain and spinal cord. In the same animals HSV could not be found in trigeminal ganglia, bone, lymph nodes, spleen, kidney, lung or liver. These data suggested that after intravenous inoculation the virus has a predilection for a variety of neural tissues among which sensory ganglion cells are the most frequently involved.

A number of investigators have attempted to explore the mechanism(s) whereby the virus, once established in its latent state, may be reactivated, presumably a prerequisite to production of peripheral disease from travel back down the axon to the periphery. Studies by Walz et al. [7] demonstrated that after mice were infected on the footpad, the latent virus could be reactivated within the sensory ganglia by sciatic neurectomy. This model did not permit the reappearance of a lesion at the periphery. Nesburn and Green [8] and associates, in a series of painstaking experiments, demonstrated that in the rabbit latently infected in the trigeminal ganglia, mechanical stimulation of the ganglia resulted in shedding of virus in the tear film within 48 hours in 80% of stimulated animals. This model closely paralleled the neurosurgical experience in humans [9] in which HSV lesions in or about the mouth are seen with great regularity after neurosurgical manipulation of the trigeminal root. Recent prospective studies in humans [10] have demonstrated reactivation of HSV within the mouth after microneurosurgical decompression of the trigeminal sensory root performed for trigeminal neuralgia. Such reactivation took place with increased frequency if the patient had a history of recurrent herpes labialis. Hill and associates have recently utilized inoculations of HSV into the ear of mice [11]. Reactivation can be provoked by the minor trauma of stripping the ear skin with cellophane tape. This model offers conveniences of simplicity, a precisely timed reactivating stimulus, a visible cutaneous lesion signifying recurrence, and reasonable analogy to human situations in which skin is traumatized either mechanically or by ultraviolet irradiation resulting in recurrent HSV lesions.

Despite the considerable attempts to devise systems in which the process of reactivation could be triggered, the actual reactivating events taking place within the ganglia and whether they are necessary for recurrence of infection at the periphery remains a mystery. Among the diverse clinical and experimental manipulations that seem to have resulted in reactivated lesions (eg. sunlight, fever, mechanical trauma, epinephrine injection, irradiation, immunosuppression), whether there is a common denominator remains unknown. Though it might be suspected that there is a biochemical sine qua non for the process of reactivation, such has not been identified.

Price and associates [12] have explored the latent infection of the superior cervical ganglia after ocular inoculation of HSV. They have demonstrated that administration of virus to resistant animals, or administration of antibody at appropriate times, serves to reduce the amount of active infection and enhance the tendency to latent infection in ganglia; post-ganglionic neurectomy in contrast augments the acute phase of viral replication and reduces latency. These experiments suggest that during the course of ganglionic infection a balance of factors may predispose to the establishment of an acute or latent infection of ganglia.

One experimental model that seems to differ significantly from those previously used is the model of footpad inoculation with HSV-2 employed by Scriba [13]. She has demonstrated that after inoculation of HSV-2 into footpad of guinea pigs, virus can be recovered from the footpad, from the sciatic nerve, from the dorsal root ganglion and the spinal cord. With HSV-1, virus can be recovered from the footpad. While it may be that the biology of HSV infection is entirely different in the guinea pig than in other animals, such would

seem unlikely. These findings warrant a careful reexamination of the possibility that small amounts of virus in peripheral tissues of mouse and rabbit may be found on more careful search, and that the differences between the guinea pig and other rodent models are more of a quantitative than qualitative nature.

The occurrence of HSV 1 in the trigeminal ganglia of humans was first demonstrated by Bastian [14] and later documented by our own group [15]. Subsequent studies established that sacral ganglia harbored HSV-2, though in a lesser frequency [16]. These observations have recently been augmented by the observations of Lonsdale et al. [17] in which HSV isolates from the trigeminal, superior cervical, and vagus ganglia were compared using restriction endonuclease techniques. These studies have shown that the viral HSV DNAs are unique to individuals who are epidemiologically unrelated, and that within one individual isolates from various ganglia are genetically identical. This would suggest that either as a result of a primary infection of multiple ganglia or a primary infection of one followed by reinfection of other ganglia, individuals tend to colonize multiple ganglia by the same virus. It would be of great interest to know whether a sensory ganglia or a sensory ganglion cell, once colonized by one strain of HSV, becomes resistant to infection and latency by a second type.

The longstanding question of the mechanism by which virus is maintained within nervous system or other tissue, first posed by Roizman [18], has not been answered with certainty. Studies by Puga [19] and associates utilizing liquid hybridization techniques demonstrated that while HSV DNA was present at the level of 0.1 genome equivalents per cell in latently infected ganglia, HSV mRNA was not detectable at a sensitivity of 0.0005 genomes per cell. Subsequently, Galloway and associates [20] used in situ hybridization with an HSV DNA fragment to demonstrate HSV mRNA in sacral and thoracic ganglion cells from one patient and in sacral, thoracic and lumbar ganglion cells from another. These studies, while preliminary, might suggest that HSV mRNA might be localized to a single or only a few ganglion cells and thus escape detection by the liquid hybridization methods. This work should be clarified by careful studies of animal models in which latent infection of known sites can be produced and analyzed. Preliminary data from Dr. Richard Tenser's laboratory [21] suggests that HSV mRNA can be detected in ganglia from experimental animals at the time of latent infection. The possibility of free viruses present in small amounts during what has been regarded as a latent infection is raised by the recent studies of Schwartz and co-workers [22]. They have utilized a presumably more sensitive detection system, namely fetal dorsal root ganglion explants, for detection of HSV in ganglia removed from mice inoculated on a footpad. They were able to demonstrate, using the dorsal root ganglia embryo cultures as the indicator, that virus was present in the homogenates of dorsal root ganglia up to 8 months after infection of the mouse but that when the same homogenates were placed on HeLa cells, cytopathic effect was not demonstrable. These results call attention to the fact that we have used an operational definition of latency, i.e. that latency depends upon the ability of virus to be demonstrated by explantation or co-cultivation of infected ganglia at a time when free virus cannot be detected using susceptible cell lines. The findings of Schwartz et al suggest that it may be necessary to revise our ideas about the usual duration that free virus can be detected within ganglia and as well that it may be necessary to revise our concepts about the nature of the persistent infection due to HSV. It is evident from the foregoing discussion that the capability of HSV to reside in sensory ganglion cells after peripheral or intravenous inoculation is quite well established in experimental animals. A similar latent infection of sensory and/or autonomic ganglia may take place in man where it is in all likelihood responsible for the recurrent peripheral, oral or genital infections by the virus. Though latency of the virus within the CNS has been established for animals, whether CNS latency takes place in man and what relationship this may have to herpes simplex encephalitis or other encephalic syndromes is still unknown. In this regard, it may be of considerable importance to carefully study the genetics of viruses of HSV isolates at autopsy from patients succumbing to HSV encephalitis and compare these with the viruses isolated from ganglia.

A number of questions concerning the basic biology of HSV remain unexplained.

We have incomplete and sometimes conflicting information concerning the mechanism by which the virus is able to maintain itself within ganglia (and presumably within ganglion cells) without destroying the ganglia. The central question posed by Roizman in 1965 concerning the nature of the latent infection, viz, whether the virus is present in a dynamic or static state, remains unanswered. Similarly, while there has been much work directed towards establishing model systems in which reactivation of virus from its latent ganglionic site can be provoked, these have not yet led us to a basic understanding of the reactivation process. One would like to think that among all of the stimuli which are recognized to provoke recurrent cutaneous HSV infections, there is a final or common pathway, activation of which is necessary for virus to be reexpressed. An understanding of these factors may contribute not only to our further knowledge of the biology of this virus and its relationship to nervous system tissue, but may enable us to devise ways in which recurrent infection may be diminished or abolished.

*Varicella zoster latency:* The facts that varicella zoster virus (VZV) is related to HSV and that it is notorious for producing eruptions in a radicular distribution would suggest that the virus may be harbored within sensory ganglion cells from which it has the capacity to erupt to produce the typical zosteriform rash. Studies by Bastian [23] and Shibuta [24] have established that from patients dying near the time of a zoster eruption, VZV can be isolated from the relevant dorsal root ganglion. However, studies by Plotkin [25] and in our laboratory attempting to recover VZV from thoracic and other ganglia of individuals dying with no history of shingles have been uniformly unsuccessful. Whether this is because the virus is not there during the latent phase or simply more recondite is unknown. The well recognized cell-associated nature of VZV may render it more difficult to recover from latently infected ganglion cells than the more easily recoverable HSV. The clinical observations [25] that irradiation of renal transplant patients results in a high incidence of zoster eruptions in the irradiated segments suggests that VZV may lie dormant in many sensory ganglia or nearby sites, from which it can be activated by local X-ray as well as other stimuli.

**Acknowledgment.** The author would like to acknowledge the help of Mrs. Nancy Torelli, Mrs. Judy Rohrer and Miss Prima Conde in preparation of the manuscript and helpful discussions with Drs. Richard Dix and Harry Openshaw.

## References

1. Goodpasture EW (1929) Medicine 8:223
2. Plummer G, Hollingsworth DC, Phuangsab A, Bowling CP (1970) Infect Immun 1:351
3. Stevens JG, Gook ML (1970) Science 173:843
4. Stevens JG (1975) Curr Top Microbiol Immunol 70:31
5. Knotts FB, Cook ML, Stevens JG (1973) J Exp Med 138:740
6. Cook ML, Stevens JG (1976) J Gen Virol 31:75
7. Walz MA, Price RW, Notkins AL (1974) Science 184:1185
8. Nesburn AB, Green MT (1976) Invest Ophthalmol Visual Sci 15:515
9. Carton CA (1953) J Neurosurg 10:463
10. Pazin GJ, Ho M, Jannetta PJ (1978) J Infect Dis 138:405
11. Hill TJ, Blyth WA, Harbour DA (1978) J Gen Virol 39:21
12. Price RW, Schmitz J (1979) Infect Immun 23:373
13. Scriba M (1977) Nature 267:529
14. Bastian FO, Rabson AS, Lee CL, Tralka TS (1972) Science 178:306
15. Baringer JR, Swoveland P (1973) N Engl J Med 288:648
16. Baringer JR (1974) N Engl J Med 291:818
17. Lonsdale DM, Brown SM, Subak-Sharpe JH, Warren KG, Koprowski H (1979) J Gen Virol 43:151
18. Roizman B (1965) An inquiry into the mechanisms of recurrent herpes infections in man. In: Pollard M (ed) Virology, vol IV. New York: Academic, New York, pp 283–301
19. Puga A, Rosenthal JD, Openshaw H, Notkins AL (1978) Virol 89:102
20. Galloway DA, Fenoglio C, Shevchuk M, McDougall JK (1979) Virol 95:265
21. Tenser R, Dawson M (1980) Neurology 30:427
22. Schwartz J, Whetsell WO, Elizan TS (1978) J Neuropath Exp Neurol 37:45
23. Bastian FO, Robson AS, Lee CL, Tralka TS (1974) Arch Pathol 97:331
24. Shibuta H, Ishikawa T, Hondo R, Aoyama Y, Kurata K, Matumoto M (1974) Arch Ges Virusforsch 45:382
25. Plotkin SA, Stein S, Snyder M, Immesoete P (1977) Ann Neurol 2:249
26. Rifkind D (1966) J Lab Clin Med 68:463

## Discussion on the Contribution pp. 27–31

D. Epstein (Stockholm)
You mention that the virus, the HSV, thrives in the ganglion and does not destroy it. I was under the assumption that the virus, in order to replicate, must destroy, or am I confusing the issue?

R. Baringer (San Francisco)
I didn't mean to imply that the virus doesn't destroy some cells. If you look at a ganglionic infection which has ascended from a peripheral infection, e.g. in a rabbit eye, there is an acute ganglionic infection with a surrounding inflammatory infiltrate. There may be a few ganglionic cells which become infected. What happens to those, I don't think anybody knows. Whether a ganglionic cell can recover from such an insult or not is, as far as I know, not known.

D. Epstein (Stockholm)
Could you mention any other system elsewhere with other viruses that behave in the same way?

R. Baringer (San Francisco)
In terms of ganglionic infection? No, I don't know of any others.

D. Epstein (Stockholm)
This leaves a very open question, right?

T.J. Hill (Bristol)
I would like to comment, Dick, on attempts which have been made to detect HSV messenger RNA in latently infected ganglion. In their successful attempts Galloway and McDougal looked at human ganglia whereas Notkins' group, who were unsuccessful, used ganglia from Balb/c mice. It may be significant that in our experience Balb/c is a strain of mice in which it is difficult to induce recurrent skin lesions. There may turn out to be some connection between this and the state of latency in the ganglion of these animals.

R. Baringer (San Francisco)
Yes, but there is another difference that is important. Notkins and coworkers performed their study by liquid hybridization which means that a single, isolated ganglionic cell which contained RNA might not have been detected by these methods, whereas it might have been in situ hybridization that Drs. Galloway and McDougal used. So there are differences in technique as well as in species, and I think the point is that we really don't know much about the way in which the virus is maintained in the ganglionic cells. The evidence is conflicting, and yet, incomplete; and I think that it's still a very open question about the biological mechanisms.

H. zur Hausen (Freiburg)
It appears to me that the obvious problem is that we still lack a suitable tissue culture system for studying HSV latency.

W. Jaeger (Heidelberg)
Your interesting experimental investigations have some clinical implications. I mean the difficult situation when you are asked by an insurance company whether or not there exists a causal relationship between a peripheral trauma and herpetic ocular disease. Can you give us some more exact rules for this decision?

R. Baringer (San Francisco)
I found that in the United States those problems are settled by juries rather than doctors. No, I think it is very difficult to determine whether or not a relationship between peripheral trauma and herpes exists. I think the most direct evidence relates to blow-out fractures of the orbit. Hoyt has reported on two or three patients who have had blow-out fractures of the orbit which were followed by the recurrence of herpes on the face within a few days after the event. That makes some kind of sense in terms of what we know about trauma to the nerve and recurrence of HSV. As far as the other kind of relationship of injuries and herpes is concerned in which the local injury is not directly traumatizing the nervous structures, it's anybody's guess as to what the relation is.

Y.C. Cheng (Chapel Hill)
I am quite intrigued that Herpes simplex viruses pick up neurons as the site for latency. May this be due to the fact that neurons under normal conditions could not serve as a host for virus replication and that HSV replication requires some host enzyme participation? Is there any information about it? Could it be possible that something in the neurons inhibits virus growth or do the neurons not support enough material for virus replication?

R. Baringer (San Francisco)
I just don't have an answer to that question. I think that better minds than mine have tried to think about the problem; why is it that the neurons seem to be the cells which are capable of sustaining a prolonged infection with the virus. There isn't a very good biochemical or other answer, at least none I know of.

Y.C. Cheng (Chapel Hill)
If you explant a neuron cell and infect it with HSV, will the virus multiply?

R. Baringer (San Francisco)
If you explant neuronal tissue and get neurons to survive in vitro and then put herpes virus into that system, the neurons are destroyed like any other cells would be destroyed, so that in vitro they behave entirely different than they appear to behave in vivo. I think the answer is somewhere in that.

Sundmacher, R. (Hrsg.):
Herpetische Augenerkrankungen
© J.F. Bergmann Verlag, München 1981

# Trigeminal Nerve Lesions After Corneal HSV Infection: Cellular Responses

J.J. Townsend, San Francisco

**Key words.** HSV – ganglionic colonization and latency, trigeminal root, demyelination

**Schlüsselwörter.** HSV – ganglionäre Infektion und Latenz, Trigeminuswurzel, Demyelinisierung

**Summary.** Corneal inoculation in mice with Herpes simplex type 1 virus leads to a demyelinative encephalitis of the trigeminal root entry zone. The demyelination occurs only on the central nervous system (CNS) side of the junctional zone. The reasons for this marked difference in response between the CNS and peripheral nervous system (PNS) is not known. Schwann cells and ganglion cells contain viral particles but neither Schwann cell lysis nor demyelination is seen in the PNS. By days 7 to 9 post infection (PI), the demyelination and cellular response are pronounced in the CNS. Immunosuppression with cyclophosphamide before infection decreases the severity of the lesion. In nude (athymic) mice there is only mild CNS myelin splitting, while immune competent Balb c litter mates show dramatic demyelination with numerous mononuclear cells. These studies suggest a prominent role for cell mediated immunity. However, ultrastructural studies of the early junctional lesion 60–70 hours PI reveal a predominant astrocytic infection at the junction with cell lysis. Scattered mononuclear cells appear at this early stage suggesting an initial non-specific response to cell lysis or viral release. This may be responsible for triggering the cell mediated immune response by day 7. The greater vulnerability of the astrocyte to productive HSV infection when compared to the Schwann cell may be an important difference leading to the CNS lesion.

**Zusammenfassung.** Die korneale Einimpfung von Herpes simplex-Virus Typ 1 führt bei Mäusen zu einer Enzephalitis mit Demyelinisierung im Bereich der Trigeminuswurzel. Die Demyelinisierung erfolgt ausschließlich auf der zentralnervösen Seite der Übergangszone. Es ist unbekannt, warum das zentrale Nervensystem und das periphere Nervensystem derart unterschiedlich reagieren. Obwohl Schwannsche Zellen und Ganglienzellen Viruspartikel enthalten, kommt es im peripheren Nervensystem weder zu einer Zytolyse der Schwannschen Zellen noch zu einer Demyelinisierung. Vom 7. bis 9. Tag post infectionem findet man hingegen im zentralen Nervensystem eine deutliche Demyelinisierung mit zellulärer Reaktion. Eine vor der Infektion einsetzende Immunsuppression mit Zyklophosphamid mildert diese Reaktion. Bei nackten (athymischen) Mäusen findet man nur eine geringe Myelinaufsplitterung im zentralen Nervensystem, während immunkompetente Balb-c-Mäuse eine dramatische Demyelinisierung mit zahlreichen mononukleären Entzündungszellen erleiden. Diese Untersuchungen deuten auf eine ausschlaggebende Rolle der zellulären Immunität für diese Veränderungen hin. Auffällig ist, daß elektronenmikroskopische Untersuchungen der Entzündungsherde in der Übergangszone 60 bis 70 Std. nach der Infektion vorwiegend eine astrozytäre Infektion mit Zytolyse in der Übergangszone zeigen. Zu dieser Zeit erscheinen vereinzelte mononukleäre Zellen, was auf eine ursprünglich unspezifische Reaktion auf den Zelluntergang oder die Virusfreisetzung hindeutet. Als Reaktion hierauf kommt es dann vielleicht zu der zellulären Immunantwort vom 7. Tag an. Der entscheidende Grund für die Ausbildung von zentralnervösen entzündlichen Defekten liegt vielleicht darin, daß die Astrozyten im Vergleich zu den Schwannschen Zellen für eine zytolytische Herpes simplex-Virus-Infektion anfälliger sind.

Corneal infection with Herpes Simplex Virus (HSV) in rabbits and mice causes an ascending infection of the trigeminal nerve [1, 2]. Approximately seven days after corneal infection a demyelinating lesion on the central nervous system (CNS) side of the trigeminal root entry zone can be seen [3–5]. The lesion occurs on the inferior medial portion of the entry zone corresponding to the ophthalmic division of the trigeminal nerve. The transition or junction zone divides the peripheral nervous system (PNS) from the CNS. At this point the Schwann cell which is responsible for myelinating the PNS gives way to the oligodendroglial cell which is responsible for central myelination. On the CNS side the astrocyte has its foot process on the junctional node of Ranvier. The basal lamina of the Schwann cell turns back at the junctional node of Ranvier and covers the terminal astrocytic process [6].

After corneal infection with HSV the major transport of viral particles is in the axoplasm of the trigeminal nerve to the brainstem [7, 8]. In the PNS both ganglion cells and Schwann cells are infected. However, no loss of myelin occurs until the CNS is reached [3–5]. Approximately seven days after corneal infection numerous mononuclear cells are found on the CNS side of the junction and denuded axons are present. The axons although swollen are preserved and separated by extracellular edema. This demyelination begins at the junctional node of Ranvier and extends into the CNS.

If the cell mediated immune response is removed with cyclophosphamide, the amount of demyelination is markedly decreased [9]. Preliminary studies with Nude (athymic) mice also show a marked decrease in demyelination when compared to their immune competent litter mates [10]. Because cyclophosphamide decreases the T cell compartment and Nude (athymic) mice have no T cells, these studies would suggest a role for the T cells in the demyelination of the CNS compartment. Although oligodendroglial cells are infected, their infection does not appear to cause significant demyelination seven days after infection.

Seventy 4–6 week old Swiss mice were infected on the right scarified cornea with 0.05cc of HSV ($1 \times 10^7$pfu/ml.) The animals were sacrificed with intracardiac perfusion of Karnovsky's solution at various time intervals (48–96 h) after infection. Ultrastructural studies of the junctional region 2 to 3 days after infection demonstrate that there is an early nonspecific mononuclear cell response present. Although no demyelination has occurred at this early stage, astrocytes are already infected with virus and eventually undergo lysis. The early mononuclear cells are found around vessels and in a perineural distribution. Schwann cells contain viral particles during this early stage of the disease but

no Schwann cell lysis has been seen and no subsequent demyelination occurs in the PNS. Hill and Field have suggested that Schwann cells do not create a productive infection with enveloped infective viral particles [11]. This contrasts to the astrocytes in the CNS which do contain enveloped viral particles in the cytoplasm.

Normally oligodendroglial cells are sparse at the junction but scattered infected oligodendrocytes are seen early in the disease process. Retraction of CNS terminal loops at the junctional node of Ranvier was observed and could have been secondary to oligodendroglial infection. This may lead to mild early myelin disruption.

These morphological studies of the early lesion after corneal infection with HSV in Swiss mice demonstrate on overwhelming infection of junctional astrocytes with lysis. The non-specific mononuclear cell infiltrate seen at this early stage may be in response to release of virus by these dying cells. These non-specific cells may then transfer antigenic information to the cell mediated immune system which then responds causing significant demyelination seven days after corneal infection.

## References

1. Cook ML, Stevens JG (1973) Pathogenesis of herpetic neuritis and ganglionitis in mice: evidence for intra-axonal transport of infection. Infect Immun 7:272
2. Baringer JR, Griffith JF (1970) Experimental herpes simplex encephalitis: Early neuropathologic changes. J Neuropath Exp Neurol 29:89
3. Townsend JJ, Baringer JR (1976) Comparative vulnerability of peripheral and central nervous tissue to herpes simplex virus. J Neuropath Exp Neurol 35:100
4. Kristensson K, Vahlne A, Persson LA, Lyche E (1978) Neural spread of herpes simplex virus Types 1 and 2 in mice after corneal or subcutaneous (footpad) inoculation. J Neurol Sci 35:331
5. Townsend JJ, Baringer JR (1978) Central nervous system susceptibility to herpes simplex infection. J Neuropath Exp Neurol 37:255
6. Carlstedt T (1977) Observations on the morphology at the transition between the peripheral and the central nervous system in the Cat I–V. Acta Physiol Scand suppl 446

7. Kristensson K, Lycke E, Sjostrand J (1971) Spread of herpes simplex virus in peripheral nerves. Acta Neuropathol (Berl) 17:44

8. Hill TJ, Field HJ, Roome APC (1972) Intra-axonal location of HSV particles. J Gen Virol 15:253

9. Townsend JJ, Baringer JR (1979) Morphology of CNS disease in immunosuppressed mice after peripheral HSV inoculation. Lab Invest 40:178

10. Townsend JJ (1980) Demyelination in athymic mice following herpes simplex infection. International Conference on Human Herpes Virus, Atlanta, Georgia

11. Hill TJ, Field HJ (1973) The interaction of herpes simplex virus with cultures of peripheral nervous tissue: An electron microscopic study. J Gen Virol 21:123

## Discussion on the Contribution pp. 33–35

W.A. Blyth (Bristol)
Could you tell us whether the animals were doomed to die or were you taking care of the animals so that they would continue to live?

J.J. Townsend (San Francisco)
Most of the Swiss mice were sacrificed during the first week. Approximately 60% of those that were not sacrificed died during the acute phase and 40% went on to live. After several months these animals demonstrated remyelination by Schwann cells at the junction. The Nude mice were all sacrificed acutely and no attempt made to keep them alive for long periods.

J.R. Baringer (San Francisco)
What do you think makes the virus escape? The virus apparently travels up the axon and doesn't seem to do much at all until it hits the junction between the PNS and the CNS. It then explodes into a very dramatic infection. Do you have any ideas as to how the virus gets out at this point?

J.J. Townsend (San Francisco)
In general, although I don't know, I can speculate. There are two things that occur at the junction which may make viral escape more likely. One thing, the basement membrane or basal lamina covering the Schwann cell ends at the junctional node of Ranvier and turns back to cover the astrocytic cell border. At this point there is no basal lamina separating the axoplasmic entrance from the CNS. Perhaps the basal lamina acts as a barrier to the virus in the PNS.

Sundmacher, R. (Hrsg.):
Herpetische Augenerkrankungen
© J.F. Bergmann Verlag, München 1981

# Infection With Herpes Simplex Virus in the Eye and Trigeminal Ganglion of Mice

T.J. Hill, K. Ahluwalia, W.A. Blyth, Bristol

**Key words.** Recurrent HSV disease, latency, immunosuppression, reactivation

**Schlüsselwörter.** HSV – Rezidiverkrankungen, Latenz, Immunsuppression, Reaktivierung

**Summary.** Swiss white mice were infected in the right eye with herpes simplex virus (HSV) type 1. During the subsequent latent infection HSV could be isolated after in vitro culture from the right trigeminal ganglion of 95% of the animals. Neither spontaneous recurrence of ocular disease nor shedding of virus in eye secretions were detected in such animals. Various stimuli were tested for their ability to induce recurrent ocular disease or reappearance of infectious virus in eye secretions, the cornea or trigeminal ganglion of latently infected animals. Trauma to the cornea failed to induce recurrent disease and reappearance of virus in the cornea and ganglion. After direct trauma to the ganglion infectious virus was detected there one day later, but no clinical disease or infectious virus was produced in the eye.

Infectious virus was detected in the trigeminal ganglion on the 6th day after commencement of treatment with immunosuppressive drugs (cyclophosphamide, prednisolone or antithymocyte serum). None of these treatments induced recurrent ocular disease and only cyclophosphamide induced reappearance of virus in the cornea.

**Zusammenfassung.** Die rechten Augen von Schweizer weißen Mäusen wurden mit Herpes simplex-Virus (HSV) Typ 1 infiziert. Im Verlauf der folgenden latenten Infektion konnte HSV aus dem rechten Trigeminalganglion der Tiere zu 95% mittels in vitro-Kultur gewonnen werden. Die Tiere zeigten aber weder spontane Rezidive der Augenerkrankung noch schieden sie Virus in die Tränenflüssigkeit aus.

Mit verschiedenen Auslösereizen wurde bei latent infizierten Tieren versucht, Rezidive einer Augenerkrankung zu provozieren oder das Wiederauftreten infektiösen Virus in der Tränenflüssigkeit, der Kornea oder dem Trigeminalganglion hervorzurufen. Verletzungen der Hornhaut führten zu keiner Rezidiverkrankung und zu keinem Wiederauftauchen des Virus in der Hornhaut und dem Ganglion. Nur unmittelbare Verletzung des Ganglion selbst führte einen Tag später zu isolierbarem Virus, aber weder zu einer klinischen Erkrankung noch zur Isolierung von Virus aus Augenstrukturen.

6 Tage nach dem Beginn einer immunsuppressiven Therapie (Cyclophosphamid, Prednisolon oder Antithymozyten-Serum) konnte Virus im Trigeminalganglion gefunden werden. Keine dieser Therapieformen führte aber zu einer Augenerkrankung, und nur nach Cyclophosphamid fanden wir Herpesvirus in der Hornhaut.

## Introduction

A suitable animal model would be of great value in experiments on the elucidation of the pathogenesis of recurrent ocular herpetic disease in man. Experiments involving the rabbit eye have made some advances in this direction. In particular direct stimulation of the trigeminal ganglion [10], the site of latency, or iontophoresis of epinephrine into the cornea [8] both induce shedding of virus in eye secretions. However such shedding does not appear to be associated with clinical disease in the cornea.

The present report describes attempts to establish recurrent clinical herpetic disease in the mouse eye. The experimental approach was influenced by our successful development of a mouse model, in which recurrent clinical lesions can be induced in the skin of the ear by the application of a variety of stimuli e.g. trauma or UV irradiation to the originally infected site [1, 4].

## Materials and Methods

### Latently Infected Mice

Male, 8 week old outbred Swiss white mice were anaesthetised with sodium pentobarbitone. After scarification of the right cornea with a 26 gauge needle in a grid pattern (20 strokes in each direction), 5 µl of HSV type 1 strain SC16 [5] containing $5 \times 10^4$ pfu were dropped onto the surface of the cornea.

At least 4 weeks elapsed between primary infection and use of mice for subsequent experiments. Mice whose right eyes were then abnormal were excluded.

### Isolation of Virus From Eye Washings

Mice were anaesthetised and 8 µl maintenance medium [5] was dropped onto the right cornea. The medium was sucked up and down five times with an automatic pipette and then inoculated onto cultures of Vero cells.

### Isolation of Virus From the Cornea and Trigeminal Ganglion

The cornea or ganglion were ground in 0.4 ml maintenance medium in a glass grinder. In the case of the ganglion the homogenate was frozen and thawed three times. Assay of infectious virus was done in Vero cells [4]. In some experiments virus was detected in the cornea by culture of whole explants. Individual corneas were cultured freely floating in 5 ml of Liebowitz L-15 medium in 5 cm diameter petri dishes containing a confluent monolayer of Vero cells. The Vero cells were observed daily for evidence of cytopathic effect characteristic of HSV.

### Detection of Latent Infection in the Trigeminal Ganglion

Mice were killed by i.p. injection with sodium pentobarbitone and the right trigeminal ganglion was removed. After culture for 3 days at 35° in 0.5 ml growth medium, the ganglion was ground in a tissue grinder and 50 µl samples were inoculated onto Vero cells to detect the presence of HSV.

### Trauma to the Trigeminal Ganglion

A 30 gauge injection needle was inserted through the right side of the cranium at a point on the perimeter of the dorso rostral quadrant of the external auditory meatus. Insertion of the needle to a depth of 6 mm ensured that the point just transfixed the right trigeminal ganglion.

### Treatment With Immunosuppressive Drugs

Cyclophosphamide (Koch-Light Ltd) was injected i.p., 0.5 ml/mouse at 200 mg/kg, 150 mg/kg or 100 mg/kg on days 1 and 3 of the experiment and at 15 mg/kg on day 5. Prednisolone (Koch-Light Ltd) was suspended in 0.5% methyl cellulose in PBSA. Mice were injected i.p. with 0.5 ml at 60 mg/kg on days 1, 3 and 5 of the experiment.
Antithymocyte serum (ATS) was prepared in rabbits [2]. Mice were injected s.c. with 0.35 ml ATS on the 1st, 2nd, 3rd and 5th days of the experiment.

### Detection of Lesions in the Corneal Epithelium

Mice were anaesthetised and examined daily under a dissecting microscope for evidence of corneal lesions. Corneal ulceration was detected by staining with 1% Rose Bengal solution (Smith and Nephew Pharmaceuticals Ltd).

## Results

### Primary Disease in the Eye

Ulcerative lesions in the cornea were seen in nearly all animals within 1–2 days after infection. Infectious virus reached peak titres in the cornea by day 3 and in the trigeminal ganglion by day 4 after infection. About 20% of animals died with infection spreading to the CNS. In animals surviving the primary disease infectious virus was not detected in eye washings or corneal explants over a period of 10–55 days after infection. Latent infection was demonstrated in the right trigeminal ganglion of 95% of mice tested at least 4 weeks after primary infection.

## Attempts to Induce Recurrent Ocular Disease

### Trauma to the Cornea

The right eyes of groups of latently infected

**Table 1.** Trauma to the cornea

| Stimulus | Days after stimulus | Virus isolated from | |
| --- | --- | --- | --- |
| | | Cornea (by explant culture) | Trigeminal ganglion (by grinding, freezing and thawing) |
| Scarifi-cation of cornea | 2 | $\dfrac{0^*}{21}$ | $\dfrac{0}{21}$ |
| | 4 | $\dfrac{0}{15}$ | $\dfrac{0}{15}$ |
| UV irradia-tion of cornea | 2 | $\dfrac{1}{27}$ | $\dfrac{0}{27}$ |
| | 4 | $\dfrac{0}{13}$ | $\dfrac{0}{13}$ |
| No treat-ment | | $\dfrac{0}{35}$ | $\dfrac{0}{35}$ |

In a further group of 18 mice no infectious virus was detected in daily eye washings taken for 10 days after scarification of the cornea.

* $\dfrac{\text{No. with virus}}{\text{total tested}}$

mice were scarified in a similar manner to that used in establishing the primary infection.

In other groups the right eye was irradiated for 60 seconds with UV light under conditions similar to those used for the skin of the ear [1]. Control groups were anaesthetised but received no treatment to the cornea. On days 2 and 4 after irradiation or scarification, mice were killed and the right trigeminal ganglion and cornea were tested for infectious virus (Table 1). No virus was isolated except from the cornea of 1 of 27 mice tested 2 days after irradiation with UV light.

*Trauma to the Trigeminal Ganglion*

At various times after trauma to the right ganglion the right corneas and ganglion from groups of mice were tested for infectious HSV (Table 2). No virus was detected in the corneas. HSV was isolated from the ganglion

**Table 2.** Trauma to the trigeminal ganglion

| Days after trauma to the ganglion | Virus isolated from | |
| --- | --- | --- |
| | Cornea (by explant culture) | Trigeminal ganglion (by grinding, freezing and thawing) |
| 1 | $\dfrac{0^*}{11}$ | $\dfrac{3}{11}$ |
| 2 | $\dfrac{0}{10}$ | $\dfrac{0}{10}$ |
| 4 | $\dfrac{0}{7}$ | $\dfrac{1}{7}$ |
| 9 | $\dfrac{0}{11}$ | $\dfrac{0}{11}$ |

* $\dfrac{\text{no. with virus}}{\text{total tested}}$

**Table 3.** Treatment with immunosuppressive drugs

| Treatment | Virus isolated 6 days after beginning of treatment | |
| --- | --- | --- |
| | Cornea (by explant culture) | Trigeminal ganglion (by grinding, freezing and thawing) |
| Cyclophosphamide: | | |
| a) 200 mg/kg days 1, 3 | 1* | 6 |
| 15 mg/kg day 5 | 25 | 25 |
| b) 150 mg/kg days 1, 3 | 2 | 3 |
| 15 mg/kg day 5 | 21 | 21 |
| c) 100 mg/kg days 1, 3 | 0 | 0 |
| 15 mg/kg day 5 | 14 | 14 |
| Antithymocyte serum days 1, 2, 3 and 5 | 0 / 14 | 2 / 14 |
| Prednisolone 60 mg/kg days 1, 3, 5 | 0 / 23 | 2 / 23 |

* no. with virus
total tested

of 3/11 mice tested one day after trauma and 1/7 after 4 days.

In another group of 35 latently infected mice infectious HSV was not isolated from the untraumatised ganglion.

### Treatment With Immunosuppressive Drugs

Treatment of normal 8 week old male mice with the highest dose of cyclophosphamide produced a 70% reduction in circulating lymphocytes by day 1 after start of treatment. A single dose of 100 mg/kg produced a similar effect [2].

ATS depressed blood lymphocyte counts by an average of about 70% by the 5th day of treatment [2].

Groups of latently infected mice were treated with prednisolone, ATS or three different doses of cyclophosphamide (Table 3). Six days after the start of the treatment mice were killed and the right coreas and trigeminal ganglion were tested for infectious HSV.

After treatment with the two highest doses of cyclophosphamide HSV was isolated from the cornea (from about 6% of mice) and ganglion (from about 20% of mice) but not with the lowest dose.

After treatment with ATS or prednisolone HSV was also isolated from the ganglia of about 14% of mice treated with ATS and 9% of those treated with prednisolone. Virus was not isolated from the cornea after these treatments.

None of the above treatments, trauma to the cornea or ganglion or treatment with immunosuppressive drugs, produced evidence of recurrent clinical disease in the corneal epithelium.

### Discussion

The establishment of primary infection with HSV in the mouse eye and subsequent latency in the trigeminal ganglion confirms the observations of Knotts et al. [7]. These workers like ourselves did not see shedding of virus in eye secretions or development of ocular disease in latently infected mice. In man [6] and rabbits [11] HSV can be isolated from eye secretions and spontaneous recurrent disease develops. Whether this represents a significant difference between species and/or between different strains of virus (see Kaufman and Centifanto this symposium) remains to be established.

Agents which have proved successful in inducing recurrence of HSV in the skin of the mouse viz, trauma [4] and irradiation with UV light [1] failed to do so in the eye. With UV light only 1 of 27 mice showed virus in the cornea 2 days after irradiation. As in the skin [1] assessment of recurrent clinical disease was difficult owing to the long lasting inflammatory response in the irradiated eye. The failure of these stimuli to induce significant recurrence of virus or clinical disease in the eye may reflect differences between the response of the cornea and skin to injury. Healing of the corneal epithelium is very rapid and may involve less inflammatory response and release of mediators than in the skin where the release of such mediators, particularly prostaglandins, may be important in the induction of recurrent disease [3, 4].

In the rabbit direct stimulation (mechanical or electrical) of the trigeminal ganglion causes shedding of virus in the tears in a large proportion of animals within 2 days of the stimulation [10]. In the mouse trauma to the ganglion induced reactivation of virus in the ganglion within 1 day but no shedding of virus or clinical disease in the cornea. This reactivation in the ganglion may be analogous to that produced by the trauma involved in culture of ganglion explants for the demonstration of latency. The observations in the rabbit and the mouse suggest that induction of clinical disease in the eye may require changes in addition to those in the ganglion e.g. a trigger which produces changes in the susceptibility of the peripheral tissues [3].

Treatment with immunosuppressive drugs although not inducing clinical disease in the eye or skin [2] was the most effective means of inducing the appearance of infectious virus in the ganglion and in some cases (the highest doses of cyclophosphamide) in the cornea. Similar results on the effects of cyclophosphamide have been reported by Openshaw et al. [12].

The mechanisms underlying these effects of the immunosuppressive drugs are not clear. It is extremely unlikely that such short term immunosuppression would significantly affect levels of circulating antibody. Stevens and Cook [13] and Lehner et al. [9] have suggested that antiviral antibody bound to the neuronal surface might be important in controlling latency in the ganglion. Whether short term immunosuppression would affect such cell bound antibody is unknown.

As yet there is no evidence that cell mediated immunity has a role in controlling ganglionic latency. The results with ATS in particular might be interpreted that some such control is important. However it is also possible that ATS could produce membrane changes in neurones by binding to the theta antigens which neurones and lymphocytes have in common. Such membrane changes might then lead to reactivation of HSV. Similar arguments could be made for the induction of non-specific changes in neuronal membranes induced by prednisolone through the known effects of steroids on cell membranes.

With regard to cyclophosphamide Openshaw et al. [12] have pointed out that its ability to induce reactivation of HSV in the ganglion may be related to the ability of the drug to damage neuronal DNA rather than its immunosuppressive activity.

Thus although immunosuppressive drugs induce reactivation of HSV in the ganglion they may be acting through mechanisms other than by immunosuppression. It is therefore dangerous to conclude from the drugs activity that immune reactions control latency.

**Acknowledgment.** This work was supported in part by a grant from Parke-Davis Ltd.

# References

1. Blyth WA, Hill TJ, Field HJ, Harbour DA (1976) Reactivation of herpes simplex virus infection by ultraviolet light and possible involvement of prostaglandins. J Gen Virol 33: 547–550

2. Blyth WA, Harbour DA, Hill TJ (in press) Effect of immunosuppression on recurrent herpes simplex in mice. Infect Immun

3. Hill TJ, Blyth WA (1976) An alternative theory of herpes simplex recurrence and a possible role for prostaglandins. Lancet 1:397–399

4. Hill TJ, Blyth WA, Harbour DA (1978) Trauma to the skin causes recurrence of herpes simplex in the mouse. J Gen Virol 39:21–28

5. Hill TJ, Field HJ, Blyth WA (1975) Acute and recurrent infection with herpes simplex virus in the mouse: a model for studying latency and recurrent disease. J Gen Virol 28:341–353

6. Kaufman HE, Brown DC, Ellison EM (1967) Recurrent herpes in the rabbit and man. Science 156:1628–1629

7. Knotts FB, Cook ML, Stevens JG (1974) Pathogenesis of herpetic encephalitis in mice after

ophthalmic inoculation. J Infect Dis 130:16–27

8. Kwon BS, Gangarosa LP, Hill JM (in press) Induction of ocular herpes simplex virus shedding by epinephrine iontophoresis in rabbits.

9. Lehner T, Wilton JMA, Shillitoe EJ (1975) Immunological basis for latency, recurrences and putative oncogenecity of herpes simplex virus. Lancet 2:60–62

10. Nesburn AB, Dickinson R, Radnotti M, Radnotti MT (1976) Experimental reactivation of ocular herpes simplex in rabbits. Surv Ophthalmol 21:185

11. Nesburn AB, Elliott JH, Leibowitz HM (1967) Spontaneous reactivation of experimental herpes simplex keratitis in rabbits. Arch Ophthalmol 78:523

12. Openshaw H, Asher LVS, Wohlenberg C, Sekizawa T, Notkins AL (1979) Acute and latent infection of sensory ganglia with herpes simplex virus: immune control and virus reactivation. J Gen Virol 44:205–215

13. Stevens JG, Cook ML (1974) Maintenance of latent herpetic infection: an apparent role for antiviral IgG. J Immunol 113:1685–1693

Sundmacher, R. (Hrsg.):
Herpetische Augenerkrankungen
© J.F. Bergmann Verlag, München 1981

# Mechanisms of Control of Latent Herpes Simplex Virus Infection in the Skin and Eye

W.A. Blyth, T.J. Hill, D.A. Harbour, Bristol

**Key words.** Latency, reactivation, recurrent HSV disease – in the skin, in the eye

**Schlüsselwörter.** Latenz, Reaktivierung, Herpesrezidive in der Haut, im Auge

**Summary.** The sensory ganglia are probably the primary site of latency in herpes simplex virus (HSV) infections but infectious virus can be isolated from them only after cultivating the ganglia in vitro. Various systemic stimuli (treatment with cyclophosphamide, experimental infection with pneumococci) reactivate the virus in the ganglion but there is no direct evidence that this is significant in causing recurrent disease in the skin. Similarly after primary infection in the eye, treatment with cyclophosphamide or trauma to the trigeminal ganglion reactivates virus in the ganglion and can be followed by infectious virus being present in tears or cornea. Again the relationship between this reactivation and recurrent corneal disease has not been demonstrated.

In experimental animals stimuli applied to the skin in the area of primary infection (for instance trauma, inflammation, UV irradiation) induce recurrent disease. Observations in man confirm these findings but it cannot be assumed that the stimuli act only in the skin. In infection of the eye such "triggers" of recurrent disease have not yet been defined. Thus comparisons between herpes infection in the skin and the eye may be valuable, but it is not known how closely the infections are analogous.

**Zusammenfassung.** Wir berichten über die Kontrollmechanismen einer latenten Herpes simplex-Virus-(HSV-)Infektion sowie die Ursachen für die Entstehung von Rezidiverkrankungen in der Haut und im Auge. Die primären Latenzorte sind wahrscheinlich sensible Ganglien, aus denen man infektiöses Virus aber nur nach einer in vitro-Kultur der Ganglien gewinnen kann. Verschiedene systemische Reize (Behandlung mit Cy-clophosphamid, experimentelle Pneumokokkeninfektion) reaktivieren das Virus in den Ganglien; es gibt aber keinen Beweis dafür, daß dieser Schritt wichtig für die Erzeugung einer Rezidiverkrankung in der Haut ist. Auch nach einer primären Augeninfektion führen eine Cyclophosphamidbehandlung oder ein direktes Trauma des Trigeminalganglion zur Wiedervermehrung des Virus im Ganglion, und man kann auch infektiöses Virus in der Tränenflüssigkeit oder der Hornhaut finden. Aber auch in diesem Fall ist eigentlich unklar, was eine Reaktivierung für die Auslösung einer rezidivierenden Hornhauterkrankung bedeutet.

In Tierexperimenten kann man mit Reizen, die auf das Hautareal der Primärinfektion gesetzt werden (z.B. Verletzung, Entzündung, UV-Bestrahlung) eine Rezidiverkrankung erzeugen. Klinische Beobachtungen beim Menschen gehen in die gleiche Richtung; man kann aus ihnen aber nicht ohne weiteres schließen, daß die Stimuli nur auf die Haut wirken. Bei Augeninfektionen hat man solche "Trigger" einer Rezidiverkrankung noch nicht eindeutig identifizieren können. Deshalb könnten Vergleiche der Herpesinfektionen der Haut und des Auges wertvoll sein, obwohl nicht genau bekannt ist, wie sehr sich beide Infektionen entsprechen.

## The Site and Nature of the Latent Infection

There is abundant evidence from observation in humans [1] and experimental animals [12, 24] that sensory ganglia are important sites of latent infection with herpes simplex virus (HSV) and that neurons within the ganglia harbour the virus [5]. The siting of the original infection determines which ganglia (or parts of ganglia) are involved and this in turn controls the site of recurrent lesions. During latent infection virus cannot be isolated from disrupted ganglion cells. However if intact ganglia are cultivated in vitro for some days or weeks HSV can be isolated [24]. These observations led to the suggestion that during latency the virus exists in a non-infectious form, for example as viral DNA, perhaps integrated into the host cell genome [22]. However the possibility cannot be excluded that small numbers of infective virions are always present in nervous tissue and that only inefficiencies of techniques preclude their recovery.

## Reactivation of the Latent Infection

Stimuli that "reactivate" virus so that it can be isolated immediately after tissue is removed from the host have been found experimentally in the mouse. These include cyclophosphamide in doses of about 200 mg/kg [21], pneumococcal infection [26] and section of the nerves distal to the ganglia [29]. By interpreting such results some authors [6, 18] have suggested that recurrence of herpetic disease involves the following steps: stimulation in the nervous tissue resulting in production of infectious virus (or amplification of the amount present), transfer of virus along axons to the skin, and multiplication of the virus in skin cells to produce a lesion. In this sequence it is implicit that the major site of control of the infection is in the ganglion and that if virus escapes from this control and invades the skin a lesion results.

However evidence for this sequence is difficult to find. Clinical lesions in the skin have not been recognised in animals subjected to the stimuli known to reactivate virus in the ganglia. Thus even though it is very probable that they are connected, the significance of reactivation of latent infection in the nervous system to development of lesions in the skin is not yet known.

It is also clear that the sequence of events described above cannot fully explain the development of recurrent lesions in the skin. This was argued previously [11], but in summary a different sequence is needed to explain the following points. The interval between stimulus and development of lesions in some people undergoing fever therapy can be as short as 1 day [30] and HSV can occur in the skin without production of disease [13]. Moreover some well known factors that induce recurrent lesions, particularly trauma and irradiation by U.V. light directly affect the

**Table 1.** Induction of recurrent clinical disease in the mouse ear

| Ineffective agents | Effective agents |
| --- | --- |
| Cyclophosphamide | |
| Anti-thymocyte serum | U.V. Light |
| Azathioprine with prednisolone[a] | Sellophange tape stripping |
| Methyl mercury acetate | Xylene (50% in ethanol) |
| Cadmium chloride | Acetic acid |
| DMSO on ear[a] | Tetra phorbol acetate |
| Ethanol (50%) on ear | Trauma of injection |
| Acetone on ear | $PGE_2$ |
| | Retinoic acid (in acetone) |

[a] About 10% of mice had recurrent lesions after these treatments

skin (though this does not preclude effects in the ganglia or elsewhere). In this connection stimuli that efficiently induce recurrent lesions in mice are those that affect the skin in the site of primary infection (Table 1), often to cause some degree of inflammatory or regenerative activity. These observations led us to propose the "skin trigger" theory [11]. It was proposed that virus is frequently released from the ganglion but recurrent disease does not develop every time the virus invades the skin. Usually this virus is removed by host defence mechanisms and only when conditions in the skin particularly favour virus multiplication (i.e. after some triggering factor) does a clinical lesion develop.

The part played by the immunological reaction against HSV in controlling the development of recurrent herpes is not clear though it has been suggested that immunoglobulins on the surface of neurons control latency in the ganglion [17, 25]. There is conflicting evidence whether lesions are more frequent in immunocompromised people [19, 23, 31] (though they are undoubtedly severe and long lasting). Immunosuppression alone was shown to induce recurrent lesions in one experimental study [28] but in others the skin was almost certainly altered by plucking the hair so that interpretation is difficult [15]. In our own studies immunosuppression induced very few recurrent lesions and increased their incidence after trauma to the skin only slightly if at all [3]. It is difficult to see how minor sunburn or trauma to the skin could induce generalized immunosuppression. However, localized suppression, perhaps mediated by prostaglandins released in the skin after these stimuli [10, 27], might temporarily allow sufficient virus multiplication to cause a clinical lesion.

### The Recurrent Lesion

Whatever the mechanisms involved the recurrent lesion in the skin is relatively well defined. After a prodromal stage with some inflammation a vesicle develops and after 1 or 2 days is infiltrated with cells to form a pustule. At this stage the amount of virus that can be isolated from the contents of the lesion is decreasing rapidly and there is evidence that even the infectious virus is complexed with antibody [7]. Thus it is likely that by the time that scabs form, active infection is already controlled and that the duration of the scabbed lesion merely reflects the time taken to heal the tissue damage that developed in the first 2 days.

In ocular infection there is a greater chance for more varied pathology if only because all the different types of tissue which make up the eye can become involved. At the lid margins lesions exactly analogous to those around the mouth occur but in the conjunctiva vesicles are probably transient or absent. The conjunctival mucous membrane might withstand the pressure of liquid within a vesicle less well than keratinized skin, and the constant movement of the opposed surfaces of the conjunctiva might lead to early ulceration. Acute conjunctivitis is sometimes the only sign [8]. In its early stages at least the corneal dendritic ulcer appears as a simple lesion with relatively little inflammation. In most cases the ulcer heals without involvement of tissues other than the surface layers of the cornea but disease in the stromal layer and chronic inflammation are serious complications. It is likely that much of the pathology in this deep seated or chronic disease arises only indirectly from the viral infection of the cornea and may involve immune reactions within the tissue [9]. It is also difficult to decide to what extent such complications are affected or even to some extent induced by therapy [9].

The typical dendritic morphology of the corneal ulcer is remarkable and its pathogenesis requires explanation. If there is one original centre of infection in the cornea epithelial cells particularly susceptible to viral infection must occur in dendritic patterns or some other mechanism must force the spreading infection into the characteristic shape. It appears more likely that multiple sites of simultaneous virus infection join to form the dendritic pattern, an interpretation supported by the scanning electron microscopy study of Harnisch and Hoffmann [14]. Their pictures show "ballooned" (and presumably therefore infected) cells in clumps along the lines of the developing dendritic pattern. These infected cells slough off to give shallow ulcerated areas which quickly heal, presumably by the well known ability of the epithelial cells to spread across the surface.

What is the origin of the virus particles that start the lesion? Since infectious virus can occur in eye secretions these provide a possible source. The virus may arise from nodes of occasional or even chronic infection in cells of the lacrimal gland. However both in experimental animals [20] and in humans [16] HSV can be isolated from eye secretions in the absence of manifest corneal disease, so that this virus may be irrelevant to the development of corneal lesions. If this is so it may be that corneal lesions develop only if virus is delivered directly from nerve ending to cells in the surface of the cornea.

In this case it is tempting to suggest that the dendritic shape develops because virus is seeded into epithelial cells along the underlying path of a nerve. However Baum [2] has argued against this suggestion following his observation that in rabbit corneas infected with HSV 14 days after transplantation, dendritic ulcers developed even though there was no evidence of re-growth of epithelial nerves. The question is further complicated by the observation by Colin et al. [4] that dendritic ulcers can develop in the conjunctiva though the importance or frequency of this occurrence is not known. In one of Colin's cases the cornea remained clinically normal, and in another corneal ulcers developed the day after those in the conjunctiva were seen. This report underlines the fact that the cornea is not the only site of development of ophthalmic herpes and may not be a particularly important one for the initiation of disease.

Factors that precipitate recurrent herpes lesions in the skin are well known, but with the exception of fever little is known of those factors that might induce corneal lesions. So far in our experimental studies, UV light and trauma have failed to induce corneal lesions in latently infected mice even though they efficiently induce lesions in the skin. In order to understand the mechanisms underlying development of recurrent disease it is important to establish whether fever acts on cells harbouring latent infection in the nervous system or at the periphery (or at both sites).

Triggers that appear to act in the skin by producing inflammatory responses may not be so important in the cornea because of this tissue's adaptation to transparency which requires that inflammatory response is minimised. This does not of course apply to the conjunctiva and here inflammation may well increase the chance of development or recurrent lesions which may then spread to involve the cornea. If this interpretation has value it might be expected that herpetic lesions of the conjunctiva might even be more common than those in the cornea but that they are often overlooked because of their relatively trivial nature. Thus it is difficult to decide how closely mechanisms underlying control of latency or recrudescence of disease in the cornea are analogous to those that act on disease in the skin.

# References

1. Baringer JR, Swoveland P (1973) Recovery of herpes simplex virus from human trigeminal ganglions. N Engl J Med 288:648–650
2. Baum JL (1970) Morphogenesis of the dentritic figure in herpes simplex keratitis. Am J Ophthalmol 70:722–724
3. Blyth WA, Harbour DA, Hill TJ (1980) Effect of immunosuppression on recurrent herpes simplex in mice. Infect Immun 29:902–907
4. Colin J, LeGrignou A, Baikoff G, Chastel C (1980) Three cases of dendritic ulceration of the conjunctiva Am J Ophthalmol 89:608–609
5. Cook ML, Bastone VB, Stevens JG (1974) Evidence that neurons harbor latent herpes simplex virus. Infect Immun 9:946–951
6. Cook ML, Stevens JG (1973) Pathogenesis of herpetic neuritis and ganglionitis in mice: evidence for intraaxonal transport of infection. Infect Immun 7:272–288
7. Daniels CA, Legoff SG, Notkins AL (1975) Shedding of infectious virus/antibody complexes from vesicular lesions of patients with recurrent herpes labialis. Lancet 2:524–528
8. Darougar S, Hunter PA, Viswalingam M, Gibson JA, Jones BR (1978) Acute follicular conjunctivitis and keratoconjunctivitis due to HSV in London. Br J Ophthalmol 62:843–849
9. Easty DL, Carter C (1979) Mechanisms of resistance and hypersensitivity in herpes simplex keratitis. Trans Ophthalmol Soc UK 99:126–133
10. Greaves MW, Sondergaard J (1970) Pharmacologic agents released in ultraviolet inflammation studies by continuous skin perfusion. J Invest Dermatol 54:365–367
11. Hill TJ, Blyth WA (1976) An alternative theory of herpes simplex recurrence and a possible role for prostaglandins. Lancet 1:397–398
12. Hill TJ, Field HJ, Blyth WA (1975) Acute and recurrent infection with herpes simplex virus in the mouse: a model for studying latency and recurrent disease. J Gen Virol 28:341–353
13. Hill TJ, Harbour DA, Blyth WA (1980) Isolation of herpes simplex virus from the skin of clinically normal mice during latent infection. J Gen Virol 47:205–207
14. Harnisch JP, Hoffmann F this vol
15. Hurd J, Robinson TWE (1977) Herpes simplex: aspects of reactivation in a mouse model. J Antimicrob Chemother 3:99–106
16. Kaufman HE, Brown DC, Ellison EM (1967) Recurrent herpes in the rabbit and man. Science 156:1628–1629
17. Lehner T, Wilton JMA, Shillitoe EJ (1975) Immunological basis for latency, recurrences, and putative oncogenicity of herpes simplex virus. Lancet 2:60–62
18. Merigan TC (1974) Host defenses against viral disease. N Engl J Med 290:323–329
19. Montgomerie JZ, Becroft DMO, Croxson MC, Doak PB, North JDK (1969) Herpes simplex virus infection after renal transplantation. Lancet 2:867–871
20. Nesburn AB, Dickinson R, Radnotti M, Radnotti MT (1976) Experimental reactivation of ocular herpes simplex in rabbits. Surv Ophthalmol 21:185
21. Openshaw H, Asher LVS, Wohlenberg C, Sekizawa T, Notkins AL (1979) Acute and latent infection of sensory ganglia with herpes simplex virus: immune control and virus reactivation. J Gen Virol 44:205–215
22. Roizman B (1965) An inquiry into the mechanisms of recurrent herpes infections of man. Perspectives in Virology 4:283–304
23. Russell AS (1974) Cell mediated immunity to HSV in man. J Infect Dis 129:142–146
24. Stevens JG, Cook ML (1971) Latent herpes simplex virus in spinal ganglia of mice. Science 173:843–845
25. Stevens JG, Cook ML (1974) Maintenance of

latent herpetic infection: an apparent role for anti-viral IgG. J Immunol 113:1685–1693

26. Stevens JG, Cook ML, Jordan MC (1975) Reactivation of latent herpes simplex virus after pneumococcal pneumonia in mice. Infect Immun 11:635–639

27. Trofatter KF, Daniels CA (1979) Interaction of human cells with prostaglandins and cyclic A.M.P. modulators. J Immunol 122:1363–1370

28. Underwood GE, Weed SD (1974) Recurrent cutaneous herpes simplex in hairless mice. Infect Immun 10:471–474

29. Walz MA, Price RW, Notkins AL (1974) Latent ganglionic infection with herpes simplex virus types 1 and 2: Viral reactivation in vivo after neurectomy. Science 184:1185–1187

30. Warren SL, Carpenter CM, Boak RA (1940) Symptomatic herpes, a sequela of artificially induced fever. J Exp Med 71:155–168

31. Wheeler CEJ (1975) Pathogenesis of recurrent herpes simplex infections. J Invest Dermatol 65:341–346

## Discussion on the Contributions pp. 37–47

Y. Centifanto (New Orleans)
Did you use only one strain of herpes that does not shed or produce recurrence? Did you use several strains? Or is it that, in mice, recurrences and shedding are not common or characteristic?

In the rabbit, you can pick up a virus which will give you the corneal disease and shedding and recurrences, while other strains do not produce disease, although they do shed virus. In other words, we see a variety of manifestations according to the virus strain used.

T.J. Hill (Bristol)
We certainly appreciate, as shown by your own work, that the virus strain could be important in determining recurrence of disease. The one strain we used in the experiments was chosen because we have a lot of information about it, particularly as regards its behaviour in skin infections in the mouse.

H.E. Kaufman (New Orleans)
If I got it right you are making the case that recurrences in the eye might be controlled by different mechanisms from that in the skin?

W.A. Blyth (Bristol)
We are not trying to make cases, we are just asking questions. I was very interested that you mentioned fever as a trigger in the eye. That is possibly a central trigger and could be acting differently from the local stimuli we find active in the skin.

H.D.M. Völker-Dieben (Leyden)
I would like to ask Dr. Blyth what he thinks about the difference in recurrence in male and female mice? Could pregnancy be a precipitating factor of recurrent disease?

W.A. Blyth (Bristol)
We did one experiment where we took latently infected female mice and mated them and watched them through pregnancy and lactation and they showed no clinical disease. But we would not say we had studied this completely.

Sundmacher, R. (Hrsg.):
Herpetische Augenerkrankungen
© J.F. Bergmann Verlag, München 1981

# Do Suppressor Lymphocytes Have a Role in Herpes Simplex Virus Latency and Recurrence?

A.A. Nash, H.J. Field, Cambridge

**Key words.** Latency, delayed hypersensitivity, suppressor B cells

**Schlüsselwörter.** Latenz, Immunität vom verzögerten Typ, Suppressor-B-Zellen

**Summary.** Draining lymph node (DLN) cells obtained from mice at various times after infection with HSV 1 were adoptively transferred into syngeneic recipients (either normal or presensitized with HSV) and the delayed-type hypersensitivity (DTH) response measured. Draining LN cells obtained 6 to 9 days post infection transferred DTH, whereas beyond this period the DLN contained suppressors of established DTH. The suppressor cells were Ig positive, thy 1.2 negative – B cells and were prominent only in the DLN, but not the contralateral lymph node, several months after the primary infection. The possible role these suppressor cells play in regulating immune responses during latency and recrudescences is discussed.

**Zusammenfassung.** Die intrazerebrale Inokulation von Herpes simplex-Virus (HSV) bei Mäusen führt zu einer Erkrankung, die viele Ähnlichkeiten mit der HSV-Infektion bei Menschen hat. Während der ersten Tage nach der Infektion entwickeln die Mäuse eine Immunität vom verzögerten Typ gegenüber HSV-Antigenen. Diese Immunität persistiert lebenslang und kann durch Inokulation von abgetötetem HSV in die Haut an der entsprechenden Reaktion gemessen werden. Die verzögerte Immunität kann frühzeitig im Verlaufe der Primärinfektion von Maus zu Maus dadurch übertragen werden, daß man Lymphozyten aus den ableitenden Lymphknoten entnimmt und diese auf nichtimmune Mäuse überträgt. Tut man dies jedoch deutlich später im Verlaufe der Infektion (mehr als 16 Tage p.i.), dann findet man einen ganz anderen Effekt der Transfer-Experimente, wenn man die Lymphozyten auf *vorimmunisierte* Tiere überträgt. In diesem Fall unterdrücken nämlich die übertragenen Zellen den verzögerten Immunitäts-effekt in den Empfängermäusen. Die Zellen, die für diese Suppression verantwortlich sind, scheinen HSV-spezifische B-Lymphozyten zu sein. Reine HSV-Antikörper ohne Zellen führen nicht zu diesem Unterdrückungseffekt. Die Bedeutung dieser Immunzellpopulation für die Regulation der klinischen Reaktion auf Reaktivierung latenten Herpes simplex-Virus in Mäusen wird diskutiert.

It is well established that cell mediated immunity (CMI) is important in the recovery and protection of a host against virus infections. An important component of this type of immunity is delayed-type hypersensitivity (DTH). We have been interested in the induction and regulation of the DTH response to herpes simplex virus type 1 (HSV 1) infected mice, as this response reflects most directly CMI events occurring in our particular model. As we have an interest in the functional properties of lymphoid cells present during the period of HSV latency, we used a mouse ear model in which latency and recrudescences have been observed [1].

Balb/c mice were inoculated with $10^5$ p.f.u. HSV 1 (SC$_{16}$C1) into the pinna of one ear. The lymph nodes draining the infected ear were removed at various times p.i., and approximately $2 \times 10^7$ cells injected intravenously into syngeneic recipients. Approximately 60 mins later the recipients were inoculated with $10^4$ p.f.u. HSV 1 (SC$_{16}$C1) into the ear pinna and daily ear thickness measurements made using a screw-gauge micrometer. The uninfected ear was used as a control. (In several experiments BHK cell sonicates or heat killed HSV 1 preparations produced only a marginal increase in ear thickness (2 to $4 \times 10^{-2}$ mm) 24 h after inoculation into normal recipients.)

In Table 1 the effect of transferring draining lymph node (DLN) cells at different times after infection is shown. DLN cells taken 6 to 9 days p.i. transfer a good DTH response

**Table 1.** Detection of DTH cells in the draining lymph node at various times after infection

| [b]Time after infection (days) | [c]Increased ear thickness (mm x $10^{-2}$) at 48 hrs | |
|---|---|---|
| | [a]Transfer (DLN cells) | Control (no cells) |
| 6 | *21 ± 4* | 11 ± 2 |
| 8 | *21 ± 3* | 14 ± 1 |
| 9 | *25 ± 1* | 13 ± 2 |
| 13 | 13.5 ± 2 | 13 ± 1 |
| 28 | 14 ± 4 | 12.5 ± 6 |
| 56 | 13.6 ± 2 | 11.7 ± 2 |

[a] $2 \times 10^7$ DLN cells transferred to each recipient
[b] Donor mice received $10^5$ p.f.u. HSV-1 (SC16) into left ear
[c] Mean ± SD of 3 to 4 mice/group

Figures *in italics* indicate significant differences when compared to control values (P <0.001)

which reached maximum intensity after 48 to 72 h. This response is similar to the classical tuberculin DTH response, which is characterized histologically by an infiltration of mononuclear cells and is not transferred by antiserum. During the time when the DTH response is transferable, there is also an accelerated reduction in the titres of infectious HSV in the ears of recipient mice [2]. Both the DTH response and reduction of virus titres are dependent on a T cell population.

Beyond day 9 the ability to transfer DTH declines rapidly. This is somewhat paradoxical since the infected donor produces a vigorous DTH response (24–48 hrs following a skin test), for up to 2 years after the primary infection. In view of this failure to transfer DTH at late times experiments were carried out to determine whether DTH cells could be suppressed in the DLN environment. DLN cells obtained from donors 1 to 4 months after infection were transferred into recipients presensitized to HSV 10 to 20 days previously. The recipients were then skin tested with either $10^4$ p.f.u. HSV 1 (SC$_{16}$C1) or $10^6$ erstwhile p.f.u. heat killed HSV and the ear thickness response measured 24–72 hrs later. As shown in Table 2 recipients receiving DLN cells had a suppressed ear swelling response when compared with the no cell control or with $2 \times 10^7$ transferred contralateral lymph node (CLN) cells. The suppressed DTH response was specific for HSV, since HSV-immune DLN cells failed to suppress a vaccinia DTH response [3]. The nature of cell type involved in the suppression is shown in Table 3. After DLN cells were separated into Ig positive or Ig negative fractions on antimouse-poly Ig coated dishes [4], only the Ig positive fraction produced suppression. In addition DLN cells pretreated with anti-thy 1.2 serum and complement also transferred the suppression. This indicates that a Ig positive, thy 1.2 negative − B cell-population is involved in the suppression of the established DTH response to HSV.

One possible mechanism by which B cells mediate this suppression is via anti-HSV antibody. This seemed unlikely as the HSV 1 presensitized recipients already produced a good neutralizing antibody response. However, the addition of more antiserum from

**Table 2.** Comparison of contralateral LN cells and draining LN cells on the suppression of DTH responses

| Expt. | Previously infected (months) | Increased ear thickness (mm x $10^{-2}$) after 24 hrs | | Control (no cells) |
|---|---|---|---|---|
| | | CLN | DLN | |
| 1 | 3 | 23 ± 2 | *14.6 ± 2* | 22.5 ± 1 |
| 2 | 4 | 19 ± 4 | *12.6 ± 3* | 21 ± 5 |
| [a]3 | 1 | 36 ± 4 | *19.5 ± 6* | 37 ± 2 |
| 4 | 2 | 14.5 ± 0.7 | *10.0 ± 1* | 18.6 ± 4.5 |

[a] $5 \times 10^4$ p.f.u. HSV-1 inoculated
1.6 to $2 \times 10^7$ CLN or DLN cells transferred/mouse
mean ± SD of 3 to 4 mice/group

Figures *in italics* denote significant differences compared to control values (P between 0.025 and 0.001)

**Table 3.** Nature of the cell transferring suppression

| | [a]Increased ear thickness after 24 hrs |
|---|---|
| Effect of Ig +ve cells | |
| Control (no cells) | 23 ± 3 |
| Ig +ve cells | *16 ± 2* |
| Unseparated cells | *14.5 ± 2* |
| | |
| Effect of anti thy 1.2 serum + c′ | |
| Control (no cells) | 37 ± 2 |
| Anti thy 1.2 + c′ treated | *22 ± 2* |
| Untreated | *19.5 ± 6* |

[a] mean ± SD of 3 to 4 mice/group

Figures *in italics* denote significant differences compared to control values (P between <0.01 to <0.001)

latently infected mice did not suppress the DTH response. This does not totally exclude a high concentration of anti-HSV antibody being produced by B cells at the site of infection, resulting in a feedback suppression via antigen blockage. However, B suppressors could act directly on T-DTH cells via anti-idiotype antibodies producing a suppression of DTH. It is certainly curious that the suppressor B cells should be predominantly localised to the lymph node draining the inoculation site. We believe such a localisation can only occur following a constant or periodic stimulation of the nodal environment by HSV. In other words, HSV recurrences are responsible for this localised B cell effect. Such recurrences most likely occur at a sub-clinical level, since we have never observed a clinical recurrent disease with our mouse model. We are currently investigating whether suppressor B cells arise following infection with a virus that does not produce a latent infection, e.g. vaccinia.

The other major question is how important are B suppressor cells in regulating the balance of the immune response in latently infected mice. A possible explanation is that B suppressors serve to dampen the T cell surveillance mechanism sufficient to allow expression of virus antigens. As the antigen load increases the suppressor system becomes inactivated and then the effector system becomes activated eventually reducing the virus load below the suppressor threshold. Such a mechanism would serve to allow a low level release of virus sufficient to activate an immunological suppressor system, which could in turn regulate local inflammatory cell responses.

It is well known that hypersensitivity reactions are an important cause of tissue damage in recurrent herpes lesions. This is particularly true of deep stromal eye disease caused by HSV. Our findings in mice suggest that the interplay between the mediators of delayed-type hypersensitivity and the cells which regulate these responses have an important role in determining the pathogenesis of such infections.

### References

1. Hill TJ, Field HJ, Blyth WA (1975) Acute and recurrent infection with herpes simplex virus in the mouse: a mouse model studying latency and recurrent disease. J Gen Virol 28:341–353
2. Nash AA, Field HJ, Quartey-Papafio R (1980) Cell mediated immunity in herpes simplex virus-infected mice: induction, characterization and antiviral effects of delayed type hypersensitivity. J Gen Virol 48:
3. Nash AA, Gell PGH (1980) Cell mediated immunity in herpes simplex virus infected mice: suppression of delayed hypersensitivity by an antigen-specific B lymphocyte. J Gen Virol 48:
4. Nash AA (1976) Separation of lymphocyte sub-populations using antibodies attached to staphylococcal protein A coated surfaces. J Immunol Methods 12:149–161

Sundmacher, R. (Hrsg.):
Herpetische Augenerkrankungen
© J.F. Bergmann Verlag, München 1981

# Aesthesiometrie bei Herpes corneae

J. Draeger, M. Lüders, R. Winter, Bremen

**Key words.** Keratoplasty after herpes, corneal sensitivity, aesthesiometry

**Schlüsselwörter.** Keratoplastik nach Herpes, Hornhautsensibilität, Ästhesiometrie

**Summary.** Sensitivity of the cornea is a main diagnostic criteria in herpetic keratitis.

With a recently developed electronic instrument, a quantitative reproducable aesthesiometry of the cornea is achieved. With this instrument it was proven that the threshold value of the corneal sensitivity does not primarily depend on the size of the tactile probe, but mainly on the applied pressure.

Morever, topographical and age correlations were studied.

In herpetic keratitis, a typical change of the topographical threshold values occures. The corneal center shows a marked disturbance of sensibility over a long period. The change in sensitivity correlates with the clinical stage of the keratitis, which was also shown in follow-up studies.

**Zusammenfassung.** Die Sensibilitätsprüfung der Hornhaut ist ein wichtiges Diagnostikum bei der Herpeskeratitis.

Mit einem kürzlich von uns entwickelten elektronischen Gerät ist jetzt eine quantitative reproduzierbare Hornhaut-Aesthesiometrie möglich. Die Empfindlichkeitsschwelle hängt dabei nicht von der Dicke des Testkörpers ab, sondern ausschließlich von der Größe des applizierten Druckes.

Mit dieser Methode untersuchten wir topographisch die Schwellen bei verschiedenen Altersgruppen.

Bei der Herpeskeratitis zeigt sich eine typische Umkehr des topographischen Schwellenprofils, indem die Hornhautmitte unverhältnismäßig stärker und länger beeinträchtigt ist. Änderungen der Sensibilität korrelierten mit dem klinischen Bild, wie sich auch bei Verlaufsstudien zeigte.

Die Störung der Hornhaut-Sensibilität als frühes Leitsymptom des Herpes simplex ist seit fast 100 Jahren bekannt. Krückmann hat schon auf die Möglichkeit zur Differentialdiagnose des Herpes simplex mit Hilfe der Sensibilitätsstörung hingewiesen.

Seither ist immer wieder versucht worden, die Messung der Hornhaut-Sensibilität zur Verlaufskontrolle sowie zur Differentialdiagnose nutzbar zu machen. Vor allem Severin [4] ist dieser Frage mit besonderer Gründlichkeit nachgegangen und hat versucht, eine klinische Klassifizierung herauszuarbeiten. Die Schwierigkeit war jedoch immer das Fehlen einer wirklich quantitativ reproduzierbaren Meßmethode. Alle bisherigen Verfahren waren von den äußeren Untersuchungsbedingungen wie Temperatur, Luftfeuchtigkeit oder der Fertigkeit des Untersuchers in hohem Maße abhängig [3]. Die Ergebnisse waren daher nicht verläßlich reproduzierbar oder miteinander vergleichbar. Dies ist der Hauptgrund, warum die Aesthesiometrie bisher nicht den ihr aus pathophysiologischen Gründen an sich zukommenden Platz in der Diagnostik des Herpes simplex gefunden hat.

Mit einem modernen optisch elektromagnetischen Instrument ist es nun aber möglich, wirklich quantitativ reproduzierbar zu messen [1, 2] (Abb. 1). Die erwähnten Umgebungsparameter spielen praktisch keine Rolle mehr.

Neben der präzisen Messung der Reizkraft kam es uns vor allem auf optische Kontrolle des Kontaktes zwischen Meßkörper und Hornhautoberfläche an, um den Ort und Zeitpunkt festlegen zu können. Eine rasche automatische Annäherung des Tastkörperchens an die Hornhautoberfläche mit definierter Geschwindigkeit vermeidet jeglichen ballistischen Effekt.

Die Handhabung des Gerätes sollte so einfach wie möglich sein, mit ständiger Anzeige der gerade ausgeübten Reizkraft.

Vor der klinischen Verwendung des

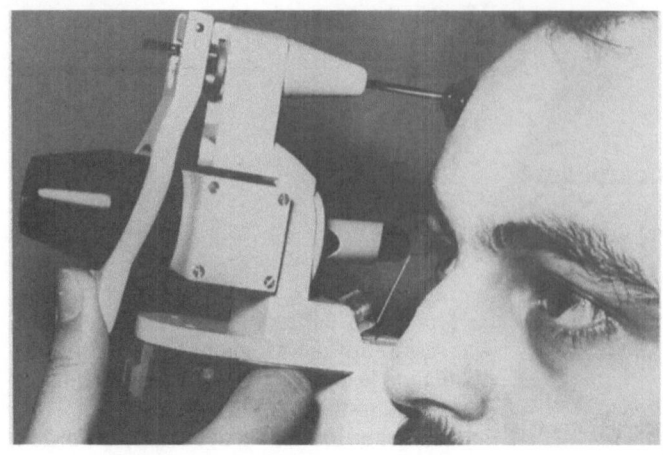

**Abb. 1.** Meßgerät, am Patienten-auge angesetzt

Gerätes bei Herpes simplex wurde zunächst das normale topographische Schwellenwert-profil ermittelt. Einen sehr niedrigen Mittelwert im Zentrum zwischen 0,8 und 2,5 $\times$ 10$^{-5}$ N entsprechen etwa zehnmal höhere Schwellenwerte im Limbusbereich.

Außerdem untersuchten wir die Altersab-hängigkeit der Hornhaut-Sensibilität, um auch hier die physiologischen Normwerte

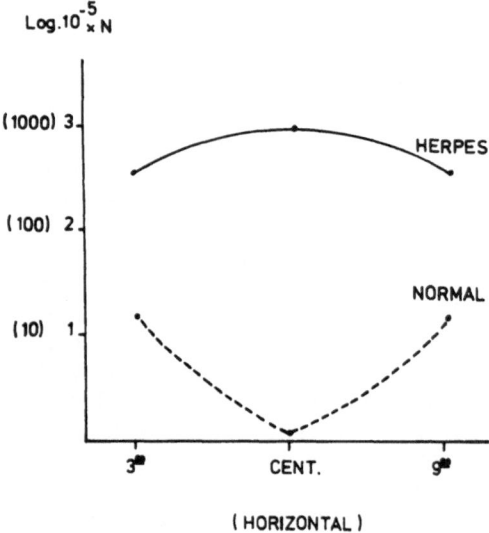

**Abb. 2.** Vergleich der Schwellenwertprofile normaler und herpetischer Hornhaut

festzulegen. Während bei Jugendlichen z.B. in 12 h Position am Limbus Schwellenwerte von 17,7 $\times$ 10$^{-5}$ N zu messen sind, benötigt der Kornealreflex bei den über 60jährigen 81 $\times$ 10$^{-5}$ N.

Für die Sensibilitätsmessungen bei Patienten mit Keratitis herpetica wurde das Schwellenwertprofil in fünf Positionen auf-genommen (limbusnah bei 3, 6, 9, 12 und zen-tral), nach Keratoplastiken noch vier zusätz-liche Positionen im Bereich der Wirtshorn-haut.

Wir unterteilten die Patienten nach dem klinischen Schweregrad:
1. rein epithelialer Herpes (Dendritica),
2. rezidivierender epithelialer Herpes, mit evtl. beginnender Stromabeteiligung,
3. schwere interstitielle Keratitiden.

Allen herpetischen Keratitiden gemein-sam war eine auffallende Umkehr der topo-graphischen Schwellenwertprofile (Abb. 2).

Während normalerweise das Hornhaut-zentrum am empfindlichsten ist, liegt hier häufig die Reizschwelle am höchsten. Gleichzeitig erhöhen sich auch die Schwellen am Limbus, jedoch nicht im gleichen Maße wie im Hornhautzentrum (Abb. 3).

Bei anderen Keratitiden, z.B. einer bak-teriellen Keratitis, bei der auch eine gewisse Sensibilitätsbeeinträchtigung zu beobachten ist, sehen wir nicht diese typische Profilum-kehr. Vielmehr finden wir bei bakteriellen Prozessen häufig eine umschriebene, mehr herdförmige, nämlich dem infizierten Areal entsprechende Sensibilitätseinschränkung, während die Umgebung völlig unbetroffen ist.

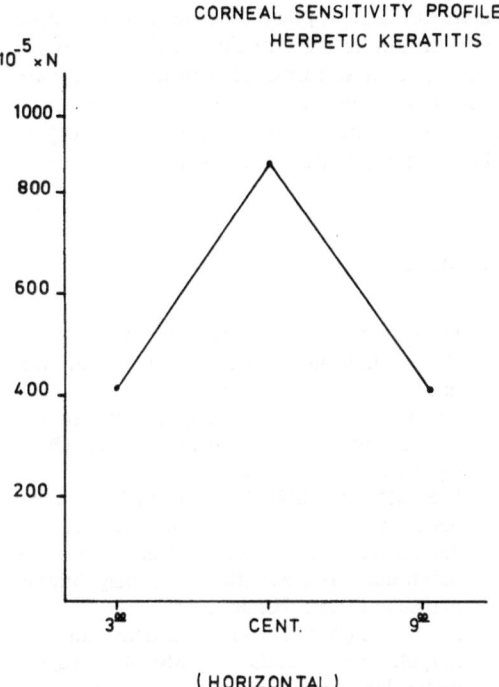

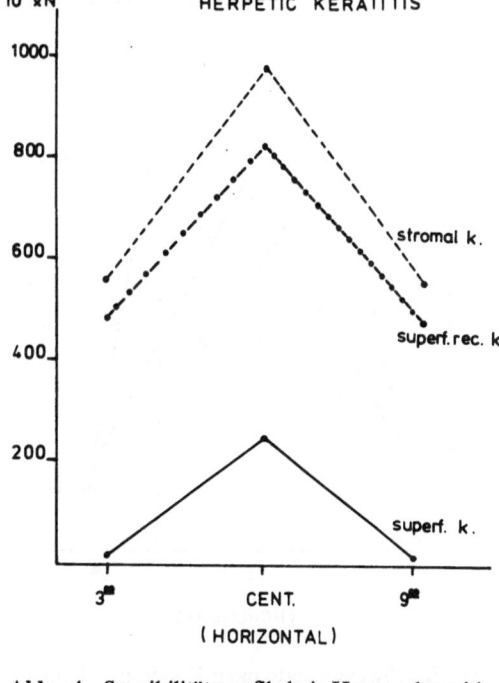

**Abb. 3.** Topographisches Schwellenprofil aller Herpesfälle

**Abb. 4.** Sensibilitätsprofil bei Herpes keratitis (epithelial, rez. epithelial, schwere interstitielle)

Das Ausmaß der Sensibilitätsstörung ist dem klinischen Bild gewissermaßen korreliert (Abb. 4), als nämlich bei der einfachen „Dendritica" zwar immer eine Schwellenerhöhung zu finden ist, diese aber stets wesentlich geringer ausfällt als bei schweren interstitiellen Prozessen.

Auffallend ist jedoch, daß auch bei einigen klinisch noch relativ harmlosen Erscheinungsformen die Schwellenwertkurven fast der schwersten Verlaufsform entsprachen: Hier handelte es sich stets um mehrfach rezidivierende Erkrankungen, bei denen also offensichtlich die Schädigung der Hornhautnerven dem Erscheinungsbild an der Spaltlampe vorauseilte, die Sensibilitätsstörung also eine bessere, insbesondere prognostische Beurteilung zuließ!

Die Dauer der Sensibilitätsstörung hängt nun wieder vom Ausmaß der Erkrankung ab. Heilt die rein epitheliale Läsion ab, so bildet sich auch eine normale Sensibilität wieder aus; und zwar in der Peripherie rascher als im Zentrum.

Die Normalisierung des zentralen Schwellenwertes und Wiederumkehr der Kurve in die Ausgangslage dauert bis zu 2 Jahren.

Bei herpetischen Keratitiden der Gruppe II (rezidivierende Epithelläsionen und evtl. Stromabeteiligung) kommt es zwar zu einer Besserung der Sensibilität, aber die typische Kurvenumkehr mit zentraler Hyposensibilität bleibt sehr lange oder dauernd bestehen. Bei einer Patientin sahen wir über 3 Jahre eine vollständige Asensibilität des Zentrums, obwohl der Prozeß klinisch mit Narben abgeheilt war.

Das Sensibilitätsprofil nach einer Keratoplastik bedarf des Vergleichs mit einer „nichtherpetischen Keratoplastik" (Abb. 5).

Normalerweise besteht direkt postoperativ eine zentrale Asensibilität entsprechend den zirkulär durchtrennten Hornhautnerven. Erst nach 2 bis 3 Jahren tritt mit dem Vorwachsen der Nervenendigung eine Reinnervierung auf. Nach ca. 7 Jahren ist die Schwelle im Zentrum wieder geringer als peripher, das typische topographische Sensibilitätsprofil ist wiederhergestellt, jedoch auf einem höheren Niveau. Anders ist der Verlauf bei der Keratoplastik nach herpetischen

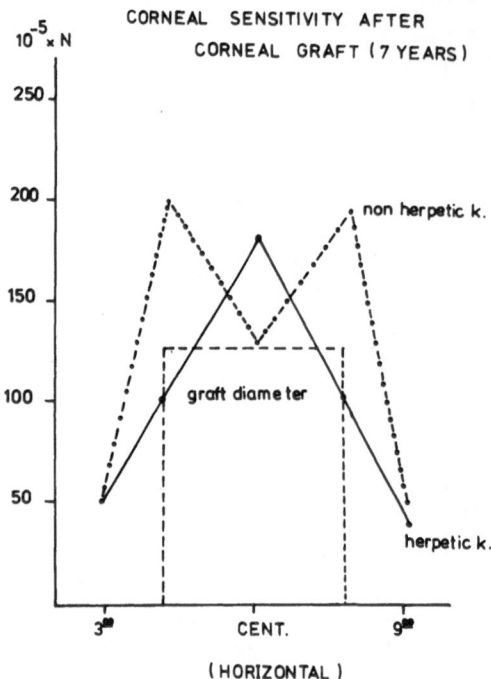

CORNEAL SENSITIVITY AFTER
CORNEAL GRAFT (7 YEARS)

$10^{-5} \times N$

non herpetic k.

graft diameter

herpetic k.

3ᵐ    CENT.    9ᵐ

( HORIZONTAL )

**Abb. 5.** Schwellenwerte nach Keratoplastik, nicht herpetisch, herpetisch

Keratitiden. Das Ansteigen der zentralen Empfindlichkeit geht langsamer vonstatten und nach mehreren Jahren ist der zentrale Schwellenwert noch höher als der periphere, die Umkehr der Schwellenwertkurve bildet sich gar nicht oder nur unvollständig zurück.

Die quantitative Aesthesiometrie mit reproduzierbaren Meßdaten ist eine wertvolle Hilfe in der Differentialdiagnostik und Verlaufskontrolle der herpetischen Keratitis. Der Unterschied zu anderen Keratitiden besteht darin, daß sich nicht nur eine allgemeine Sensibilitätsabnahme, sondern eine typische Umkehr der topographischen Schwellenwertkurve mit enormen zentralen Schwellenanstiegen auftritt. Nach unseren Messungen korreliert das klinische Erscheinungsbild nach Schwere der Erkrankung und Rezidivhäufigkeit mit dem Ausmaß der Sensibilitätsstörung.

Der zeitliche Verlauf in der Normalisierung der Schwellenwertkurven bestätigt die Schwere des Krankheitsbildes und ermöglicht es, die Rezidivgefahr vorauszuschätzen. Durch die genaue Quantifizierbarkeit der Schwellenwerte kann man auch bei der relativen Hyposensibilität, die ja vor allen Dingen

nach der Keratoplastik vorhanden ist, noch eine graduelle weitere Sensibilitätsabnahme meßbar erfassen und hat somit eine bessere Verlaufsbeurteilung nach einer Keratoplastik, insbesondere im Hinblick auf Herpes-Rezidive im Transplantatbereich.

## Literatur

1. Draeger J, Koudelka W, Lubahn E (1976) Zur Aesthesiometrie der Hornhaut. Klin Monatsbl Augenheilkd 169:407–421
2. Draeger J (1979) Klinische Ergebnisse der Aesthesiometrie der Hornhaut. Ber Dtsch Ophthalmol Ges 76:389–395
3. Frey MV von (1894) Beiträge zur Physiologie der Schmerzsinne. In: Berichte über die Verhandlungen der königlich sächsischen Gesellschaft der Wissenschaften zu Leipzig. Mathematische Klasse. Hirzel, Leipzig
4. Severin M (1965) Die Hornhautsensibilität bei herpetischer Keratitis. Klin Monatsbl Augenheilkd 146:683–695

### Diskussion zu den Beiträgen S. 53–56

W.A. Blyth (Bristol)
Did I understand you correctly that the sensitivity of the cornea returned to normal inbetween bouts of the disease?

R. Winter (Bremen)
Yes.

W.A. Blyth (Bristol)
So one could interpret it that some nerve endings were re-generating.

R. Winter (Bremen)
That is likely.

G.O. Waring III (Atlanta)
Have you used your observations to predict the clinical course of herpes? Have you taken people with known recurrent herpes simplex keratitis, performed aesthesiometry on them, and followed the subsequent clinical course to see if the state of corneal sensation gives any information about recurrences? As I understand it now, your observations are retrospective?

R. Winter (Bremen)
We followed 43 patients for different times from 1 year to 7 years. First we started a retrospective study

but presently we follow up patients prospectively and see that there is a marked decrease of sensitivity in those patients who developed recurrencies.

H.D.M. Völker-Dieben (Leyden)
I am not surprised that you find the biggest difference in sensitivity in the centre of the cornea. Because the cornea is most sensitive in the centre, it is easy to measure differences in sensitivity in the centre and it is hard to measure differences in sensitivity on the periphery, because it is less sensitive.

R. Winter (Bremen)
The normal topographic sensitivity profile of the cornea is so characteristic, that the decrease of sensitivity in the center and the less decrease in the periphery is without any doubt. With this precise measuring instrument we are sure that an increase in threshold of 10 to 20 times and more is easily to discriminate.

G.O.H. Naumann (Erlangen)
Haben Sie die Hornhaut-Sensibilität eines an Herpes simplex erkrankten Auges mit der Sensibilität der gesunden Seite verglichen? Did you study the sensitivity of the contralateral eye in herpetic corneal disease?

R. Winter (Bremen)
In our patients the sensitivity was only disturbed in the herpetic eye, in nearly all patients we controlled the contralateral eye and there was a normal sensitivity profile.

# Vaccination

Sundmacher, R. (Hrsg.):
Herpetische Augenerkrankungen
© J.F. Bergmann Verlag, München 1981

# Prospects for an Effective Vaccination Against Herpesviruses

H. zur Hausen, Freiburg

**Key words.** HSV – vaccines, oncogenicity

**Schlüsselwörter.** HSV – Vakzinen, Onkogenität

**Summary.** Herpes virus vaccines should prevent the symptoms of primary infections and should abolish or at least reduce recurrent herpetic lesions. The present state of the development of vaccines against herpes simplex virus and other herpes group viruses is briefly reviewed and the prospects for an effective control of herpesviruses by vaccination are discussed. Recent data indicating reinfection with different virus strains in previously infected individuals resulting in herpes simplex virus latency stress the problems in controlling herpetic diseases.

**Zusammenfassung.** Herpesvirus-Vakzinen sollten in der Lage sein, eine Primärinfektion zu verhüten und rezidivierende Herpeserkrankungen zu unterbinden oder zumindest im Verlauf zu mildern. Auf den gegenwärtigen Entwicklungsstand bei den Vakzinen gegen Herpes simplex-Virus und andere Viren der Herpesgruppe wird kurz eingegangen und die Aussichten für eine wirkungsvolle Kontrolle der Herpesviren mittels Schutzimpfung werden diskutiert. Neuere Befunde zeigen, daß auch vorinfizierte Individuen noch mit verschiedenen anderen Virusstämmen re-infiziert werden können, die alle wieder latent verbleiben. Dies zeigt die Schwierigkeiten bei der Kontrolle herpetischer Erkrankungen auf.

In the previous discussions we concentrated at large on the latency of herpes simplex viruses and possible modes for regulation.

By turning now to the prospects for an effective vaccination against herpesviruses we have to consider briefly the objectives of a vaccination program: they should be aimed at two directions: (i) the prevention of symptoms of primary herpetic infections and the prevention of uptake of viral genomes in susceptible target cells resulting in genome latency and (ii) in those individuals already harbouring latent genomes, in the prevention of recurrent herpetic affections.

Primary infections with herpes simplex viruses may occur inapparently but more frequently result in characteristic symptoms depending on the site of viral entry. Stomatitis aphthosa, keratitis herpetica represent frequent primary lesions in HSV 1 infections whereas cervicitis, vulvitis and balanitis are common manifestations of HSV 2. Primary infection, particularly if occurring in newborn babies or in severely immunosuppressed individuals, may result in generalized herpetic infections. Additional complications are herpes encephalitis and eczema herpeticum, although both of these latter conditions may not necessarily result from primary infections.

For the majority of patients recurrent attacks of painful and sometimes defacing herpetic inflammations represent a more significant problem when compared to the primary lesions. This accounts in particular for those patients suffering from recurrences at frequent intervals. Any immunological procedure preventing recurrences or at least prolonging their intervals would be of major clinical importance. It appears to be highly questionable, however, whether this group of individuals represents a suitable target for a vaccination program: all of these patients clearly reveal measurable titers of antibodies against the virus, some of them show a high humoral reactivity [1] and, in addition, cellular immune functions do not appear to be significantly reduced [2–4].

At this point it seems to be important to look into the regulation of viral genome persistence and to try to find an answer to the question whether immune mechanisms play at all a role or whether other factors, for instance hormonal dysbalance, may contribute to the obviously labile state of viral latency and reactivation. In addition, of course, it is important to know whether preimmune individuals are susceptible to reinfection and whether this reinfection may result in increase of latent infected cells.

The first part of these questions is presently difficult to resolve (as already indicated by the previous discussion). The replication of the virus at the site of its entry leads to uptake of viral DNA via the axon fibres into the sensory part of the trigeminal ganglion, the spinal ganglia, or the sacral ganglia depending on the primary manifestation [5–7]. It has not yet been settled whether the viral DNA persisting in the neuronal cells remains there in a genetically silent form without being transcribed or whether at least a partial transcription resulting in the synthesis of virus-specific proteins occurs. Suggestive evidence for some genetic activity originates from *in situ* hybridization experiments [8] but should await further confirmation by different procedures.

At the moment there exists no suitable tissue culture system for herpes simplex latency. The only available information on regulation of persisting herpesvirus DNA originates from studies on Epstein-Barr virus which persists in human B-lymphoblasts which are readily propagated in tissue culture. From this system we know that the viral DNA is present as a circular episome, usually in multiple copies per cell. This DNA is partially expressed resulting in the appearance of a nuclear antigen, EBNA [9] which is a reliable indicator for the EBV-DNA carrier state of the respective cell. We also do know that there exists a balanced intracellular control of viral genome reactivation which depends (among other factors) on the number of genome copies per cell, on hormonal influences and most probably on cellular mediator molecules which may be activated by different groups of chemical inducers [10–12]. Here humoral or cellular immune functions do not appear to interfer with the rate of reactivation, although a very specific inducing mechanism exists for these regularly immunoglobulin-producing cells, if treated with anti-immunoglobulins [13].

It may not be justified to correlate the mode of persistence of a clearly lymphotropic herpesgroup virus with the obviously neurotropic herpes simplex virus. The preceding discussion showed, however, that there do not exist too many hard facts which would underline an immune regulation of HSV latency. It should be emphasized, in addition, that even the severity and rapid spread of local lesions in immunosuppressed individuals provides no indication for an immune control of viral latency. Subclinical reactivation of persisting genomes may occur at constant frequency, becoming apparent, however, only under conditions of a failing immune control of virus spread of a rare virus-producing cell. In this sense it is therefore important to differentiate between the rate of recurrences and the severity of an individual attack [14, 15]. There exist some suggestions that hormonal factors interfer with the intracellular balance of persisting herpesvirus DNA. Increased incidence of recurrent manifestations during menstruation, in stress situations and particularly during skin irradiation and skin trauma, resulting for instance in the release of prostaglandins and possibly also in the activation of other endocrine factors, could support this view. This stresses the limitations of our knowledge on the regulation of HSV genome persistence and does not provide us with an optimistic outlook for an effective immune control of recurrent disease in previously infected individuals.

What about reinfection of immune patients with homologous or heterologous HSV isolates? There are two lines of evidence available that such reinfections are possible and even occur at a certain frequency in man: Blank and Haines reported in 1976 experimental human reinfection with an oral isolate of HSV at a different site resulting in subsequent recurrences also at the site of inoculation. Buchman et al. [16] reported last year the strain-specific analysis of repeated isolates from the same patients by restriction endonuclease cleavage patterns. In at least two patients, two genetically distinct strains of HSV 2 were demonstrated, respectively, during different periods of HSV recurrence, strongly suggesting that infection with HSV 2 in the same or nearby site can occur in spite of a prior infection with a genetically different strain of the same serotype. This again raises the question whether recurrent herpetic lesions can be subject of an immunization scheme or whether they rather represent a research issue for chemotherapy and possibly also for interferon treatment.

Let us now briefly turn to attempts which were made in the past and are pursued more intensively today on vaccine development against HSV (see also reviews by [17, 18]). In first attempts around 1930 [19–23] killed virus vaccines were applied which were prepared from emulsified tissues of infected animals. The low concentration of the effective antigens and the complex impurities of such preparations did not permit successful immunization after injections of these materials into animals and man. Similar approaches were continued until recently without convincing evidence of successful application in man [17, 18].

Experimental approaches in animals, however, provide some hope that vaccination of non-immune individuals may not only result in the prevention of clinical symptoms of primary infections but also in a significant reduction of latently persisting viral genomes. The group of Baringer recently showed [24] that humoral antibodies appear to play a surprisingly important role in reducing morbidity and mortality in preimmunized Balb c mice, that there is a clear-cut protective effect of passive immunization with monoclonal antibodies and that specifically the Fc-moiety of immunoglobin molecules appears to be important in an antibody-dependent cytotoxicity reaction directed against virus-producing cells.

Additional groups showed that inactivated viral lysates and subunit vaccines were able to provide considerable protection against subsequent infection and reduced significantly the uptake of viral DNA by neuronal cells.

Most of these studies show, however, a rather rapid decrease in protection with time and stress the necessity of simultaneous application of non-specific adjuvants.

Relatively little effort has been expanded on attempts to produce live attenuated strains of herpes simplex virus until recently. The availability of temperature-sensitive (ts) mutants which may even be defective in viral genome persistence could change this in the future. A number of problems associated with the use of live HSV vaccines, however, remain to be resolved. Some of them will be analyzed subsequently.

If we try to summarize the potential benefit of vaccinations against herpes simplex viruses, we can state that we probably will be able to prevent the symptoms of primary her-

pesvirus infections. This could be a remarkable benefit in a number of herpetic infections since it could include up to 10% of cases of viral encephalitis in moderate climates which do have a rather poor prognosis. It would also prevent primary eye, oral and genital manifestations and it may lead to a reduction in the number of patients with recurrent herpes infections.

Let us now turn to a specific risk associated with the application of specific herpesvirus vaccines: A major obstacle in applying herpesvirus vaccines to a larger proportion of exposed individuals is the potential oncogenicity of viral DNA-containing herpesvirus preparations. For approximately 10 years the role of HSV (particularly of HSV 2) in the induction of human genital cancer has been discussed (see review) [25]. Patients with cervical carcinomas have been demonstrated to reveal a higher ratio of HSV 2 to HSV 1 neutralizing antibodies when compared to appropriately matched controls. In addition, transforming properties of partially inactivated HSV 2 and HSV 1 have been demonstrated by Duff and Rapp [26] in different types of rodent cells, resulting in malignant cells which produce metastasizing tumors upon reinjection into the syngeneic host. No reproducible transformation of human cells has yet been obtained.

Despite these data it remains entirely unclear whether HSV is a potential oncogen for man. It is unclear whether it transforms rodent cells by a mechanism which conforms with our "conventional" understanding of tumor viruses. It proved to be extremely difficult or impossible to demonstrate persistence of virus-specific DNA or of HSV-coded products in human tumor cells or even in HSV-transformed rodent cells (see review [25]). This is in marked contrast to all other well-established tumor virus-host cell systems and still awaits clarification. Moreover, inactivated HSV and even purified herpesvirus DNA has been shown recently to induce endogenous C-type viruses [27, 28] which following reactivation may be responsible for the eventual outcome of transformation. Such viruses have not yet been convincingly demonstrated in human cells and further analysis is required to justify a statement that difficulties in the transformation of human cells in vitro by inactivated HSV could be attributed to the possible lack of such endogenous genomes within human tissue. It thus remains an open question whether a function of a persisting HSV gene is essential for the maintenance of the transformed state of rodent cells exposed to partially inactivated HSV.

It should not be ignored, however, that there could exist an alternative pathway by which HSV could exert its oncogenic potential: it was established more than 10 years ago that these viruses efficiently induce chromosomal aberrations which are also demonstrated after UV-inactivation of the virus [29, 30]. It seems likely, although not proven, that this effect of HSV infection correlates to mutagenic activity. In this instance an oncogenic role of HSV could be mediated by a similar mechanism by which most chemical and physical carcinogens (initiators) seem to interact with target cells which are effective mutagens. This would imply a different type of risk when compared to other DNA- and RNA-tumor viruses which implant at least one functioning gene into the host cell.

For these reasons oncogenicity of herpes simplex viruses represents a risk for vaccination which at present is difficult to evaluate. There exists the possibility that inactivation procedures render a previously lytic virus into a potential oncogen. Latency periods of 2 to 4 decades, frequently encountered in man between exposure to a carcinogen and eventual appearance of the induced tumor [31], certainly add to the difficulties in evaluating the risk of herpesvirus vaccine.

Let me now briefly summarize these considerations: Animal experiments with vaccines against herpes simplex viruses suggest that we can expect a reduction of "takes" under conditions of previous immunization. Taking into account the specific virus host-cell relationship in herpesvirus infections and the present epidemiologic situation, the success of a vaccination program against HSV is difficult to predict and requires further experimentation.

Vaccination against animal herpes simplex viruses has been successful in those instances where primary infection represents the most serious problem, as e.g. in pseudorabies and in Marek virus lymphomatosis of chicken. In some analogy it seems to be easier to cope with acute infections induced by herpes group viruses in man (e.g. varicella-chickenpox, Epstein-Barr virus − infectious mononucleosis) by a vaccination program than with recurrent manifestations of HSV.

A realistic evaluation of prospects in immunization against HSV infections certainly requires much more experimentation. It will be definitely a more difficult task than previous studies, performed largely with viruses which do not persist within their hosts for a life-time.

**Acknowledgment.** This study was supported by the Nationales Referenzzentrum für Herpesviren, funded by the Bundesministerium für Jugend, Familie und Gesundheit.

# References

1. Douglas RG, Couch RB (1970) A prospective study of chronic herpes simplex virus infection and recurrent herpes labialis in humans. J Immunol 104:289–295
2. Wilton JMA, Ivanyi L, Lehner T (1972) Cell-mediated immunity in herpesvirus hominis infection. Br Med J 1:723–726
3. Russel AS, Percy SJ, Kovithavongs T (1975) T-cell − mediated immunity to herpes simplex in humans: lymphocyte cytotoxicity measured by $^{51}$Cr release from infected cells. Infect Immunol 11:355–359
4. Steele RW, Vincent MM, Hensen SA, Fucillo DA, Chapa IA, Canales J (1975) Cellular immune responses to herpes simplex virus type 1 in recurrent herpes labialis: in vitro blastogenesis and cytotoxicity to infected cell lines. J Infect Dis 131:528–534
5. Bastian FO, Rabson AS, Yee CL, Tralka TS (1972) Herpes-virus hominis: isolation from human trigeminal ganglion. Science 178:306–307
6. Blank H, Haines GH (1976) Viral diseases of the skin, 1975; a 25-year perspective. J Invest Dermatol 67:169–176
7. Baringer JR (1974) Recovery of herpes simplex virus from human sacral ganglions. N Engl J Med 291:828–830
8. Jones KW, Fenoglio CM, Shevchuk-Chaban M, Maitland WJ, McDougall JK (1978) Detection of herpes simplex virus type II mRNA in human cervical biopsies by insitu cytological hybridization; in: Oncogenesis and Herpesviruses III (G. de-Thé, W. Henle and F. Rapp eds.) part II, international agency for research on cancer, Lyon, pp 917–926
9. Reedman BM, Klein G (1973) Cellular localization of an Epstein-Barr virus-associated com-

plement-fixing antigen in producer and non-producer lymphoblastoid cell lines. Int J Cancer 11:499–520

10. zur Hausen H, O'Neill F, Freese UK, Hecker E (1978) Persisting oncogenic herpesvirus induced by the tumor promoter TPA. Nature 272:373–375

11. Bister K, Yamamoto N, zur Hausen H (1979) Differential inducibility of Epstein-Barr virus in cloned Raji cells. Int J Cancer 23:818–825

12. Yamamoto N, Bister K, zur Hausen H (1979) Inhibition of Epstein-Barr virus induction by retonoic acid. Nature 278:553–554

13. Tovey MG, Lenoir G, Begon-Lours J (1978) Activation of latent Epstein-Barr virus by antibody to human IgM. Nature 276:270–272

14. Müller AS, Hermann EC, Winkelmann RK (1972) Herpes simplex infections in haematologic malignancies. Am J Med 52:102–114

15. zur Hausen H, Bornkamm GW, Schmidt R, Hecker E (1979) Tumor initiators and promoters in the induction of Epstein-Barr virus. Proc Natl Acad Sci USA 76:2

16. Buchman TG, Roizman B, Nahmias AF (1979) Demonstration of exogenous genital reinfection with herpes simplex virus type 2 by restriction endonuclease fingerprinting of viral DNA. J Infect Dis 140:295–304

17. Hilleman MR (1976) Herpes simplex vaccines. Cancer Res 36:857–858

18. Wise TG, Pavan PR, Ennis FA (1977) Herpes simplex virus vaccines. J Infect Dis 136:706–711

19. Urbain A, Schaeffer W (1929) Contribution à l'étude expérimentale d'un virus herpétique (Souche Marocaine). Ann Inst Pasteur 43:369–385

20. Holden M (1932) The nature and property of the virus of herpes. J Infect Dis 50:218–236

21. Martin N, Caneja D (1933) Tratamiento biologico herpes ocular. Arch Ottal 33:367–369

22. Brain RT (1936) Biological therapy in virus diseases. Br J Derm 48:21–26

23. Frank SB (1938) Formolized herpesvirus therapy and the neutralizing substance in herpes simplex. J Invest Dermatol 1:267–282

24. McKendall RR, Baringer R (1980) Evidence for B-cell effectiveness on peripheral challenge by HSV-1 in mice. Abstract, International Conference on Human Herpesviruses Atlanta, March 17–21, 1980

25. zur Hausen H (1975) Oncogenic herpesviruses. Biochim Biophys Acta 417:25–53

26. Duff R, Rapp F (1971) Oncogenic transformation of hamster cells after exposure to herpes simplex type 2. Nature 233:48–50

27. Hampar B, Lenoir G, Nonoyama M, Derge JG, Chang S-Y (1976) Cell cycle dependence for activation of Epstein-Barr virus by inhibitors of protein synthesis or medium deficient in arginine. Virology 69:660–668

28. Boyd AL, Derge JG, Hampar B (1978) Activation of endogenous type C virus in Balb/c mouse cells by herpesvirus DNA. Proc Natl Acad Sci USA 75:4558–4562

29. Rapp F, Hsu TC (1965) Viruses and mammalian chromosomes. IV. Replication of herpes simplex virus in diploid Chinese hamster cells. Virology 25:401–411

30. Waubke R, zur Hausen H, Henle W (1968) Chromosomal and autoradiographic studies of cells infected with herpes simplex virus. J Virol 2:1047–1054

31. Hiatt HH, Watson JD, Winsten JA (eds) (1977) Origins of Human Cancer. Cold Spring Harbor Laboratory

## Discussion on Contribution pp. 59–65

C. Ohrloff (Bonn)
Some years ago a vaccine was available, but it has disappeared from the market in the meantime. We used it in our clinic without success and I would like to ask for your opinion of this vaccine.

H. zur Hausen (Freiburg)
You are referring to a vaccine which has been prepared from inoculated chorionallantoic membranes of chickens and then heat-inactivated. This vaccine had to be withdrawn from the market because a HSV strain was used which, originally, had been propagated in Hela cells, and Hela, as you know, is a malignant cell line. So the disappearance of this vaccine is unrelated to the problem of whether or not it was effective. The question of efficacy of herpes vaccines is a major issue and I cannot address myself to this problem at length, but I can say as much that double blind studies performed under appropriate conditions (i.e. using a proper placebo vaccination) have failed to show any efficacy of this vaccine. This was not unexpected, taking into account the small amount of antigen present in this vaccine which cast some doubt anyway on its immunogenic potential.

Sundmacher, R. (Hrsg.):
Herpetische Augenerkrankungen
© J.F. Bergmann Verlag, München 1981

# Vaccination Against Herpes Simplex Virus: Animal Studies on the Efficacy Against Acute, Latent and Recurrent Infections

M. Scriba, Wien

**Key words.** Primary herpetic disease, recurrent herpetic disease, vaccines

**Schlüsselwörter.** Primärer Herpes, Herpesrezidive, Vakzinen

**Summary.** Vaccination against herpes simplex virus (HSV) may be attempted either before primary infection or during the latent phase of the infection. The efficacy of both vaccination schedules was tried in an HSV type 2 (HSV 2) infection of guinea pigs, employing extracts of HSV 2 infected cells as vaccines.

Vaccination before infection: The efficacy of vaccination on the various phases of HSV infection – primary, latent, and recurrent – was dependent on the route of challenge infection. The most effective protection was observed against intradermal infection.

Vaccination after infection: A vaccine applied in latently infected animals was not able to influence frequency or severity of recurrent lesions, although this vaccination did increase the titers of neutralizing antibodies significantly.

**Zusammenfassung.** Eine Schutzimpfung gegen Herpes simplex-Virus kann man entweder vor der Primärinfektion oder während der latenten Infektion versuchen. Beide Möglichkeiten wurden an einem Meerschweinchenmodell mit HSV Typ 2 untersucht, wobei als Vakzinen entweder inaktiviertes HSV 2 oder Lysate von HSV 2-infizierten Zellen verwandt wurden.

Schutzimpfung vor der Infektion: Beide Vakzinen konnten die akute Primärerkrankung verhindern oder zumindest erheblich mildern und Rezidive seltener machen. Aber nur die Lysat-Vakzine konnte – vermischt mit Freund'schem Adjuvans – auch die Entwicklung einer latenten Infektion und damit Rezidiverkrankungen vollständig verhindern.

Schutzimpfung nach der Infektion: Der zuletzt erwähnte Vakzine-Typ (Lysat + Adjuvans) hatte bei latent infizierten Tieren keinen Einfluß mehr auf die Häufigkeit und die Schwere der Rezidiverkrankungen, obwohl nach dieser Schutzimpfung der Titer der neutralisierenden Antikörper signifikant höher war.

In the course of HSV infections three distinct phases can be discriminated: *acute primary* infection, followed by the probably life-long *latent* infection which can be interrupted by *recurrent* infections, caused by a reactivation of the latent virus. The major goal of vaccination against HSV infections should be the prevention of recurrent herpes. This effect may be attempted to be brought about by two different time schedules of immunization: 1). Vaccination before primary infection to prevent the establishment of latent infections and thus the later development of recurrent lesions, and 2). vaccination during the latent phase of infection in order to prevent recurrent eruptions. The efficacy of both immunization schedules was tried in an animal model, i.e. HSV 2 infection of guinea pigs.

Details of the animal model have been described previously [2–4]. Briefly, the animals are inoculated with HSV 2 either subcutaneously (s.c.) or intradermally (i.d.) into one hind footpad or vaginally. All three routes of infection lead to the development of primary lesions (inflammation and vesiculation) at the inoculation site, which disappear after 2–3 weeks. After vaginal infection in a proportion of the animals, symptoms of myelitis are observed with usually lethal consequences. In surviving animals, virus remains latent in the corresponding sensory ganglia and in addition, persists, probably in a low level productive form, in the originally inoculated epithelial area. Frequent spontaneously recurring lesions develop at the inoculation site, the majority of which is apparently due to reactivation of the latent ganglionic infection. The locally persisting virus, on the other hand, is probably not responsible for any clinical symptoms and so far its relevance to the human infection is dubious (unpublished results).

The vaccines used in these studies consisted of crude extracts from HSV infected cells. Two types of vaccines were prepared: first, Hep 2 cells infected with HSV 2 were extracted in a hypotonic phosphate buffer ($10^{-3}$M, pH 7.2) by ten strokes in a Dounce homogenizer. 0.1% formol was added to the extract to inactivate the virus and cell debris was removed by low speed centrifugation. This vaccine was used for the studies on immunization prior to infection. For the later studies, i.e. immunization after infection, we used another vaccine, which had been found to be more immunogenic in the guinea pigs: HSV infected guinea pig fibroblasts were extracted in a buffer containing 5% Triton X 100. Undissolved cell material, particularly the nuclei, were then removed by low speed centrifugation. This vaccine was mixed with incomplete Freund's adjuvant.

### Vaccination Before Primary Infection

Groups of animals were immunized twice within 3 weeks s.c. with 0.2 ml of vaccine. One week after boosting, animals were challenged by infection with $10^4$ plaqueforming units (pfu) of HSV 2. The animals were observed for clinical symptoms for various time periods. Ganglia and skin were then assayed for persistent infection by cultivation of these organs on primary rabbit kidney cells as described previously [2].

In the first experiment we compared the effect of vaccination on the clinical symptoms after s.c. footpad and vaginal challenge infection (Table 1). The vaccination had no effect on the number of animals developing primary lesions after footpad infection. It did, however, reduce significantly the rate of animals developing recurrent lesions later on. In contrast, the same vaccine was effective against the primary vaginal infection. In the vaccinated group, the number of animals which were successfully infected, as assessed by virus isolation from vaginal swabs 3–5 days after infection, was significantly reduced (8/19 as compared to 13/15 in the control group). Only one out of the eight vaccinated animals which were successfully infected developed mild clinical signs of the infection, whereas all successfully infected control animals showed clinical symptoms of various degrees, and seven even died. All of the surviving controls developed recurrent genital lesions. In contrast only three of the eight vaccinated animals which had "taken" the infection developed recurrent lesions.

In the next experiment (Table 2) we determined the effect of vaccination on the establishment of the persistent infection in ganglia and footpad skin. In the control group five out of ten animals had developed recurrent lesions until day 31 after infection, seven harboured latent virus in their dorsal root ganglia and all of them harboured virus at the site of inoculation. None of the vaccinated animals showed recurrent lesions in the observation period and concurrently, none of them harboured virus in their ganglia. However, persistent footpad skin infection was still found in all animals of this group.

The third experiment compares the establishment of persistent infection after s.c. and i.d. footpad infection. In contrast to the previous experiments, the vaccine was ap-

**Table 1.** Efficacy of vaccination against s.c. footpad and vaginal infection

| Group | Footpad infection | | Vaginal infection | | | |
|---|---|---|---|---|---|---|
| | | | Primary infection | | | Recurrent infection |
| | $I^0$ lesions | Recurrent lesions | Virus isolation[a] | $I^0$ lesions | Deaths | |
| Control | 7/20[b] | 10/20 | 13/15 | 13/13 | 7/13 | 6/6 |
| Vaccinated | 8/20 | 1/19 | 8/19 | 1/8 | 0 | 3/8 |

[a] Number of animals successfully infected as assessed by virus reisolation from vaginal swabs, day 3–5 p.i. Only animals positive in this assay were included in the further study

[b] Number of animals positive/number tested

**Table 2.** Efficacy of vaccination against s. c. footpad infection

| Group | I$^{o}$ lesions | Recurrent lesions (d21–32) | Persistent infection[a] in Footpad | Ganglia |
|---|---|---|---|---|
| Control | 6/10 | 5/10 | 10/10 | 7/10 |
| Vaccinated | 1/10 | 0/10 | 10/10 | 0/10 |

[a] Assayed day 32 p.i.

**Table 3.** Efficacy of vaccination against s.c. and i.d. footpad infection

| Group | S.c. infection Persistent infection[a] in Footpad | Ganglia | I.d. infection Persistent infection[a] in Footpad | Ganglia |
|---|---|---|---|---|
| Control | 4/4 | 4/4 | 6/6 | 5/6 |
| Vaccinated | 4/4 | 0/4 | 0/7 | 0/7 |

[a] Assayed day 25–30 p.i.

plied in incomplete Freund's adjuvant. Again, the vaccination prevented the establishment of latent ganglionic infection after s.c. challenge, but did not prevent the virus from persisting locally. In contrast, the vaccine protected the animals from both ganglionic and local persistent infection after i.d. challenge (Table 3).

In conclusion, the data presented demonstrate that vaccination prior to primary HSV infection can effectively influence not only the acute disease, but also the chronic phase of infection. However, the degree of protection obtained against acute, latent and recurrent infection is largely dependent on the route of the challenge infection. These findings are in agreement with studies by Price et al. [1] on the effect of immunization on the acute and latent HSV infections of mice. It is remarkable that protection against primary lesions and against recurrent lesions is not necessarily related, as particularly demonstrated in the s.c. footpad model.

**Vaccination During the Latent Phase of Infection (Post-Infectious Immunization)**

The second approach, the attempt to vaccinate individuals who already carry a latent infection and suffer from recurrent herpetic lesions, poses one salient question: Can an inactivated or subunit vaccine stimulate any parameter of the host's immune response above the levels which are reached by the boosts produced by frequent recurrent infection?

Figure 1 demonstrates that, surprisingly enough, this is the case. Titers of neutralizing antibodies increase after infection up to about 2 months, a time when most animals have developed several eruptions of recurrent lesions. Titers then reach a plateau, which remains more or less stable for the rest of the animal's lifetime, irrespective of the animal's frequency of recurrent lesions. Vaccination, applied once during the early phase of infection, i.e. day 7 (acute phase), or more pronounced, day 20 after infection (early latent phase) leads not only to a faster increase of antibodies, but to considerably higher titers. Also, vaccination later during the latent phase of infection (day 63) can increase neutralizing antibody titers above the level reached by infections alone. These data clearly show, that the immune response can be stimulated by a vaccine, applied after primary infection, to a higher level than by recurrent infections.

In spite of the influence of post-infectious vaccination on the antibody titers, we have so far seen no effect on the frequency or severity

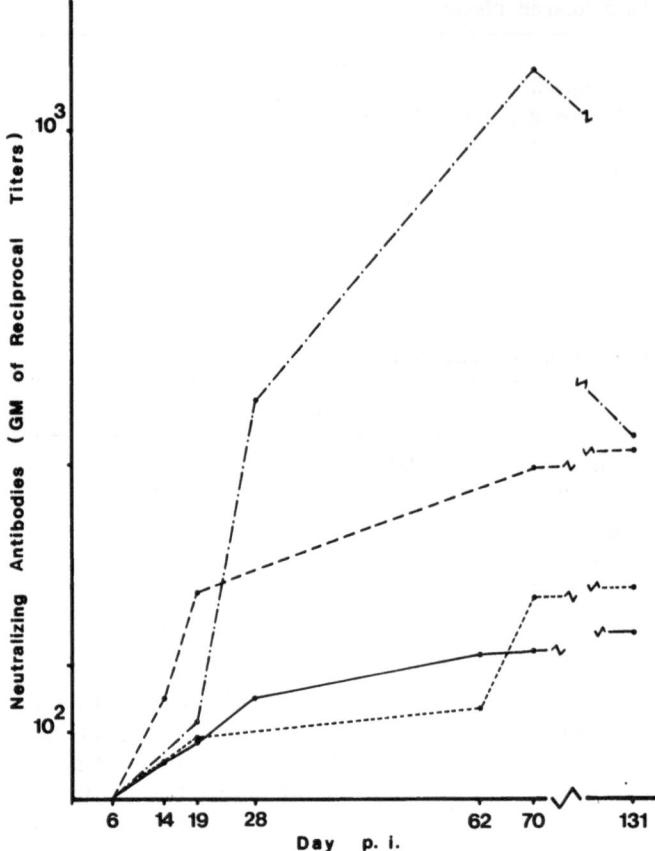

**Fig. 1.** Neutralizing antibodies after s.c. footpad infection and post-infectious vaccination. •——• control •– – –• vaccinated day 7 •–·–• vaccinated day 20 •·····• vaccinated day 63

of recurrent lesions developing in vaccinated animals. Table 4 shows that a vaccine, which was effective if it was applied before infection, had no effect on clinical symptoms if it was applied 20 days after infection, although again it raised antibody titers to significantly higher levels than the antibody titers of controls or of animals vaccinated before infection.

In the next experiment, not only one dose of post-infectious vaccination was applied but a total of nine doses, injected between day 25 and 57 (Table 5). The number of animals developing recurrent lesions was not reduced during the time period in which the vaccine was applied. In the 40 days after the vaccination, the rate of animals with recurrent

**Table 4.** Efficacy of vaccination, applied before or after s.c. footpad infection

| Group | Neutralizing antibodies[a] | | | Number of animals with | |
| | | | | I⁰ lesions | Recurrent lesions |
| | d–1 | d 10 | d 28 | (d 0–20) | (d 21–50) |
|---|---|---|---|---|---|
| Control | < 10 | 76 | 329 | 17/20 | 17/20 |
| Vaccinated before infection (d–28, –7) | 481 | 512 | 444 | 9/20 | 2/20 |
| Vaccinated after infection (d 20) | < 10 | 140 | 1573 | 15/20 | 13/20 |

[a] Geometric mean of reciprocal titers

**Table 5.** Efficacy of vaccination *after* infection

| Group | Number of animals with lesions | | |
|---|---|---|---|
| | d 0–25 | d 26–60 | d 61–102 |
| Control | 11/19 | 10/18 | 5/18 |
| Vaccinated[a] | 15/20 | 11/20 | 11/20 |

[a] 9 doses of vaccine, applied day 25–57 p.i.

lesions was even slightly higher in the vaccinated group than in the control group, although the difference is not statistically significant.

In conclusion: post-infectious vaccination can considerably stimulate the host's immune response as measured by neutralizing antibodies. This effect is, however, not accompanied by any beneficial influence on the development of recurrent herpes.

## References

1. Price RW, Walz MA, Wohlenberg C, Notkins AL (1975) Latent infection of sensory ganglia with herpes simplex virus: efficacy of immunization. Science 188:938–940
2. Scriba M (1975) Herpes simplex virus infection in guinea pigs: an animal model for studying latent and recurrent herpes simplex virus infection. Infect Immun 12:162–165
3. Scriba M (1976) Recurrent genital herpes simplex virus infection of guinea pigs. Med Microbiol Immunol (Berl) 162:201–208
4. Scriba M (1977) Extraneural localization of herpes simplex virus in latently infected guinea pigs. Nature 267:529–531

## Discussion on the Contribution pp. 67–72

R. Baringer (San Francisco)
Thank you, Dr. Scriba. This is a very important contribution. Many people have wondered about whether the development of recurrence in individuals is just related to a quantitatively insufficient antibody response and you have been able to show that a very great increase in the antibody in the animal does not alter their frequency of recurrent disease.

T.J. Hill (Bristol)
Marianne, did you look at cell mediated immunity to the virus in your vaccinated animals, particularly those in which latency was already established?

M. Scriba (Wien)
We have not looked into this in animals vaccinated after infection.

J. Oh (San Francisco)
We have carried out a similar experiment in a primary skin infection model in newborn rabbits. Passive immunization of newborn rabbits with intraperitoneal anti-type 2 herpes serum as well as transplacental immunization from immunized pregnant rabbits were very effective in blocking the primary infection of the skin, dissemination to visceral organs and to corresponding sensory ganglia. So in some aspects, our results are similar to those you found in your primary infection study.

M. Scriba (Wien)
The passive immunization certainly does ameliorate the primary disease after vaginal infection. The antibodies however, certainly did not influence the rate of animals developing latent ganglionic infection. In your model this might be different, since the virus probably spreads via hematogenous routes. Here, neutralizing antibodies should clearly have an effect.

J. Oh (San Francisco)
Yes, this is a newborn model, and dissemination is largely dependent on the hematogenous route.

H. Moser (Marburg)
Did you also look for cellular immunity after vaccination of the guinea pigs?

M. Scriba (Wien)
No, not yet.

H.J. Field (Cambridge)
It was of interest that you demonstrated that when virus persisted in the skin, you showed that the ganglia didn't appear to be protected from becoming latently infected. This is consistent with our data in a very different system but again the establishment of latency is very dependent on the amount of virus replication in the skin; if there is sufficient virus in the skin then latency is established. Do you have any information about the levels of virus replication in the skin?

M. Scriba (Wien)
Well, in the guinea pig the establishment of the latent infection in ganglia is largely independent of the dose of virus inoculated, whereas the latent or persistent infection in the skin seems to be dose related. We can get latent ganglionic infection after inoculation with as little as 10–20 pfu. After such a small dose the virus does apparently not persist in the skin. Whatever this means, I don't know.

W.J. O'Brien (Milwaukee)
Could you comment further about the method of attenuation of the virus? I believe, did you say it was detergent?

M. Scriba (Wien)
It was not live virus, it was an extract of infected cells, extracted with non-ionic detergent; Triton X 100, usually 5%.

# Immunogenetics

Sundmacher, R. (Hrsg.):
Herpetische Augenerkrankungen
© J.F. Bergmann Verlag, München 1981

# HLA-Types and Herpes Simplex Ocular Infections

J. Colin, C. Chastel, G. Renard, P. Antoine, F. Colin, J.P. Saleun, Brest

**Key words.** HLA system and herpetic diseases, HLA-B5

**Schlüsselwörter.** HLA-System und Herpeserkrankungen, HLA-B5

**Summary.** HLA antigens of 131 patients with ocular herpes simplex infection were compared to those of a control population. None of the HLA-A determinants showed a significant deviation in frequency from the control population. In the locus B, HLA-B5 antigen was significantly more common in the 44 patients with recurrent stromal keratitis. Several hypotheses are discussed in order to explain a possible relationship between HLA antigens and disease severity.

**Zusammenfassung.** Die HLA-Antigen-Muster von 131 Patienten mit herpetischen Augenerkrankungen wurden mit denen einer Kontrollgruppe verglichen. Bei den HLA-A-Antigenen fand sich kein Unterschied; bei den HLA-B-Antigenen hingegen war B5 bei den 44 Patienten mit rezidivierendem Stromaherpes signifikant häufiger. Wir diskutieren verschiedene Hypothesen, die erklären könnten, wie HLA-Antigene und Krankheitsverlauf miteinander gekoppelt sind.

## Introduction

Nowadays, ocular infection with herpes simplex is one of the most important problems in ophthalmology because of its severity and frequency.

If the primary infection is subclinical, as in most cases, the severe eye disease is generally due to recurrences. Recurrent herpes simplex keratitis is characterized by repeated corneal ulcerations, without a new attack by exogenous virus. Reinfections of the corneal epithelium are caused by herpes simplex virus (HSV) which remains latent in the trigeminal ganglia [5].

The frequency of HSV ocular infections among the general population has been said to be 1 of 1653 persons [6], and serological surveys have shown that, at 15 years of age, 90% of people have been infected by HSV [3]. This relative rarity of eye infections compared to the large diffusion of general HSV infections led us to look for a possible abnormal immunologic reactivity among these patients through the study of HLA antigens.

After an attack of dendritic keratitis, the risk of recurrence is high. Recurrences in the following 2 years [3] occur in 25 to 43% of patients. The recurrences are sometimes responsible for such severe corneal alterations that keratoplasty is necessary – either to reduce the ocular inflammation, or to restore visual acuity. We are again struck by the frequency of recurrences in these grafts; in fact, after a 15 years follow-up, 47% of patients have new herpetic ulcerations on the cornea [2]. It is interesting to observe that 53% of grafted patients had no new herpetic attack during this period, and this clinical observation allows us to express the hypothesis that there is a particular susceptibility of some cells to HSV. Generally, when a keratoplasty is performed, there is no systematic study of histocompatibility; it has been demonstrated that some cellular constituents of the donor cornea survive in the recipient. After keratoplasty, there appears to be some modification of the antigenic constituents of the cornea.

## Materials and Methods

131 patients with ocular herpes simplex infection, 89 males and 42 females, were typed for HLA-A and -B antigens. These patients were examined in the ophthalmologic department of the Brest University Hospital.

Twelve patients with recurrent blepharitis, 14 patients with superficial keratitis (first

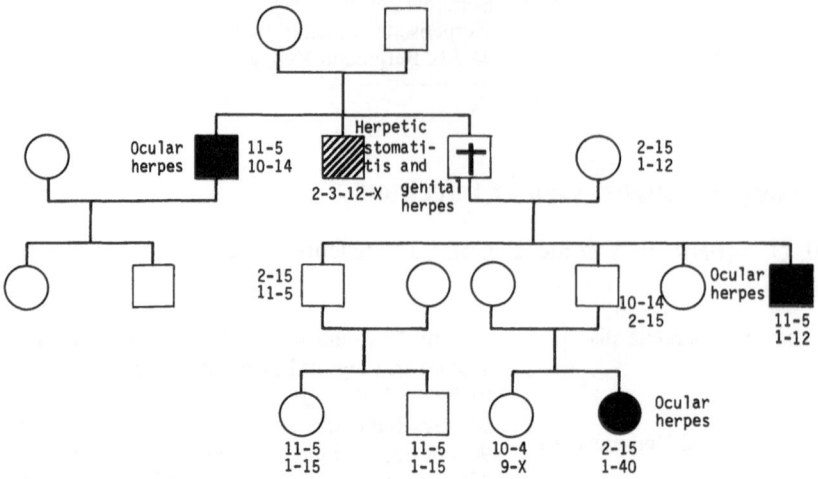

**Fig. 1.** HLA-antigens of the members of a family with high incidence of herpetic infection

attack), 61 patients with recurrent superficial keratitis and 44 patients with recurrent stromal keratitis were investigated.

We also studied the HLA antigens of the members of a family in which we found three cases of recurrent ocular herpes and one case of recurrent herpetic stomatitis with genital herpes (Fig. 1).

HLA typing for ten antigens of the A locus and 17 antigens of the B locus was performed using the microlymphocytotoxicity method described by Terasaki and McClelland [8]. The typing sera were issued by the France Transplant Association.

The antigen frequency of the control population was based on the typing, done by the same laboratory, of 200 blood donors born in Finistère.

The HLA frequencies for each of the following groups were compared with those of the control population:
– 131 ocular herpetic infections,
–  61 recurrent superficial keratitis,
–  44 recurrent stromal keratitis.

Statistical treatment of the results was performed using the chi-square test incorporating the Yates's correction factor.

The relative risk

$$\frac{\% \text{ antigen pos. patients}}{\% \text{ antigen neg. patients}} \times$$

$$\times \frac{\% \text{ antigen neg. controls}}{\% \text{ antigen pos. controls}}$$

was determined for all antigens.

## Results

The HLA-A antigens are shown in Table 1: no significant difference was observed between patients with ocular herpetic disease and control subjects.

The distribution of HLA-B antigens is shown in Table 2: HLA-B5 was significantly increased in the group with recurrent stromal keratitis:

$$X^2 = 9.7 - P = 0.001 - P \text{ corr} : 0.018 \text{ (Table 3)}.$$

The relative risk for the observed association between recurrent stromal keratitis and HLA-B5 is 3.6.

In the family study, there was no particularly noteworthy antigen among the herpetic subjects. Nevertheless two of four affected individuals had the HLA-B5 antigen.

## Discussion

In this study, we did not find an increased frequency of HLA-A1 antigen, as pointed out by Russel and Schlaut [7] in patients with recurrent labial herpes.

On the other hand, it was surprising to find the same increase in the HLA-B5 antigen, already noted by Zimmermann et al. [9], among a group of 46 patients with ocular herpes. However their results were not significant after correction for number of comparisons.

In a previous investigation of 80 patients

**Table 1.** HLA-A phenotypes and ocular herpetic infection

| HLA Phenotypes | Control Population (N = 200) | Ocular Herpetic Infections (N = 131) | | Recurrent Superficial Keratitis (N = 61) | | Recurrent Stromal Keratitis (N = 44) | |
|---|---|---|---|---|---|---|---|
| A1 | 30[a] | 35.9[a] | (1.3)[b] | 32.8 | (1.1) | 38.6 | (2.4) |
| A2 | 49.5 | 43.5 | (0.7) | 42 | (0.8) | 40.9 | (0.7) |
| A3 | 26.5 | 29 | (1.1) | 24.6 | (0.9) | 36.4 | (1.5) |
| A9 | 21.5 | 13.7 | (0.5) | 14.8 | (0.6) | 15.9 | (0.7) |
| A10 | 11.5 | 7.6 | (0.6) | 3.3 | (0.3) | 13.6 | (1.2) |
| A11 | 13.5 | 12.9 | (0.9) | 16.4 | (1.2) | 11.3 | (0.8) |
| A28 | 4.5 | 11.5 | (2.7) | 8.2 | (1.9) | 9 | (2.1) |
| A29 | 7 | 12.9 | (1.9) | 16.4 | (2.6) | 9 | (1.3) |
| Aw32 | 6 | 1.5 | (0.2) | 3.3 | (0.5) | | |
| A192 | 12 | 11.4 | (0.9) | 9.8 | (0.8) | 18.2 | (1.6) |

[a] % frequency
[b] relative risk

with recurrent ocular simplex infection of various degrees of clinical severity, we also found that HLA-B5 antigen was more common, but not significantly, in the patients group [1].

A recent study of Meyers-Elliott et al. [4] did not confirm an increased frequency of HLA-B5 in 48 patients with recurrent herpes stromal keratitis but indicated the increased frequencies of HLA-Aw30 and of HLA-DR w3 antigens.

However, our data, especially the increase in HLA-B5 in patients with recurrent herpes stromal keratitis, may support the hypothesis of an association between the major histocompatibility complex and the severity of ocular herpes infection.

The frequent recurrences of herpetic disease among some patients can be tentatively explained in two ways:

a) An abnormal response of the patient to HSV,

**Table 2.** HLA-B phenotypes and ocular herpetic infection

| HLA Phenotypes | Control Population (N = 200) | Ocular Herpetic Infections (N = 131) | | Recurrent Superficial Keratitis (N = 61) | | Recurrent Stromal Keratitis (N = 44) | |
|---|---|---|---|---|---|---|---|
| B5 | 8.5[a] | 16[a] | (2.0)[b] | 13.1 | (1.6) | 25 | (3.6) |
| B7 | 29.5 | 35.8 | (1.3) | 36 | (1.3) | 36.4 | (1.4) |
| B8 | 22 | 19 | (0.8) | 18 | (0.8) | 18.2 | (0.8) |
| B12 | 39 | 29 | (0.6) | 21.3 | (0.4) | 34 | (0.8) |
| B13 | 2.5 | 3 | (1.2) | 3.2 | (1.3) | 4.5 | (1.8) |
| B14 | 9.5 | 12.9 | (1.4) | 11.5 | (1.2) | 11.3 | (1.2) |
| Bw15 | 5 | 10.6 | (2.2) | 11.5 | (2.5) | 11.3 | (2.4) |
| B17 | 9 | 6.9 | (0.7) | 9.8 | (1.1) | 2.2 | (1.2) |
| B18 | 4 | 3.2 | (0.9) | 4.9 | (1.2) | 0 | – |
| Bw21 | 5.5 | 3.8 | (0.7) | 1.6 | (0.2) | 6.8 | (1.2) |
| Bw22 | 0.5 | 3 | – | 4.9 | – | 2.3 | – |
| B27 | 12 | 6.9 | (0.5) | 11.5 | (0.9) | 2.2 | (0.1) |
| Bw35 | 12.5 | 9.9 | (0.8) | 14.8 | (1.2) | 6.8 | (0.5) |
| B37 | 1.5 | 0.7 | – | 0 | – | 2.2 | – |
| Bw38 | 1.0 | 0.7 | – | 0 | – | 2.2 | – |
| Bw39 | 0.5 | 2.2 | – | 3.2 | – | 0 | – |
| B40 | 14.5 | 12.2 | | 11.4 | (0.9) | 15.9 | (1.1) |

[a] % frequency
[b] relative risk

**Table 3.** HLA phenotypes and recurrent herpes stromal keratitis

| HLA Phenotypes | Control Population (N = 200) % frequency | Patients (N = 44) % frequency | CHI-square | P Value | P Value with correction | Relative Risk |
|---|---|---|---|---|---|---|
| B5   | 8.5  | 25   | 9.7  | 0.001 | 0.018 | 3.6 |
| B7   | 29.5 | 36.4 | 0.8  | 0.35  | 6.4   | 1.4 |
| B8   | 22   | 18.2 | 0.31 | 0.55  | 9.9   | 0.8 |
| B12  | 39   | 34   | 0.37 | 0.52  | 9.36  | 0.8 |
| B13  | 2.5  | 4.5  | 0.54 | 0.43  | 7.74  | 1.8 |
| B14  | 9.5  | 11.3 | 0.14 | 0.67  | 12.06 | 1.2 |
| Bw15 | 5    | 11.3 | 2.53 | 0.1   | 1.8   | 2.4 |
| B17  | 9    | 2.2  | 2.27 | 0.12  | 2.16  | 1.2 |
| B18  | 4    | 0    | –    | –     | –     | –   |
| Bw21 | 5.5  | 6.8  | 0.11 | 0.11  | 12.6  | 1.2 |
| B22  | 0.5  | 2.3  | 0.6  | 0.6   | 7.2   | –   |
| B27  | 12   | 2.2  | 3.71 | 0.05  | 0.9   | 0.1 |
| Bw35 | 12.5 | 6.8  | 1.14 | 0.25  | 4.5   | 0.5 |
| B37  | 1.5  | 2.2  | –    | –     | –     | –   |
| Bw38 | 1.0  | 2.2  | –    | –     | –     | –   |
| Bw39 | 0.5  | 0    | –    | –     | –     | –   |
| B40  | 14.5 | 15.9 | 0.06 | 0.95  | 17.1  | 1.1 |

b) A particular virulence of some HSV strains.

a) The increased frequency of HLA-B5 patients suffering from recurrent stromal keratitis allows us to express the hypothesis that there is an association between this disease and an immunoreactivity gene that is linked to the HLA system. The origin of recurrences might have some relation to the dysfunction of one or more immune response genes located on chromosome 6 very close to the HLA genes. The study of the other loci, especially the D-locus, which lies in even greater proximity to the immunoreactivity genes, seems highly justified.

b) Some differences between HSV strains might explain the greater tendency in some patients toward recurrence of ocular disease.

We must, however, point out that these ideas do not explain the absence or the presence of herpetic recurrences in corneal graft after keratoplasty.

In the attempt to explain these facts one might propose two hypotheses:

– There is a possibility that HLA-molecules themselves, or molecules coded by neighboring genes, might act like HSV receptors.

– The existence of a structural similarity between HLA-molecules and some antigens of the viral envelope could lead to a cross tolerance. This, in turn, could make it impossible for the patient to generate an appropriate immune response.

The finding of HSV in the tear film of persons without any observable ocular lesions and the finding of some antigenic modifications of the cornea after keratoplasty are reasons to suggest the existence of a particular susceptibility of certain cells to herpetic infection due to their surface-antigens.

This is what we shall scrutinize in a study of the susceptibility to HSV of human corneal cells in organ cultures according to HLA-types.

**Acknowledgments.** The authors are indebted to Professor G. Richard O'Connor, San Francisco, for his kindness in manuscript preparation and to Mrs Angélique Couvin for her excellent technical assistance. This study was supported in part by a grant of INSERM 68-78-100 and by a grant of "Fondation pour la Recherche Médicale Française".

**References**

1. Colin J, Chastel C, Saleun JP, Morin JF, Renard G (1979) Herpès oculaire récidivant et

antigènes HLA; étude préliminaire. J Fr Ophthalmol 4:263–266

2. Fine M, Cignetti FE (1977) Penetrating keratoplasty in herpes simplex keratitis. Arch Ophthalmol 95:613–617

3. Leopold IH, Sery TW (1963) Epidemiology of herpes simplex keratitis. Invest Ophthalmol Visual Sci 2:298–303

4. Meyers-Elliott RH, Elliott JH, Maxwell WA, Pettit TH, O'Day DM, Terasaki PI, Bernoco D (1980) HLA antigens in recurrent stromal herpes simplex virus keratitis. Am J Ophthalmol 89:54–57

5. Nesburn AB, Cook ML, Stevens JG (1972) Latent herpes simplex virus. Isolation from rabbit trigeminal ganglia between episodes of recurrent ocular infection. Arch Ophthalmol 88:412–417

6. Ribaric V (1976) The incidence of herpetic keratitis among population. Ophthalmologica 173:19–22

7. Russel AS, Schlaut J (1975) HLA transplantation antigens in subjects susceptible to recrudescent herpes labialis. Tissue Antigens 6:257–261

8. Terasaki PI, McClelland JD (1964) Microdroplet assay of human serum cytotoxins. Nature 204:998–1000

9. Zimmermann TJ, McNeill JI, Richman A, Kaufman HE, Waltman SR (1977) HLA-types and recurrent corneal herpes simplex infection. Invest Ophthalmol Visual Sci 16:756–757

Sundmacher, R. (Hrsg.):
Herpetische Augenerkrankungen
© J.F. Bergmann Verlag, München 1981

# HLA-DR Antigens and Recurrent Herpes Simplex Virus Infections

R.H. Meyers-Elliott, J.H. Elliott, A.R. Ahmed, W.A. Maxwell, T.H. Pettit, D.M. O'Day,
P.J. Terasaki, Los Angeles and Nashville

**Key words.** Recurrent herpetic disease and HLA system, HLA-DR

**Schlüsselwörter.** Herpesrezidive und HLA-System, HLA-DR

**Summary.** The possible associations of HLA-DR antigens and predisposition to recurrent HSV infections were studied in patients with recurrent HSV 1 and HSV 2 infections. HLA-DR antigens have been determined in over 34 patients with recurrent HSV stromal keratitis (HSV type 1). An increased frequency HLA-DRw3 was found in the patient group (35%) compared to the control group (23%) but the P value was not statistically significant. HLA-DRw7 was also found with increased frequency in the patient group (38%) compared to the control group (22%). The uncorrected P value of $< 0.05$ was significant; however, after correcting for the number of variables studied the corrected P value was not significant.

The increased frequency of HLA-DRw7 in recurrent HSV keratitis prompted us to look further at possible associations with another recurrent HSV infection, that of recurrent herpes genitalis (HSV 2). A statistically significant association of HLA-DRw7 was found in 36 patients with recurrent HSV progenitalis (43%) compared to controls (20%) with P corrected to $< 0.05$.

Interestingly, no associations between the HLA-A, -B or -C antigens and recurrent HSV stromal keratitis or recurrent HSV progenitalis was found. The strong association of HLA-DRw7 with recurrent HSV genitalis suggests that the HLA-DR antigen products are involved in the predisposition to recurrent HSV disease and supports the view that the immune response genes are probably responsible for the relationship.

**Zusammenfassung.** Wir untersuchten einen möglichen Zusammenhang zwischen HLA-DR-Antigenen und dem Auftreten rezidivierender HSV 1- and HSV 2-Infektionen bei Patienten. Bei über 34 Patienten mit HSV 1-Erkrankung (rezidivierende herpetische Stromakeratitis) bestimmten wir die HLA-DR-Antigene und fanden eine größere Häufigkeit von HLA-DRw3 bei den Patienten (35%) im Vergleich zu der Kontrollgruppe (23%). Dieser Unterschied war aber statistisch nicht signifikant. Zweitens fanden wir eine größere Häufigkeit von HLA-DRw7 (35% im Vergleich mit 22%). Hier war der unkorrigierte p-Wert mit $< 0.05$ signifikant; nach Korrektur des p-Wertes für die Anzahl der Variablen ergab sich aber auch in diesem Fall kein signifikanter Unterschied.

Nachdem wir diese größere Häufigkeit von HLA-DRw7 bei rezidivierender Herpeskeratitis gefunden hatten, untersuchten wir, ob dies auch für eine HSV 2-Erkrankung zutrifft. Bei rezidivierendem Herpes progenitalis war HLA-DRw7 bei 36 Patienten signifikant häufiger als bei den Kontrollen vertreten (43% gegenüber 20%; korrigierter p-Wert $< 0.05$).

Auffälligerweise fanden wir keinerlei Beziehungen zwischen rezidivierendem Stromaherpes oder Herpes progenitalis und HLA-A, HLA-B oder HLA-C. Die signifikante Korrelation zwischen HLA-DRw7 und rezidivierendem Herpes progenitalis scheint uns aber zu zeigen, daß HLA-DR-Antigenprodukte irgendetwas mit einer Prädisposition für rezidivierende Herpeserkrankungen zu tun haben, was die Ansicht stützt, daß wahrscheinlich Immunregulationsgene für diesen Zusammenhang verantwortlich sind.

## Introduction

Many functions and capabilities of the host response to microbiologic agents may be controlled or regulated by genes in the HLA region, or in the major histocompitability complex, or in a closely linked genetic loci [2, 6, 7]. Evidence for HLA and disease association and predisposition to recurrent virus infections is very limited. There have been two conflicting reports on the association of HLA and recurrent HSV infections. Russell and Schlaut [5] have shown an increased frequency of HLA-A1 in patients with recurrent HSV labialis. Zimmerman et al. [9] found an increased prevalence of HLA-B5 in epithelial herpes keratitis. However, only the HLA-A and HLA-B specificities were determined in these reports.

Recently there has been great interest in the possibility that the HLA-D locus may be highly linked to disease susceptibility genes because of the analogy of the HLA-D locus with the mouse Ia (immune associated) locus [6, 7]. Up to now, HLA-D antigen typing was performed using the mixed lymphocyte cytotoxicity reaction. These spcificities can now be determined serologically by using B lymphocytes [8]. The antigens indentified on B lymphocytes by the cytotoxicity reaction are the antigens of the DR locus which are considered operationally equivalent to the D locus [7].

There have been no reports of viral disease associations and the HLA-DR loci. Because of the ubiquitous nature of HSV and the relative rarity of recurrent HSV infections, differences in immunoreactivity of susceptible patients has been suggested. We examined the possible genetically determined differences in predisposition to recurrent HSV 1 [3, 4] and HSV 2 infections [1].

of Medicine, and at the Corneal-External Disease Clinic of the Department of Ophthalmology, Vanderbilt University School of Medicine. Thirty-six patients with a documented recurrent herpes genitalis (HSV 2) who were seen at the Dermatology Clinic at the UCLA School of Medicine were selected for HLA-DR typing on the basis of their long-standing recurrent infections. All patients were serologically typed for six HLA-DR antigens [8]. Data were expressed as phenotypic frequency in normal Caucasians as compared to recurrent herpes patients typed in the same laboratory. The frequency of the HLA-DR antigens in the 34 herpes stromal keratitis patients was compared to 218 normal controls and in the 36 herpes genitalis patients with 197 normal controls. All HLA typing was performed in the Tissue Typing Laboratory, Department of Surgery, UCLA School of Medicine. The chi-square test with Yates continuity correction for the number of comparisons was used for statistical analysis of the results. The P values were computed by using Fisher's exact probabilities from the distribution of the chi square. The relative risk, how many times more frequent a disease is in individuals carrying the antigens compared to individuals lacking the antigen, was determined for all antigens.

## Subjects and Methods

Thirty-four patients with a history of recurrent herpes stromal keratitis (HSV 1) were typed for DR antigens. All patients were examined at the External Disease Clinic of the Jules Stein Eye Institute, UCLA School

## Results

The HLA-DR phenotypes for the 34 patients with recurrent HSV stromal keratitis are shown in Table 1. An increased frequency of HLA-DRw3 was found in the patient group (35%) compared to the Caucasian control

Table 1. HLA-DR antigen frequencies in patients with recurrent herpes simplex virus (HSV 1) stromal keratitis

| HLA Antigen | Normal Caucasians (n = 218) % frequency | Herpes Patients (n = 34) % frequency | Chi Square | P Value[a] | Relative Risk |
|---|---|---|---|---|---|
| DRw1 | 19 | 18 | 0.05 | .82 | 0.9 |
| DRw2 | 28 | 21 | 0.48 | .49 | 0.7 |
| DRw3 | 23 | 35 | 1.98 | .16 | 1.8 |
| DRw4 | 30 | 24 | 0.36 | .55 | 0.7 |
| DRw5 | 22 | 24 | 0.00 | .97 | 1.09 |
| DRw7 | 22 | 38 | 3.64 | .06 | 2.19 |

[a] Uncorrected for the number of variables studied

**Table 2.** HLA-DR antigen frequencies in patients with recurrent herpes (HSV 2) genitalis

| HLA Antigen | Normal Caucasians (n = 193) % frequency | Herpes patients (n = 36) % frequency | Chi Square | P Value[a] | Relative Risk |
|---|---|---|---|---|---|
| DRw1 | 20 | 14 | 0.28 | 0.59 | 0.6 |
| DRw2 | 28 | 14 | 2.21 | 0.14 | 0.4 |
| DRw3 | 19 | 6 | 2.75 | 0.10 | 0.3 |
| DRw4 | 28 | 26 | 0.02 | 0.90 | 0.9 |
| DRw5 | 21 | 29 | 0.64 | 0.42 | 1.4 |
| DRw7 | 20 | 43 | 7.61 | 0.006 | 3.2 |

[a] Uncorrected for the number of variables studied

group (23%) but the P value was not statistically significant. HLA-DRw7 was also found with increased frequency in the patient group (38%) compared to the control group (22%). The relative risk was 2.2. The uncorrected P value of < 0.05 was significant; however, after correcting for the number of variables studied (probability of 0.05 × 6 antigens studied at the DR locus), the corrected value was not significant. In Table 2 are shown the HLA-DR phenotypes of 36 patients with recurrent HSV progenitalis. A statistically significant association of HLA-DRw7 was found in patients (43%) compared to Caucasian controls (20%) with P corrected of < 0.05 and a relative risk of 3.2. No significant differences in other DR antigen frequencies could be detected.

**Discussion**

The greatest source of error in attributing an association between HLA and disease is in the statistical analysis. The number of parameters (HLA specificities) should be accounted for and the final P value should be multiplied by this number to give a corrected P value. An uncorrected P value in our study would have led to a significant association between HLA-DRw7 and herpes stromal keratitis.

Our finding of a significant association of HLA-DRw7 with recurrent HSV 2 and a higher frequency of HLA-DRw7 in patients with recurrent stromal keratitis may be of special significance in explaining genetic predisposition of selected individuals to recurrent HSV infections. Data [3, 4] not presented here on over 48 patients with recurrent herpes

stromal keratitis failed to support the reported significance of the HLA-B5 antigen and recurrent herpes keratitis [9]. No HLA-B5 antigens were found in the patients with HSV 2 genitalis. Also no significant associations between the HLA-A, -B or -C antigens and recurrent stromal keratitis [3, 4] or progenitalis were observed in our previous studies. The added significance of the HLA-DRw7 and recurrent HSV disease is that this is the first reported association of a human disease of viral etiology with an HLA-DR antigen. Since the immune response genes in man are closely linked to the HLA genetic loci, individuals with HLA-DRw7 may be genetically selected or predisposed to HSV recurrence by virtue of some coded and predetermined immunologic deviation of their host defense mechanisms.

**Acknowledgment.** Supported by research grants EY02646 and 00331 from the National Eye Institute.

**References**

1. Ahmed AR, Meyers-Elliott RH, Terasaki PI (1981) HLA-DRw7 and recurrent herpes genitalis. Lancet submitted
2. Bodmer WF (ed) (1978) The HLA system. Br Med Bull 34:213–216
3. Meyers-Elliott RH, Elliott JH, Maxwell WA, Pettit TH, O'Day DM, Terasaki PI (1979) HLA antigens associated with recurrent herpes simplex keratitis. Invest Ophthalmol Visual Sci (ARVO Suppl) 19:70
4. Meyers-Elliott RH, Elliott JH, Maxwell WA, Pettit TH, O'Day DM, Terasaki PI, Bernoco D (1980) HLA antigens in recurrent stromal her-

pes simplex virus keratitis. Am J Ophthalmol 89:54–57

5. Russell AS, Schlaut J (1975) HLA-A transplantation antigens in subjects susceptible to recrudescent herpes labialis. Tissue Antigens 6:257–261

6. Svejaard A, Jersild C, Nielsen LC, Bodmer WF (1974) HLA-A antigens and disease. Statistical and genetic considerations. Tissue Antigens 4:95–105

7. Svejaard A, Ryder LP (1977) Associations between HLA and disease. In: Dausset J, Svejaard A (eds) HLA and disease. Williams and Wilkins, Baltimore, pp 46–316

8. Terasaki PI, Bernoco D, Park MS, Ozturk G, Iwaki Y (1978) Microdroplet testing for HLA-A, -B, -C, and -D antigens. Am J Clin Pathol 69:103–120

9. Zimmerman TJ, McNeill JI, Richman A, Kaufman HE, Waltman S (1977) HLA type and recurrent corneal herpes simplex infection. Invest Ophthalmol Visual Sci 15:756–758

Sundmacher, R. (Hrsg.):
Herpetische Augenerkrankungen
© J.F. Bergmann Verlag, München 1981

# Natural Killer Activity and HLA Phenotypes in Patients With Herpes Simplex Keratitis

C.S. Foster, D.P. Dubey, S. Stux, E. Unis, Boston

**Key words.** HLA system and herpetic diseases, HLA-DR

**Schlüsselwörter.** HLA-System und Herpeserkrankungen, HLA-DR

**Summary.** Natural killer cell assays were performed in eight herpes patients and in four controls. The number of patients is still too small for statistical analysis; the preliminary results indicate, however, that non-recurrent HSK patients may have a greater NK activity than patients with frequently recurring HSK.

The results of HLA-A, B, and C typing on 24 patients showed no significant changes of phenotypic frequencies for the HSK patients as a total group or as separate groups of recurrent vs non-recurrent HSK.

Fifteen patients have been typed for HLA-DR. There was a suggestive though as yet not significant trend of increased DRw3 in herpes patients (47% vs 22%).

**Zusammenfassung.** Bei acht Herpespatienten und vier Kontrollpatienten bestimmten wir die Aktivität der „natürlichen Killerzellen" im Blut. Die Fallzahl ist noch zu klein, um gültige Schlüsse zu ziehen; es scheint sich aber abzuzeichnen, daß Patienten mit selten rezidivierender Herpeserkrankung eine höhere Killerzell-Aktivität haben als Patienten, bei denen Rezidive häufig sind.

Bei 24 Patienten, bei denen wir HLA-A, B und C bestimmten, fanden wir weder im Vergleich zum Normalkollektiv noch beim Vergleich von Patienten hoher mit Patienten geringer Rezidivhäufigkeit einen Unterschied.

Fünfzehnmal typisierten wir HLA-DR ohne signifikantes Endergebnis; HLA-DRw3 scheint aber bei Herpes-Patienten häufiger als bei Kontrollpersonen zu sein (47% gegenüber 22%).

HLA antigens are glycoproteins present on the cell surface membrane of most human nucleated cells. They comprise one of the most complex immunogenetic systems yet studied, with identifiable multiple alleles. The synthesis of the glycoproteins is controlled by genetic loci mapped on the chromosome 6 [2, 10]. The biologic significance of these glycoproteins is incompletely understood; but evidence points to a role in membrane directed cell-cell interaction as well as a role in immune defense mechanisms detecting foreignness in the form of chemical or viral modifications of cells. Studies have shown that certain diseases appear to be associated with certain specific HLA phenotypes [4, 93]. The basis for this association is unclear, although several hypotheses have been proposed, including molecular mimicry [7] and HLA-immune response gene associations [13]. Our study of HLA phenotypes in the context of immune response parameters in patients with herpes simplex keratitis (HSK) was a sequel to the foregoing observations. It also seemed appropriate to assess the natural killer (NK) lymphocyte activity of HSK patients, considering the viral etiology of this disease, since it is now established that normal individuals have this subpopulation of lymphoid cells that destroy spontaneously transformed tumor cells and/or virally modified cells [5]. Many patients with an attack of HSK never experience clinical evidence of recurrent HSK episodes. Some experience few recurrent attacks. And yet others will have many recurrent attacks of HSK. It is the recurrent episodes, each producing sequentially more corneal scarring, which commonly result in corneal blindness due to HSK. We investigated whether differences in HLA phenotypes and/or in natural killer lymphocyte function could be correlated between our patients with recurrent HSK when compared to a group of patients with non-recurrent HSK, using normal individuals as controls.

## Materials and Methods

HLA-A, B, C, and DRw typing was performed on peripheral blood lymphocytes of 24 patients with a history of herpes simplex keratitis. The patients ranged in age from 12 to 68 years with a mean age of 46 years. Twelve of the patients were male and 12 were female. Patients were categorized as having "non-recurrent infectious HSK" if they experienced three episodes of infectious keratitis per year, or less, and as having "recurrent infectious HSK" if they experienced more than three episodes of infectious keratitis per year.

Five of the patients experienced episodes of stromal disciform edema periodically; all of these patients were part of the "non-recurrent infectious HSK" group. None of the patients had infectious stromal herpetic keratitis. All patients received their primary ophthalmic care longitudinally at the Cornea Service of the Massachusetts Eye and Ear Infirmary.

HLA-A, B, and C typing for lymphocytes was done by the Amos method [1]. Each individual was tested against a panel of 142 well characterized anti HLA-A, B, C sera defining 18, 27, and 5 antigens at the loci A, B, and C respectively. The HLA-DRw typing for nylon wool T cell-depleted B lymphocytes was done on 15 patients by the standard complement dependent microcytotoxicity NIII technique [16]. A total of 70 platelet absorbed alloantisera detecting seven B cell DR or Ia-like antigen determinants on B cells were used with each sample.

Data were expressed as phenotypic frequency in normal causasians as compared to the HSK patients typed in our laboratory. The P values were computed by using the Fisher's exact probabilities from the distribution of the Chi-square.

Natural killer (NK) activity was assayed in eight HSK patients by the modified method of West [17]. Target cells from the myeloid leukemia cell line K562 were incubated with 0.2 ml radioactive sodium chromate ($Na_2$ $^{51}CrO_4$, 292 mCi/mg. New England Nuclear, Boston, MA) for 45 min at 37 °C. Following labelling, cells were washed three times in Hanks' Balanced Salt Solution (HBSS) at 4 °C. The natural killer assay was carried out in Linbro roundbottom microtiter plates with three different concentrations of lymphoid effector cells ranging from $10^5$ - $5 \times 10^5$ and a fixed number of $10^4$ target K562 cells per well in a total volume of 0.2 ml. After 4 h of incubation the plates were centrifuged at 1500 rpm for 10 min at 4 °C and 0.1 ml of supernatant from each well was removed and counted for released radioactivity. Total counts were derived by counting an aliquot of target cells after resuspension in 0.2 ml media in the microtiter cells. Spontaneous release was determined by culturing $^{51}Cr$-labeled target cells alone. Percent specific chromium release or percent cytotoxicity was determined from the relation:

$$\% \text{ Lysis} = \frac{\text{experimental release (cpm)} - \text{spontaneous release (cpm)}}{\text{total counts (cpm)} - \text{spontaneous release (cpm)}} \times 100$$

Results for individual cells were expressed as percent specific chromium release at an effector/target ratio of 25 : 1.

## Results

The results of the NK assay in eight patients and in four controls are seen in Fig. 1. The number of patients tested is small and therefore meaningfull statistical analysis of the data is not possible. Nonetheless, certain interesting trends are suggested by these preliminary results. Comparison (using a one tail test) of controls with patients with non-recurrent HSK suggests that non-recurrent HSK patients may have greater NK activity than controls (p = 0.07). The data spread in the recurrent HSK group is great; no statistically significant differences in NK activity are detected between this group and controls or non-recurrent HSK patients. Two of the patients tested had previously had penetrating keratoplasties. One of these patients had high NK activity; his transplant had been rejected 2 years prior to NK testing. The other patient had low NK activity; his transplant was clear and free of any rejection episodes 2 years after grafting.

The results of HLA-A, B, and C typing on 24 patients show no significant changes of phenotypic frequencies for the HSK patients as a total group or as separate groups of recurrent vs non-recurrent HSK.

The results of DRw typing on 15 of the patients are seen in Table 1. No statistically

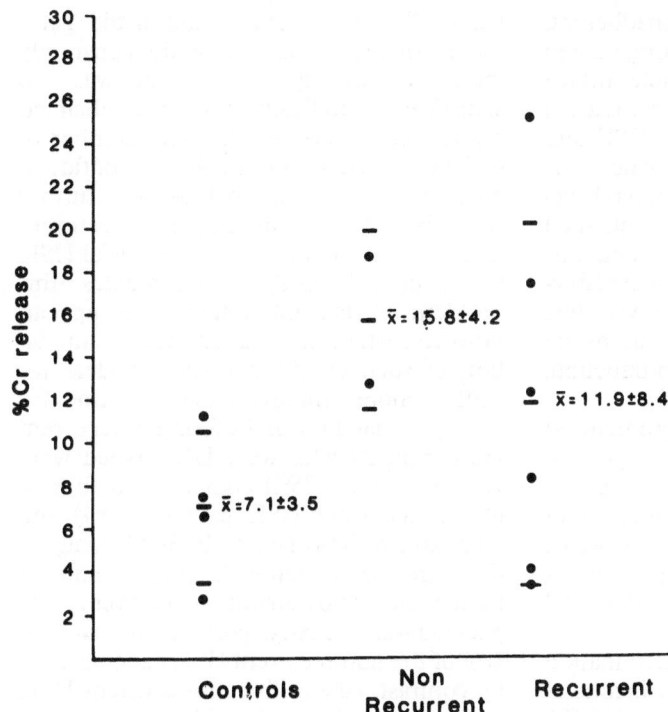

**Fig. 1.** NK activity, expressed as % $^{51}$Cr release from target cells exposed to nonsensitized lymphocytes from controls or from patients with history of herpes simplex keratitis (either recurrent or non-recurrent). × = mean of group

significant differences between the study groups were found. However a suggestive trend of increased DRw3 frequency (47% vs 22%) in HSK patients (PR 3.1) was observed.

## Discussion

Normal individuals have a subpopulation of lymphoid cells, currently designated as natural killer (NK) cells, that spontaneously destroy (without priming or prior contact)

transformed tumor cells and/or virally modified cells [5]. Although the origin of NK cells is not yet well understood, and their actual biological significance is still unclear, there is general agreement that this subpopulation is an important component of the immune surveillance mechanism, since these cells can destroy tumor cells (and thus by extension possibly allografts as well) and virally transformed cells [3, 14].

Some evidence suggests that NK cells may arise from promonocytemacrophage

**Table 1.** Herpes simplex virus – patients tested – 15

| DRw Antigen | Control Population MSFCI (81%)[a] | US (255)[b] | HSV Patients No | % | RR | X$^2$ | P |
|---|---|---|---|---|---|---|---|
| 1 | 22.2 | 16.1 | 1 | 7 | – | – | |
| 2 | 28.4 | 27.1 | 3 | 20 | – | – | |
| 3 | 22.2 | 22.0 | 7 | 47 | 3.10/3.14 | 4.21 | p < .05 |
| 4 | 22.2 | 24.7 | 3 | 20 | – | – | |
| 5 | 21.0 | 18.0 | 3 | 20 | – | – | |
| 6 | 14.8 | 6.3 | 1 | 7 | – | – | |
| 7 | 30.9 | 23.1 | 3 | 20 | – | – | |

a Combined Minnesota and Sidney Farber Cancer Institute panel
b US 7 panel of 255 individuals. Histocompatibility testing 1977. Munngard Copenhagen

precursors [6]. They are small, nonadherent, nonphagocytic lymphocytes that originate in the bone marrow and lack detectable surface immunoglobulins [5]. It is of more than casual interest, with respect to recurrent HSK and recurrence triggers, that NK cytolytic function is markedly suppressed by dibutyryl cyclic AMP or by C-AMP-elevating agents such as prostaglandin $E_1$, theophylline and histamine [11] and this suppression is at the effector (i.e. NK cell) level. Similarly, in vivo NK activity is stimulated by interferon or by agents that stimulate interferon production, and is suppressed by estrogens [15].

In this context it seemed appropriate to assess the NK activity of HSK patients, considering the viral etiology of this disease. Moreover, since corneal transplant is one of the clinical options in managing the disease, the question of transplant outcome versus patient NK activity might provide additional clues in assessing prognosis.

The results of NK activity determination in eight of our HSK patients are inconclusive, but suggest that our non-recurrent HSK patients have relatively high NK activity. It may be possible that high NK activity in HSK patients is protective as a first line of defense against recurrent disease. The fact that of the two HSK patients with corneal transplants who had NK activity determined, the one with high NK activity had a rejected transplant and the one with normal or low NK activity had successful transplant is intrigueing. It is possible that NK activity might be an important prognostic feature for corneal transplantation in HSK patients. Our data obviously do not definitively answer any of these questions, but they suggest the importance of more extensive study of these parameters. Greater numbers of patients more carefully characterized clinically, and studied sequentially, in a longitudinal fashion should be investigated. The same may be said of the HLA typing data.

Russell and Schlaut [12] reported an increased prevalence of HLA-A1, in patients with recurrent HSV labialis, and Zimmerman et al. [18] reported an increased prevalence of HLA-B5 in 46 patients with recurrent infectious epithelial HSK. We did not find increased frequencies of these phenotypes in our study sample. Meyers-Elliot [8] found an increased frequency of HLA-DRw3 in 25 patients with "recurrent herpes stromal keratitis"; but with application of the Yates correction to the data analysis, this apparently increased phenotypic frequency was not statistically significant. We have obtained remarkedly similar results. The number of patients tested is too small for confident, meaningful statistical analysis, and further subdivision of the study sample into recurrent and non-recurrent infectious epithelial HSK for subgroup analysis accentuates this problem. Certain interesting trends appear, however, when this is attempted. Examination of such trends may suggest ideas for further, more definitive studies. We find, for example, that three of the four non-recurrent HSK patients who were DRw typed were DRw3 positive (75%) compared to four to eleven recurrent HSK patients (35%) and compared to 20% of controls. Similar suggestive trends were seen with HLA-A2 and A3 frequencies. Thus, 36% of the recurrent HSK patients were HLA-A3 positive, compared to 20% of the non-recurrent HSK patients. And by contrast, 80% of the non-recurrent HSK patients were HLA-A2 positive, compared to 45% of controls and 60% of recurrent HSK patients.

We believe these data suggest ideas for further, more definitive HLA and immune function studies on patients with herpes simplex keratitis. We would emphasize the importance of precise definition of the form of HSK (infectious epithelial, non-infectious "trophic" (metaherpetic) epithelial, infectious stromal, immune "disciform" (non-infectious) stromal, uveitis, keratouveitis) and the importance of precise definition of the frequency of recurrent attacks of disease manifestations. The need for large numbers of patients representing each subgroup of HSK manifestations is clear. And the desirability to study immune function parameters (NK activity) longitudinally, relating results to clinical status should likewise be obvious. We are currently attempting these kinds of studies.

Acknowledgment. Supported in part by Grant EY03063 (Foster) and CA27063 (Dubey) from the National Institute of Health. Reprint requests to Dr. Foster, 20 Staniford Street, Boston, MA 02114, USA.

## References

1. Amos DB, Bashir H, Boyle W et al in Ind Med

(1969) A simple micro cytotoxicity test. Transplantation 7:220–223

2. Amos DB, Batchelor R, Bodmer WF et al (1976) WHO-IUTS terminology committee: Nomenclature for factors of the HLA system. Transplantation 21:353–358

3. Azocar J, Dubey D, Stux S, Yunis E, Essex M (1979) Human Natural Killer eventually kill RNA tumor virus infected lymphoid cells. Ed. Boris-Latin, Boris-Latin, Presented at Proc International Assoc Competitive and Related Diseases in Titsunba, USSR

4. Dausset J, Degos L, Hors J (1974) The association of the HLA antigens with diseases. Clin Immunol Immunopathol 3:127–149

5. Herberman RB, Djeu J, Kay HD, Ortaldo JR, Riccardi C, Bonnard GD, Holden HT, Fagnani R, Santoni A, Puccetti P (1979) Natural killer cells: Characteristics and regulation of activity. Immunol Rev 44:43–70

6. Lohmann-Matthes ML, Domzig W, Roder J (1979) Promonocytes have the functional characteristics of natural killer cells. J Immunol 123:1883–1886

7. Lyampert IM, Danilova TA (1975) Immunological phenomena associated with cross-reactive antigens of micro-organisms and mammalian tissues. Prog Allergy 18:423–477

8. Meyers-Elliott RH, Elliott JH, Maxwell WA, Pettit TH, O'Day DM, Terasaki PI, Bernoco D (1980) HLA antigens in recurrent stromal herpes simplex keratitis. Am J Ophthalmol 89: 54–57

9. Oh JH, MacLean JD (1975) Diseases associated with specific HLA antigens. Can Med Assoc J 112:1315–1318

10. Pierres M, Fradelizi D, Neauport-Sautes C et al (1975) Third HLA segregant series: Genetic analysis and molecular independence on lymphocyte surface. Tissue Antigens 5:266–279

11. Roder JC, Klein M (1979) Target-effector interaction in the natural killer cell system. IV. modulation by cyclic nucleotides. J Immunol 123:2785–2790

12. Russell AS, Schlaut J (1975) HLA transplantation antigens in subjects susceptible to recrudescent herpes labialis. Tissue Antigens 6: 257–261

13. Sachs DH, Dickler HB (1975) The possible role of I region determined cell surface molecules in the regulation of immune responses. Transplant Rev 23:159–175

14. Santoli D, Trinchieri G, Lief FS (1978) Cell-mediated cytotoxicity against virus-infected target cells in humans. I. Characterization of the effector lymphocyte. J Immunol 121:526–531

15. Seaman WE, Merigan TC, Talal N (1979) Natural killing in estrogen-treated mice responds poorly to poly I-C despite normal stimulation of circulating interferon. J Immunol 123:2903–2905

16. Terasaki PI, Bernoco D, Park MS, Ozturk G, Iwaki Y (1978) Microdroplet testing for HLA-A, -B, -C, and -D antigens. Am J Clin Pathol 69:103–120

17. West WH, Cannon GB, Kay HD, Bonnard GD, Herberman RB (1977) Natural cytotoxic reactivity of human lymphocytes against a myeloid cell line: Characterization of effector cells. J Immunol 118:355–361

18. Zimmerman TJ, McNeill JI, Richman A, Kaufman HE, Waltman SR (1977) HLA types and recurrent corneal herpes simplex infection. Invest Ophthalmol Visual Sci 16:756–757

Sundmacher, R. (Hrsg.):
Herpetische Augenerkrankungen
© J.F. Bergmann Verlag, München 1981

# HLA Antigens in Recurrent Corneal Herpes Simplex Virus Infection

H.J. Völker-Dieben, C.C. Kok-van Alphen, I. Schreuder, J. D'Amaro, Leyden

**Key words.** HLA system and herpetic diseases, HLA-A3

**Schlüsselwörter.** HLA-System und Herpeserkrankungen, HLA-A3

**Summary.** 115 patients with recurrent herpetic keratitis and 123 controls were studied for the distribution of HLA-A, B, and C antigens. HLA-A3 was found to be significantly more frequent in the herpes population (corrected p value <0.042). Also, males were nearly twice as frequently affected as females (p < 0.001). Females seem to be less susceptible for HSV keratitis between the age of 15 to 45.

**Zusammenfassung.** Bei 115 Patienten mit herpetischen Augenerkrankungen und bei 123 Kontrollpersonen untersuchten wir das HLA-A-, B- und C-Muster. HLA-A3 war bei den Herpespatienten signifikant häufiger (korrigierter p-Wert < 0.042). Auch fanden sich fast zweimal häufiger Männer als Frauen unter den Erkrankten (p < 0.001). Frauen zwischen 15 und 45 scheinen weniger zu rezidivierender Herpeskeratitis zu neigen.

The human histocompatibility complex, HLA, plays an important role in immune responsiveness and in susceptibility to disease and its subsequent clinical course [5]. Two reports on the association of HLA and recurrent Herpes Simplex Virus (HSV) infection have been published. Zimmerman et al. reported an increased frequency of HLA-B5 in recurrent HSV keratitis. Meyers-Elliott et al. [3] reported that HLA-Aw 30 occurred three times more frequently in patients with HSV keratitis than in normal whites. However, the P value was not significant after correction. The almost universal human infection by HSV makes it all the more remarkable that corneal HSV infection is relatively rare.

Corneal HSV keratitis is not a very serious infection in its initial phase. The recurrent version develops in 25% of the patients. Because of its recurrent nature, the eventual condition of the cornea may become so bad that corneal transplantation is indicated. One third of our corneal transplantation patients have the diagnosis of recurrent HSV keratitis.

## Subjects and Methods

Patients (N = 115) and healthy controls (N = 123) were all selected from the Dutch population in order to avoid spurious associations due to ethnic differences or mixtures. The HLA antigens of the 115 patients were analysed for a possible association between the HLA-A, -B and -C antigens and the predisposition to recurrent HSV keratits.

Typing for 8 HLA-A, 16 HLA-B and 6 HLA-C antigens was performed by using the microlymphocytotoxicity test [4]. The HLA frequencies of the patient group were compared to those of a control group of 123 normal persons typed in the same laboratory in Leyden. The Woolf-Haldane analysis [2, 6] was used to access the significance of the different antigen frequencies in these patients and controls. All P values were corrected for a total of 30 antigens studied using the procedure suggested by Edwards [1].

## Results

### HLA and Disease Association

The HLA-A phenotype frequencies for the patients with recurrent HSV keratitis and the controls are shown in Table 1. HLA-A3 was found to be significantly increased. The corrected P value was 0.042. There were no

**Table 1.** Woolf-Haldane analysis of the HLA antigen frequencies in 115 patients with recurrent corneal herpes and in 123 healthy controls

| Antigen | Patients Pos | Neg | Controls Pos | Neg | Relative Risk | Chi Square | Corr p |
|---------|------|-----|------|-----|--------|--------|--------|
| A1   | 34 | 81  | 41 | 82  | 0.842 | 0.389  | n.s.  |
| A2   | 54 | 61  | 63 | 60  | 0.844 | 0.432  | n.s.  |
| A3   | 45 | 70  | 24 | 99  | 2.621 | 10.819 | 0.042 |
| A9   | 21 | 94  | 24 | 99  | 0.924 | 0.059  | n.s.  |
| A10  | 2  | 113 | 12 | 111 | 0.196 | 6.187  | n.s.  |
| A11  | 8  | 107 | 18 | 105 | 0.451 | 3.477  | n.s.  |
| A28  | 16 | 99  | 10 | 113 | 1.793 | 2.021  | n.s.  |
| Aw19 | 24 | 91  | 28 | 95  | 0.897 | 0.123  | n.s.  |

p values have been corrected for a total of 30 comparisons

significant differencies in any of the other HLA antigen frequencies.

The HLA-B and HLA-C phenotype frequencies for the patients and controls are shown in Tables 2 and 3. There were no significantly increased frequencies for the HLA-B or HLA-C antigens.

*Sex Rate in Recurrent HSV Keratitis*

We found a remarkable sex incidence. In 131 patients with recurrent HSV keratitis (of which 115 were HLA typed) we found almost two times more males than females i.e. 85

male patients and 46 females. This differential sex distribution was highly significant (chi-square = 11.61, $p < 0.001$).

The ages of onset of the primary HSV infection are shown in Fig. 1. It was found that 56% of the male patients incurred their primary HSV infection between the ages of 15 and 45 years. Only 26% of the female patients incurred their primary infection in that age span.

*Duration of the Recurrent HSV Keratitis*

The 131 patients with recurrent HSV keratitis

**Table 2.** Woolf-Haldane analysis of the HLA antigen frequencies in 115 patients with recurrent corneal herpes and in 123 healthy controls

| Antigen | Patients Pos | Neg | Controls Pos | Neg | Relative Risk | Chi Square | Corr p |
|---------|------|-----|------|-----|--------|--------|--------|
| B5   | 17 | 98  | 20 | 103 | 0.984 | 0.002 | n.s. |
| B7   | 27 | 88  | 20 | 103 | 1.720 | 2.849 | n.s. |
| B8   | 36 | 79  | 29 | 94  | 1.471 | 1.785 | n.s. |
| B12  | 26 | 89  | 28 | 95  | 0.992 | 0.001 | n.s. |
| B13  | 6  | 109 | 6  | 117 | 1.073 | 0.016 | n.s. |
| B14  | 3  | 112 | 2  | 121 | 1.512 | 0.285 | n.s. |
| B15  | 16 | 99  | 16 | 107 | 1.080 | 0.044 | n.s. |
| Bw16 | 13 | 102 | 10 | 113 | 1.424 | 0.690 | n.s. |
| B17  | 7  | 108 | 12 | 111 | 0.617 | 1.063 | n.s. |
| B18  | 7  | 108 | 15 | 108 | 0.484 | 2.560 | n.s. |
| Bw21 | 4  | 111 | 7  | 116 | 0.627 | 0.637 | n.s. |
| Bw22 | 2  | 113 | 10 | 113 | 0.238 | 4.662 | n.s. |
| B27  | 10 | 105 | 13 | 110 | 0.815 | 0.232 | n.s. |
| Bw35 | 18 | 97  | 20 | 103 | 0.958 | 0.015 | n.s. |
| B37  | 1  | 114 | 4  | 119 | 0.348 | 1.555 | n.s. |
| B40  | 20 | 95  | 15 | 108 | 1.503 | 1.278 | n.s. |

p values have been corrected for a total of 30 comparisons

**Table 3.** Woolf-Haldane analysis of the HLA antigen frequencies in 115 patients with recurrent corneal herpes and in 123 healthy controls

| Antigen | Patients Pos | Neg | Controls Pos | Neg | Relative Risk | Chi Square | Corr p |
|---------|-------|-----|--------------|-----|---------------|------------|--------|
| Cw1 | 5 | 110 | 11 | 112 | 0.487 | 1.934 | n.s. |
| Cw2 | 14 | 101 | 12 | 111 | 1.274 | 0.362 | n.s. |
| Cw3 | 35 | 80 | 29 | 94 | 1.413 | 1.421 | n.s. |
| Cw4 | 22 | 93 | 22 | 101 | 1.086 | 0.063 | n.s. |
| Cw5 | 10 | 82 | 11 | 112 | 1.245 | 0.246 | n.s. |
| Cw6 | 10 | 49 | 26 | 97 | 0.780 | 0.389 | n.s. |

p values have been corrected for a total of 30 comparisons

were all grafted in the corneal department of the Leyden University Hospital. The average duration of the recurrent HSV keratitis was 17.7 years (2–65 years) at the time of transplantation. The age of the patients varied from 5 to 81 years, average 51.2 years.

**Discussion**

*Ad 1.*

Our findings of a significantly increased frequency of HLA-A3 in 115 patients with recurrent HSV keratitis when compared to their controls (corr. P value = 0.042) does not agree with the findings of Zimmerman et al. [7] who studied 46 patients, nor with the findings of Meyers-Elliott et al. [3] who studied 48 patients.

Zimmerman et al. [7] reported an increased frequency of HLA-B5 in 46 patients with recurrent corneal HSV as compared to 282 normal controls. However, the increase is not significant when the P value is corrected for the 32 antigens which were studied. In addition, there is uncertainty about the patient and control populations which are referred only as "white" and "normal" respectively. Even if the subjects were all Caucasoids, that would not exclude population heterogeneity, which could be the reason for the differential antigen frequencies in patients and controls.

Meyers-Elliott et al. [3] reported HLA-Aw 30 increased but not significantly after correction.

Incidentally, these authors corrected the P value only for the 14 antigens in the HLA-A locus instead of for the total 40 antigens in the HLA-A, -B, -C and DR loci. If they had done so, they would have obtained a corrected P

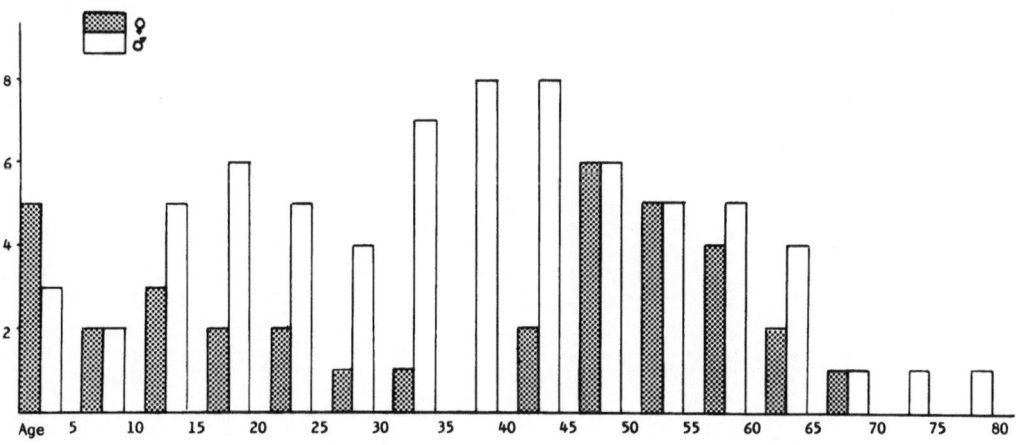

**Fig. 1.** Ages of onset of the primary HSV infection

93

value of 1.20 using the method which they cited. The proper correction is $1 - (1 - 0.3)^{40} = 0.70$. Finally a precise description of the populations is not found in their report. They speak of patients and normal whites. Therefore, as in the Zimmerman report we are confronted again with the possibility of population heterogeneity as a possible explanation for the differential antigen frequencies in patients and controls.

## Ad 2.

The highly significant difference in the numbers of male and female patients (85 ♂ : 46 ♀) with recurrent HSV keratitis, and the fact that 56% of the male patients as compared to 26% of the female patients incurred their primary HSV infection between the age of 15 and 45 years, can not be explained at this time. One possibility is that females between 15 and 45 demonstrate a beneficial effect of hormonal factors during their reproductive period. Further studies are necessary to test this hypothesis.

## Conclusions

HLA -A, -B and -C typing of patients with recurrent HSV keratitis revealed a significantly increased frequency of HLA-A3 (p = 0.042).
- Almost twice as many male patients (N = 85) as female (N = 46) were found in the group of patients with recurrent HSV keratitis. This differential sex distribution was highly significant (P < 0.001).
- Female patients seem to be less susceptible for the HSV keratitis between the age of 15 to 45.
- Using matched homogenous patients and control population would facilitate the comparisons of findings in different studies.

## References

1. Edwards JH (1974) HLA and disease. The detection of associations. J Immunogenet 1: 249
2. Haldane JBS (1955) The estimation and significance of the logarithm of a ratio of frequencies. Ann Hum Genet 20:30
3. Meyers-Elliott RH, et al. (1980) HLA antigens in herpes stromal keratitis. Am Ophthalmol 89:54–58
4. Ray JG, et al. (1977) Nih lymphocyte microcytotoxicity technique. Niaid Manual of Tissue Typing Techniques 77–545:22
5. Rood JJ van, (1980) The genetics and biology of the HLA system. In: Benacerraf B, Dorf ME (eds) The role of the Major Histocompatibility Complex in immunology. Garland, New York
6. Woolf B (1955) On estimating the relation between blood groups and disease. Ann Hum Genet 19:251
7. Zimmerman TJ, et al. (1977) HLA type and recurrent corneal herpes simplex infection. Invest Ophthalmol Visual Sci 15:756

Sundmacher, R. (Hrsg.):
Herpetische Augenerkrankungen
© J.F. Bergmann Verlag, München 1981

# HLA Phenotypes in Patients With Herpetic Keratitis

V. Lenhard, P. Haug, H. Kirchner, C. Hallermann, A. Mattes, R. Sundmacher, Heidelberg, Freiburg

**Key words.** HLA system and herpetic diseases

**Schlüsselwörter.** HLA-System und Herpeserkrankungen

**Summary.** Typing for HLA-A, B, and C antigens was performed in 81 patients with herpetic keratitis, 23 of them were typed for DR antigens. The antigen frequencies of patients and healthy controls were compared. A significant association between HLA and herpetic keratitis was not detected. Nevertheless the frequencies of some HLA antigens such as A1, A3, B7, B8 and particularly DR2 and DR3 showed a remarkable increase. The small number of DR typed patients should be increased to answer the question of genetic predisposition to herpetic keratitis definitely. In addition, it would be useful to perform family studies in order to analyse haplotype frequencies.

**Zusammenfassung.** Bei 81 Patienten mit herpetischer Keratitis wurden die HLA-A-, B-, C-Antigene, bei 23 Patienten zusätzlich die HLA-DR-Antigene bestimmt. Die Antigenfrequenzen von Patienten und gesunden Kontrollpersonen wurden verglichen. Eine signifikante Assoziation zwischen HLA und herpetischer Keratitis konnte nicht nachgewiesen werden. Allerdings waren die Frequenzen einiger HLA-Antigene, wie z.B. A1, A3, B7, B8 und insbesondere DR2 und DR3, deutlich erhöht. Die bisher noch geringe Zahl DR-typisierter Patienten sollte erweitert werden, um die Frage einer genetischen Prädisposition bei herpetischer Keratitis definitiv zu klären. Außerdem wären Familienuntersuchungen, die eine Analyse der Haplotypfrequenzen ermöglichen, sinnvoll.

## Introduction

An increasing number of HLA associated diseases has been reported in the recent years. However, evidence for HLA dependent predisposition to diseases with known viral aetiology is limited. Conflicting results on the association of HLA and herpes simplex virus infection have been published. Russell and Schlaut have reported an increased frequency of HLA-A1 in patients with recurrent herpes simplex virus labialis [1]. Zimmerman et al. found a significant association of HLA-B5 with recurrent epithelial herpes keratitis [2]. Recently, Meyers-Elliott et al. noted increased frequencies of the HLA antigens AW30 and DR3 in patients with recurrent stromal herpes simplex virus keratitis [3]. The purpose of the present study was to reanalyse the possible relationship between HLA and herpes simplex virus keratitis.

## Patients and Methods

Eighty-one patients with herpes virus keratitis diagnosed at the Department of Ophthalmology, Freiburg, were studied. The diagnosis was based on clinical findings as well as on virus detection. Typing for all HLA-A, B, and C specificities as defined at the Seventh International Histocompatibility Workshop was performed. The antigen frequencies of patients were compared to those in 800 healthy controls. Additionally, 23 patients were typed for HLA-DR antigens by using a modified B cell cytotoxicity technique [4]; 248 healthy individuals served as controls. The statistical comparisons of the HLA antigen frequencies among diseased and healthy individuals were done by the chi$^2$-test with Yates' correction introduced for discontinuity in small samples. The relative risk (RR) values for the deviating antigens were computed according to the method of Woolf [5].

## Results

The HLA-A antigen frequencies for the patients with herpetic keratitis and the controls are shown in Table 1. HLA-A1 was found in 37% of the patients as compared to only 27% of the controls. The P value was 0.1, the relative risk was calculated as 1.6. The increase of HLA-A1 therefore is not statistically significant and may only indicate a trend. HLA-A3 was slightly increased (28% in patients vs. 23% in controls, $P = 0.4$, $RR = 1.3$). In the B locus series HLA-B7 (35% vs. 25%, $P = 0.1$ $RR = 1.5$) and HLA-B8 (24% vs. 18%, $P = 0.3$, $RR = 1.4$) showed an increase, but not to a significant degree (Table 2). No remarkable deviation of HLA-C antigen frequencies was observed. The DR antigen frequencies are depicted in Table 3. DR2 was defined in 39% of herpetic keratitis patients (controls: 22%, $P = 0.1$, $RR = 2.2$), and DR3 was detected in 34% (controls: 19%, $P = 0.2$, $RR = 2.2$). Probably due to the small patient sample size typed for DR antigens these differences were not statistically significant. The highest RR values, however, were found for DR2 and DR3.

## Discussion

No significant HLA association could be found so far in patients with herpes simplex keratitis. However, it is noteworthy that a series of A, B, and DR antigens are increased in this disease, namely A1, A3; B7, B8; DR2, DR3. The relative risk values for DR2 and DR3 were higher than those for the A or B locus antigens, indicating a position of a possible disease susceptibility gene more closely to the DR locus. The increase of A and B locus antigens mentioned above might be explained as secondary to the increase of DR antigens, reflecting the marked degree of linkage disequilibrium between these antigens. On the other hand, it can be speculated that herpetic keratitis is associated with the typical Caucasian haplotypes A1-B8-DR3 and A3-B7-DR2.

Our data are partially consistent with those of Meyers-Elliott and coworkers [3], who described an increased frequency of HLA-DR3. An increase of HLA-AW30 or HLA-B5, as reported by other groups [3, 4], was not found by us. The different findings may be explained by the heterogeneity of the patient groups studied. Further studies are needed to answer definitely the question of genetic factors in predisposition to herpetic keratitis. Particular attention should be paid to the DR antigen frequencies. An association between the disease and HLA haplotypes has to be analysed by family studies.

**Table 1.** HLA-A antigen frequencies in patients with herpetic keratitis and in healthy controls

| HLA Antigens | Controls (n = 800) | | Patients (n = 81) | | Chi-square | P-Value* | Relative Risk |
|---|---|---|---|---|---|---|---|
| | n | % | n | % | | | |
| A1 | 217 | 27 | 30 | 37 | 3.12 | 0.1 | 1.6 |
| A2 | 395 | 49 | 39 | 48 | 0.11 | 0.7 | 1.0 |
| A3 | 186 | 23 | 23 | 28 | 0.81 | 0.4 | 1.3 |
| A9 | 171 | 21 | 20 | 25 | 0.30 | 0.6 | 1.2 |
| AW23[a] | 51 | 6 | 4 | 5 | 0.50 | 0.5 | 0.8 |
| AW24[a] | 120 | 15 | 16 | 20 | 1.06 | 0.3 | 1.4 |
| A10 | 103 | 13 | 11 | 14 | 0.00 | 1.0 | 1.1 |
| A25[b] | 34 | 4 | 4 | 5 | 0.00 | 1.0 | 1.1 |
| A26[b] | 69 | 9 | 7 | 9 | 0.08 | 0.8 | 1.0 |
| A11 | 73 | 9 | 6 | 7 | 0.52 | 0.5 | 0.8 |
| A28 | 59 | 7 | 5 | 6 | 0.39 | 0.6 | 0.8 |
| A29 | 42 | 5 | 6 | 7 | 0.31 | 0.6 | 1.4 |
| AW30 | 32 | 4 | 5 | 6 | 0.41 | 0.5 | 1.5 |
| AW31 | 49 | 6 | 3 | 4 | 1.27 | 0.3 | 0.6 |
| AW32 | 58 | 7 | 3 | 4 | 2.04 | 0.2 | 0.5 |
| AW33 | 10 | 1 | 1 | 1 | 0.29 | 0.6 | 1.0 |

* Uncorrected for the number of antigens tested   [a] included in A9   [b] included in A10

**Table 2.** HLA-B antigen frequencies in patients with herpetic keratitis and in healthy controls

| HLA Antigens | Controls (n = 800) | | Patients (n = 81) | | Chi-Square | P-Value* | Relative Risk |
|---|---|---|---|---|---|---|---|
| | n | % | n | % | | | |
| B5 | 94 | 12 | 9 | 11 | 0.12 | 0.7 | 0.9 |
| B7 | 204 | 25 | 28 | 35 | 2.67 | 0.1 | 1.5 |
| B8 | 143 | 18 | 19 | 24 | 1.05 | 0.3 | 1.4 |
| B12 | 182 | 23 | 18 | 22 | 0.06 | 0.8 | 1.0 |
| B13 | 56 | 7 | 3 | 4 | 1.86 | 0.2 | 0.5 |
| B14 | 42 | 5 | 7 | 9 | 1.03 | 0.3 | 1.7 |
| B15 | 115 | 14 | 10 | 12 | 0.44 | 0.5 | 0.8 |
| BW16 | 63 | 8 | 6 | 7 | 0.13 | 0.7 | 0.9 |
| BW38[a] | 34 | 4 | 5 | 6 | 0.26 | 0.6 | 1.5 |
| BW39[a] | 29 | 4 | 2 | 2 | 0.73 | 0.4 | 0.7 |
| B17 | 61 | 8 | 8 | 10 | 0.25 | 0.6 | 1.3 |
| B18 | 82 | 10 | 4 | 5 | 2.99 | 0.1 | 0.5 |
| BW21 | 49 | 6 | 4 | 5 | 0.45 | 0.5 | 0.8 |
| BW22 | 30 | 4 | 2 | 2 | 0.80 | 0.4 | 0.6 |
| B27 | 67 | 8 | 7 | 9 | 0.01 | 0.9 | 1.0 |
| BW35 | 115 | 14 | 11 | 14 | 0.13 | 0.7 | 0.9 |
| B37 | 25 | 3 | 1 | 1 | 1.69 | 0.2 | 0.4 |
| B40 | 86 | 11 | 6 | 7 | 1.27 | 0.3 | 0.7 |
| BW41 | 11 | 1 | 2 | 2 | 0.08 | 0.8 | 1.8 |
| BW53 | 14 | 2 | – | – | – | – | – |

* Uncorrected for the number of antigens tested  [a] BW38 and BW39 are included in BW16

**Table 3.** HLA-DR antigen frequencies in patients with herpetic keratitis and in healthy controls

| HLA Antigens | Controls (n = 248) | | Patients (n = 23) | | Chi-square | P-Value* | Relative Risk |
|---|---|---|---|---|---|---|---|
| | n | % | n | % | | | |
| DR1 | 41 | 16 | 4 | 19 | 0.03 | 0.9 | 1.1 |
| DR2 | 56 | 22 | 9 | 39 | 2.31 | 0.1 | 2.2 |
| DR3 | 49 | 19 | 8 | 34 | 2.02 | 0.2 | 2.2 |
| DR4 | 62 | 26 | 5 | 21 | 0.35 | 0.6 | 0.8 |
| DR5 | 43 | 18 | 5 | 21 | 0.05 | 0.8 | 1.3 |
| DRW6 | 18 | 7 | 2 | 9 | 0.02 | 0.9 | 1.2 |
| DR7 | 54 | 21 | 5 | 21 | 0.07 | 0.8 | 1.0 |

* Uncorrected for the number of antigens tested

## References

1. Russell AS, Schlaut J (1975) HL-A transplantation antigens in subjects susceptible to recrudescent herpes labialis. Tissue Antigens 6:257
2. Zimmerman TJ, McNeill JI, Richman A, Kaufman HE, Waltman S (1977) HLA type and recurrent corneal herpes simplex infection. Invest Ophthalmol Visual Sci 15:756
3. Meyers-Elliott RH, Elliott JH, Maxwell WA, Pettit TH, O'Day DM, Terasaki PI, Bernoco D (1980) HLA antigens in recurrent stromal herpes simplex virus keratitis. Am J Ophthalmol 89:54
4. Terasaki PI, Bernoco D, Park MS, Ozturk G, Iwaki Y (1978) Microdroplet testing for HLA-A, -B, -C, and D antigens. Am J Clin Pathol 69:103
5. Svejgaard A, Ryder LP (1977) Associations between HLA and disease. In: Dausset J, Svejgaard A (eds) HLA and Disease. Williams and Wilkins, Baltimore, pp 46–316

## Discussion on the Contributions pp. 75 – pp. 97

**W. Böke (Kiel)**
I would like to open the general discussion on these posters and papers, Dr. Kaufman:

**H.E. Kaufman (New Orleans)**
We did find an association between HLA-B5 and ocular disease. However, I think that a great many studies on HLA typing are not good because the controls are not correctly chosen. This was summarized beautifully in Costa-Hoffman's paper. We know that blacks have a normal frequency of HLA tissue types different from that of the white population, Swedes are different from Finns, and one ethnic group within the United States is different from other ethnic groups in the same country. Unless the controls closely mirror the patient population and are matched in terms of race, site of origin and general socio-economic group, we really do not know what we have when we measure HLA types. Separating races alone is not sufficient.

In the typical HLA study, 10, 20, or 30 patients are compared with 200 controls that are not really representative of the patients, and the differences found don't mean anything. In our study, we did choose the controls very carefully, and found a small, but significant difference in the frequency of HLA types. This work has been confirmed by Dr. Colin. Also, in our study, statistical correction was made for all variables. Dr. Völker-Dieben is not correct about the Zimmerman statistics. When the Gainesville and St. Louis data were considered together, the difference was clearly significant using the statistical corrections. Similarly, apparent differences with the published work of Meyers-Elliot are not real, because we measured epithelial recurrences and she measured stromal recurrences. This was pointed out to the authors before publication, but unfortunately was not mentioned in their paper.

At any rate, the important question is, what does such a difference in the frequency of HLA tissue types mean? If you find 30% in the normal population and maybe 40 or 45% in the study population, it is very interesting, but it's hard to believe that the HLA association is causing the disease, as it does in rheumatoid arthritis, where you find 8% in the normal population and 90% in the affected population. Our conclusion in our original study, which showed much the same results as Dr. Colin's work, was that the difference is probably real, but very likely does not mean much. I would suspect that the predominance of a given HLA type is so small that, even if it is real and not a sampling artifact, it is hard to believe that this association determines whether or not you have the disease.

**H.D.M. Völker-Dieben (Leyden)**
Thank you for the explanations of the HLA type and disease response, but I would like to remind you that the number of patients was not limited to 50, compared to 73 controls. We studied the HLA phenotypes of 115 patients and 123 controls. Secondly, I think it is necessary, especially for American investigators, to discriminate between normal whites and caucasoids. This should solve a lot of problems.

**E. Bloch-Michel (Paris)**
I would like to add to the general remarks made by Dr. Kaufman, of which I approve totally. In our experience, HLA typing is useful in uveitis for two alleles only: B 27 and B 5. Yet, as this method is being more and more widely developed for the diagnosis of the disease, some discrepancies are observed. In the results given, concerning the same patient, by two different laboratories. Is this finding due to the difficulty of the technique? Or to the use of non-purified antisera? By the way, it is puzzling to notice that it is particularly for B 5 that the majority of conflicting results appear in the literature regarding HLA typing, as well as for Behcet's disease and for HSV. These difficulties may be possibly due to the fact that HLA B 5 is still not well defined.

**H.D.M. Völker-Dieben (Leyden)**
I think it is not very worthwhile to speak so much about the significance of the HLA-B5 because this was not a significant finding after correction for the *total* number of antigens studied.

**J. Colin (Brest)**
Our study was performed in Brittany, which is particularly interesting for epidemiological investigations because of its largely homogenous population. All the typings were performed in the same laboratory. At the same time, I agree with Dr. Bloch-Michel's comment. There may be some cross reactions with analogous reactive genes of HLA B5: B15; B21; and Bw35.

**G. Smolin (San Francisco)**
I will address this question to Dr. Colin. The histocompatibility antigen B5 has been demonstrated to be associated with a variety of immunologic diseases. Is it possible that there is a common denominator or defect in the immune system that leads not only to herpetic disease but to the other diseases as well?

**J. Colin (Brest)**
Subjects with HLA B5 might have some predisposition to several immunological diseases. Up to now, we can only speculate on the possible relationship.

**W.A. Blyth (Bristol)**

I am a coward. I do not know anything about HLA but I would like to ask Dr. Colin a question about the patients who were given a corneal transplant because of their severe herpes and then 50% of them did not recur for 15 years. Can you give us an estimate of their incidence of recurrence had they not had a corneal transplant and secondly, do you know the HLA type of the transplanted cornea?

**J. Colin (Brest)**

Some investigations have shown that more than 40% of herpes simplex keratitis recurred after recurrent ulcers over a 2 year follow-up.

We did not know the HLA types of the transplanted corneas.

**W. Böke (Kiel)**

Thank you. We have to conclude this very interesting discussion, but I would not like to do so without saying what I felt when I listened to these papers. My first impression was: Has HLA any meaning in the pathogenesis of ocular herpetic disease? I think we may say it does. Secondly, which HLA type? One says it is B, the other says A, the next says D. I think the whole topic is still very much open for discussion and further research, and I feel that is the only conclusion we can draw at the present time.

**H.D.M. Völker-Dieben (Leyden)**

That may well be true. There is still one point we did not discuss. That is the highly significant difference in the numbers of female and male patients with recurrent HSV and the possibility that females between 15 and 45 demonstrate a beneficial effect of hormones during their reproductive period. Do you have the same findings?

**B.R. Jones (London)**

We have the same sort of distribution in London.

Sundmacher, R. (Hrsg.):
Herpetische Augenerkrankungen
© J.F. Bergmann Verlag, München 1981

# Atopy and Herpetic Keratitis

E. Bloch-Michel, D. Vamvoukos, R. Campinchi, F. Niessen, Paris

**Key words.** Atopy and HSV disease, hyposensitization

**Schlüsselwörter.** Atopie und Herpeserkrankungen, Hyposensibilisierung

**Summary.** 15 patients with multi-recurrent acute and/or corticodependant forms of herpes of the cornea were found to be atopic. The hyposensitization treatment with house-dust and mites extract to which these patients were allergic seemed to be effective on both frequency of the recurrences and the level of corticodependance.

The explanation for such favourable findings remains unclear. But these results seem to indicate that the association to an atopic state should be cautiously evaluated in all cases of chronic herpetic keratitis since the allergologic treatment may be a useful and inoffensive means for improving those patients.

**Zusammenfassung.** Wir fanden 15 Patienten mit chronisch rezidivierendem oder steroidabhängigem Herpes corneae and gleichzeitiger Atopie. Die Desensibilisierungsbehandlung mit Hausstaub- und Milben-Antigenen, auf die diese Patienten allergisch reagiert hatten, scheint sich sowohl auf die Häufigkeit der Rezidive als auch auf den Grad der Cortisonabhängigkeit günstig ausgewirkt zu haben.

Eine Erklärung für dieses günstige Resultat ist nicht einfach zu geben. Wir schließen aber aus unseren Ergebnissen, daß man bei allen Patienten mit chronischer Herpeskeratitis einen allergologischen Status erheben sollte, weil man mit einer Desensibilisierungsbehandlung u.U. ein nützliches und gefahrloses Therapiemittel in der Hand hat.

## Introduction

There has been so far little information regarding the possible relationship between herpes and atopy. In our experience one out of four cases of chronic herpes in the cornea may be assumed to be an atopic patient.

Desensitization treatment to house-dust and mites, to which fifteen patients were allergic, seemed to improve the course of the disease markedly in most cases.

## Material and Methods

Fifteen patients were selected for suffering from both chronic herpetic keratitis and atopic diseases.

### Herpetic Keratitis

The 15 cases included:
4 kerato-uveitis,
6 interstitial (or stromal) keratitis,
5 disciform keratitis.

In all cases the diagnosis of herpes could be confirmed either from a previous dendritic ulcer or from the presence of antibodies to HSV in the aqueous (Witmer' quotient $\geq 4$) or from both.

The mean duration of the disease was 2.2 years (Fig. 1) ranging from 6 months to 6 years.

In ten cases there were recurrent attacks (Fig. 2.), with an average of 4.8 recurrences per year. In 11 cases the disease was corticodependant, with a daily dose of oral Prednisone up to 10 mg/day in seven cases and a topical therapy up to six instillations/day of Prednisolone in four other cases (Fig. 3).

The visual acuity was known before treatment in 14 out of 15 cases: it did not exceed 0.2 in any of them.

### Allergic Data

Seven patients had a past history of at least one major allergic manifestation (asthma, hay

101

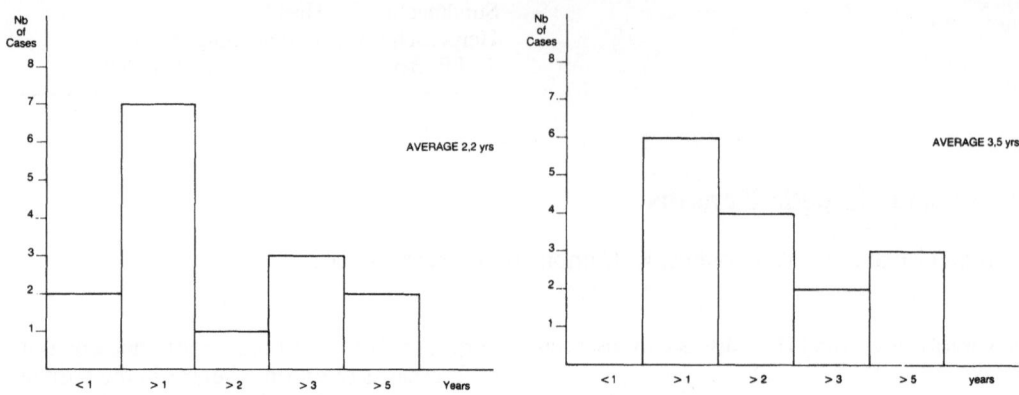

**Fig. 1. a** Duration of the disease prior to hyposensitization treatment and **b** duration of the follow-up after hyposensitization treatment

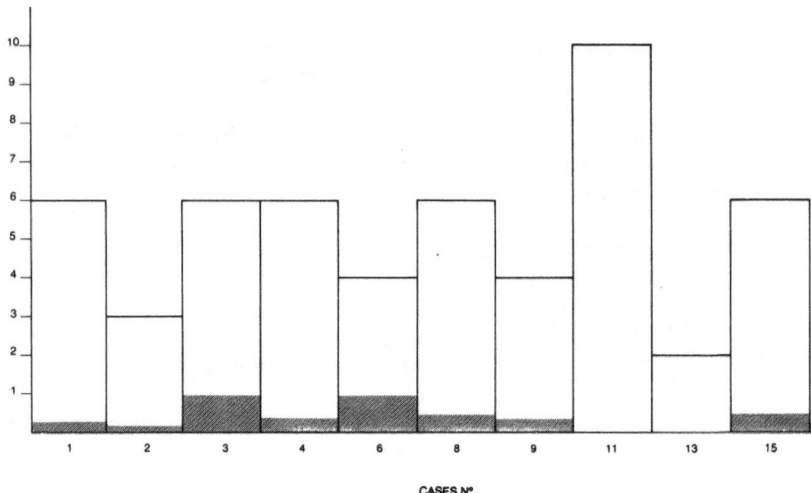

**Fig. 2.** Recurrences per year (10 cases). □ prior to hyposensitization treatment ■ after hyposensitization treatment. average □ 4.8 ■ 0.5

fever, eczema, spasmodic tracheitis or spasmodic coryza). In three other cases there was a family history of atopy (including one of the above symptoms in at least two relatives).

On skin testing with house-dust and mites' extracts, 12 of 12 patients displayed a strong intradermal response. Moreover a local (ocular or extraocular) response was observed within 48 h following allergenic challenge in 7 cases of 12. In the remaining three cases the atopic state was demonstrated by Rast and/or Rist test, and by the past history of the patient. In one case IGE plasma cells were markedly present in the adjacent papillary conjunctiva [1].

On slit lamp examination there was a papillary conjunctivitis in 7 of 15 cases. In the other cases the conjunctiva was apparently normal.

### Desensitization Treatment

This treatment was carried out with soluble allergenic extracts injected subcutaneously according to a technique currently used for allergic conjunctivitis [2, 3].

This treatment was carried out for over 1 year in all the cases, and for more than 2 years in eight cases with an average follow-up of 3.5 years. (Fig. 1)

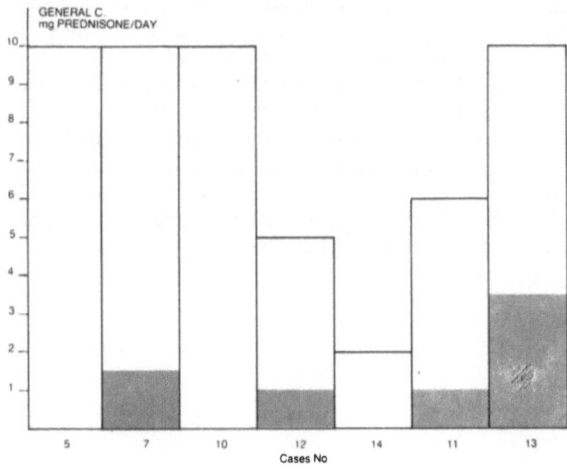

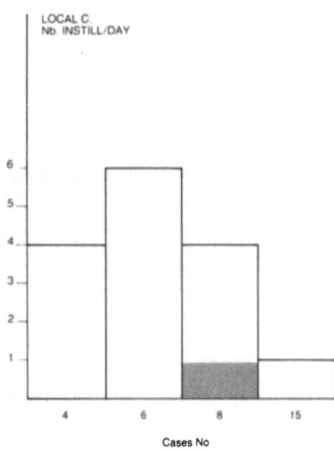

**Fig. 3.** Decrease of corticodependance (11 cases) □ prior to hyposensitization treatment ■ after hyposensitization treatment

## Results

In the ten recurrent forms (Fig. 2) there was a marked decrease in the incidence of the attacks, ranging from 4.8 attacks/year before treatment to 0.5 attacks/year after it was initiated.

In the 11 corticodependant cases, the improvement was easier to quantify (Fig. 3.) since there was a strong decrease in the daily dose of steroids.

In three of seven corticodependant cases with systemic cortisone and in three of four topically corticodependant cases, corti-

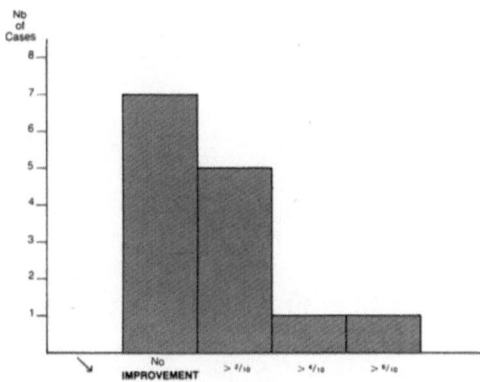

**Fig. 4.** Visual improvement (14 cases)

cotherapy could be completely discontinued after a certain time.

Visual acuity decreased in none of the cases. There was no visible improvement in half the cases and some improvement (from 0.2 to 0.6) was observed in seven other cases (Fig. 4).

## Discussion

The reason why an atopic state of hypersensitivity might enhance the chronic course of a herpetic disease in the cornea remains unknown. From our findings it is obvious that the treatment of the atopic background had a favourable effect on our herpetic cases. Since most of these forms seemed to be related to an immunologic local disturbance, it may be assumed that the desensitization treatment somehow modified the local immunologic status by acting either on the production or the type of immunocompetent cells, in particular on those present in the adjacent allergic conjunctiva. In addition, the accumulation of mast cells, eosinophils, and plasma cells in this allergic mucosa may have enhanced the release of mediators, by facilitating vasodilatation and finally have increased the inflammatory course of the herpetic disease. This explanation could account for a better effect of the hyposensitizing treatment on the inflammatory symptoms of the herpetic disease than on its consequences.

## References

1. Bloch-Michel E, Audouin-Berault J, Diebold S, Herman D, Dry J, Campinchi R (1977) Etude en Immunofluorescence des plasmocytes de la conjonctive allergique en particulier des cellules formatrices des immunoglobulines E (IGE). Arch Ophthalmol (Paris) 37:89
2. Wolfromm R, Miller HA, Campinchi R, Valery-Radot C, Laroché MA, Bloch-Michel E (1976) Diagnostic et traitement des conjonctivites allergiques. XXII$^e$ Concilium Ophthalmologicum Acta, Paris 1974. Masson, Paris, p 807
3. Bloch-Michel E (1975) L'allergie oculaire. Ouest Medical 28:869

Sundmacher, R. (Hrsg.):
Herpetische Augenerkrankungen
© J.F. Bergmann Verlag, München 1981

# Interference Between Ocular Herpes and Allergic Diseases.
# An Epidemiologic Approach

J. Roussos, J. Denis, Paris

**Key words.** Ocular herpes, allergy, epidemiology

**Schlüsselwörter.** Herpeskeratitis - Allergie, Epidemiologie

**Summary.** An epidemiological survey, limited to questions concerning personal clinical history of allergy, was carried out on 100 patients suffering from ocular herpes and on 100 control subjects. Ocular herpes was twice as frequent in atopic individuals. Similarly, the tendency towards Mucocutaneous herpes and ocular herpes was more frequent in allergic subjects than in non-allergic. However, there was no correlation between the type of ocular herpes and allergy. The atopic area would seem to favour the herpetic infection, without doubt due to a defect of cell mediated immunity which is perhaps influenced by prostaglandins.

**Zusammenfassung.** Bei 100 Herpespatienten und 100 Kontrollpersonen führten wir eine epidemiologische Befragung in Hinblick auf die allergische Situation durch. Ein okulärer Herpes fand sich bei Atopikern zweimal häufiger. Auch die Neigung zu muko-kutanen Herpeserkrankungen war bei den Allergikern häufiger als bei den Kontrollpersonen. Zwischen der Art der okulären Herpeserkrankung und der Allergie fand sich hingegen keine Korrelation. Bei Atopikern wird eine Herpesinfektion offenbar durch einen Defekt in der zellulären Immunreaktion gefördert, der wiederum möglicherweise unter dem Einfluß einer Prostaglandinwirkung steht.

The interrogation of patients consulting at the Hôtel-Dieu hospital in Paris for an ocular herpes, revealed that a surprising number of these patients had a previous clinical history of allergy. To confirm this observation we undertook a survey of 100 cases of confirmed herpes and 100 control patients.

## Inquiry Method

Ocular herpes was diagnosed for the 100 patients on the basis of one or several of the following three criteria:
- corneal dendritic ulcer
- isolation of the viral strain
- coefficient of antiherpetic antibody activity in the aqueous humor to that in the serum superior or equal to two (see chapter 24). The different clinical aspects of ocular herpes in these patients were divided as follows:

17 Superficial keratitis
8 Both interstitial and superficial keratitis
23 Disciform Keratitis
52 Anterior segmentitis

The members of the second group of 100 control subjects had the following disorders:

24 Ocular traumatism
20 Corneal disorders not due to herpes
17 Cataracts
15 Retineal involvement
8 Disorders of the conjunctiva and adjoining tissues
5 Glaucoma
5 Neuro-ophthalmologic diseases
2 Uveitis
4 Diverse

The control group was chosen in such a fashion that the distributions of age and sex were rigorously parallel to that of the herpes patients.

The allergological survey only concerned, as do most of the epidemiological studies of the same type, personal clinical history of allergy and familial clinical history. This survey allows a direct comparison with french epidemiological studies [1, 3, 11]. It consisted of the following questions:

a) Personal allergic diseases
- Rhinitis: seasonal or perennial
- Asthma

- Eczema
- Drug allergy
- Other allergy
  b) Familial allergic diseases
Nature of disease and relationship to patient
in question

## Results

The global result (Table 1) shows that there
are twice the number of atopic subjects in the
group of patients with ocular herpes than in
the control group. This figure only concerned
personal clinical history of allergy, the familial
clincal history being more disputable.

Similarly, the association with cutaneo-
mucous herpes and ocular herpes (Table 2)
is more frequent in allergic subjects than in
non-allergic patients.

The comparison of these results with
epidemiological studies carried out in France
(Table 3) with several different groups of
individuals, confirms that the control group in
this present study is an average sample of the
population. Three such studies have been
performed on a large number of cases:
- 8140 students [3]
- 3015 manual workers [11]
- 12 018 subjects undergoing a routine
  medical check-up [1]
in all, a total of 23 173 individuals. The percentage of allergic subjects was 15.06%. This fig-

**Table 1.** Frequency of allergic diseases in patients
with ocular herpes

|  | Ocular herpes 100 | Controls 100 |
|---|---|---|
| With allergy | 37 | 17 |
| Without allergy | 63 | 83 |

Dependence: $X^2 = 0.05$ and $X^2 0.05 [99] = 3.84$

**Table 2.** Association of muco-cutaneous and ocular
herpes interaction with allergic disease

| Ocular herpes N = 100 |
|---|
| With allergy 21/37 |
| Without allergy 21/63 |

Dependence: $X^2 = 2.07$ and $X^2 0.05 [99] = 3.84$

**Table 3.** Other investigations of allergies in France

|  | Allergic individuals | Non-allergic individuals | % |
|---|---|---|---|
| Students [3] | 1 141 | 6 999 | 14.01 |
| Workers [11] | 230 | 2 785 | 7.5 |
| "Sécurité Sociale" Indi- viduals [1] | 2 021 | 9 997 | 16.81 |

In the general population, a mean of 15.06% of individuals suffer from allergic diseases

**Table 4.** No correlation between herpetic ocular lesions and allergies. 100 ocular herpes

| Clinical form | With allergy |
|---|---|
| Superficial K. | 5/17 |
| Interst. + Superf. K. | 2/8 |
| Disciform K. | 11/23 |
| Ant. Segmentitis | 19/52 |

ure is comparable to the percentage of allergic
persons in the control group of this present
study, i.e. 17%. The different forms of allergy
are also comparable – respiratory allergy represents 38.24% of all these cases and 40.54%
of the controls of this study.

It is interesting to note that the clinical
form of ocular herpes is not related to allergy
(Table 4) and that the atopic area does not
seem to affect either the frequency of relapses
or their severity. The eventual role of the antigenic type of the infecting viral strain remains
unknown, since all the strains isolated from
the patients in this study were found to be of
type 1 by seroneutralization; only the study of
thermosensitivity revealed two varieties,
types 1 and intermediate, which were distributed similarly in allergic and non-allergic
patients.

## Discussion

The increase in the frequency of ocular
herpes in allergic subjects raises the question
of the role of the herpetic virus in the etiology
of an allergic infection, but above all the question of the role of the atopic area on the
development of the herpetic infection.

At the present state of knowledge, it is not possible to affirm the existence of a common HLA type. During an herpetic infection, the haplotype B5 was found to be predominant [2, 8], although only a certain relationship between pollen allergies and the haplotype A1.B8 [5] is known with regard to allergic diseases. Furthermore, the antigenicity of the herpes virus does not seem to be involved in the majority of the allergic phenomena described, especially during respiratory allergies.

The role of the allergic area as a favorable element for the development of the herpetic infection seems much more plausible. The atopic subject has an abnormal predisposition for bacterial and especially viral infections [9, 4]. A herpes infection can become generalised in patients with eczema. The stimulation of lymphocytes from atopic patients by phytohemagglutinin is usually diminished. This deficiency essentially involves the thymus-dependent lymphocytes and more particularly T-suppressor lymphocytes, thus explaining the increase in IgE.

The allergic area also seems capable of favoring the development of the herpes infection if one accepts the pathogenic mechanism proposed by Hill and Blyth [6]; changes at the skin level, perhaps induced by prostaglandins, would allow the multiplication of the herpetic virus. The more recent experimental studies of Trofatter and Daniels [10] tend to show that the prostaglandins can favor the herpetic infection by suppression of antibody dependent cell-mediated cytolysis (ADCC).

Finally, attempts at specific desensitization have been proposed and have given interesting clinical results for the prevention of herpetic recurrences (Chapter 17).

In this same line of thought, one of our patients desensitized to *candida albicans* showed an increase in ocular herpes every time the threshold of 60 units was reached during an injection of desensitization.

## Conclusions

If the increase in frequency of ocular herpes in atopic subjects seems to be an established fact, the pathogenesis of the herpetic infection has not been totally clarified. The accentuated susceptibility of an allergic subject with regard to a viral infection is very probable, the development of the herpes virus being favored by an immune deficiency or by the intervention of intermediary substances. This pathogenic schema allows complementary treatment to be envisaged. The lymphocytic deficiency could be corrected by immunostimulants such as levamisole or by the injection of a transfer factor. Furthermore a desensitization has been shown to be capable of stimulating the generation of T-suppressor lymphocytes [7].

## References

1. Brégevin B, Denis J, Herman D, Wolfin R (1975) Etude de la morbidité asthmatique dans trois populations différentes. Congrès Intern. asthme, allergies respiratoires et environnement socio-écologique, Le Mont-Dore, 29 mai 1975.
2. Colin J, Chastel C, Saleun JP, Morin JF, Renard G (1979) Herpès oculaire récidivant et antigènes HLA: étude préliminaire. J Ophtalmol 2:263–266
3. Denis J, Bussutil R, Vie A, Lacourbe R, Wolfromm R (1970) Fréquence des maladies allergiques dans la population étudiante. Enquête auprès de 8 000 sujets. Rev Franc Allergol 10:177–189
4. Guilhou JJ, Meynadier J, Clot J (1979) Les troubles immunitaires au cours de l'eczema atopique. Nouv Presse Méd 8:2967–2970
5. Gwynn CM, Mackintosh P (1979) HLA haplotypes and hayfever: a possible prospective role. Clin Allergy 9:425–427
6. Hill TJ, Blyth WA (1976) An alternative theory of herpes simplex recurrence and a possible role for prostaglandins. Lancet 1:397–399
7. Ishizaka K (1977) Cellular mecanisms of the IgE antibody response. In: Mathov E, Sindo T, Naranjo P (ed) Allergy and clinical immunology. Excerp. Med., Amsterdam, p 75–84
8. Rahi AHS (1979) HLA and eye disease. Br J Ophthalmol 63:283–292
9. Rogge JL, Hanifin JM (1976) Immuno deficiencies in severe atopic dermatitis. Arch Dermatol 112:1391–1396
10. Trofatter KF, Daniels CA (1979) Interaction of human cells with prostaglandins and cyclic AMP modulators. I. Effects on complement – mediated lysis and antibody – dependent cell – mediated cytolysis of herpes simplex virus – infected human fibroblasts. J Immunol 122: 1363–1370
11. Wolfin R, Denis J (1974) Morbidité allergique dans une population de travailleurs. Rev Franç Allergol 14:131–134

## Discussion on the Contributions pp. 101–107

**C. Kok van Alphen (Leyden)**

I saw your poster and you mentioned drug allergies, too. I would say that those herpes patients have already had so many drugs that they nearly all have a drug allergy. I do not understand why you count those patients.

**J. Denis (Paris)**

The problem of eye-drops allergy certainly exists, but in our work, we counted patients having a general reaction with drugs and mostly antibiotics.

**B.R. Jones (London)**

I want to ask either Dr. Denis or Dr. Bloch-Michel whether in their series of atopic patients with herpes there has been a higher incidence of secondary infection with bacterii or fungi than in similar herpes not associated with atopy. As you will hear in our presentation later in this meeting, on people who have had corneal grafting for herpetic keratitis, there was a substantially high prevalence of infection in grafts in the atopic patients.

**E. Bloch-Michel (Paris)**

I'd like to answer this question. In our study, there was no prevalence of infection due to candidins in our patients. Besides I must point out the fact that these (Dr. Denis's and mine) two studies were completely independent and did not include the same patients.

**D. Easty (Bristol)**

I'd just like to re-enforce Dr. Bloch-Michel's comments about this association which we found particularly in patients with extreme elevation in IgE when real problems occur especially in adults. I think there is a number of factors contributing. I don't think these people appear to be immuno-deficient in our experience. They have a tremendous number of mast cells in their tarsal plates, and one wonders whether a degranulation and production of pharmacologically active substances has more to do with it than anything else. They're also occasionally on systemic steroids, and have had topical steroids so this is another factor. I suspect these topical treatments are important.

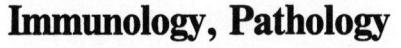

**Immunology, Pathology**

Sundmacher, R. (Hrsg.):
Herpetische Augenerkrankungen
© J.F. Bergmann Verlag, München 1981

# The Influence of Antiviral Immunity in Epithelial Herpetic Keratitis

C.A. Carter, D.L. Easty, Bristol

**Key words.** Herpetic keratitis – immunologic aspects, dendritic keratitis

**Schlüsselwörter.** Herpeskeratitis – immunologische Aspekte, Keratitis dendritica

**Summary.** The Jones and Al-Hussaini rabbit model for ulcerative herpetic keratitis was adapted to study both the initial susceptibility of the cornea to herpes simplex virus (HSV) infection, and also the subsequent progress of ulcerative disease. This method was used to investigate the influence of prior skin or eye infection with HSV on corneal resistance to ulcerative herpetic disease. Systemic cellular and humoral immune responses to HSV, assayed by the lymphocyte transformation (LT) and complement-fixing (CF) antibody tests were examined in relation to the development of corneal infection in normal rabbits (primary) and in rabbits with previous skin infection (secondary).

The results indicated that prior skin infection with HSV confers a high degree of protection on the cornea. This was exemplified by a considerable initial resistance to infection, greatly reduced spread of ulceration, and earlier commencement of healing. A similar degree of corneal protection resulted from previous infection of the opposite eye, while a cornea which had itself recovered from herpetic disease exhibited greater resistance. It is suggested that secondary corneal HSV infection in rabbits is a better model for human ulcerative herpetic keratitis than is primary corneal disease.

Systemic LT and CF antibody responses were observed following primary and secondary corneal infection. Both responses were accelerated in secondary disease, and CF antibody reached higher titres.

The timing of the systemic immune responses in relation to the progress of corneal ulcerative disease revealed that the commencement of healing of primary and secondary ulcerative herpetic keratitis in the rabbits was more closely correlated with the LT than with the CF antibody response.

**Zusammenfassung.** Jones und Al-Hussaini entwickelten eine Methode, mit der man die Empfänglichkeit der Hornhaut gegenüber Herpes simplex-Viren studieren und den weiteren Infektionsverlauf quantitativ bewerten kann. Mit dieser Methode untersuchten wir den Einfluß einer vorhergegangenen Haut- oder Hornhautinfektion mit Herpes simplex-Virus (HSV) auf eine nachfolgende HSV-Inokulation. Sowohl bei nicht-immunisierten Kaninchen als auch bei Tieren, die via die Haut vorimmunisiert worden waren, untersuchten wir die zelluläre und humorale Immunantwort nach kornealer Herpesinfektion mittels des Lymphozytentransformations-Testes (LT) und der Komplementbindungsreaktion (CF-Antikörper).

Wir fanden, daß eine vorhergegangene Hautinfektion der Hornhaut einen erheblichen Schutz gegenüber einer späteren Virusinfektion vermittelt. Dies zeigte sich sowohl in einer erheblich gesteigerten Resistenz gegen das Angehen der Infektion als auch in einem geringeren Schweregrad der manifesten Erkrankung, die zudem noch schneller abheilte. Eine vorhergegangene Infektion des Partnerauges vermittelte einen ähnlich guten Schutz. Hatte hingegen das gleiche Auge schon einmal eine Herpesinfektion durchgemacht, war der Schutz noch höher. Wir schließen hieraus, daß Kaninchenmodelle mit Infektionen vorimmunisierter Tiere den Verhältnissen beim Menschen wahrscheinlich besser entsprechen als die üblichen Modelle mit primären Infektionen.

Sowohl nach primärer als auch nach sekundärer kornealer Infektion beobachteten wir eine Immunantwort im LT- und CF-Test. Beide Reaktionen war bei sekundären Infektionen schneller, und die CF-Antikörper erreichten bei sekundären Reaktionen auch höhere Titer.

Wenn man hingegen den zeitlichen Verlauf dieser Immunreaktionen mit dem klinischen Bild korrelierte, kam heraus, daß bei beiden Infektionsarten das Einsetzen der Heilung stärker mit der zellulären als mit der humoralen Immunantwort korreliert war.

Most of the adult human population possesses serum antibody to herpes simplex virus (HSV) [10] and has presumably experienced a clinical or subclinical herpetic infection. The influence of such a previous contact with the virus on corneal susceptibility to infection is therefore of interest, especially since most animal models used to study ulcerative herpetic keratitis employ normal rabbits, which have not had previous infections with HSV, and so do not exhibit specific immune responses.

Previous work using rabbits as experimental animals has indicated that an eye which has itself recovered from a herpetic keratitis is relatively resistant to reinfection [5, 8]. The effect of previous HSV infection at a distant non-ocular or ocular site was less clear, being considered negligible by some authors [4, 9], while others found evidence of some corneal protection [3, 5].

In the present study, we wished to determine firstly, whether systemic cell-mediated and humoral immune responses could be detected following primary corneal disease, and also after corneal infection of previously skin-infected rabbits ('secondary corneal infection'); and secondly, whether the susceptibility of the cornea to ulcerative herpetic keratitis can be modified by previous skin infection, and by previous infection of the same, or the opposite eye.

**Methods**

HSV type 1, strain PH, was used, the stock titre being $4 \times 10^8$ pfu/ml. The rabbits were 2 to 4 kg. New Zealand Whites. The individual groups of rabbits used to study LT and CF antibody responses respectively contained six to seven and two to four animals. Virus dose-response curves were calculated from data obtained from 50 corneas in all, while the progress of corneal ulcerative disease was followed using four to five corneas in each group. *Skin infection* was induced by intradermal injection of $1.25 \times 10^6$ pfu. virus in 0.05 ml. saline, in the right ear pinna. The resulting erythema resolved within a few days, and the rabbits were rested for 6 weeks to 6 months before corneal virus inoculation.
*Immune responses:* The parameters studied were lymphocyte transformation in response to HSV antigen (LT), and complement-fixing (CF) antibody to HSV. LT was determined using triplicate cultures of whole blood incubated in medium with HSV antigen, control

antigen, phytohaemagglutinin (PHA), or no stimulant [2]. 1 uCi of $^3$H-thymidine was added for the last 6 h of the 3 days' incubation, and the DNA-containing material was extracted and assayed for B-radioactivity (expressed in disintegrations per minute: dpm).

The transformation index (TI) for each rabbit at each date was calculated as

$$\frac{\text{mean dpm. from cultures with HSV antigen}}{\text{mean dpm. from unstimulated cultures.}}$$

The micro-complement-fixation test [1] was used to assay serum from peripheral blood for antibody to HSV antigen.

*Corneal inoculation of virus* employed the same procedure for primary and secondary corneal infections, but various ranges of virus concentration were used to suit the experiment. The Jones and Al-Hussaini [6] microtitration method was used, in which four different virus concentrations are each inoculated into four sites on the cornea. Serial four-fold virus dilutions were used, the ranges of virus concentration being $6.25–0.10 \times 10^6$ and $25.00–0.39 \times 10^6$ pfu/ml. respectively for primary and secondary corneal infection in experiments to test initial susceptibility to HSV, and $1.56–0.39 \times 10^6$ and $10.00–0.16 \times 10^6$ pfu/ml. in experiments to study the progress of ulcerative disease.

*Assessment of corneal infection* employed two techniques. Firstly, on day 2 post-infection, the results of the virus microtitrations were read, and the numbers of positive infected sites for each virus concentration were used to draw a virus dose-response curve and calculate the concentration of virus required to produce infection in 50% of inoculated sites ($CID_{50}$).

These data were compared between the groups of rabbits or corneas, a high $CID_{50}$ denoting good resistance to initial infection. Secondly, to study the progress of ulcerative disease, accurate scale diagrams of the corneal ulcers were made at intervals, and the total area of ulceration on each cornea measured by densitometry [7].

**Results**

*Immune Responses*

LT, and CF antibody, responses were seen following primary skin, and primary and sec-

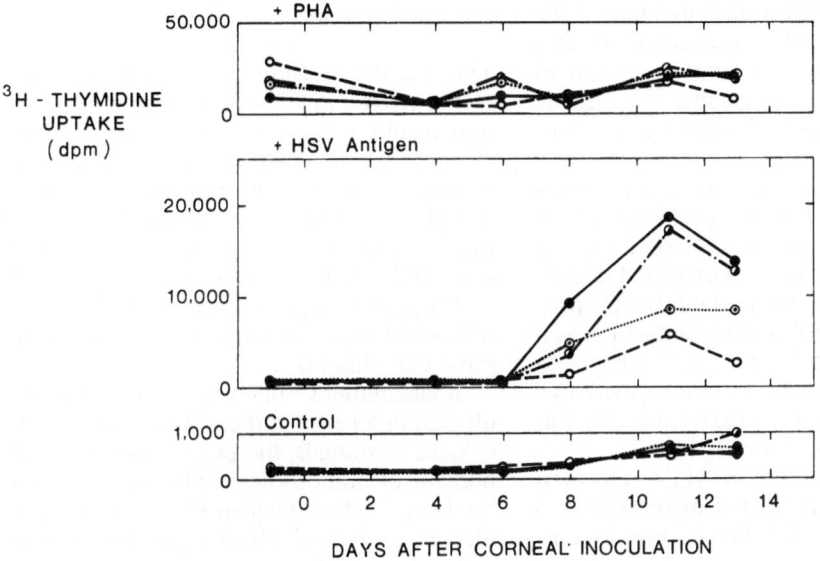

**Fig. 1.** Lymphocyte transformation in triplicate whole blood cultures following primary corneal infection

ondary corneal infections in all the rabbits studied.

The time of initiation of the *LT response* after injection of virus into the skin was variable, occurring between day 4 and day 9. The initiation of an LT response, as signified by a rise in transformation index (TI), occurred on day 8 in all rabbits with a primary corneal infection, and on day 6 in rabbits with

secondary corneal infection, with one exception (P < 0.01)*. The commencement of the LT response therefore occurred earlier after secondary than after primary corneal infection, although evaluation of data as dpm. showed a slightly less clearcut difference. The rise in TI following secondary corneal infec-

_____

* exact 2 × 2 test

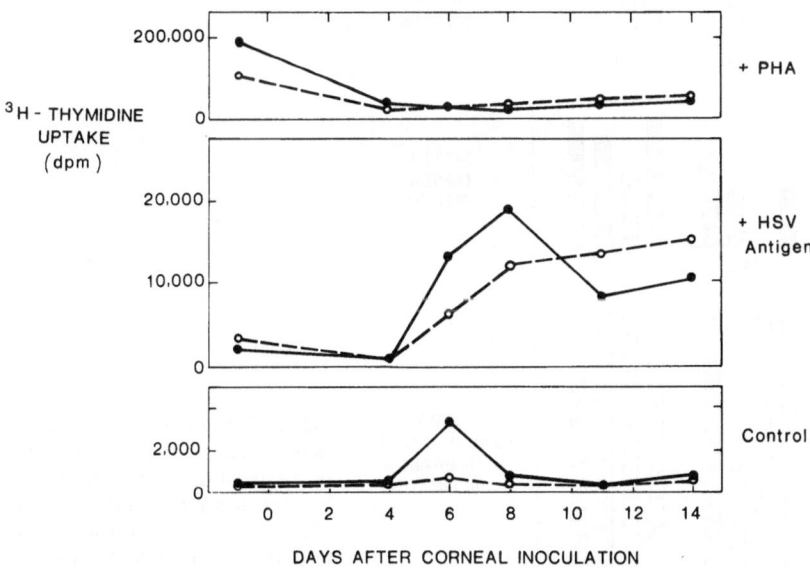

**Fig. 2.** Lymphocyte transformation in triplicate whole blood cultures following secondary corneal infection

113

tion was preceded by a drop in TI from the resting level 4 days after inoculation of virus in all animals. The subsequent pattern of development of the LT response was variable in all three groups of animals: some rabbits exhibited a peak at 8 to 11 days, while others showed a continuing increase until the experiment was ended at day 13 or 14 (Figs. 1, 2). The levels of TI demonstrated are indicated by the maximum responses observed in each animal: the mean levels reached after primary skin, primary corneal, and secondary corneal infections were $35.3 \pm 19.7$, $21.8 \pm 8.9$, and $60.3 \pm 39.4$ respectively. Therefore, there was a tendency for a high level to be observed following secondary infections.

*Serum CF antibody* to HSV appeared between days 8 and 13 following primary skin infection, and by day 13 following primary corneal infection. Secondary corneal inoculation of virus induced no change in antibody titre until day 8, which was significantly earlier than after primary corneal infection (P < 0.02)*. The primary skin and corneal infections induced comparable mean titres, of 1/24 and 1/36 respectively, while secondary corneal infection caused a dramatic rise in titre to more than 1/512 (Fig. 3).

———————————

* exact 2 × 2 test

*Corneal Infection*

The virus dose-response curves showed that a great increase in corneal resistance to infection results from a previous skin infection (Fig. 4). Previous infection of one eye induced a greater protection of that cornea, and the opposite cornea showed a similar resistance to those of previously skin-infected animals (Log. $CID_{50}$ values were –1.31 and –1.74 respectively, compared to –2.80 for normal and –1.68 for skin-infected controls in the same experiment).

Measurement of the total area of ulceration on each cornea demonstrated that in normal animals, the progressive phase of herpetic ulceration ('active phase') continued until day 8, when the phase of recovery from ulcerative disease ('healing phase') began with a sharp decline in the areas of ulceration. In secondary corneal infection, a much lower peak in area of ulceration was reached in spite of the 16-fold increase in concentration of virus inoculated, and the healing phase commenced on day 6. Corneas of previously-infected eyes showed very restricted ulceration, which nevertheless was not quickly eradicated. The opposite corneas of these rabbits developed similar degrees of ulceration to those seen in secondary corneal

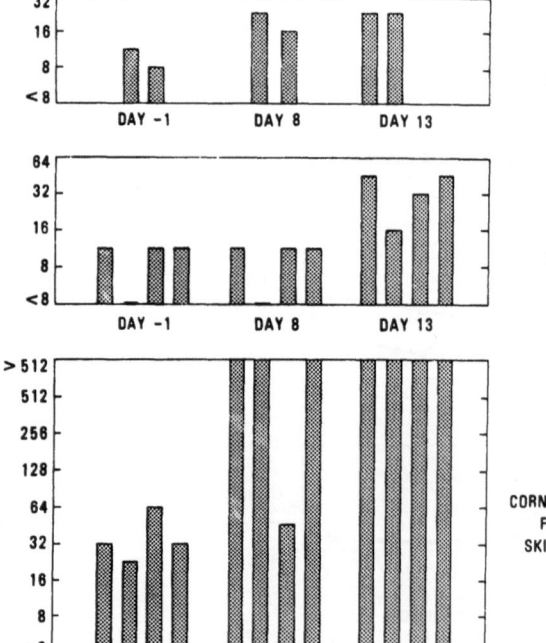

AFTER 1° SKIN INFECTION

AFTER 1° CORNEAL INFECTION

AFTER CORNEAL INFECTION FOLLOWING SKIN INFECTION

Fig. 3. Complement-fixing antibody titres, on days 1, 8 and 13 post-infection. Note the great increase in antibody titre at day 8 after secondary corneal infection: titres at day 6 had not risen above resting levels (data not shown)

114

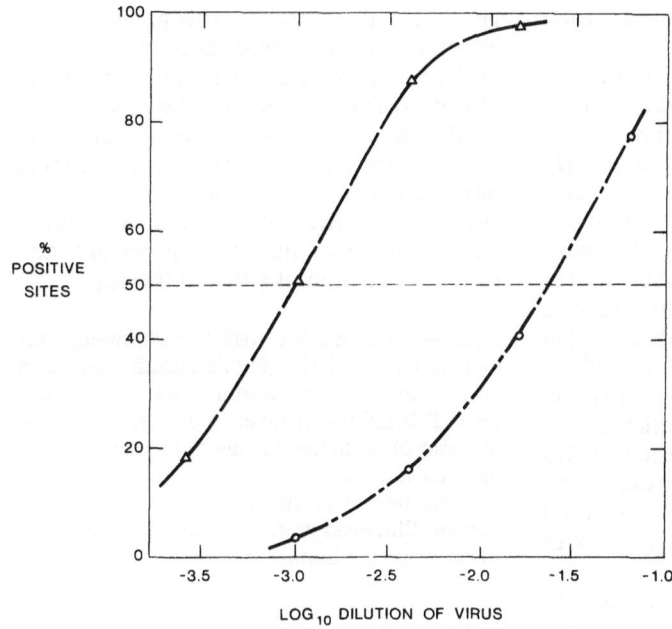

**Fig. 4.** Virus dose-response curves for primary and secondary corneal inoculation: data accumulated over several experiments. $-\triangle-$ primary infection; log. $CID_{50} =: -3.08$ $--O--$ secondary infection; log. $CID_{50} = -1.66$

infection, except that the active phase of disease continued until day 8. The times taken to complete healing were not markedly different between groups (Fig. 5).

### Discussion

It may be concluded from the above results that primary and secondary corneal HSV infection, as well as primary skin infection, induce cellular and humoral immune responses in the blood. Also, corneal susceptibility to herpetic ulceration is considerably reduced following prior infection of the animal at a distant site (skin or opposite eye).

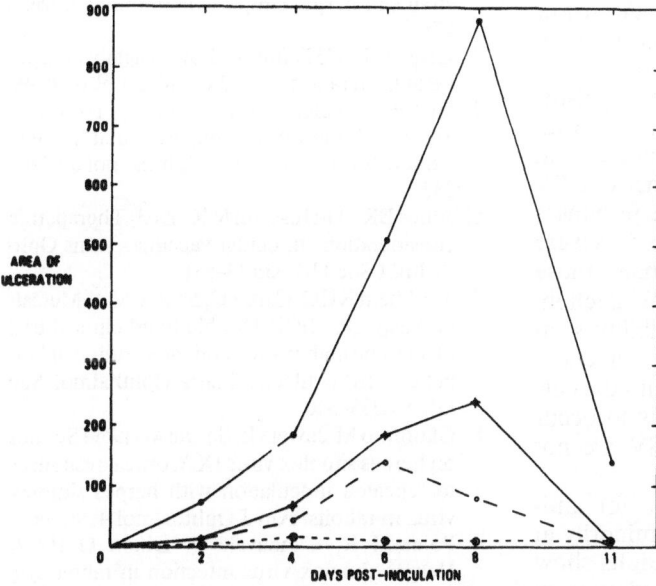

**Fig. 5.** Mean areas of corneal ulceration following infection of corneas of normal rabbits (low virus inoculum) $-●-$; corneas of rabbits with previous skin infection $--O--$; previously infected corneas $---\ ◑\ ---$; and the opposite corneas of rabbits with previous unilateral ocular infection $-+-$

A previously-infected cornea shows a greater resistance to infection.

The rise in LT levels after primary and secondary corneal infection in the rabbit follows the pattern seen in patients with primary or recurrent ulcerative herpetic keratitis [2], although the experimental disease represents an exogenous, rather than a recurrent infection. The fall in LT found at the early stage of secondary corneal infection in rabbits indicates that proliferation of virus can induce a decrease in LT levels; this indicates that similar findings in the human should be treated with caution when relating recurrences to transient immunodeficits.

The particular parameters tested in this study do not necessarily represent the immune responses which are most important in protecting the cornea. However, it is of interest that the initiation of the LT response coincides with the initiation of healing in both primary and secondary corneal infections, while CF antibody titres do not rise until after the disease has begun to resolve. It is, therefore, possible that the activation of mechanisms operating locally to halt the spread of corneal infection may correlate with the development of the systemic LT response. A significant role for specific antibody in tears or corneal tissue is not suggested by our current studies which indicate that levels of neutralising antibody to HSV are low in tears and undetectable in corneas of animals with previous skin infection.

Whatever the precise mechanisms involved, the experimental findings with regard to corneal disease indicate that individuals with previous experience of HSV infection and possessing immune responses to the virus, are less susceptible to severe ulcerative herpetic keratitis than those without prior clinical or nonclinical infection. The dramatically reduced susceptibility, seen in rabbits with previous herpetic infection, suggests that the spread of virus into the corneal stroma would be more likely to occur where immune responses to HSV are not present or are deficient.

Although people seronegative for anti-HSV antibody form a significant minority in the population, the majority of adults show immune responses to the virus and primary herpetic keratitis is, therefore, rare. The experimental model used in this study is not one of recurrence, but we feel that ulcerative herpetic keratitis in rabbits with previous HSV infection provides a more accurate reflection of the human disease than does the corneal infection of normal rabbits. The modification of the Jones and Al-Hussaini method to involve secondary corneal infection should be a useful model for the study of topical and systemic agents which induce immunomodulation or immunosuppression, and for the evaluation of antiviral therapy.

**Acknowledgments.** We wish to acknowledge the help of Dr. S. Clarke (Public Health Laboratory Service, Bristol) in performing the CF tests and of Dr. G.R.B. Skinner (University of Birmingham) for the assay of neutralising antibody in samples of rabbit tears and cornea.

This work was supported by a Research to Prevent Blindness grant from the Royal National Institute for the Blind.

## References

1. Bradstreet CM, Taylor CED (1962) Techniques of complement-fixation test applicable to the diagnosis of virus disease. Monthly Bull Min Health and PHLS 21:96–104
2. Easty DL, Carter CA, Funk A, Entwhistle C (1980) Factors influencing spread of HSV into the corneal stroma. This vol.
3. Florman AL, Trader FW (1947) A comparative study of pathogenicity and antigenicity of four strains of herpes simplex. J Immunol 55:263–275
4. Gispen R (1957) Immunization against herpes keratitis in rabbits. Am J Ophthalmol 44:88–90
5. Hall FL, MacKneson RG, Ormsby HL (1955) Studies of immunity in experimental herpetic keratitis in rabbits. Am J Ophthalmol 39:226–233
6. Jones BR, Al-Hussaini MK (1963) Therapeutic considerations in ocular vaccinia. Trans Ophthalmol Soc UK 83:613–631
7. Markham RHC, Carter C, Scobie MA, Metcalf C, Easty DL (1977) Double blind clinical trial of adenine arabinoside and idoxuridine in herpetic corneal ulcers. Trans Ophthalmol Soc UK 97:333–340
8. Okumoto M, Jawetz E, Sonne M (1959) Studies on herpes simplex virus IX. Corneal responses to repeated inoculation with herpes simplex virus in rabbits. Am J Ophthalmol 47:61–66
9. Pollikoff R, Cannavale P, Dixon O (1972) Herpes simplex virus infection in rabbit eye. Arch Ophthalmol 88:52–57
10. Smith IW, Peutherer JF, MacCallum FO (1967) The incidence of *Herpesvirus hominis* antibody in the population. J Hyg (Camb) 65:395–408

Sundmacher, R. (Hrsg.):
Herpetische Augenerkrankungen
© J.F. Bergmann Verlag, München 1981

# Factors Influencing the Spread of Herpes Simplex Virus Into the Corneal Stroma

D.L. Easty, C. Carter, A. Funk, C. Entwhistle, Bristol

**Key words.** Immune responses in herpetic keratitis, lymphocyte transformation, macrophage migration inhibition

**Schlüsselwörter.** Immunreaktionen bei Herpeskeratitis, Lymphzytentransformation, Makrophagen-Migrationshemmung

**Summary.** Groups of patients with dendritic ulcers, persistent stromal disease, together with a group of controls were investigated for humoral and cell mediated immune responses in order to find whether correlation exists between disease severity and these in vitro tests. Kinetic studies of cell mediated immune responses were also carried out in a small group of patients. Using a whole blood test of lymphocyte transformation to HSV antigen, there was some evidence of a depression of specific response in patients with stromal disease. Primary herpetic keratitis was associated with a considerable positive response in lymphocyte transformation and in the production of macrophage migration inhibition factor. Recurrent disease was associated with elevation of specific lymphocyte transformation during active disease, which fell to a normal resting level during convalescence. Although there was a tendency towards increased frequency in HL-A 1 in patients with dendritic ulcers which was not apparent in stromal disease, this trend did not reach statistical significance. Since lymphocyte transformation using specific virus antigen was the only in vitro correlate of clinical severity, it is concluded that it can be recommended as a useful test to determine patients at risk of developing the more serious forms of keratitis.

**Zusammenfassung.** Wir untersuchten die zelluläre und humorale Immunantwort bei Patienten mit Keratitis dendritica, persistierendem Stromaherpes und bei Kontrollpersonen, um herauszufinden, ob sich zwischen diesen immunologischen in-vitro-Testen und dem Krankheitsbild eine Korrelation herstellen läßt. Bei einzelnen Patienten wurden auch Verlaufskorrelationen versucht. Im Lymphozytentransformations-Test mit HSV-Antigen zeigte sich bei Verwendung von Vollblut ein Hinweis, daß bei Patienten mit Stromaherpes die spezifische Immunantwort auf Herpesantigene verringert sein könnte. Eine primäre Herpeskeratitis hingegen war mit einer erheblich gesteigerten Reaktion im Transformationstest und im Makrophagen-Migrations-Hemmungstest verbunden. Bei wiederholten Infektionen waren die Reaktionen im Transformationstest während der akuten Erkrankungsphase erhöht und sanken im Verlauf der Heilung auf normales Niveau ab.

Patienten mit Keratitis wiesen etwas häufiger das HLA-A1 auf. Dies war aber nicht statistisch signifikant.

Der Lymphozytentransformationstest war der einzige in-vitro-Test, der sich mit dem klinischen Schweregrad korrelieren ließ. Er wird von uns deshalb als nützlicher Test dafür empfohlen, ob bei Herpes-Patienten die Gefahr besteht, daß sie eine der schwereren Keratitisformen entwickeln.

There are a number of factors which may influence the spread of the herpes simplex virus HSV into the corneal stroma (Table 1). It would be expected that where virus proliferates in an uninhibited way in the epithelium there would be an increased chance of it entering the stroma. We have

**Table 1.** Factors influencing penetration of HSV into the stroma or uvea

Mode of infection; primary
                     secondary
                     recurrent
Virulence of virus
Type of virus
Nature of trigger in recurrence
Immune responses in the host
Associated diseases
Immunodeficiency
Immunosuppression
Genetic susceptibility
Therapeutic management

been able to show in laboratory animals that systemic immune responses induced by previous exposure to the virus at another site inhibits the rate of virus proliferation in the epithelium when compared with animals in which there has been no previous exposure to the virus. Although this model is not one of true recurrence we interpret that this indicates that systemic immune responses can influence virus proliferation in the clinical disease. This is supported by evidence such as the increased risk of suffering severe attacks of herpetic infections in patients who have undergone organ transplantation [15] and we have noted that patients may develop particularly severe ocular herpetic keratitis following renal transplantation.

The pattern of disease in herpes simplex keratitis is unique in that the penetration of virus or its antigen into the deep tissues is a serious complication because of the effect which this may have on vision. There does not appear to be a parallel in other medical disciplines, which therefore makes comparison between data collected from differing disease entities caused by the HSV difficult to interpret.

Because there might be a connection between the extension of epithelial disease into stroma and systemic immune responses, we have assessed patients for humoral and cell-mediated responses who have suffered keratitis of two distinct types – epithelial or persistent stromal disease – and compared them with a group of control subjects, some of whom were sero-positive and others were sero-negative for HSV infections. We have previously noted that epithelial herpetic disease may be more severe in patients with severe atopic disease, and so this group has been assessed as a separate group. This paper reports the results of these studies, together with changes in cell mediated responses over a period of time in a patient with primary disease, and a small group with recurrent disease. A subsidiary study investigating the frequency of the HL-A antigens in the same groups of patients and controls is also reported.

## Methods

Twenty seven patients with dendritic ulcers were selected with and without minimal stromal involvement, and compared with a group of 30 patients with active stomal disease of disciform, limbal or diffuse type. A separate group with severe atopic disease and active epithelial or stromal disease were also investigated. The control group was composed of normal subjects with or without antibody to herpes simplex virus (16 and 15 subjects respectively).

Kinetic studies of cell mediated immune responses were performed in two patients with primary herpes simplex keratitis, nine patients with recurrent dendritic ulcers, and two patients with severe keratouveitis.

Serum immunoglobulins were assessed using Partigen immunodiffusion plates (Hoechst). Serum antibody to HSV was measured by complement fixation [1].

Lymphocyte transformations were carried out in cultures of whole blood using the method of Junge, Hoekstra, Wolfe and Deinhardt [11]. 0.1 ml of heparinised blood was cultured in 1 ml Eagles MEM containing HSV type 1 antigen at a final dilution of 1 : 200 v/v of a lyophilised stock preparation of viral culture, 50 $\gamma$ phytohaemagglutinen (PHA; purified; Wellcome Reagents), or no stimulant (control cultures). Cultures were set up in triplicate and incubated in 5% $CO_2$, 100% humidity for 7 days. Tritiated thymidine, $1_\mu Ci$ per tube was added for the last 18 hours of culture. The trichloracetic acid insoluble material, containing DNA, was recovered from each culture tube and the Beta radioactivity counted as disintegrations per minute (DPM).

In smaller groups of subjects macrophage migration inhibition factor was measured following challenge by HSV antigen. Lymphocytes were cultured for 7 days in Eagles MEM with HSV in the test cultures, and without in the control cultures. The supernatants were then removed and assayed for macrophage migration inhibition factor (MIF). Antigen was added to the control supernatants, and foetal calf serum to both test and control media. Guinea pig macrophages, stimulated by intra-peritoneal injection of paraffin oil 5–7 days earlier were recovered and centrifuged into small glass tubes. These were placed in wells each of which was then filled with test or control supernatant and incubated in 5% $CO_2$. The areas covered by macrophages migrating on the floors of the wells was measured 18 h later. The migration index was calculated from the mean migration area in the test supernatants expressed as a percentage of the mean migration area in control supernatants. The groups of patients with herpetic keratitis were assessed for their HL-A antigen distribution using standard techniques [14].

## Results

### Group Studies

Serum immunoglobulin levels were within normal limits for IgA and IgG but a proportion of patients with stromal disease demonstrated elevation of IgM (30%). IgE levels were normal in patients with epithelial and stromal herpetic keratitis, but were elevated in 50% of patients with concurrent atopic disease. Antibody of HSV did not show any difference between controls and patients (Fig. 1).

The whole blood lymphocyte transformation response to PHA showed no evidence of a difference between the groups of patients and controls (Fig. 2). The responses to HSV antigen expressed as transformation indices are demonstrated in Fig. 3. A transformation index of 8.5 separates the controls with and without antibody from each other, and can be taken for the upper level of normal in the sero-negative group, or a lower level of normal in the sero-positive group. 40% of patients with stromal disease had transformation indices lower than 8.5 compared with only 8% of patients with epithelial disease. Mean levels in sero-positive controls and in patients with epithelial disease were significantly higher than the mean level in the group with stromal disease ($p < 0.05$ and $< 0.01$ respectively*). There is therefore some tendency for patients with stromal disease to have depression of CMI to HSV antigen when the whole blood technique of lymphocyte transformation is employed. Figure 4 compares the mean uptake of 3 H Thymidine in DPM using HSV and PHA antigens and highlights the reduction in transformation using specific antigen in contrast to mitogenic challenge.

Macrophage migration inhibition factor was produced in significant quantities in all nine patients with stromal disease, six out of nine patients with epithelial keratitis, and five out of twelve controls. They did not dis-

*Wilcoxon rank sum test

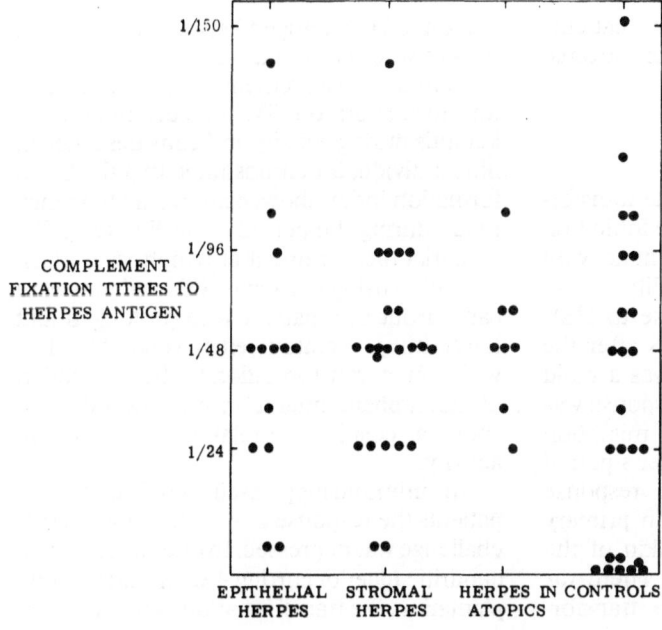

HERPES SIMPLEX COMPLEMENT - FIXATION
TITRES IN PATIENTS AND CONTROLS

COMPLEMENT FIXATION TITRES TO HERPES ANTIGEN

EPITHELIAL HERPES    STROMAL HERPES    HERPES IN ATOPICS    CONTROLS

Fig. 1. Complement fixing antibody in patients with epithelial and stromal keratitis compared with a group of control subjects. Patients with herpetic keratitis in association with severe atopic disease are shown as a separate group

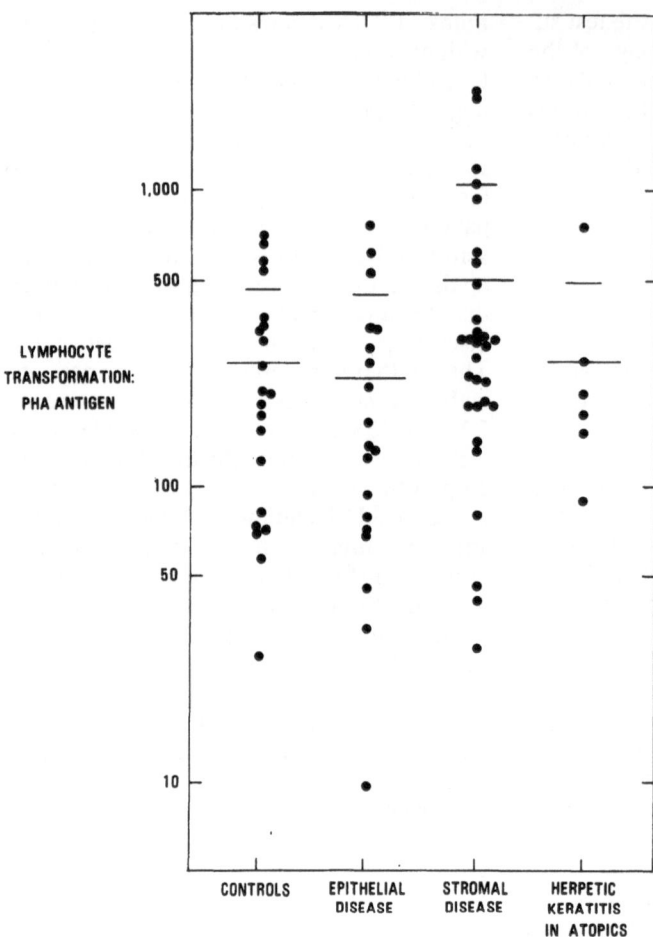

LYMPHOCYTE
TRANSFORMATION:
PHA ANTIGEN

CONTROLS    EPITHELIAL    STROMAL    HERPETIC
            DISEASE       DISEASE    KERATITIS
                                     IN ATOPICS

**Fig. 2.** Lymphocyte transformation expressed as the transformation index using PHA as antigen in patients compared with a group of controls. Mean levels and standard deviations are shown

tinguish group differences between patients with either epithelial disease or stromal disease (Table 2).

*Kinetic Studies*

Serial measurement of lymphocyte transformation and macrophage migration inhibition were made in a 28 year old female with primary herpetic keratitis. The ability of lymphocytes to transform in response to HSV antigen was first detected 10 days after the onset of the disease, and there was a rapid resolution when the maximum response was achieved (Fig. 5). Macrophage migration inhibition factor was produced after a period of 10 days (Fig. 6). A similar response occurred in an atopic female with primary herpetic infection affecting the skin of the face, and causing bilateral keratitis. There was a sharp increase in lymphocyte transfor-

mation to HSV antigen between the 2nd and the 4th weeks of the disease.

Paired measurements of lymphocyte transformation to HSV in recurrent herpetic keratitis during activity and convalescence in nine individuals demonstrated that the transformation index showed an overall tendency to fall during the period of healing (Fig. 7).

Serial measurement of lymphocyte transformation using PHA and HSV antigens were carried out in a patient with prolonged and unremitting kerato-uveitis (Fig. 8). The variation in transformation or the production of macrophage migration inhibition did not show a positive correlation with disease activity.

In immunosuppressed renal transplant patients the response of lymphocytes to HSV challenge was depressed. In one patient with a dendritic ulcer occurring 4 weeks after transplantation, the transformation index was 1.76,

120

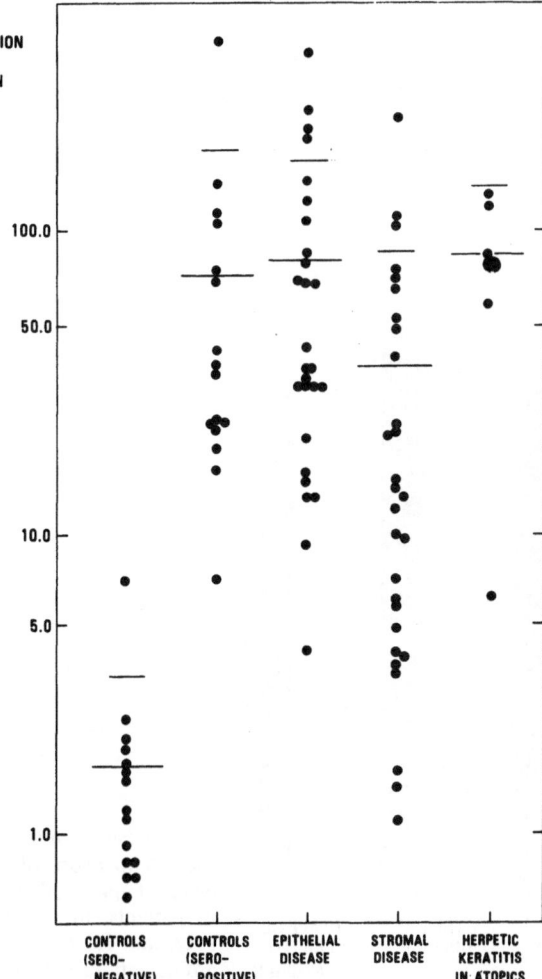

TRANSFORMATION
INDEX:
HS ANTIGEN

100.0

50.0

10.0

5.0

1.0

CONTROLS
(SERO-
NEGATIVE)

CONTROLS
(SERO-
POSITIVE)

EPITHELIAL
DISEASE

STROMAL
DISEASE

HERPETIC
KERATITIS
IN ATOPICS

**Fig. 3.** Lymphocyte transformation to herpes simplex antigen in patients and controls. Mean levels and standard deviations are shown

and in a second patient with severe stromal disease the index was 2.00.

*HL-A Antigen Frequency*

Figure 9 demonstrates the frequencies of the HL-A antigens in patients and controls, and shows that there was a tendency for HL-A 1 to be increased above a normal frequency in patients with dendritic ulcers, this trend not being apparent in subjects with persistent and unremitting stromal disease.

**Discussion**

In the study of group differences between patients and controls, there was little to indicate that there was a difference using specific

complement-fixing antibody, the production of macrophage migration inhibition factor, or lymphocyte transformation using the mitogen phytohaemagglutinin. The results of the test of specific lymphocyte responses to challenge with HSV antigen show that in a proportion of patients with stromal keratitis, there is evidence of a deficit in cell-mediated immunity. This is not apparent using the production of macrophage migration inhibition factor as a test of cell-mediated immunity, and it would seem that there is no deficit in the production of this particular lymphokine. Patients with dendritic figures showed no difference in their lymphocyte response when compared with the control group, but in sequential studies, there is evidence of a fall in this response in the period of convalescence   following the dendrite

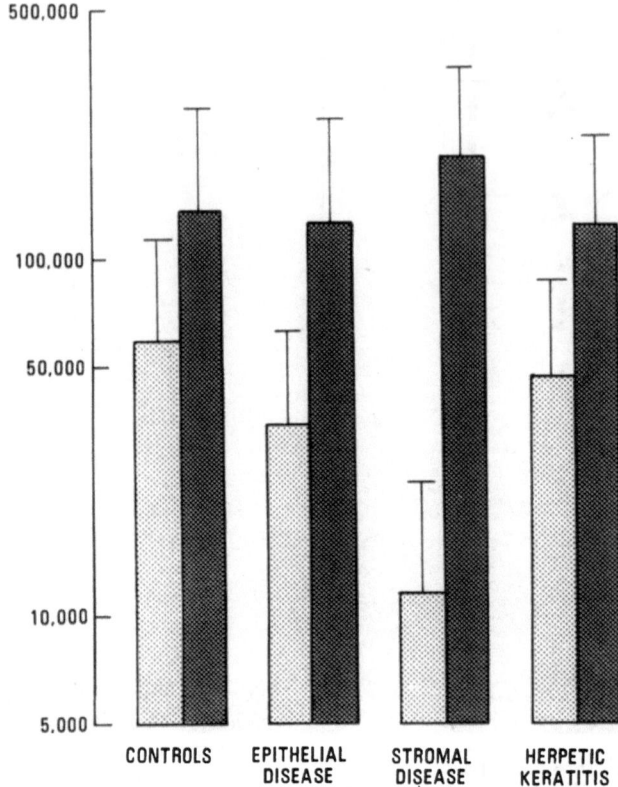

MEAN UPTAKE
OF 3 H THYMIDINE
(DPM)

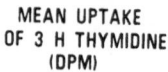 HS ANTIGEN

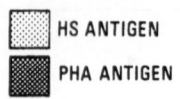 PHA ANTIGEN

500,000 —

100,000 —

50,000 —

10,000 —

5,000 —

CONTROLS   EPITHELIAL   STROMAL   HERPETIC
           DISEASE      DISEASE   KERATITIS
                                  IN ATOPICS

**Fig. 4.** Histogram demonstrating the comparison of the mean levels of uptake of 3 H thymidine in patients and controls using PHA and HSV antigens. Standard deviations are shown

which might indicate a transient elevation of response during the active phase of the disease. In discussing the relevance of our findings to the reported results in the literature, it should be remembered that each disease which has been investigated is likely to show immunological abnormalities which might not necessarily be expected to agree with those found in other disease processes known or thought to be caused by the herpes

**Table 2.** Macrophage migration inhibition factor production in epithelial disease, stromal disease and controls

| Group | No. of patients | No. of patients producing MIF | Mean % inhibition ± ISD |
|---|---|---|---|
| Epithelial Disease | 9 | 6 | 34.2 ± 33.0 |
| Stromal Disease | 9 | 9 | 64.4 ± 29.2 |
| Controls (Seropositive) | 12 | 5 | 16.6 ± 19.9 |

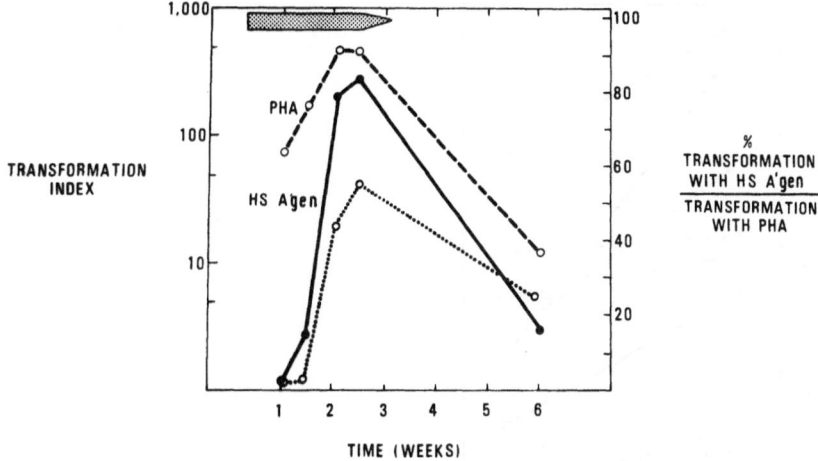

**Fig. 5.** Serial lymphocyte transformation studies in a patient with primary herpetic keratitis, using PHA (O---O) and HSV (●—●) antigens. The hatched block indicates the period of disease activity. The transformation levels of HSV stimulated lymphocytes have been expressed as a percentage of the PHA stimulated lymphocytes (O·····O)

simplex virus. Studies in patients with recurrent herpes labialis, progenitalis, or herpetic corneal infection not surprisingly give somewhat conflicting results, although positive results are regularly observed using tests of lymphocyte transformation [5, 16, 19, 26, 27]. When lymphocyte cytotoxicity tests are employed varying results are obtained [23, ]. An increase of cytotoxicity was reported during active disease compared with the quiescent phase [25]. Interferon production by lymphocytes was found to be high immediately after active herpes labialis and subsequently declined [8, 16, 17]. Macrophage migration inhibition factor production was reported to be impaired in patients with active recurrent herpes labialis by Wilton et al. [27], and similar findings were reported by Gange et al. [6] for virus-specific leukocyte migration inhibitory factor synthesis in patients with

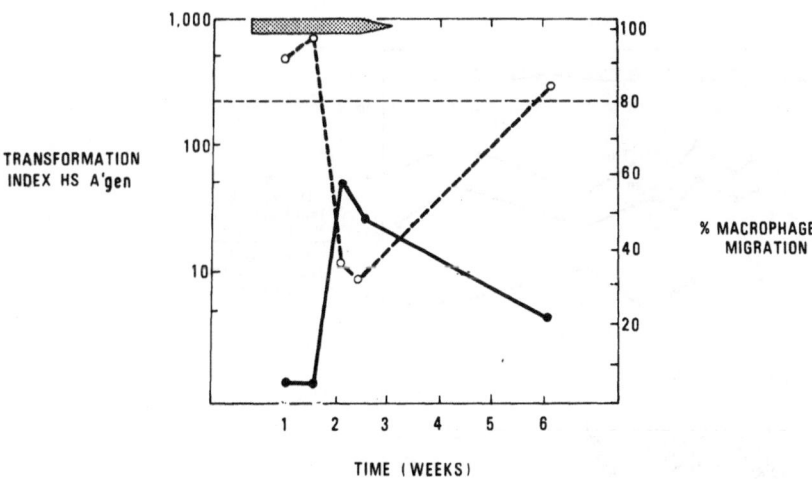

**Fig. 6.** Macrophage migration inhibition factor production (0---0) and lymphocyte transformation using separated lymphocytes (●—●) in a patient with primary herpetic keratitis. The hatched block indicates the period of disease activity

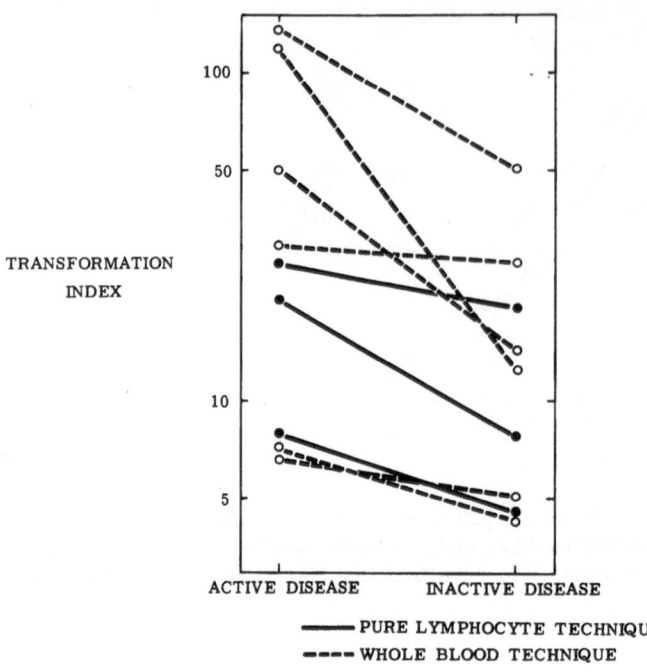

TRANSFORMATION
INDEX

ACTIVE DISEASE    INACTIVE DISEASE

———— PURE LYMPHOCYTE TECHNIQUE

----- WHOLE BLOOD TECHNIQUE

**Fig. 7.** Lymphocyte transformation during active dendritic ulcers and convalescence in a group of patients subject to recurrent disease

active disease. These findings were not confirmed by Russell et al. [21] who found no deficit with this method. Rosenburg et al. [20] reported increased lymphotoxin by virus-challenged lymphocytes 7 days after the appearance of vesicles. Grabner et al. [7] reported a significantly reduced production of leucocyte migration inhibitory factor in primary and recurrent ocular infections caused by the herpes simplex virus. On the other hand, patients with stromal disease did not demonstrate evidence of reduced migration inhibitory factor, and were similar to the control group. The results of the present study confirm our preliminary results [5], and suggest that simple tests of lymphocyte function using the whole blood technique of lymphocyte transformation may show

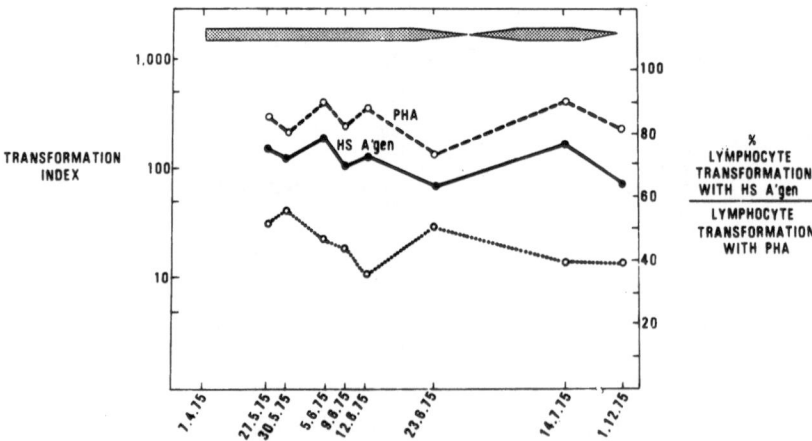

**Fig. 8.** Lymphocyte transformation to PHA and HSV antigen in a patient with prolonged keratouveitis. Disease activity is demonstrated with hatched blocks. The lymphocyte response to HSV antigen is also expressed as a percentage of the response to PHA (O·····O)

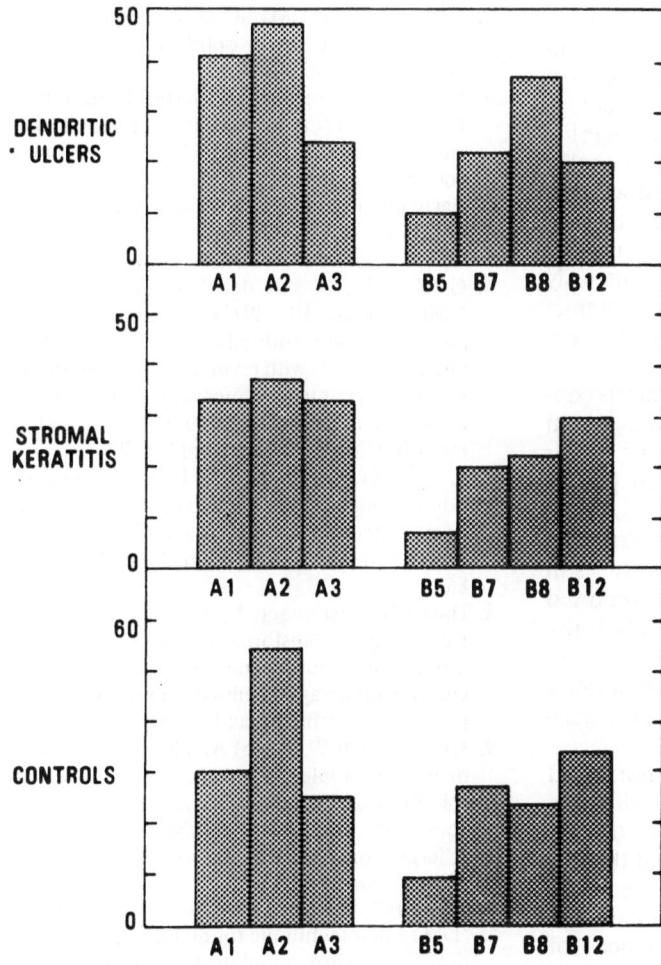

**Fig. 9.** The frequency distributions of the common HL-A antigens in 51 patients with dendritic ulcers, 27 patients with stromal disease and 350 controls

a closer and more reproducible correlation with the in vivo manifestations of herpetic keratitis. The production of macrophage migration inhibition factor did not demonstrate evidence of a deficit in primary disease, but the response was variable in recurrent disease so that no valid conclusions could be made from kinetic studies. In patients with stromal disease, levels of lymphocyte transformation and macrophage migration inhibition demonstrated considerable variation which highlights the difficulties which are encountered in the interpretation of data from patients with chronic disease processes.

It is our impression at a clinical level that many patients with persistent stromal keratouveitis have had topical corticosteroid early in the disease, often during the period of dendritic ulceration. Such erroneous use of topical steroids leads to enhancement of virus

spread in the epithelium and it is likely that this leads to virus penetration into the stroma with the consequent production of persistent stromal keratitis. Nevertheless in a proportion of patients with stromal disease our data suggests that there is evidence of a deficit in cell mediated immunity which is confirmed by the similar deficits which may be found in patients who have undergone organ transplantation with immunosuppression [18], who suffer from severe herpetic infections, including persistent stromal disease [3].

Though no signs of immunodeficiency were located in patients with herpetic keratitis in association with atopic disease, there is other evidence that cell-mediated reactions in such patients are abnormal [2, 10, 12, 17, 24]. However it must also be remembered that many patients with atopic disease have allergic responses occurring in their conjunctiva which is known to be crowded with mast cells [4], together with many other types of inflammatory cells. It therefore remains possible that local mediator production such as prostaglandins [9] may play a role in triggering the frequent attacks of persistent epithelial keratitis from which these unfortunate patients may suffer. It is interesting that recurrences of herpetic keratitis cease once the allergic conjunctivitis has spontaneously resolved. An additional factor is the systemic and topical use of corticosteroid which many atopic subjects undergo.

There have been a number of reports concerning the frequency of the HLA antigens in patients with recurrent cutaneous or ocular herpetic keratitis. Russell and Schlaut [22] reported increased prevalence of HL-A 1 in patients with herpes labialis, while Zimmerman et al. [28] found significant increases in Hl-A B5. Meyers-Elliott et al. [13] reported increased HL-A w3. Our studies confirm the studies of Russell et al. [23] as a trend only in the patients with dendritic ulcers, this trend not being apparent in the group with persistent stromal disease.

From this investigation of humoral and cell-mediated immunity in patients with dendritic ulcers and persistent stromal disease due to the HSV, it is concluded that there is some evidence of a correlation between clinical disease and lymphocyte transformation to specific antigen, but no evidence of correlations between antibody levels and disease severity. It is considered that lymphocyte transformation can be used to identify those who may be at risk of developing severe and persistent stromal disease, but is also considered that the use of topical corticosteroids early in the disease during dendritic ulceration may adversely influence the prognosis to a greater extent.

# References

1. Bradstreet CM, Taylor CED (1962) Technique of complement-fixation test applicable to the diagnosis of virus diseases. Monthly Bulletin of the Ministry of Health and Public Health Laboratory Service 21:96
2. Buckley RH, Wray BB, Belmaker EZ (1972) Extreme hyperimmunoglobulinaemia E and unknown susceptibility to infection. Pediatrics 49:59
3. Easty DL (1977) Manifestations of immunodeficiency diseases in ophthalmology. Trans Ophthalmol Soc UK 97:8
4. Easty DL, Birkenshaw M, Merrett T, Merrett J, Madden P (1979) Immunology of vernal disease. In: Pepys T, Edward AM (eds) The mast cell. Pitman, London
5. Easty DL, Maini RN, Jones BR (1973) Cellular immunity in herpes simplex keratitis. Trans Ophthalmol Soc UK 93:171
6. Gange RW, Bats A de, Park JR, Bradstreet CMP, Rhodes EL (1975) Cellular immunity and circulating antibody to herpes simplex virus in subjects with recurrent herpes simplex lesions and controls as measured by the mixed leucocyte migration inhibition and complement fluction. Br J Dermatol 97:539
7. Grabner G, Jarisoh R (1979) Leucocyte migration inhibitory factor in primary and recurrent ocular infections by herpes simplex virus. Albrecht von Graefe Arch Klin Ophthalmol 211:85
8. Haahr S, Rasmussen L, Merigan TC (1976) Lymphocyte transformation and interferon production in human mononuclear cell microcultures for assay of cellular immunity to herpes simplex virus. Infect Immunol 14:47
9. Hill PJ, Blyth WJ (1976) An alternative theory of herpes simplex recurrence and a possible role for prostaglandins. Lancet 1:397
10. Jones HE, Lewis CW, MacMarlin SL (1973) Allergic contact sensitivity in atopic patients. Arch Dermatol 107:217
11. Junge NP, Hoekstra J, Wolfe L, Deinhardt F (1976) Microtechnique for quantitative evaluation of in vitro lymphocyte transformation. Clin Exp Immunol 7:431
12. Lobitz WC, Honeyman JF, Winkler NW (1972) Suppressed cell-mediative immunity in two adults with atopic dermatitis. Br J Dermatol 86:317
13. Meyers-Elliott RH, Elliott JH, Maxwell WA, Pettit TH, O'Day DM, Terasaki PI, Bernoco DVM (1980) HL-A Antigens in recurrent stromal herpes simplex virus keratitis. Am J Ophthalmol 89:54
14. Mittal KK, Mickey MR, Singhal DP, Terasaki PJ (1968) Serotyping for homotransplantation. XVIII. Refinement of microdroplet lymphocyte cytotoxicity test. Transplantation 6:913
15. Montgomerie JZ, Becroft DMO, Croxson MC, Doak PB, North JDK (1969) Herpes simplex virus infection after renal transplantation. Lancet 2:867
16. O'Reilly RJ, Chibaro A, Anger E, Lopez C (1977) Cell mediated immune responses in patients with recurrent herpes simplex infections. 11. Infection-associated deficiency of lymphokine production in patients with re-

current herpes labialis or herpes progenitalis. J Immunol 118:1095

17. Palacious J, Fuller EW, Blaycock WK (1966) Immunological capabilities of patients with atopic dermatitis. J Invest Dermatol 47:484
18. Rand KH, Rasmussen LE, Pollard RB, Arvin A, Merigan TC (1976) Cellular immunity and herpes virus infections in cardiac transplant patients. N Eng J Med 296:1372
19. Rasmussen LE, Jordan GW, Stevens DA, Merigan TG (1974) Lymphocyte interferon production and transformation after herpes simplex infections in humans. J Immunol 112: 728
20. Rosenburg GL, Snyderman R, Notkins AL (1974) Production of chemotactic factor and lymphotoxin by human leukocytes stimulated with herpes simplex virus. Infect Immun 10:111
21. Russell AS, Konsei J, Lad VS (1976) Cell mediated immunity to herpes simplex in man IV A correlation of lymphocyte stimulation and inhibition of leukocyte migration. J Immunol Methods 9:273
22. Russell AS, Schlaut J (1975) HL-A Transplantation antigens in subjects susceptible to recrudescent herpes labialis. Tissue Antigens 6:257
23. Russell AS, Percy JS, Kovithavongs T (1975) Cell mediated immunity to herpes simplex in humans. Lymphocyte cytotoxicity measured by [51]cr release from infected cells. Infect Immun 11:355
24. Thestrup-Pederson K, Ellegard J, Thulin H, Zachariae H (1977) PPD and mitogen responsiveness of lymphocytes from patients with atopic dermatitis. Clin Exp Immunol 27:118
25. Thong YH, Vincent MM, Hensen SA, Fucillo DA, Rola-Plesczynski M, Bellanti JA (1975) Depressed specific cell mediated immunity to herpes simplex virus type 1 in patients with recurrent herpes labialis. Infect Immun 12:76
26. Tokumary TY, Shimiza Y, Sabety Y (1975) Herpetic epithelial keratitis: A radioassay evaluation of the hosts humoral and cellular responsiveness. Ophthalmic Res 7:345
27. Wilton JMA, Ivanyi L, Lehner T (1972) Cell mediated immunity in herpes virus hominis infections. Br Med J 1:723
28. Zimmerman TJ, McNeill JI, Richman A, Kaufman HE, Waltman S (1977) HL-A type and recurrent corneal herpes simplex infection. Invest Ophthalmol Visual Sci 15:756

## Discussion on the Contributions pp. 111–127

G. Smolin (San Francisco)
Carlos Lopez reported a decreased number of natural killer cells in patients who have a susceptibility to stromal or recurrent herpetic disease. He also demonstrated that patients with chronic stromal disease tend to have decreased numbers of suppressor macrophages whereas the patients who don't develop chronic disease have adequate numbers. Do you have any experience in this matter?

D. Easty (Bristol)
We haven't got into that type of work. In fact, most of our tests involve the whole blood technique which really is a bit of a blunderbuss method, but we felt that it pulled out the levels and allowed us to see these changes between populations. When we used isolated lymphocytes it was more difficult to show these differences. We have not actually separated the killer-cells or looked at macrophages specifically; we've just found that macrophage migration inhibition does seem to vary between the groups.

C. Kok van Alphen (Leyden)
I would like to ask Mr. Easty something. A rabbit is not a human being. Have you had any experience with patients who have had muco-cutaneous herpes? As an "old" ophthalmologist I have the idea that human beings who have had muco-cutaneous herpes really never have ocular herpes. Do you have any figures?

D. Easty (Bristol)
That's not been our experience actually. In fact its a question I always ask: 'have you had a recent attack of cutaneous herpes' and the answer is quite often in the affirmative, so I think a patient quite often has had cutaneous herpes prior to the disease.

C. Kok van Alphen (Leyden)
Well, but we have the experience of many people having muco-cutaneous herpes and not ocular herpes.

B.R. Jones (London)
Could I ask Dr. Carter what were the intervals between the first infection and the second infection in the cornea in the experiments in which she showed resistance to second infections?

C. Carter (Bristol)
Infecting first one cornea and then both; the difference was 8 weeks. With the skin infection prior to corneal challenge it was at least 6 weeks.

Sundmacher, R. (Hrsg.):
Herpetische Augenerkrankungen
© J.F. Bergmann Verlag, München 1981

# The Turnover of Lysosomal Particles During Corneal Herpetic Infection. Morphometric Study

J. Francois, O. Miraglia, V. Victoria-Troncoso, Gent

**Key words.** Dendritic keratitis, pinocytosis vacuoles, lysosomes

**Schlüsselwörter.** Keratitis dendritica, Pinozytose-Vakuolen, Lysosomen

**Summary.** The first manifestation at the level of the corneal epithelium after inoculation with herpes virus is the loss of the microvilli, which may fuse together. Subsequently, one observes (1) rounded foci of the punctate type, consisting of detached cells, (2) linear lesions consisting of strings of detached cells, (3) branched linear lesions, forming three-pointed stars and (4) typical dendritic lesions. In addition, a cycle of pinocytosis vacuoles lasting about 60 h and a cycle of lysosomes lasting about 48 h are observed. The defensive cycle is shorter than the infectious cycle, which lasts about 6 days, and this fact might explain the survival of the virus in the latent state. The morphometric studies of the vacuoles and the particles of the lysosomal type are discussed.

**Zusammenfassung.** Als erstes Zeichen einer Infektion des Hornhautepithels durch Herpes simplex Virus zeigt sich ein Verlust und ein Verklumpen von Mikrovilli. Dann beobachtet man (1) kleine Rundherde, in deren Bereich Zellen herausgelöst sind, (2) gestreckte Läsionen, die durch erkrankte Zell-Ketten gebildet werden, (3) verzweigte lineare Herde, die ein Sternmuster ausbilden und (4) typische Dendritika-Läsionen. Darüber hinaus beobachtet man einen Reaktionszyklus von Pinozytose-Vakuolen, der ungefähr 60 Std dauert, und einen Zyklus von Lysosomen-Reaktionen, der ca. 48 Std anhält. Da diese Abwehr-Zyklen erheblich kürzer als der Infektions-Zyklus sind, der ca. 6 Tage anhält, kann man mit diesen Beobachtungen vielleicht ein längeres latentes Verbleiben des Virus erklären. Die morphometrischen Befunde bzgl. der Pinozytose- und Lysosomen-Partikel werden diskutiert.

## Introduction

We have already described the changes in the corneal epithelium after experimental infection with type 2 herpes virus, "in situ", as well as in tissue culture [2, 3]. In rabbits we were able to determine the duration and the evolution of the corneal lesions after herpetic primo-infection. In this study, we compared the duration of the infectious cycle to that of the lysosomal cycle, and we discuss the part played by the latter in the evolution of the cell infection.

## Materials and Methods

We used male Flanders Giant rabbits, weighing about 2 kg. Their nictating membranes were removed. Both eyes were infected after a slight scarification of the center of the cornea. We used 0.5 ml of a suspension of type 1, KOS strain, herpes simplex virus, of titre 1 LD50 : $10^{-4}$.

For the study of the lysosomal cycle, we dissected the corneal epithelium, together with a very thin layer of stroma, by way of support. After having located the epithelial lesions at the biomicroscope, the specimen was divided into two parts, each containing some of the lesions. A flat preparation was treated by Takeuchi and Tanoue's method [2] and was immediately photographed. The other part was fixed and treated for examination by the electron microscope, according to the following method:

1. Fixation by glutaldehyde and osmic acid, buffered with 0.2 M phosphate at pH 7.2

2. Dehydration and inclusion in Epon

3. After having determined the proper orientation on thick sections, we made seriated fine sections which were then photographed. It was on these photographs that the morphometric measurements were made,

both for the pinocytosis vacuoles and for the lysosomes.

We used two series of rabbits. One series was used for the scanning microscopy, whereby the evolution of the changes in the corneal epithelium was observed, the corneas having been treated by the critical-drying-point method. The other series was used for the morphometric study of the lysosomes, which were located by their markers, the acid phosphatases.

For the morphometry, we employed the MOP-Digiplan (Kontron) system, which comprises of:

1. A measuring table, upon which the photograph to be analysed is placed. Each particle is outlined with a precision of 0.1 mm by means of a pencil.

2. A computer, which enables various morphometric programs to be employed.

At first, we located each particle to be analysed on the photographs of the seriated sections. The biggest image was chosen, because it represented the cross-section of the particle at the level of its greatest diameter. Three measurements were made simultaneously, following the outline of each particle: the maximum diameter, the area and the length. The computer storage then made it possible to establish a histogram, wherein the analysed elements were classified according to their dimensions.

The method of recording the coordinates in the MOP system is based on the principle of measuring the propagation time of magnetostrictive pulses in magnetised parallel wires located beneath the surface of the plate and arranged as the X and Y axes.

Magnetostriction is based on the property of ferromagnetic materials slightly changing their shape under the influence of an external magnetic field (produced, in this case, by a coil). By the Joule effect, a variation in length occurs in a direction perpendicular to the applied magnetic field and a mechanical tension wave in the wires is produced. This wave, by the Villari effect, engenders a variation of the magnetic permeability and, because the wires are premagnetised, a momentary modification of the magnetic flux along the wire. This modification of the flux can be utilised to indicate the passage of a tension wave.

The animals were killed after the following intervals: 0, 6, 12, 18, 24, 30, 36, 42, 48, 54, 60, 66 and 72 h and 5, 6, 7, 8, 9 and 10 days.

## Results

*Appearance of the Corneal Surface After Inoculation With Herpes Virus*

The most characteristic features were observed during the first 24 to 48 h for the initial lesions and on the 4th day for the evolved lesions. Spontaneous healing set in on the 6th day.

Scanning Microscopy 48 Hours After the Inoculation

The first manifestation was the loss in places of the microvilli. At low magnification, several rounded spots were observed, in some cases confluent, which had lost their brightness. Several cells of the corneal surface were affected. There could be up to 10 or 15 such dark spots, formed of a smooth surface containing some isolated and atrophied villi of 8 to 10 µm in length. This surface was surrounded by a collar-shaped bulging part, produced by the fusion of a large number of microvilli. Apart from the lesions, the appearance was normal, although there could be some diminution of the microvilli. There were, in addition, some double lesions, that is to say, that two surfaces could be seen, rounded and surrounded by microvilli, which, by fusion, produced irregular folds. Lesions of another type consisted of the fusion of some microvilli, which took tuberous or irregular shapes. These structures, which measured 1 to 3 µm, were very clearly separated from the normal microvilli that surrounded them.

Lesions of a third type were constituted by the association of these two previous types. The bulging part surrounding the smooth surface was more prominent. In the center of the lesion, there was a raised formation, in some cases sessile, formed by the fusion of microvilli. It was also possible to see a few isolated microvilli. The areas where the microvilli were absent were prominent and had a perfectly spherical shape.

Lesions of a fourth type were punctate and more evolved. They consisted of a rounded group of several cells comprising of two areas:

a) A central area, where the cells were separated from each other. These cells, which were of an irregular polyhedral shape, were attached to the base of the lesion and in parts also to neighbouring cells. These lesions measured from 0.15 to 0.20 mm. The surface of the cell generally displayed some microvilli, which might, nevertheless, be absent in some places. At higher magnification, it was possible to see some cells bristling with small microvilli.

b) A marginal area, where the cells were still attached but were located at a lower level relative to the surrounding normal surface. This depressed area was separated from the normal corneal surface by a line representing the intercellular spaces between the normal cells and the pathological cells.

## Scanning Microscopy 4 Days After the Infection

We observed (1) rounded foci of the punctate type, consisting of detached cells, (2) linear lesions consisting of strings of detached cells, (3) branched linear lesions, forming three-pointed stars and (4) typical dendritic lesions.

At higher magnification, it was possible to observe irregular polyhedral cells, with and without microvilli. Those microvilli might be hypertrophic, ending in bulbous dilations. There were also rounded cells, displaying many microvilli and consequently having a very bright appearance. These cells were attached to the underlying cells at a single point.

In the deeper lesions, we observed keratocytes which had migrated toward the surface. These keratocytes were spindle-shaped and were attached to the epithelial cells by fine pseudopods.

The most characteristic feature was the presence of numerous rounded particles of about 1 μm, located on the smooth cells, as well as on the cells having microvilli.

At the point of branching of a linear lesion, we observed clearly that certain superficial elements were detached, making it possible to see the typical polyhedral and rounded elements that we have described. The lesion had a main branch, from one side of which a new branch sprang, to produce a complete dendritic figure.

At high magnification, the polyhedral cells displayed cytoplasmic filaments, which connected the cells to each other and which in fact represented desmosomes.

In conclusion, the cycle of the infectious lesions lasted in general for 6 days, although it could in some cases continue up to the 8th day.

## Morphometrical Study of the Cytoplasmic Particles

Immediately after the virus infection, we saw a large number of vacuoles developing in the most superficial layers of the corneal epithelium. An increasing number of particles of the lysosomal type then formed at the level of the basal and middle layers. There are two cycles, which develop at the level of this vacuolar system (Fig. 1 and 2):

a) The *cycle of the pinocytosis vacuoles,* which begins during the first 6 h after the infection. The number of vacuoles reached its maximum by the 12th h and thereafter diminished progressively until the 60th h (Fig. 1).

b) The *cycle of the particles of the lysosomal type,* which are histochemically found in a region highly positive for acid phosphatase and between 1.2 and 1.7 mm wide. The number of these particles increased progressively up to the 48th h and thereafter diminished very rapidly after the 50th h (Fig. 2 and 3).

Neither the vacuoles nor the particles of the lysosomal type changed in size during their respective cycles. Their morphometrical measurements are reproduced in Fig. 7 to 9.

The *pinocytosis vacuoles* aligned themselves in such a fashion that the greatest diameter of most of them was parallel to the surface of the cornea. Their greatest diameter was between 0.28 and 0.90 μm, while some isolated particles measured between 0.72 and 0.76 μm, or even 0.90 μm in exceptional cases (Fig. 4).

The greatest area measured between 0.50 and 1.45 μm$^2$, with maximum values attaining in some cases 1.60 to 2.45 μm$^2$. The apparent disparity between certain values of the maximum diameter and those of the maximum area resulted from the different degrees of flattening of the vacuoles (Fig. 5).

The lengths ranged from 0.84 to 1.60 μm. The distribution showed two peaks, one of them between 0.90 and 1.14 μm and the other at 1.40 μm. Maximum values between 1.75 and 2.05 μm were observed in some cases (Fig. 6).

The *particles of the lysosomal type* were sometimes flattened in the same sense as the

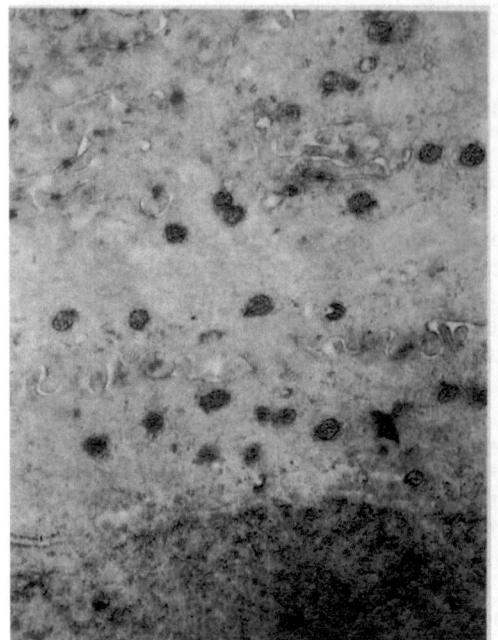
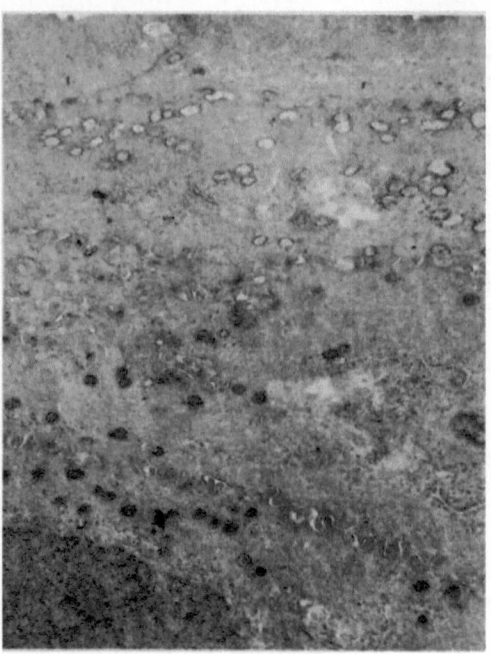

1

2

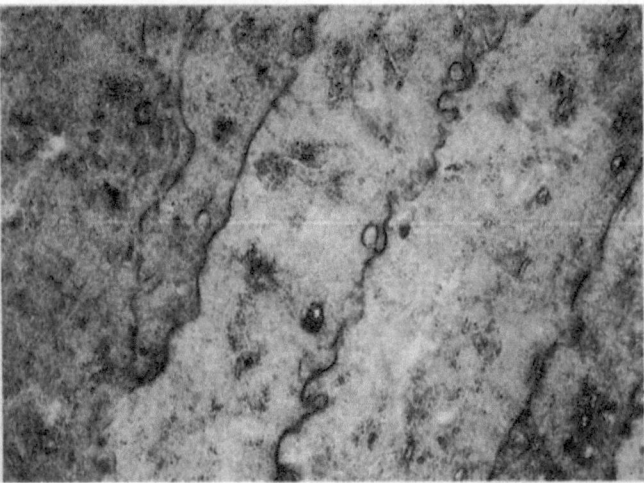

3

**Fig. 1.** At the moment of the infection (0 hour) only one particle of the lysosomal type is seen in the middle cellular layers of the corneal epithelium. There are many ribosomes. Transmission electron microscope (× 31.000)

**Fig. 2.** Development of pinocytosis vacuoles in the superficial layers of the corneal epithelium and of particles of the lysosomal type in the middle and deep layers, 48 h after the infection. Transmission electron microscope (× 34.000)

**Fig. 3.** Most of the particles of the lysosomal type are enveloped by a membrane, a few are not. Transmission electron microscope (× 15.000)

pinocytosis vacuoles. This effect is probably due to the tension of the cytoplasmic tonofibrils.

The greatest diameter of the particles varied from 0.23 to 0.54 µm, the model values occurring between 0.37 and 0.41 µm. A diameter of 0.68 µm was attained in exceptional cases (Fig. 7).

The maximal areas varied between 0.24 and 1.20 µm$^2$. The distribution showed two peaks, one between 0.56 and 0.63 µm$^2$, and another at 0.90 µm$^2$. Values of 1.37 or even of

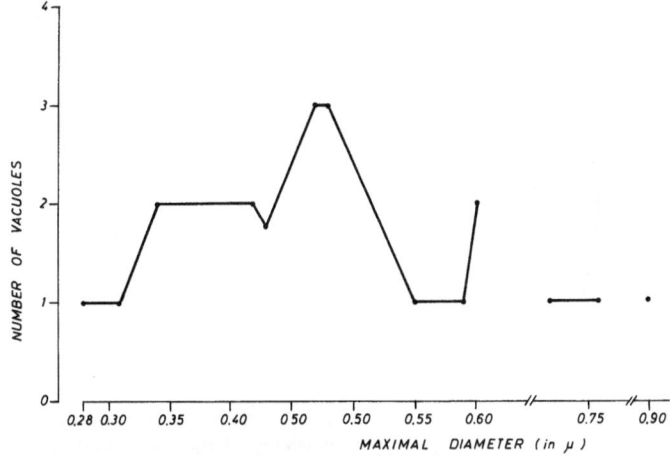

**Fig. 4.** Distribution curve of the pinocytosis vacuoles. Maximal diameter 48 h after infection

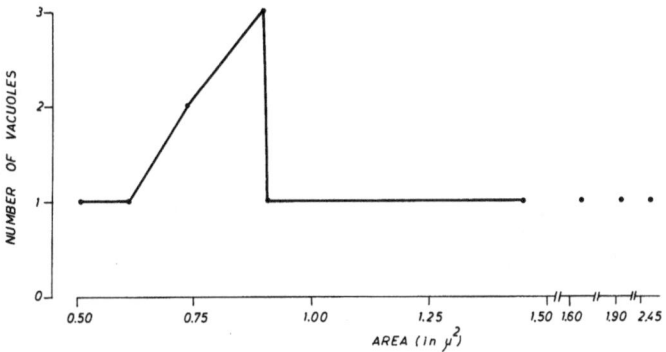

**Fig. 5.** Distribution curve of the pinocytosis vacuoles. Maximal area 48 h after infection

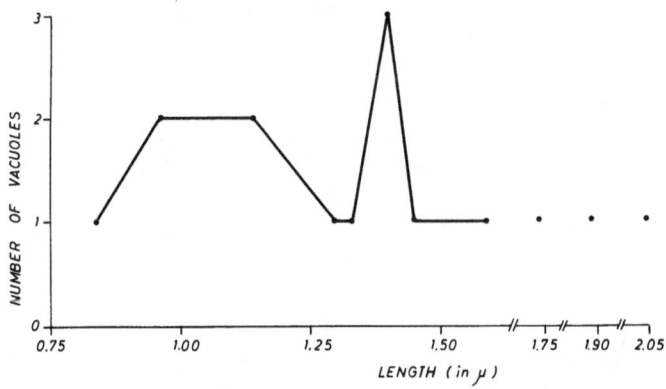

**Fig. 6.** Distribution curve of the pinocytosis vacuoles. Maximal length 48 h after infection

1.45 $\mu m^2$ were obtained in exceptional cases (Fig. 8).

The lengths ranged from 0.61 to 1.60 $\mu m$, with a peak in the distribution curve at 1.14 $\mu m$ (Fig. 9).

The histogram reproduced in Table 1, based on a very large number of particles, enables them to be classified according to their dimensions.

It must be mentioned that the measurements made on very great enlargements gave in general slightly lower figures.

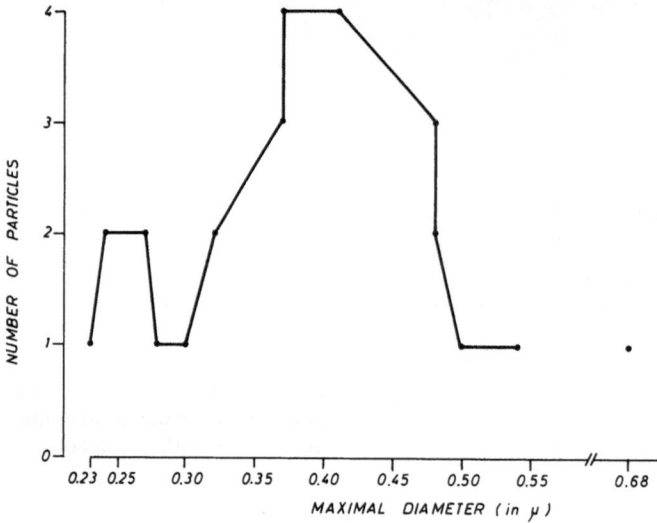

**Fig. 7.** Distribution curve of the particles of the lysosomal type. Maximal diameter 48 h after infection

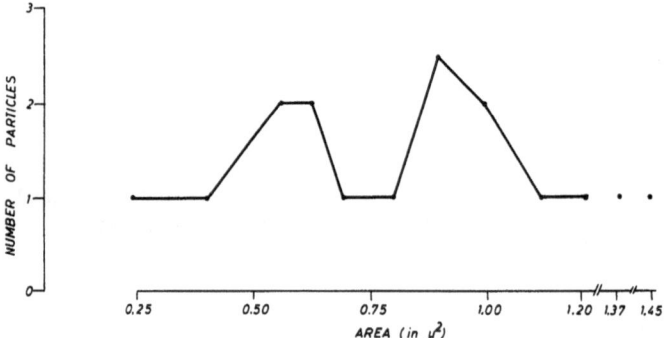

**Fig. 8.** Distribution curve of the particles of the lysosomal type. Maximal area 48 h after infection

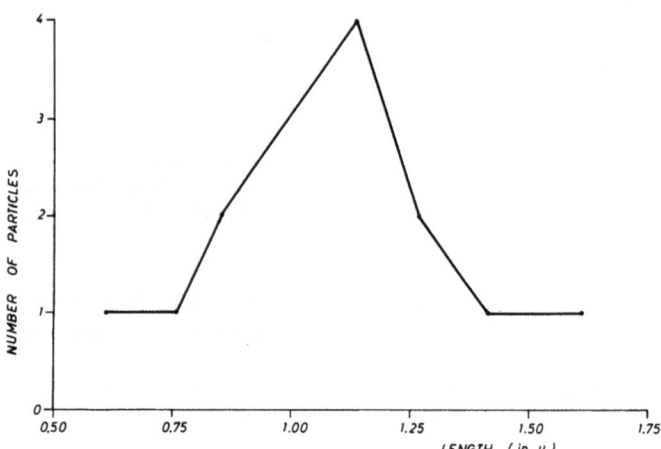

**Fig. 9.** Distribution curve of the particles of the lysosomal type. Maximal length 48 h after infection

**Table 1.** Histogram of the particles of the lysosomal type 48 h after infection

| Length classification | | | | Area classification | | | |
|---|---|---|---|---|---|---|---|
| | | 4506.5 | length | | | 12206.1 | area |
| | | 72 | count | | | 72 | count |
| | | 52.5 | median | | | 113.3 | median |
| M = | | 62.6 | S = 47.5 | M = | | 169.5 | S = 161.26 |
| | 35 | / | 10 | | 25 | / | 10 |
| Count | Perc. | Limit | No | Count | Perc. | Limit | No |
| 2 | 2.8 | .0 | 0 | 2 | 2.8 | .0 | 1 |
| 3 | 4.2 | 10 | 1 | 2 | 2.8 | 10 | 2 |
| 8 | 11.1 | 20 | 2 | 5 | 6.9 | 20 | 3 |
| 7 | 9.7 | 30 | 3 | 3 | 4.2 | 30 | 4 |
| 14 | 19.4 | 40 | 4 | 4 | 5.6 | 40 | 5 |
| 8 | 11.1 | 50 | 5 | 5 | 6.9 | 50 | 6 |
| 8 | 11.1 | 60 | 6 | 1 | 1.4 | 60 | 7 |
| 6 | 8.3 | 70 | 7 | 6 | 8.3 | 70 | 8 |
| 3 | 4.2 | 80 | 8 | 4 | 5.6 | 80 | 9 |
| 5 | 6.9 | 90 | 9 | 1 | 1.4 | 90 | 10 |
| 2 | 2.8 | 100 | 10 | 2 | 2.8 | 100 | 11 |
| 4 | 5.6 | 110 | 11 | 3 | 4.2 | 110 | 12 |
| 1 | 1.4 | 270 | 27 | 3 | 4.2 | 120 | 13 |
| 1 | 1.4 | 300 | 30 | 2 | 2.8 | 130 | 14 |
| | | | | 3 | 4.2 | 140 | 15 |
| | | | | 1 | 1.4 | 150 | 16 |
| | | | | 3 | 4.2 | 160 | 17 |
| | | | | 1 | 1.4 | 170 | 18 |
| | | | | 1 | 1.4 | 200 | 21 |
| | | | | 2 | 2.8 | 210 | 22 |
| | | | | 1 | 1.4 | 220 | 23 |
| | | | | 1 | 1.4 | 240 | 25 |
| | | | | 16 | 22.2 | 250 | 26 |

## Discussion

It is well known that viruses are introduced into cells by pinocytosis. It was for that reason that the cycle of the pinocytosis vacuoles are seen to develop from the first hours on.

The lysosomes contain enzymes capable of digesting the capside and thus disclosing the nucleic acids, which are in turn digested by the nucleases. Other liberated particles make use of the cellular ribosomes for their reduplication.

Babblar and Chowdhury [1] found that, in CAM cultures, the cell lyses obtained 18 h after the infection had no infective titres but that these reached their maximum after 18 h.

It should be again pointed out that the basal cells of the corneal epithelium normally contain some isolated lysosomal particles, at the level of which a weak acid-phosphatase positivity can be demonstrated histochemically. Not much is known about the enzymes stored by those lysosomes. Our study showed a lysosomal cycle which lasted only 48 h, the particles thereafter diminished very rapidly. If, furthermore, we compare the lysosomal cycle to the experimental infectious cycle, we find that the former is distinctly shorter. The defensive cycle is thus insufficient and therefore could explain the survival of the virus in a latent form, until some other factor disturbs the cellular equilibrium and produces a recurrence.

The morphometric study indicated a very homogenous distribution of the particles of the lysosomal type, whereas the population of pinocytosis vacuoles was more heterogeneous. The cycle of the pinocytosis vacuoles overlapped that of the lysosomes.

The corticosteroids must have a

deleterious effect, even in the presence of a relatively intact epithelium, because by strengthening the lysosomal membrane and thereby preventing the liberation of the enzymes, they prevent the destruction of the capsides, which is favourable for the persistence of the virus in the latent state and thus its resistance to treatment.

**Acknowledgment.** We thank Miss L. van Renterghem, virologist, who procured us the herpes virus.

## References

1. Babblar OP, Chowdhury BL (1976) Studies on the possible role of lytic enzymes in the intracellular viral decoating using an "in vitro" virus trimming system. Indian J Med Res 64:824–834
2. François J, Victoria-Troncoso V, Miraglia O, Lentini F (1980) Experimental herpetic keratitis. Ophthalmic Res 12:205–220
3. Victoria-Troncoso V, Miraglia O, Lentini F (1980) Kératite herpétique expérimentale. Etude de la surface cornéenne au microscope à balayage. Bull Soc Belge Ophtalmol

## Discussion on the Contribution pp. 129–136

P.C. Maudgal (Leuven)
If I understood you correctly, did you say that the nucleated epithelial cells were on the surface because the superficial cells which are non-nucleated had exfoliated?

V. Victoria-Troncoso (Ghent)
Yes.

P.C. Maudgal (Leuven)
I have been studying the flat preparations of superficial corneal epithelium by corneal replica technique. I found that every superficial cell has a nucleus.

V. Victoria-Troncoso (Ghent)
Not all the superficial cells are nucleated. In normal conditions, most of them show an altered nucleus, however.

Sundmacher, R. (Hrsg.):
Herpetische Augenerkrankungen
© J.F. Bergmann Verlag, München 1981

# Unspecific Immunostimulation in Patients With Herpes Simplex Corneae Using BCG and Levamisole

G. Grabner, R. Jarisch, P. Heilig, E. Schuster, Wien

**Key words.** Herpetic keratitis – immunostimulation, levamisole, BCG

**Schlüsselwörter.** Herpeskeratitis – Immunstimulation, Levamisol, BCG

**Summary.** In 75 patients with primary or recurrent ocular herpes simplex virus (HSV) infection, a parameter of cell-mediated immunity (Leukocyte Migration Inhibitory Factor) was investigated. As a control, 22 persons free of herpetic disease were tested. Ten of the 22 were retested after a period of 14 days and seven after 6–9 months.

In 15 patients with recurrent epithelial HSV-infection the migration inhibition (MI) $(6.0 \pm 9.44\%)$ was significantly lower than the MI of the 14 patients with stromal involvement $(34.14 \pm 22.33\%, p < 0.001)$ or the MI of the control group $(28.0 \pm 17.27\%, p < 0.0001)$.

Patients with a MI below 20% received an immunostimulating therapy in addition to topical treatment. With a negative Tine-test, a BCG-vaccination was administered; with a positive one, Levamisole was given. During the course of the disease, a significant rise of MI was observed in the 17 treated as well as in the 11 untreated control patients; however, after a mean observation time of 11.38 months, the rise in the Levamisole-treated group was found to be significantly higher (p < 0.05). In this group the frequency of recurrences was slightly lower (4/17 = 23.5%) than in the untreated group (4/11 = 36.4%). A cautious interpretation is required, however, since the mean observation time of the treated patients was shorter than the one of the control group, although the difference was statistically not significant.

BCG-vaccination did not lead to a significant rise in MI in five patients after a period of 7.9 months.

**Zusammenfassung.** Bei 75 Patienten mit primärem oder rezidivierendem Herpes simplex corneae (HSV) wurde ein Parameter der zellulären Immunität mittels des Leukozyten-Migrations-Inhibitions-Testes in vitro gemessen. Als Kontrollgruppe dienten 22 Herpes-simplex-freie Personen, von denen zehn nach 14 Tagen und sieben nach einem Zeitraum von 6–9 Monaten neuerlich getestet wurden.

Bei fünfzehn Patienten mit rezidivierender, vorwiegend epithelialer HSV-Infektion war die Migrations-Inhibition (MI) $(6,0 \pm 9,44\%)$ signifikant niedriger als die MI der 14 Patienten mit zusätzlicher Stromabeteiligung $(34,14 \pm 22,33\%, p < 0,001)$ oder der MI der 22 Kontrollpersonen $(28,0 \pm 17,27\%, p < 0,0001)$.

Patienten mit einer MI unter 20% erhielten zusätzlich zur Lokaltherapie eine immunstimulierende allgemeine Therapie. Bei negativem Tine-Test wurde eine BCG-Impfung durchgeführt, bei positivem Ausfall eine Behandlung mit Levamisol. Im Verlauf der Erkrankung kam es sowohl bei 17 behandelten als auch bei elf unbehandelten Kontroll-Patienten zu einem signifikanten Anstieg der MI, der nach einem mittleren Beobachtungszeitraum von 11,38 Monaten bei der Levamisole behandelten Gruppe signifikant größer war (p < 0,05). In dieser Gruppe war auch die Rezidivrate etwas geringer (4/17 = 23,5%) als bei den unbehandelten Patienten (4/11 = 36,4%); dieses Ergebnis muß jedoch mit Vorsicht interpretiert werden, da der mittlere Beobachtungszeitraum in der Kontrollgruppe, wenn auch nicht statistisch signifikant, so doch etwas länger war. Die BCG-Behandlung führte bei fünf Patienten über einen Zeitraum von 7,9 Monaten zu keiner signifikanten Erhöhung der MI.

## Introduction

It is widely accepted that cell mediated immunity (CMI) plays a dominant role in the defense mechanisms against viral infections [1, 10, 16, 18]. Therefore, unspecific immunostimulation using BCG and Levamisole has encountered widespread interest in recent years (for review see [15]). Several research

137

groups have reported promising results of this treatment in patients with recurrent herpes labialis and aphthous stomatitis [6, 9, 14]. In addition, Jarisch and co-workers [7] were able to demonstrate a positive correlation between the clinical success of Levamisole and BCG therapy and the in vitro results of a leukocyte migration inhibitory factor assay (LMIF). Patients responding well to this treatment responded strongly to the herpes simplex virus (HSV) antigen whereas those with unaltered recurrences developed no antigen-stimulated reaction in the LMIF.

It is the aim of our study to investigate whether

a) the results of LMIF correlate with herpetic corneal disease,

b) nonspecific immunostimulation with Levamisole or BCG has an influence on LMIF in patients with herpetic corneal disease,

c) the results of LMIF parallels the clinical result due to therapy.

## Methods and Study Populations

### Migration Inhibition Assay

A method according to Glade [4] was used as previously described in detail [6]. Briefly, a direct assay of leukocyte migration inhibitory factor was performed, using heat-inactivated herpes simplex virus (type 1) antigen, and control cultures without antigen. After an incubation of 16 h migration areas were projected on a screen (eight fold magnification) and measured by planimetry. All tests were performed in quadruplicate and were highly reproducible. Migration inhibition was then calculated using the following formula: % migration inhibition = 100 X

$$\frac{\text{mean area of migration (controls)} - \text{mean area of migration (with HSV-Ag)}}{\text{mean area of migration (controls)}}$$

An inhibition of more than 20% was considered positive and a demonstration of virus-antigen stimulated CMI response [4].

### Patient and Control Populations

Primary Ocular HSV Infection

We tested 46 patients (age: 6–81 years, mean: 44.78 years) at different times (from 2 days up to 8 weeks) after the onset of the disease. Of these patients 19 presented additional involvement of the corneal stroma (infiltration, edema) and mild anterior uveitis at the time of blood sampling. Fifteen were tested when the dendritic ulcer was already healed.

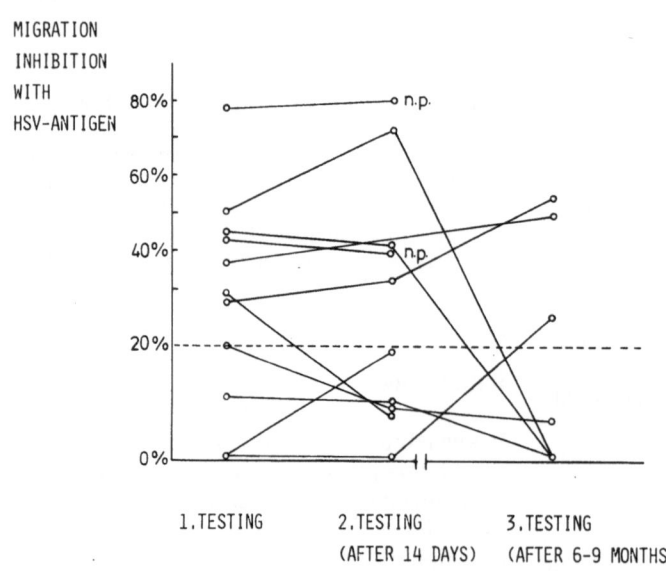

1.TESTING     2.TESTING     3.TESTING
(AFTER 14 DAYS)    (AFTER 6-9 MONTHS)

N.P.: 3RD TESTING NOT POSSIBLE

**Fig. 1.** Control group (longitudinal study) (N = 10)

138

## Recurrent Ocular HSV Infection

Of the 29 patients (age: 3–71 years, mean: 43.61 years, duration of the disease: 2 months–31 years) 20 were tested during an active and 9 during a quiescent stage. In 14 of these the corneal stroma was involved, in the 15 others the disease affected the corneal epithelium only.

## The Control Population

It consisted of 22 individuals (age: 13–84 years, mean 50.59 years); they had been free of herpetic disease for at least a year or usually more. Ten of these were retested after an interval of 14 days, in addition seven were retested after an interval of 6–9 months (Fig. 1).

### Treatment Schedules

Prior to immunostimulating therapy a Tine-test was performed on all the patients (5 IU Oldtuberculine, puncture test, classified after 48 and 72 h as − to ++++).

– In patients with a migration inhibition (MI) *below* 20%, topical treatment was combined with an *immunostimulating therapy:*
  a) whenever the Tine-test yielded a negative result, *BCG* was applied intradermally once (five patients in total),
  b) whenever the Tine-test was positive, *Levamisole* was used for treatment.
  (3 × 50 mg for 3 days, repeated every 14 days, five times. White blood count was performed before and during the treatment at monthly intervals.)

– Topical treatment only was applied in patients where the MI to HSV-Ag was *above* 20%.

*Control patients:* Eleven patients with a MI below 20% received neither immunostimulating therapy (seven of which received a placebo).

*Double-masked control trial for Levamisole-induced changes in LMIF:* A group of 18 patients received Levamisole in a coded man-

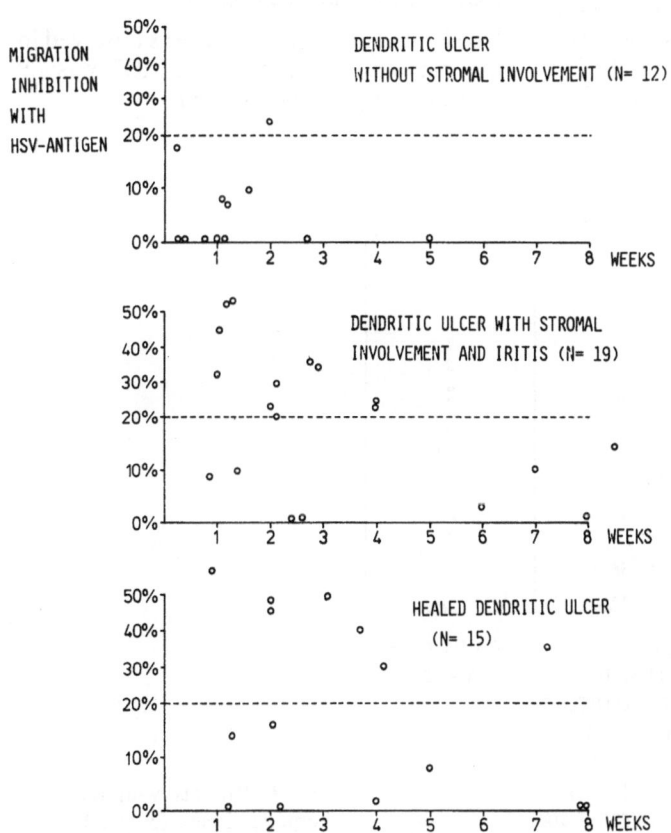

**Fig. 2.** Results of LMIF-testing, patients with primary HSV-infection (N = 46)

139

ner; LMIF was retested in 14 of those after a mean observation time of 5.1 months (2.5–11 months).

*Statistical evaluation:* The different groups were compared using the Kruskal-Wallis test. The statistical differences were discovered using the U-test; because of multiple comparisons corrections according to Bonferoni were necessary.

## Results

### Primary Ocular HSV Infections

The MI with HSV-antigen in 46 patients is shown in Fig. 2. However, a valid statistical comparison between these three groups is not possible, since the patients were tested at different times after the onset of the disease and rapid changes (within a few days) of MI were described [10].

### Recurrent Ocular HSV Infections

Results of LMIF are shown in Fig. 3. Fourteen patients with deep stromal involvement (disciform keratitis, infiltration, vascularisation, ulceration and iridocyclitis) had a mean MI of $34.14 \pm 22.33\%$ (range = 0–67%). This value is not significantly different from

the one in the control group. In contrast, 15 patients with only recurrent dendritic ulcers, without significant inflammatory signs of the corneal stroma or the anterior uvea had a mean MI of $6.0 \pm 9.44\%$ (range: 0–33%). Statistical comparison between the two groups showed this difference to be significant ($p < 0.001$). The mean MI of patients with predominantly epithelial disease also differed significantly from the MI of the control group ($28.0 \pm 17.27\%$, range: 0–78%), $p < 0.0001$.

### Double-Masked Trial (Fig. 4)

Of the 18 patients receiving Levamisole or a placebo in a coded manner, 14 (7/7) could be retested after a mean observation time (MOT) of 5.1 months (range: 2.5 to 11 months). Values of MI increased significantly in both groups (Levamisole: $p < 0.02$; placebo: $p < 0.05$), however the mean changes of both groups did *not* differ significantly. The MOT of both groups did not differ significantly either.

### BCG Treated Patients (Fig. 6)

No significant change in MI was observed in five patients treated by BCG. MOT was 7.9 months (range: 6–14 months).

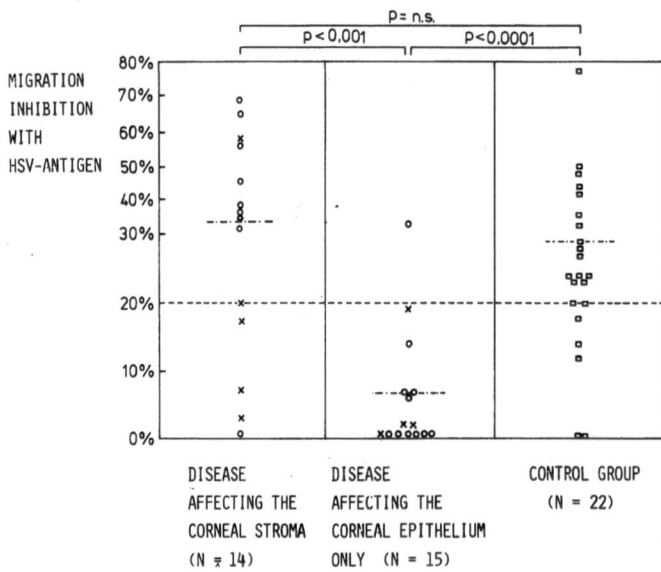

Fig. 3. Patients with recurrent herpetic disease (N = 29)

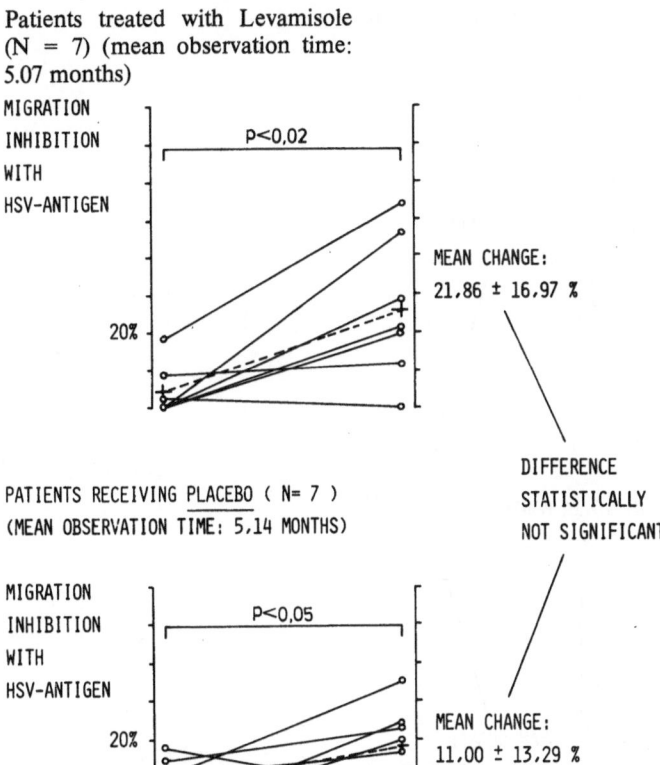

Patients treated with Levamisole (N = 7) (mean observation time: 5.07 months)

MIGRATION INHIBITION WITH HSV-ANTIGEN

p<0,02

20%

MEAN CHANGE: 21,86 ± 16,97 %

PATIENTS RECEIVING PLACEBO ( N= 7 )
(MEAN OBSERVATION TIME: 5,14 MONTHS)

MIGRATION INHIBITION WITH HSV-ANTIGEN

p<0,05

20%

MEAN CHANGE: 11,00 ± 13,29 %

DIFFERENCE STATISTICALLY NOT SIGNIFICANT

**Fig. 4.** Results of treatment. Influence of Levamisole on LMIF (double-blind study, 18 patients, 4 dropouts)

*Influence of Levamisole on LMIF and Frequency of Recurrences*

(Fig. 5) (Open *and* double masked study) The 17 patients treated with Levamisole over periods from 2.5 to 29 months (MOT: 11.38 months) showed a pronounced increase of MI after treatment (p < 0.0001). In patients where several tests were performed, values of the first and last LMIF were used for calculations. We observed four recurrences out of these 17 patients (= 23.5%) (one severe metaherpetic ulceration, one metaherpetic dystrophy with secondary glaucoma, needing enucleation and two dendritic ulcers).

The eleven patients observed over periods of 3 to 38 months (MOT: 16.14 months) without any immunostimulating therapy also showed a significant rise in MI (p < 0.02). In this group four recurrences (all dendritic ulcers) were observed (= 36.4%). The mean change of MI (23.94 ± 16.27%) of the treated patients differed significantly (p < 0.05) from the mean change of MI (10.36 ± 13.08%) of the untreated patients. The MOT ob both groups did not differ significantly.

*Side Effects of Levamisole Treatment*

Only one patient discontinued treatment because of unspecified cardiac sensations. No change in w.b.c. (e.g. leucopenia) was observed.

**Discussion**

The testing of one parameter of cell mediated immunity to HSV-antigen (the production of a leukocyte migration inhibitory factor by immunocompetent cells) in a larger group of patients with primary or recurrent ocular HSV-infections has confirmed our preliminary results [5]: patients with predominantly epithelial involvement of the cornea (primary or recurrent disease) show a significantly lower migration inhibition than those with stromal involvement or healthy controls. It has to be noted, however, that marked fluctuations of migration inhibition are observed in healthy people over prolonged periods of time and that patients with herpetic eye disease have remained free of recurrences for up to 2 years without detectable LMIF.

141

Patients treated with Levamisole (N = 17) (observation time: 2.5 to 29 months, mean: 11.38 months

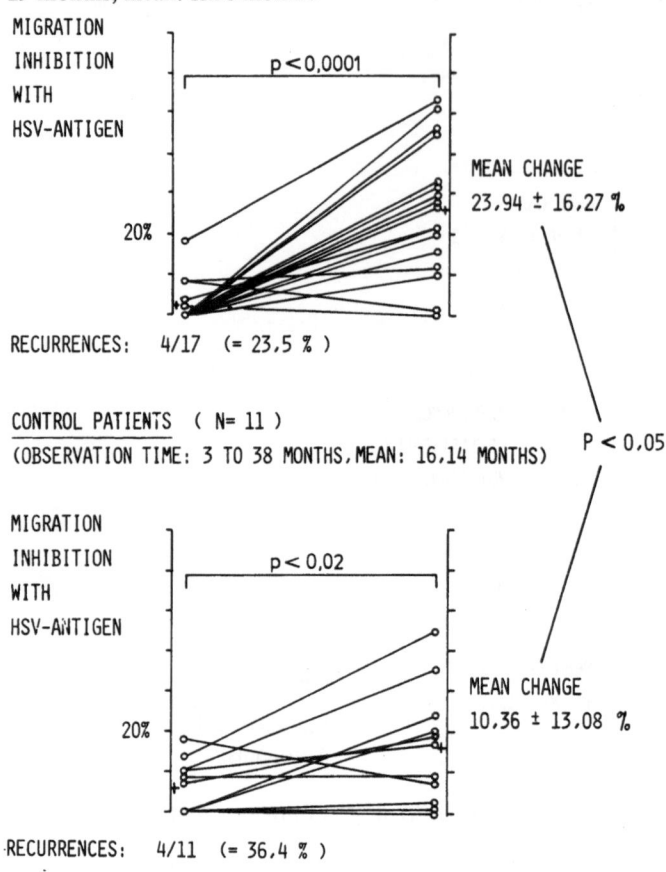

MIGRATION INHIBITION WITH HSV-ANTIGEN

p < 0,0001

20%

MEAN CHANGE 23,94 ± 16,27 %

RECURRENCES:     4/17   (= 23,5 % )

CONTROL PATIENTS  ( N= 11 )
(OBSERVATION TIME: 3 TO 38 MONTHS, MEAN: 16,14 MONTHS)

P < 0,05

MIGRATION INHIBITION WITH HSV-ANTIGEN

p < 0,02

20%

MEAN CHANGE 10,36 ± 13,08 %

RECURRENCES:    4/11   (= 36,4 % )

THE OBSERVATION TIMES DO NOT DIFFER SIGNIFICANTLY.

**Fig. 5.** Influence of Levamisole on LMIF and frequency of recurrences. All patients, open and doubleblind study

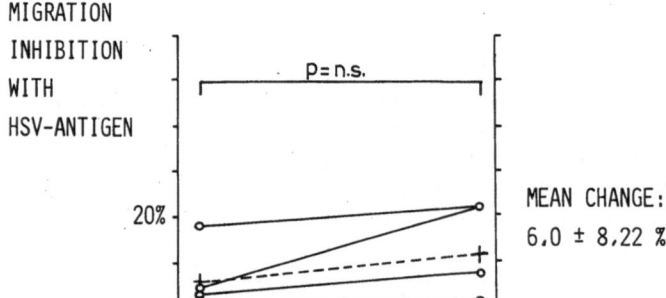

MIGRATION INHIBITION WITH HSV-ANTIGEN

P= n.s.

20%

MEAN CHANGE: 6,0 ± 8,22 %

**Fig. 6.** Influence of BCG treatment on LMIF (5 patients, mean observation time: 7.9 months)

Therefore prognostic predictions based on this in vitro assay are to be made with caution. Nevertheless we feel that patients without detectable LMIF run a greater risk of getting herpetic infections than those with an inhibition over 20%. In addition, we have observed dendritic ulcers in patients with high LMIF after topical treatment with corti-

costeroids. We conclude therefore, that LMIF, measuring activities of immunocompetent cells in the peripheral blood, does not necessarily reflect the *local* immunological situation at the priviledged site of the cornea.

It is apparent from our studies, however, that during the natural course of the disease a significant increase of LMIF occurs even in patients without additional immunostimulating therapy.

From experimental studies in guinea pigs, performed by Smolin and co-workers [12], it appears that a pretreatment with BCG does not produce a beneficial effect on the course and on the titers of virus present in the affected corneas. In contrast, a good response to this treatment was reported by Jarisch et al. [7] in patients with herpes simplex labialis. Due to our present treatment schedule, only five patients received a BCG vaccination, leaving LMIF unaffected after a mean observation time of 7.9 months. No valid conclusion on the recurrence rate is possible due to the small number. Levamisole, an antihelminthic agent and BCG nonspecifically normalize depressed CMI responses, presumably by stimulating macrophage and lymphocyte functions [2, 6, 11, 17]; for review see [15]. There is conflicting experimental evidence regarding the treatment of herpes simplex keratitis in rabbits. Whereas Kaufman and Varnell [8] observed no alteration in acute infection and recurrence rate, Smolin et al. [13] reported a more rapid healing of epithelial lesions and far less stromal opacifications in steroid-pretreated and reinfected animals [3].

We now report a significant rise in LMIF in patients treated with Levamisole in comparison to untreated patients. The frequency of recurrences was also lower in those receiving immunostimulating therapy $(4/17 = 23.5\%)$ than in control patients $(4/11 = 36.4\%)$. A very cautious interpretation is required, however, since the mean observation time of the treated group was shorter than the one of the control group, although the difference was statistically not significant. The lack of serious side-effects is encouraging for a further long-time observation, which we hope will help to definitely clarify whether our finding is a lasting success of immunostimulating therapy.

**Acknowledgment.** The authors are very grateful to Mrs. Irene Matejovsky and Mrs. Emmi Zambo (both Department of Dermatology I) for their excellent technical assistance.

# References

1. Easty DL, Maini RN, Jones BR (1973) Cellular immunity in herpes simplex keratitis. Trans Ophthalmol Soc UK 93:171–180
2. Florentin J, Huchet R, Bruley-Rosset M, Halle-Panenko O, Mathe G (1976) Studies on the mechanisms of action of BCG. Cancer Immunol Immunother 1:31–39
3. Friedlaender MH, Smolin G, Okumoto M (1978) The treatment of herpetic reinfection with levamisole. Am J Ophthalmol 86:245–249
4. Glade PR, Broder SW, Grotsiky H, Hirschhorn K (1971) The use of cultured lymphoid cells as target cells for the detection of migration inhibitory factors: In: Bloom BR, David JR (eds) In vitro methods in cell-mediated immunity. Academic, New York, pp 307–312
5. Grabner G, Jarisch R (1979) Leukocyte migration inhibitory factor in primary and recurrent ocular infections with Herpes simplexvirus. Preliminary results. Albrecht von Graefes Arch Klin Ophthalmol 211:85–93
6. Jarisch R, Sandor I (1977) MIF in der Therapiekontrolle von Herpes simplex recidivans: Behandlung mit Levamisole, BCG, Urushiol and Herpes Antigen Vaccine. Arch Derm Res 258:151–159
7. Jarisch R, Sandor I, Cerni C (1979) Der Leukozytenmigrationshemmtest (LMIT) bei Herpes simplex labialis recidivans. Vergleich der Therapieerfolge mit BCG und Levamisole. Arch Derm Res 265:15–22
8. Kaufman HE, Varnell ED (1977) Lack of levamisole effect on experimental herpes keratitis. Invest Ophthalmol Visual Sci 16:1148–1150
9. Kint A, Verlinden L (1974) Levamisole for recurrent herpes labialis. N Engl J Med 291:308
10. O'Reilly RJ, Chibbaro A, Anger E, Lopez C (1977) Cell mediated immune responses in patients with recurrent herpes simplex infections. II. Infection-associated deficiency of lymphokine production in patients with recurrent herpes labialis or herpes progenitalis. J Immunol 118:1095–1102
11. Sher NA, Poplack DG, Blaese RM, Brown TM, Chaparas SC (1977) Effect of corynebacterium parvum, methanolextraction residue of BCG and levamisole on macrophage random migration, chemotaxis and periocytosis. J Natl Cancer Inst 58:1753–1757
12. Smolin G, Okumoto M, Belfort jr R (1975) The treatment of experimental herpetic keratitis with BCG. Can J Ophthalmol 10:385–390
13. Smolin G, Okumoto M, Friedlaender M: Treatment of herpes simplex keratitis with levamisole. Arch Ophthalmol 96:1078–1081
14. Symoens J, Brugmans J (1974) Treatment of recurrent aphthous stomatitis and herpes with levamisole. Br J Med 4:592–593
15. Symoens J, Rosenthal M, Brabander M de, Goldstein G (1979) Immunoregulation with Levamisole. Springers Semin Immunopathol 2:49–68

16. Tokumary TY, Shimizu Y, Sabety Y (1975) Herpetic epithelial keratitis: a radioassay evaluation of the host's humoral and cellular responsiveness. Ophthal Res 7:345–353
17. Verhaegen H, Decree J, Cock W de (1974) Levamisole and the immune response. N Engl J Med 289:1148–1149
18. Wilton JMA, Ivanyi L, Lehner T (1972) Cell mediated immunity in herpes virus hominis infections. Br Med J 1:723–726

## Discussion on the Contribution pp. 137–144

R. Sundmacher (Freiburg)
I would like to point to a problem which you, of course, know, but of which not all participants may be aware. When a clinician speaks of "primary" dendritic keratitis, he most often means the first manifestation of this disease, which has nothing to do with a true primary infection in the course of which you observe seroconversion. As has been pointed out before, most cases of so-called "primary" dendritic keratitis in fact represent already recurrences from the pathophysiological point of view. This is because the true primary infection is mostly subclinical and noted by neither patient nor doctor. To avoid confusion, I would suggest that also the clinical ophthalmologists be reluctant in using the term "primary" which should be reserved for those cases with seroconversion. The other point I'd like to make is that things being as outlined above, you would not actually expect any differences between a "primary" dendritic keratitis in the clinical sense (i.e. the first manifestation) and a recurrent dendritic keratitis, would you? And exactly this has been your result.

G. Grabner (Wien)
I completely agree with you in regard to the pathophysiology of herpetic eye infection. We introduced the subdivisions "primary" and recurrent herpes simplex keratitis only because these terms are commonly used by ophthalmologists. Immunological findings do not show any significant differences between the two.

Sundmacher, R. (Hrsg.):
Herpetische Augenerkrankungen
© J.F. Bergmann Verlag, München 1981

# Herpetic Keratitis In Diet Deficient Animals. I. Zinc Deficiency*

G. Smolin, M. Okumoto, L. Feiler, D. Condon, San Francisco

**Key words.** Zinc deficiency, herpetic keratitis

**Schlüsselwörter.** Zinkmangel, Herpeskeratitis

**Summary.** Thirty New Zealand white adult rabbits weighing 5 to 6 pounds were divided into two groups of 15 animals each. Group I received a regular diet and group II received the identical diet from which zinc was removed. The animals were weighed weekly. After 3 weeks, sheep red blood cells (SRBC) were injected into all animals. One week later, the animals were bled to determine their zinc plasma level and antibody response to SRBC. The animals were skin-tested to oxazolone (a skin-sensitizer). One drop of a pH-strain Herpes simplex virus was placed onto the previously scarified corneas of all animals.

In group 1, half of the animals received two saline drops Q/D and the other half received two drops Q/D 1% zinc sulphate solution. In group II, the animals were similarly divided and treated.

The zinc-deficient animals weighed significantly less than the control animals after 2 weeks. Their plasma zinc levels and immune responses were depressed.

The zinc deficient untreated animals had the worst herpetic keratitis as compared to all other subgroups. Treatment of comparable rabbits with the local zinc resulted in no change herpetic keratitis.

**Zusammenfassung.** Es wurden 30 weiße Neuseelandkaninchen von 5–6 Pfund Gewicht in zwei Gruppen zu 15 Tieren eingeteilt. Die erste Gruppe erhielt ein normales Futter, die zweite hingegen eine zinkfreie Nahrung. Die Tiere wurden wöchentlich gewogen. Nach 3 Wochen wurden sie alle durch Injektionen mit Schaferythrozyten immunisiert. Eine Woche später bestimmten wir dann den Zink-Plasmaspiegel sowie die Antikörper-Titer gegenüber den Schaferythrozyten. Außerdem wurden die Tiere auf ihre Reaktion auf Oxazolon (ein Hautallergen) überprüft. Dann erhielten alle Tiere einen Tropfen des Herpes simplex-Virusstammes PH auf die skarifizierte Hornhaut.

In der ersten Gruppe erhielt die Hälfte der Tiere täglich 0.2 ml Kochsalzlösung subkonjunktival, die andere 0,2 ml einer 1%igen Zink-Sulfat-Lösung. Die Tiere in der Gruppe 2 wurden genauso aufgeteilt und behandelt.

Die Zink-Mangeltiere wogen nach 2 Wochen signifikant weniger als die Kontrolltiere und ihre Zink-Plasmaspiegel sowie die Immunreaktionen waren deutlich erniedrigt.

Die unbehandelten Zink-Mangeltiere hatten verglichen mit allen anderen Untergruppen die schwerste Herpeskeratitis.

Die Behandlung solcher Tiere mit lokalen Zink-Gaben führte dann zu einer milderen Herpeskeratitis ähnlich wie in den Kontrollgruppen.

## Discussion on the Contribution pp. 145

E. Bloch-Michel (Paris)
Your results are extremely striking. Do you know other examples of immune disease induced by zinc deficiency?

G. Smolin (San Francisco)
There are several good articles regarding zinc and the immune system. *Good* demonstrated that zinc added to lymphocytes can enhance blastogenesis in the elderly population whereas in the young, healthy population it had no effect. He concluded that zinc is effective in enhancing the immune response in a immunosuppressed population. In addition, *Golden* in *Lancet* demonstrated that an immunosuppressed population of children on a very low protein diet was anergic to common skin antigens (trichophytin, SKSD, mumps, etc.). If they rubbed zinc on the test sites the children developed normal cell-mediated immune responses at that

---

* A detailed presentation of the material has been accepted for publication by Invest Ophthalmol

site. There are many articles regarding acrodermatitis enteropathica. These people have depressed cellular immunity, but if fed zinc their immunologic status may return to normal. Patients on unusual diets or hyperalimentation may become zinc deficient and immunosuppressed. The addition of zinc may correct the defect. In the Turkish literature there was an article about Hodgkin's patients who had depressed cellular immunity and depressed zinc levels. The addition of zinc occasionally enhanced the immune status of these patients.

D. Easty (Bristol)

Did you look at specific responses in these animals, like antibody titres or cell-mediated reactions to specific virus? How do you think this depression affected your model? Did you make any measurements of humoral or cellmediated responses in these animals as a result of their infection with a herpes simplex virus? What I'm asking is: Did you find evidence of specific depression of immune responses?

G. Smolin (San Francisco)

Regarding the herpetic disease, I observed the clinical course of the disease in the cornea. I demonstrated that their cell-mediated immune response was depressed by performing skin tests to oxazolone. I also tested the animals antibody response to sheep red blood cells. The weight loss, mortality rate and poor health also reflected the depressed immune status of the zinc deficient animals.

W.H. Prusoff (New Haven)

Instead of giving the zinc topically, did you try giving the zinc systemically? If so, is there any difference in effect?

G. Smolin (San Francisco)

We are presently testing the effect of systemic zinc in this model and I do not have the results at this time.

Y.C. Cheng (Chapel Hill)

Is it possible that zinc is in some way required for the adequate absorption of food in the intestine? The observations you made may relate to malnutrition.

G. Smolin (San Francisco)

I'am sure that is partly true. In many states in which there is zinc deficiency, acrodermatitis, for example, the patients develop diarrhea; so they are loosing other elements as well, there is no question about it. As far as our experiments are concerned I can't relate to you statistically, but the animals started to die off early at a very high rate. So there's no question in my mind that zinc played a role; and that they also developed diarrhea was another factor involved. But there have been in vitro studies with purely zinc which have shown that zinc does play an active role in cell immunity and possibly in humoral immunity.

Sundmacher, R. (Hrsg.):
Herpetische Augenerkrankungen
© J.F. Bergmann Verlag, München 1981

# Coefficient of Antibody Activity in the Aqueous Humor to That in the Serum in Ocular Herpes Simplex

J. Denis, A. Rossignol, M. Langlois, C. Dorey, M. Aymard, J.P. Giraud, Paris, Lyon

**Key words.** Acqeous humour – specific antiherpetic antibody coefficient, antibody mediated immunity

**Schlüsselwörter.** Kammerwasser – spezifischer antiherpetischer Antikörper-Koeffizient, antikörpervermittelte Immunität

**Summary.** The biological diagnosis of serious intraocular herpetic infections is generally only possible due to a study of the aqueous humor either by the isolation of the viral strain, by the demonstration of viral antigens or by an elevation in the coefficient of antiherpetic antibody activity in the aqueous humor to that in the serum, which seems to correspond to a local synthesis of antibody. The study of this coefficient concerned 163 aqueous humor-serum pairs taken from patients, the majority of whom were suffering from anterior segmentitis, disciform keratitis, interstitial keratitis or uveitis.

The titration of the antiherpetic antibodies by passive hemagglutination (Ab AH, AbS) and the assay of total immunoglobulin using the Laurell technique (Ig AH, IgS) allowed the coefficient to be calculated:

$$C = \frac{Ab\,AH}{Ab\,S} \times \frac{IG\,S}{Ig\,AH}$$ which normally is equal to 1.

82 coefficients out of 163 (50.3%) were lower or equal to 1, i.e. not signifying ocular herpes. 81 were superior to 1. Statistical calculation allows, at present, a coefficient above or equal to 2 to be considered significant for a herpetic infection, that is to say 59 coefficients in this study (36.2%) leaving 22 coefficients (13.5%) which are of an uncertain diagnostic value. 91 specimens were studied in parallel with regard to measles, an ubiquitous infection of children, usually without ocular involvement. The titer of antimeasles antibody in the aqueous humor is a function of the hematocamerular barrier. The measles coefficients remained low, with one exception, and thus support the diagnostic value of a raised herpes coefficient. The comparison of herpes and measles coefficients is above all useful when the herpes coefficient is around the limiting value of 2.

Out of the 163 patients, with various different diseases, 88 ocular herpes cases were identified on the basis on the basis of well-defined clinical or biological criteria. For 38 of the latter, the increase in the herpes coefficient was the only diagnostic element. This coefficient is especially significant in diseases of the anterior chamber in the acute phase: anterior segmentitis or deep keratitis; it remains low in superficial keratitis and is exceptionally raised in isolated uveitis. The coefficient is not significant in the other 22 cases of ocular herpes diagnosed by other criteria. The cause of this failure is not always evident. It is possible that a variation in viral multiplication in the uvea is responsible.

**Zusammenfassung.** Die Diagnose eines intraokularen Herpes kann man nur durch die Virusisolierung aus dem Kammerwasser oder den Nachweis von Virusantigen aus dem Augeninnern oder schließlich durch die Bestimmung eines spezifischen Antikörper-Koeffizienten stellen, der das Verhältnis der Antikörper im Kammerwasser zu dem im Serum angibt und bei positivem Ausfall für eine lokale Antikörperproduktion spricht. Wir untersuchten 163 Kammerwasser-Serum-Paare. Die meisten Patienten litten an einer vorderen Segmentitis, einer disciformen Keratitis, einer interstitiellen Keratitis oder einer Uveitis. Wenn man die spezifischen Antikörper mit der passiven Hämagglutination und die Gesamt-Immunproteine mit der Laurell-Technik bestimmt, kann man folgenden Koeffizienten berechnen, der im allgemeinen ungefähr 1 ist:

$$C = \frac{AK\,KW}{AK\,S} \times \frac{Ig\,S}{Ig\,KW}$$

Von 163 Koeffizienten waren 82 ≦ 1 (50,3%) und sprachen gegen eine Herpes-Ätiologie, 81 waren über 1. Nach statistischen Berechnungen nehmen wir derzeit einen Koeffizienten von gleich oder größer als 2 als beweisend für eine Herpesinfektion an. Dies fanden wir 59mal (36,2%). 22 Koeffizienten waren diagnostisch grenzwertig und damit unsicher (13,5%). Bei 91 Patienten konnten wir gleichzeitig auch den spezifischen Koeffizienten für Masernantikörper bestimmen, eine Infektion des Kindesalters ohne intraokulare Komplikationen. Deshalb kann man die Menge der Masern-AK im Kammerwasser als Ausdruck der Durchlässigkeit der Blut-Kammerwasserschranke ansehen. Bis auf eine Ausnahme blieben die Masern-Koeffizienten tatsächlich niedrig und bestätigten damit den diagnostischen Wert gleichzeitig auf über 2 erhöhter Herpes-Koeffizienten.

Bei 88 von den 163 Patienten stellten wir die Herpesdiagnose aufgrund anerkannter klinischer Kriterien oder aufgrund unseres Testausfalles. Letzteres war 38mal das einzige Kriterium. Der Koeffizient erscheint uns besonders hilfreich bei Erkrankungen im Bereich der Vorderkammer wie einer akuten vorderen Segmentitis oder einer tiefen Keratitis; bei einer oberflächlichen Keratitis bleibt er niedrig; im Gegensatz hierzu ist er bei einer isolierten Uveitis ungewöhnlich hoch. 22mal fanden wir trotz der anderweitig wahrscheinlichen Herpesdiagnose keinen erhöhten Koeffizienten. Warum das so war, ist nicht immer klar. Möglicherweise sind Besonderheiten und Schwankungen der Virusvermehrung in der Uvea hierfür verantwortlich.

Ocular herpes, once considered as a benign infection, has now become a real adventure and neither the course of the disease nor the end result are known. The spread of the lesions towards the uvea occurs frequently, and the clinical aspect can be serious from the onset: disciform keratitis, interstitial or deep keratitis, uveitis or anterior segmentitis (26). Superficial keratitis sometimes only appears at a second stage and does not always have the characteristic aspect of a dendritic ulcer.

The biological diagnosis of intraocular herpetic lesions is difficult. The removal of specimens from the interior of the globe is limited; punction of the anterior chamber is the most usual method allowing aqueous humor to be collected. Iris specimens are still infrequent [31]. Thus the study of the aqueous humor is about the only means of proving an intraocular herpetic infection. Two methods are available:
– detection of viral antigens or isolation of the viral strain,
– proof of an intraocular local formation of specific antibodies.

The isolation of the viral strain has been performed with some success since the work of Cavara [3], in particular by Sundmacher and Neumann-Haefelin [25]. The detection of viral antigens in cells from the aqueous humor has been carried out in a limited number of cases by Patterson et al. [18] and Kaufman et al. [12] using immunofluorescence.

The presence of specific antibodies in the aqueous humor is not synonymous with a local formation, since these can come from the blood by crossing the hemato-camerular barrier [10, 16] and are normally at a concentration 500 times less than that in the serum. The efficiency of this barrier varies, in particular with an inflammatory state. To evaluate the local formation of antibodies, it is necessary to compare the titers of antibodies in the serum and in the aqueous humor, by referring them to the quantities of globulins in these two liquids, by use of the coefficient of Goldmann and Witmer [9]:

$$C = \frac{Ab\ AH}{Ab\ S} \times \frac{Ig\ S}{Ig\ AH}$$

Ab AH: Titer of specific antibody in the aqueous humor
Ab S: Titer of specific antibody in the serum
Ig S: Quantity of immunoglobulin in the serum
Ig AH: Quantity of immunoglobulin in the aqueous humor

This coefficient is normally equal to 1, and its increase is significant of an ocular lesion. The diagnostic value of this coefficient has been shown during various experimental [8, 23, 24, 28, 29, 32] and clinical [7, 14, 15, 30, 31] ocular infections. Its usefulness in ocular herpes infections has been known since 1967 [2]. The titration of antiherpetic antibodies by passive hemagglutination, a more sensitive technique than complement fixation, has increased the diagnostic importance of this method; thus in a previous study on 30 patients with ocular herpes, 20 had a significant coefficient [4].

This present work involves 177 aqueous humor-serum pairs, taken between 1971 and 1978. Its objective was to define the diagnostic interest of the coefficient of antiherpetic antibody activity in the aqueous humor to that in the serum, as well as its reliability and its margin of error. For this, the coefficient obtained with regard to herpes was compared to that calulated for measles, a viral infection usually at a young age, and in general without ocular involvement. In the latter case the antimeasles antibodies can only enter the aqueous humor by crossing the hemato-camerular barrier.

## Material and Methods

### Patients

These consisted of 112 men and 65 women. This male predominance is a usually found occurrence in epidemiological studies on ocular herpes. The distribution of this population according to age was approximately uniform for different age groups which ranged from 4 to 83 years, with, however, a lower number of patients under 20 years of age. Aqueous humor and serum was taken simultaneously from each patient; 7 patients were sampled two or three times, either successively or bilaterally.

In general these patients suffered from serious ocular disease:

26 disciform keratitis
20 anterior segmentitis with disciform keratitis
50 anterior segmentitis
35 anterior segmentitis with glaucoma
13 iridocyclitis
16 both interstitial and superficial keratitis
 4 superficial keratitis
 3 unknown symptoms
29 of the patients had bilateral lesions and 70% of the cases were recurrences.

At the time of sampling only 25 cases had been diagnosed as herpes, based on two criteria: dendritic corneal ulcer and/or isolation of the viral strain from a corneo-conjunctival specimen.

### Titration of Antiherpetic and Antimeasles Antibodies

Serum and aqueous humor of the same subject were studied simultaneously. Two tests of similar sensitivity were chosen:
 – Passive hemagglutination for the titration of antiherpetic antibody in the aqueous humor and serum.
 – Inhibition of the hemagglutination for the titration of antimeasles antibody, carried out simultaneously on 91 pairs of samples.

a) *Antiherpetic antibody* was titrated by passive hemagglutination, using the technique of Huraux et al. [11], on conical-bottomed microplates with an antigen of type 1. The viral strain used for the preparation of the antigen was isolated from a child's throat, then cultured on KB cells. The antigen was fixed on tanned sheep red blood cells. Serum and aqueous humor were decomplemented, and tested in doubling dilutions; the first dilutions were $\frac{1}{8}$ and $\frac{1}{2}$ respectively. A comparative titration was always carried out with serum absorbed with sheep red blood cells. The reaction was performed using several controls: serum, red blood cells, cellular antigen and by the titration of five different diluted sera, containing different levels of antibody. Two tests were read after overnight incubation at +4 °C with the plates inclined at 45°.

b) *The antimeasles antibodies* were titrated by inhibition of hemagglutination using the classical technique of Rosen [20]. The antigen was prepared by culture of the Enders virus strain on human cells, then treated with Tween 80 and ether. It was used at 4 hemagglutinating units. The samples to be tested were inactivated, treated with kaolin and absorbed with the red blood cells of *cercopithecus aethiops,* which were subsequently used in the hemagglutination reaction. Doubling dilutions were carried out, the first at $\frac{1}{2}$ for the aqueous humors and at $\frac{1}{10}$ for the sera.

### Measurement of Total Ig

The method used was the rocket immunoelectrophoretic technique of Laurell [27]. Sera diluted in a 0.013 M veronal buffer, formolised at 0.4 M, at $\frac{1}{40}$, and the aqueous humors, at $\frac{1}{2}$, were examined simultaneously for the same subject. The assay of total Ig was carried out by comparison with 3 dilutions of the same reference serum, $\frac{1}{40}$, $\frac{1}{80}$ and $\frac{1}{160}$ which were always included in each reaction plate. These plates were submitted to an electric current of 2.5 volts/cm gel, for 18 h at 12 °C. The comparison was carried out on the basis of the product of the height of the peak and the width at mid-height, which leads to a greater precision than the square of the height.

Aqueous humor-serum pairs (163) were thus studied, the volume of the 14 other aqueous humors having become insufficient after titration of the antibodies.

### Calculation of the Coefficients of Antibody Activity in the Aqueous Humor to That in the Serum

The coefficient C: $\dfrac{Ab\ AH}{Ab\ S} \times \dfrac{Ig\ S}{Ig\ AH}$

149

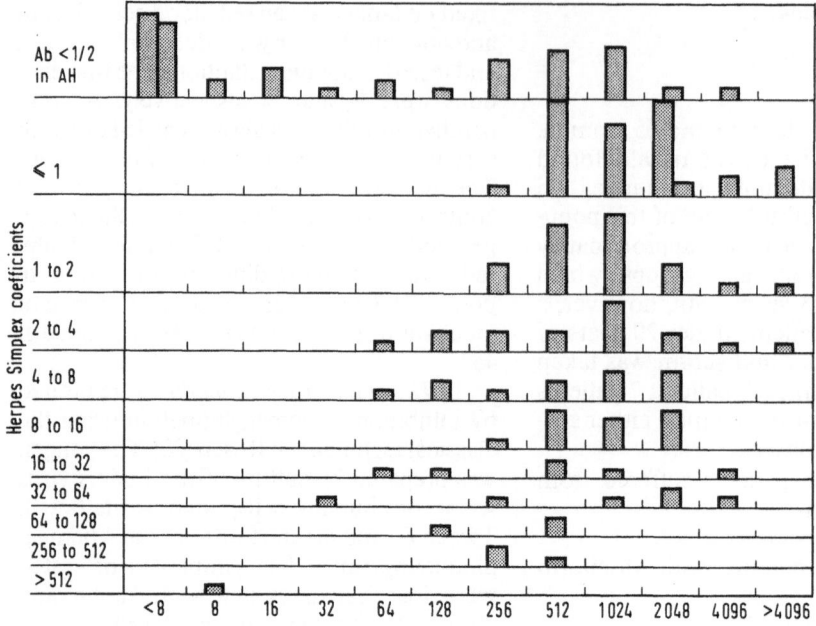

**Fig. 1.** Relation between serum antiherpetic anti bodies and coefficients in the aqueous humor. 163 paired samples of AH and serum. Antiherpetic AB in sera

is evaluated comparatively with respect to Herpes, a suspected ocular infection, and with respect to measles, a previous viral infection, whose level of antibody in the aqueous humor depends uniquely on the blood-aqueous barrier.

**Results**

*Calculation of the Coefficients of Antiherpetic Antibody Activity in the Aqueous Humor to That in the Serum*

The aqueous humor was generally low in

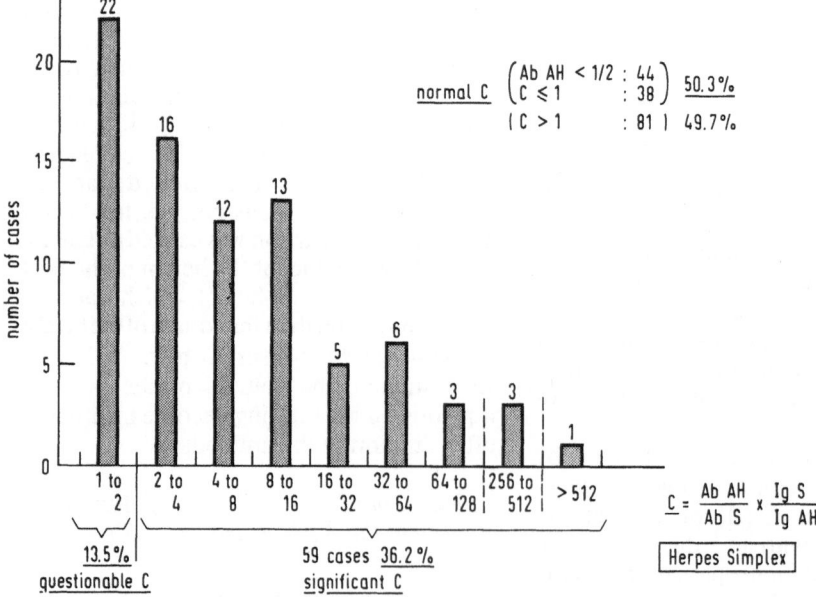

**Fig. 2.** Numerical value of the 163 coefficients

150

**Table 1.** Seven patients with AB AH ≫ AB S

| Patients | AB AH | AB S | $\dfrac{\text{IG S}}{\text{IG AH}}$ | C |
|---|---|---|---|---|
| 1 | 8 | 8 | 668,73 | 668,73 |
| 2 | 512 | 512 | 15,27 | 15,27 |
| 3 | 1024 | 1024 | 7,54 | 7,54 |
| 4 | 1024 | 1024 | 8,41 | 8,41 |
| 5 | 2048 | 2048 | 14,02 | 14,02 |
| 6 | 4096 | 4096 | 3,06 | 48,96 |
| 7 | 4096 | 512 | 34,90 | 279,18 |

Variability of $\dfrac{\text{IG S}}{\text{IG AH}}$ according to blood-aqueous barrier

antiherpetic antibody. It was absent in 44 out of 163 (27%), the titer being below two. The level in the other 119 varied between 2 and 512, sometimes reaching 1024 or even 4096.

The serum titers were the most often between 64 and 4096 (Fig. 1). 17 patients (10%) had very low levels, inferior to eight; these were of various ages, from 4 to 60 years. The absorption of the serum with sheep red blood cells only modified the titration by one dilution – with one exception out of 177 cases. The serum level was higher than that in the aqueous humor in most patients, with seven exceptions where the figures for aqueous humor were equal to or superior to those for serum (Table 1).

The assay of total Ig revealed a great diversity from one aqueous humor to another. No precipitation peak whatsoever was obtained for 5 samples, even after several repeated attempts; their concentration of Ig was evaluated at 0.1 mg p. cent, the limit of detection of the Laurell technique. The ratios of the serum Ig levels to those of the aqueous humor were thus also very variable from one patient to another (Table 1).

This reflects the function of the blood-aqueous barrier which varies, according to the inflammatory state, between approximately 500, the figure considered normal, and values lower than 0.

The coefficient of antiherpetic antibody activity in the aqueous humor to that in the serum showed no parallelism with the titer of serum antibody (Fig. 1). A high serum level was often accompagnied by a low coefficient.

Thirty-eight coefficients out of 163 (23.3%) were equal to or inferior to 1, that is to say normal (Fig. 2). If we add to this figure, that of the aqueous humors not containing antiherpetic antibodies, *82 coefficients were not significant of an ocular herpes, i.e. 50.3%*. 81 were superior to 1, up to 668, i.e. 49.7%, and can be considered significant of an ocular herpes in the absence of any technical error.

What is the margin of error? What is the diagnostic value of this coefficient? What is its reliability?

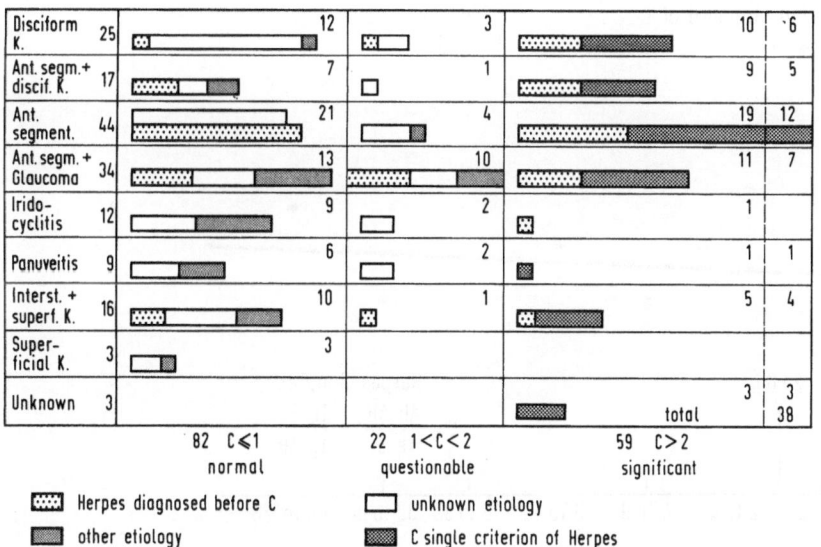

**Fig. 3.** 163 Herpes simplex coefficients

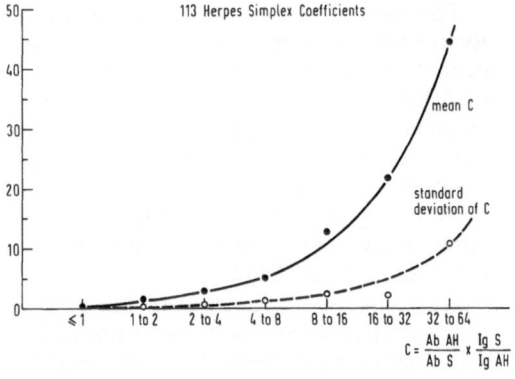

Fig. 4. Graphs of the mean and standard deviation as a function of the coefficients grouped in geometric progression

cients above 1 were grouped according to a geometric progression of base 2 (*Table 3*). *The absolute value of a coefficient should be taken less into consideration than its positioning in a group of this geometric progression.*

The mean and standard deviation of the coefficients in each of these groups were calculated (Fig. 4). The curve of the means as a function of the coefficients grouped in geometric progression has approximately the same form as that of the standard deviations. This coefficient mean/standard deviation (Fig. 5) is constant, and is approximately equal to 5. Thus *the standard deviation of a coefficient is $\frac{1}{5}$ of its value.* If a coefficient is 2: $C = 2 \pm 0.4$, it is still above 1, and can be considered as indicating an ocular herpes infection. *This coefficient value 2 can be considered at present as the limit of significance, but it must be verified by further tests and clinical and experimental observations.* Indeed, if one draws on a straight line the means surrounded by their standard deviations (Fig. 6) there is no ambiguity, the confidence intervals do not overlap.

## The Diagnostic Value and Reliability of the Coefficient

Two methods were used, one mathematical, the other biological, by comparison with antimeasles antibodies, humoral stigmas of a general viral infection at a young age.

### Statistical Calculation

The dilutions for the titration of the antiherpetic antibody were carried out by doubling dilutions. It is for this reason that the 81 coeffi-

### Comparison With the Coefficient of the Proportion Antimeasles Antibodies in the Globulins of the Aqueous Humor

This comparison was carried out for 91 pairs of aqueous humor-serum (Table 2) which

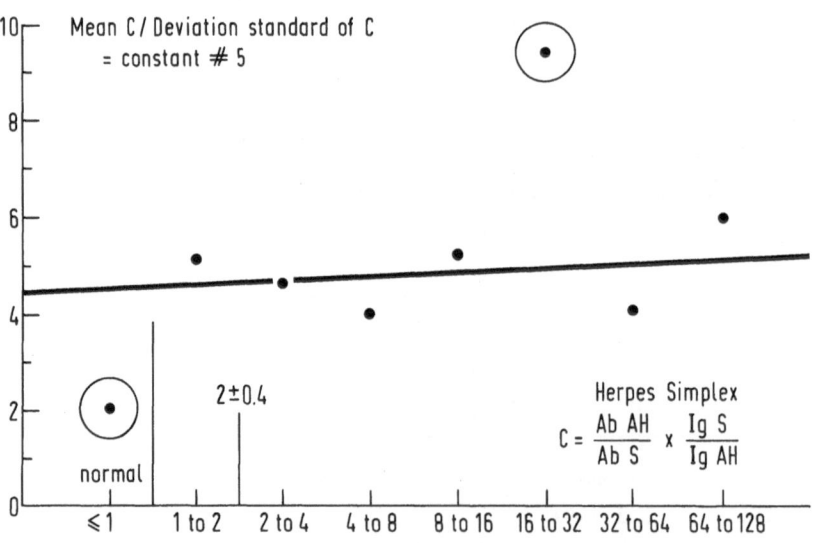

Fig. 5. Graph of the ratio mean/standard deviation as a function of the coefficients grouped in geometric progression

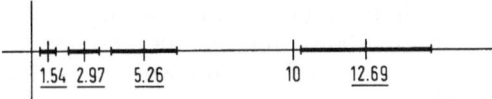

1.54  2.97    5.26        10    12.69

**Fig. 6.** Means surrounded by their standard deviations for the coefficients grouped in geometric progression: 1 to 2, 2 to 4, 4 to 8, 8 to 16

gave the following coefficients with regard to herpes:

36 with $C \leq 1$
14 with $1 < C < 2$
41 with $C \geq 2$

*The serum titers* of antimeasles antibody varied, being sometimes raised, equal to or higher than 640, and sometimes very low. If the level was lower than 2 the calculation of the coefficient was obviously impossible. Seven patients showed this peculiarity – they were all above 40 years of age.

*The titers in the aqueous humor* were nearly always below 2. Only 20 samples had a defined level, sometimes reaching 16 and in one case 64.

The calculation of the coefficient of antimeasles antibody activity in the aqueous humor to that in the serum reveals seven cases with a figure superior to 1:

- five with a coefficient between 1 and 2, which can be considered as the limit of normality
- two with a coefficient between 2 and 3, which merits further explication.

One of these patients had a herpes coefficient of 3.58 which was superior to this measles coefficient of 2.86. The diagnosis was

confirmed by the isolation of a herpes viral strain. The other patient was a 23 year-old man with a dubious herpes coefficient of 1.9 and a higher measles coefficient of 2.79 which could not be explained. The diagnosis of herpes was nevertheless retained after taking into account a previous dendritic ulcer.

*The comparison of the herpes and measles coefficients shows that all the herpes coefficients higher than or equal to 2,41 in this study, correspond to lower measles coefficients, nearly always below 2.*

*Statistical calculations and immunological comparisons between herpes and measles allow a herpes coefficient above or equal to 2 to be considered as significant of an ocular herpes. As for every biological examination, results at the limit of significance, here between 2 and 4, must be discussed and compared with clinical evidence.*

The results of the study of 163 aqueous humors and sera can be divided as follows:

a) 82 coefficients lower or equal to 1, normal, 50.3%

b) 22 coefficients between 1 and 2, doubtful, 13.5%

c) 59 coefficients equal or higher than 2, considered significant of an ocular herpes, 36.2%

### Clinical Interest of the Coefficient

From a group of 163 patients sent to the ophthalmologic clinic, most often thought to have had a herpes infection, the diagnosis appears confirmed in 88 cases (54%) on the basis of one or several of the three following criteria:

- corneal dendritic ulcer
- isolation of herpetic strain from a corneo-conjunctival sample
- coefficient of antiherpetic antibody activity in the aqueous humor to that in the serum above or equal to 2.

Among the other 75 patients, the ocular lesions were later found to be due to a different etiology in 22 cases (18%): zona, smallpox, microbial hypersensitivity to streptococcus or tuberculin or staphylococcus aureus, toxoplasmosis, ankylosing spondylarthritis, Fiessinger – Leroy – Reiter syndrome, Behcet's disease etc . . .

However, in 46 cases (28%), the etiology could not be determined.

Out of the 88 ocular herpes:

**Table 2.** 91 AH-Correlation between herpes simplex coefficient and measles coefficient

| Measles Ab | Herpes simplex | | | | |
|---|---|---|---|---|---|
| | $< \frac{1}{2}$ | $\leqslant 1$ | 1 to 2 | 2 to 4 | $\geqslant 4$ |
| Ab | | | | | |
| $< \frac{1}{2}$ | 8 | 22 | 11 | 8 | 24 |
| $\leqslant 1$ | 3 | 3 | | 4 | 3 |
| 1 to 2 | | | 2 | | 3 |
| 2 to 3 | | | 1 | 1 | |
| Total | 11 | 25 | 14 | 13 | 28 |
| | Normal C | | | Significant C | |

153

**Table 3.** Clinical results of study of 163 herpes simplex coefficients

| | |
|---|---|
| Diagnosis of herpes: 88 cases | 54% |
| by dentritic ulcer and/or | |
| viral strain isolation: 29 cases | 33% |
| by the above as well as confirmation | |
| with coefficient: 21 cases | 24% |
| by coefficient alone: 38 cases | 43% |
| Other diagnosis: 29 cases | 18% |
| Unknown diagnosis: 46 cases | 28% |

– 29 were confirmed by the presence of a dendritic ulcer and/or the isolation of a viral strain (33%)

– 21 had both of the above criteria with an elevated coefficient as well (24%)

– 38 had a coefficient superior or equal to 2 as the only diagnostic criterion (43%).

Thus the interest of the coefficient appears evident. The latter group comprised of:

6 disciform keratitis

24 anterior segmentitis (5 with disciform keratitis and 7 with glaucoma)

4 interstitial keratitis (3 with endothelitis)

3 with unknown symptomatology

1 bilateral panuveitis with only a slightly raised herpes coefficient of 2.72, probably of streptococcal orgin with 600 units ASLO.

The presence of a superficial keratitis may allow a dendritic ulcer to be seen or the isolation of a viral strain from a corneo-conjunctival specimen. It was in this way that 22 of our patients were classified as herpetic in spite of a non-significant coefficient (Table 3). The diagnostic possibilities of the calculation of the coefficient of antiherpetic antibody

activity in the aqueous humor to that in the serum are shown fully in the absence of evolutive epithelial lesions, which was the case for 23 of our patients.

The herpetic origin of the disciform keratitis, the anterior segmentitis, and the interstitial keratitis with endothelitis was affirmed in half of the cases (Table 4), especially when the disciform keratitis was associated with an anterior segmentitis. On the other hand, a herpetic infection was not proven in the cases of iridocyclitis and panuveitis. However, an observation of an iridocyclitis accompagnied by glaucoma and corneal oedema, allowed the confirmation of the herpetic etiology; the iridocyclitis marked the beginning of a bilateralisation of a known ocular herpes.

The coefficient was not significant in 22 cases of ocular herpes confirmed by other criteria. The cause of this defect is not evident. The age of the patient and the antigenic type of the infecting viral strain seem to bear no influence, as does neither the duration of the infection before removal of the test specimen. Nevertheless it seems advisable to wait a few days after the beginning of the infection before taking samples for testing, this delay being necessary for antibody synthesis. Repeated testing of the same patient has shown that it is important to perform the puncture of the anterior chamber during the acute period and especially to puncture a primary aqueous humor.

The existence or absence of a raised coefficient does not allow the prognosis of ocular herpes to be established.

In spite of these weaknesses, the comparative study of aqueous humor and serum

**Table 4.** Number of cases of herpes and diagnostic value of coefficient

| Clinical Form | Diagnosed Herpes | C ≪ 2 (with superf. K.) | C ≫ 2 Total | C ≧ 2 Without superf. K. |
|---|---|---|---|---|
| Disciform K. | 12/26 | 2 | 10 | 5 |
| Ant. Segm. + | | | | |
| Discif. K | 12/17 | 3 | 9 | 3 |
| Ant. Segmentitis | 25/47 | 6 | 19 | 6 |
| Ant. Segm. + | | | | |
| Glaucoma | 19/35 | 8 | 11 | 7 |
| Interst. + | | | | |
| Superf. K. | 8/16 | 3 | 5 | 2 |

merits a certain interest during the course of the serious forms of ocular herpes, which are often not typical. Indeed, out of the 88 cases of confirmed herpes, at the time the sample was taken, there were only 31 cases of superficial keratitis, including ten dendritic ulcers. Certain clinical cases are particularly difficult and our diagnostic criteria have permitted the identification of:

– 15 anterior segmentitis, from the first onset
– 3 corneal abscesses
– 2 hypopyons

The differential diagnosis of herpes from zona is sometimes difficult. One of our observations illustrates this problem. Eight months after the beginning of an ophthalmic zona, the patient had a dendritic ulcer on an anterior segmentitis. The herpes coefficient was 0.62, but the zona coefficient, after titration of the antizosterian antibodies by an immunoenzymatic technique (ELISA) was 10. The uveitis thus seemed to be of zosterian origin; however, a doubt remains about the etiology of the dendritic ulcer since the isolation of virus from a corneo-conjunctival sample was not attempted.

## Discussion

### Diagnostic Reliability of an Increase in the Coefficient

In this study, statistical calculation on 163 cases and the comparison of 91 herpes coefficients with the measles coefficients calculated for the same samples, presently allows *a herpes coefficient which is higher than or equal to 2 to be considered as significant of an ocular herpes.* The 91 measles coefficients were lower than 2, with the exception of two cases which were between 2 and 3. A comparison with the measles coefficient does not seem to be indispensable for diagnosis, but it remains desirable as a control for the assay of the immunoglobulins and becomes very useful when the herpes coefficient has a borderline value, around the figure 2, which still remains, however, superior to the measles coefficient. A comparison with the clinical signs is always necessary. It is of capital importance to take both serum and aqueous humor simultaneously from the patient and to carry out the titration of antibodies and measurement

of Ig during the same experimental manipulations.

These results are parallel to those of Bloch-Michel [1] who compared the herpes and toxoplasmosis coefficients in 44 uveitis of various etiology.

In effect, the applications of such a comparative immunological study of aqueous humor and serum to uveitis have become numerous since the first work by Witmer [28] on the periodic ophthalmia of the horse to Leptospira Pomona. Witmer [30, 31] has used this method in various intraocular infections: tuberculosis, toxoplasmosis, streptococcal infections, leptospirosis and phaco-antigenic uveitis. Using the same techniques, Martenet [14, 15] recognised a viral etiology, the most often herpes, in 5 to 10 percent of the uveitis she studied. In France the evaluation of the coefficient is applied, by Desmonts [7], to the diagnosis of ocular toxoplasmosis; it allows one third of posterior uveitis to be linked to this etiology.

The use of this diagnostic method has been widened to other biological liquids e.g antiherpetic antibodies have been shown to be present in *tears* [2]. Liotet et al. [13] have compared tears and serum, using the same methods as for aqueous humor, and show the proof of superficial corneo-conjunctival herpetic infections.

The study of the *vitreous* is possible. But the vitreous which we have been able to take were very modified. The presence of antiherpetic antibodies was always linked to a low coefficient.

This immunological technique has also been used for the cerebro-spinal fluid [21, 22]. The ocular globe and the central nervous system have many embryological and anatomical analogies, in particular the absence of lymphatics. The cerebro-spinal fluid, whose composition and low levels of Ig recall the aqueous humor, was compared immunologically to serum. The measurement of viral antibodies was carried out during the course of encephalitis.

### Diagnostic Interest of the Coefficient During an Ocular Herpes

In 59 of 88 ocular herpes diagnosed in the study, that is 67%, have a coefficient of antiherpetic antibody activity in the aqueous humor significant of an infection. In 38 cases of these 88, this criterion is shown to its full value since it is the only etiological element. *The comparative study of the aqueous humor and the serum, taken in preference during the acute phase, is of special interest during disciform keratitis, anterior segmentitis, and deep or interstitial keratitis with endothelitis.* On the other hand, the coefficient remains low in superficial keratitis. It should also be noted that it is exceptional that an isolated uveitis shows a raised coefficient.

This last remark confirms the data of Martenet [15] who observed only 23 significant coefficients of ocular herpes of 774 cases of uveitis, most of them without an associated keratitis. This small proportion of diagnosed herpes is without doubt due to the recruitment of the patients and perhaps to the techniques used, which were different to ours.

In certain cases this method is the only means of diagnosis, when the usual clinical and biological criteria fail, in particular in the most serious forms of ocular herpes with attack of the anterior chamber without a superficial keratitis. Even the dendritic ulcer has lost its absolute specificity for the herpetic lesion and can appear during an ophthalmic zona, as has been proven by the isolation of the zosterian virus [19].

*The isolation of a viral strain from a corneoconjunctival specimen* is in general only possible in the presence of active epithelial lesions. This technique, invaluable for the diagnosis of superficial keratitis, is thus shown to be complementary to the increase in the coefficient of antibody activity in the aqueous humor to that in the serum which becomes interesting in the most posterior forms.

*The isolation of a viral strain from the aqueous humor* was performed by Sundmacher and Neumann-Haefelin [25] in 9 of 33 ocular herpes cases. A secondary glaucoma is a good indication for the detection of a virus by isolation. The clinical forms known are the focal uveitis, peripheral endothelitis and prolonged disciform keratitis. The proportion of positive specimens seems to be approximately equal to that of the few cases diagnosed by the detection of viral antigens by immunofluorescence in the cells of the aqueous humor: two times out of eight for Patterson et al [18], five times out of ten for Kaufman et al. [12].

*The titration of serum levels of antibody by*

*itself* is of little interest during herpetic recurrences. Low titers often coexist with high coefficients in the aqueous humor. The eye is immunologically isolated from the rest of the organism.

Nevertheless, the study of the coefficient has its weaknesses, since in our results 22 herpes cases, identified by other criteria, have a very low non-significant coefficient which we cannot explain. The following hypotheses are possible: the infecting viral agent might be eliminated by the defence mechanisms and the immunological response would remain feeble or the antibodies could enter into the formation of immunocomplexes [5]. *As is the case with all virological examinations, a positive result corresponds to an etiological proof whereas a negative result remains an uncertain element.*

*Pathogenic Significance of the Coefficient*

We have shown in 59 ocular herpes out of 88 that in proportion to the total Ig, there are more antiherpetic antibodies in the aqueous humor than in the serum, whereas the antimeasles antibodies are approximately equal. These antimeasles antibodies have reached the aqueous humor by crossing the hemato-camerular barrier. The increase in antiherpetic antibody would seem to correspond to an intraocular synthesis, significant of a local infection.

The histological proof of the synthesis of antibodies in the plasmocytes of the uvea was obtained using immunofluorescence as long ago as 1955 by Witmer [29] in rabbits injected with ovalbumin, then by Dieckhues [8] with Escherichia Coli. This formation of antibody in the uvea has also been shown in vitro using the typhoid bacillus by Wolkowitz et al. [32]. Plasmocytosis, always present in the normal state in uveal tissue, increases markedly during inflammatory states. The origin of these immune competent cells which infiltrate the uvea has been the object of many studies [23, 24, 29].

What is the nature of the immunoglobulins synthesized? In this study, we measured the total Ig. Dernouchamps and Michiels [6] have indicated a selective augmentation of several immunoglobulins in the aqueous humor of uveitis: IgG, IgA or IgM. For Martenet [15] the IgA, as well as $C_3$, are frequently at high levels in the aqueous humors of uveitis, both anterior and posterior; this statement suggests a local production of IgA.

The local production of antibody implies the presence of antigen at the uveal level. Experimentally, in rabbits, Oh [17] has shown that whereas the active herpes virus is necessary for the induction of a primary uveitis, the secondary uveitis can be equally provoked by inactive viral antigens. Does the herpes virus remain in the uveal tissue, or does it persist in the form of inactive antigens, or does it completely disappear? Are the inflammatory lesions sustained by an autoimmune process? These hypotheses could perhaps explain some diagnostic failures in the study of the coefficient.

## Conclusions

The aqueous humor is the easiest biological material to remove during uveitis and posterior infections of the globe. The immunological results of these specimens would seem to be essential for the diagnosis of ocular herpes.

An increase in the coefficient of antiherpetic antibody activity in the aqueous humor to that in the serum allowed 59 serious herpes infections out of 88 (67%) to be diagnosed during ocular lesions of the anterior chamber: anterior segmentitis, disciform keratitis, and interstitial or deep keratitis.

The statistical calculation and the comparison with the measles coefficient, which always stays low, allows, at present, a herpes coefficient above or equal to 2 to be considered as significant of a herpetic infection.

This method detects a local synthesis of specific antibodies, signifying an intraocular infection. It is of greater interest than a simple serological study even if the latter should show a rise in the concentration of antibodies. In spite of the failures (33%) this method is a precious diagnostic tool which should be used while adhering to certain rules:
- a minutious clinical examination which orientates the diagnosis towards suspicion of herpes
- simultaneous sampling of the aqueous humor and the serum, in the acute phase
- titration of specific antibodies and assay of the Ig carried out at the same time
- utilisation of a sensitive technique for titration of antiherpetic antibodies, passive hemagglutination in this study

- measurement of the total Ig, by studying the complete spectrum of Ig which could by synthesized
- numerical and diagnostic evaluation of the coefficient, taking into account the geometric progression of the dilutions
- comparison with the measles coefficient and with the clinical data especially for borderline values around 2.

**Acknowledgment.** This work has been supported by Grants INSERM U-86 − (Prof. Y. Pouliquen).

## References

1. Bloch-Michel E (1979) Immunologie de l'humeur aqueuse. Journées d'ophtal Chibret
2. Campinchi R, Denis J, Virat J, Marsetio M, Offret G (1967) Apport de l'immunologie au diagnostic de l'herpès oculaire. Etude du sérum, de l'humeur aqueuse et des larmes. Bull des Soc d'ophtal France 10:856–865
3. Cavara V (1955) The role of viruses in the etiology of uveitis. Acta XVII Concilium ophthalmologicum (1954), vol 2. University of Toronto Press, Toronto, p 1232–1483
4. Denis J (1976) Immunological study of the aqueous humor in ocular herpes simplex: Proc. 1st Int. Symp. on Immunol. and Immunopathol. of the Eye (1974). Mod Probl Ophthalmol 16:220–224
5. Dernouchamps JP, Michiels J (1978) Circulating antigen-antibody complexes in the aqueous humor. Proc. 2nd Int. Symp. on Immunol. and Immunopathol. of the Eye (1978). Masson, New York p 40–45
6. Dernouchamps JP, Michiels J (1977) Molecular sieve properties of the blood-aqueous barrier in uveitis. Exp Eye Res 25:25–31
7. Desmonts G (1966) Definitive serological diagnosis of ocular toxoplasmosis. Arch Ophthalmol 76:839–851
8. Dieckhues B (1965) Endogene Uveitis als Ausdruck eines bakteriell-allergischen Geschehens am Auge. Vortrag VI − Europ. Allerg. Kongr., Stockholm (1965)
9. Goldmann H, Witmer R (1954) Antikörper im Kammerwasser. Ophthalmologica 127:323–330
10. Grabner G, Zehetbauer G, Bettelheim H, Hönigsmann C, Dorda W (1978) The blood-aqueous barrier and its permeability for proteins of different molecular weight. Albrecht von Graefes Arch Klin Ophthalmol 207:137–148
11. Huraux JM, Bouvier A, Bricout F (1971) Le titrage des anticorps antiherpès par hémagglutination indirecte au cours des gingivo-sto-

matites de l'enfant. Rev Eur Etud Clin Biol 16:474–476

12. Kaufman HE, Kanai A, Ellison ED (1971) Herpetic iritis: Demonstration of virus in the anterior chamber by fluorescent antibody techniques and electron microscopy. Am J Ophthalmol 7:465–469

13. Liotet S, Huet JF, Massin M, Chatellier PH (in press) Diagnostic des kératites herpétiques par dosage des anticorps des larmes par immunofluorescence. Soc d'ophtal. de Paris (15 décembre 1979). Bull des Soc d'ophtal de France

14. Martenet AC (1971) Virus et uvéites. Doin, Paris

15. Martenet AC (1979) Immunology of the aqueous humor. II. XXIII Concilium ophthalmologicum (1978) Acta Pars I. Excerpta Medica, Amsterdam Oxford, p 117–125

16. Michiels J, Dernouchamps JP (1976) Quantitation of specific antibodies in the aqueous humor. Mod Probl Ophthalmol 16:131–136

17. Oh JO (1979) Role of immunity in the pathogenesis of herpes simplex uveitis. Proc. 2nd Int. Symp. on Immunol. and Immunopathol. of the Eye (1978). Masson, New York p 248–255

18. Patterson A, Sommerville RG, Jones BR (1969) Herpetic keratouveitis with herpes virus antigen in the anterior chamber. Trans Ophthalmol Soc UK 88:243–249

19. Pavan-Langston D, McCulley JP (1973) Herpes Zoster. Dentritic keratitis. Arch Ophthalmol 89:25–29

20. Rosen L (1961) Hemagglutination and hemagglutination-inhibition with measles virus. Virology 13:139–141

21. Schuller E (1979) Les immunoglobulines du liquide céphalo-rachidien. I. Nature et origine. Nouv Presse Méd 8:351–357

22. Schuller E (1979) Les immunoglobulines du liquide céphalo-rachidien. II. Variations dans les diverses situations pathologiques. Nouv Presse Méd 8:427–432

23. Silverstein AM (1963) Effect of X-irradiation on the development of immunogenic uveitis. Invest Ophthalmol Visual Sci 2:58–62

24. Smith RE, Jensen AD, Silverstein AM (1969) Antibody formation by single cells during experimental immunogenic uveitis. Invest Ophthalmol Visual Sci 8:373–380

25. Sundmacher R, Neumann-Haefelin D (1979) Herpes-simplex-Virus Isolierung aus dem Kammerwasser bei fokaler Iritis, Endotheliitis und langdauernder Keratitis disciformis mit Sekundärglaukom. Klin Monatsbl Augenheilkd 175:488–501

26. Thygeson P, Spencer WH (1973) The changing character of infectious corneal disease: emerging opportunistic microbial forms (1928–1973). Trans Am Ophthalmol Soc 71:246–253

27. Weeke B (1973) Rocket immunoelectrophoresis. Scand J Immunol (Suppl 1) 2:37–46

28. Witmer R (1954) Periodic ophthalmia in horses. Am J Ophthalmol 37:243–253

29. Witmer R (1955) Antibody formation in the rabbit eye studied with fluorescein labeled antibody. Arch Ophthalmol 53:811–816

30. Witmer R (1967) The significance of ocular antibodies in endogenous inflammatory disease of the eye. Mod. Trends Ophthalmol 4:117–129

31. Witmer R (1979) Immunology of the aqueous humor. I. XXIII Concilium ophthalmologicum (1978) Acta Pars I. Excerpta Medica, Amsterdam Oxford, p 111–116

32. Wolkowitz MI, Hallett JW, Leopold IH (1960) Studies on antibody production in the rabbit eye. I. Antibody formation in vitro after intraocular injection of typhoid bacilli. Am J Ophthalmol 50:126–138

Sundmacher, R. (Hrsg.):
Herpetische Augenerkrankungen
© J.F. Bergmann Verlag, München 1981

# Changes of Immune Globulins in Different Herpetic Diseases

I. Tapasztó, Kecskemét

**Key words.** Tears - content of antibodies, IgA, IgG, herpetic keratitis, iritis, adenovirus conjunctivitis

**Schlüsselwörter.** Tränenflüssigkeit - Immunoglobulingehalt, IgA, IgG, Herpeskeratitis, Iritis, Adenoviruskonjunktivitis

**Summary.** Changes in levels of immune globulins IgA and IgG in human tears were investigated in 22 patients suffering from herpetic dendritic keratitis, in 6 patients with herpetic disciform keratitis, in 3 patients with herpetic iridocyclitis, in 62 patients with adenovirus conjunctivitis and in 100 healthy persons. It appeared that in the case of herpetic dendritic keratitis, the level of IgA decreased and that of IgG increased in human tears. In herpetic disciform keratitis, IgA increased and IgG slightly increased. In herpetic iridocyclitis, IgA slightly increased while IgG increased considerably. Adenovirus conjunctivitis caused a high increase in both IgA and IgG levels of human tears. It is inferred that in herpetic diseases of the eye the levels of immune globulins in human tears increase only if the herpetic disease spreads over tissues with good blood supply while in diseases of the cornea, there is little change in the levels of immune globulins.

**Zusammenfassung.** Schwankungen des Immunglobulin-A und Immunglobulin-G-Gehalts in der Tränenflüssigkeit wurden bei 22 Patienten mit Keratitis dendritica, 6 Patienten mit Keratitis disciformis, 3 Patienten mit herpetischer Iridocyclitis, 62 Patienten mit Adenoviruskonjunktivitis und 100 gesunden Kontrollpersonen untersucht. Dabei zeigte sich, daß bei der Keratitis dendritica der Ig-A-Spiegel erniedrigt und der Ig-G Spiegel in der Tränenflüssigkeit erhöht war. Bei der Keratitis disciformis fanden wir Ig-A erhöht und Ig-G leicht erhöht. Bei der herpetischen Iridocyclitis war Ig-A leicht erhöht, während Ig-G beträchtlich erhöht war. Eine Adenoviruskonjunktivitis führte sowohl zu einem hohen Anstieg des Ig-A als auch des Ig-G-Spiegels in der Tränenflüssigkeit. Wir schließen hieraus, daß bei herpetischen Augenerkrankungen die Immunglobulinspiegel in den Tränen nur dann ansteigen, wenn Gewebe mit guter Blutversorgung erkrankt sind, während es bei Hornhauterkrankungen nur geringe Schwankungen im Immunoglobulinspiegel gibt.

Research on the biochemistry of tears began only a few years ago as stated in the literature. Immune globulins and immune chemistry have only been dealt with in detail for the last 15 years. Investigations were carried on partly to find out which of the antibodies produced by the organism penetrated the eye and could be detected there, and partly to detect the antibodies produced by the eye and its adnexa themselves, which in their part control different eye diseases. Present investigations show a certain similarity between immune globulins found in the tears and antibodies of the serum with some difference, however, in their structure. We cannot tell yet whether certain immune globulins in the tears are fully identical with immune globulins of the serum, or only some structural parts (in the case of closer similarity some determinant groups) are identical with structural parts or determinant groups of the serum immune globulins.

Chodirker and Tomasi [9] found 7 mg % IgA in tears. Bonavida et al. [7] discovered 5% IgG and 30% IgA in tears 4 h after intravenous injection of IgA and IgG marked with $J^{125}$ into rabbits.

It was a very important event when Josephson and Weiner [12] and Thompson et al. [24] found a characteristic substance in the tears, which was named secretion component. Later its presence was discovered in other secretions such as in the saliva, bronchial mucous membrane and colostrum. That component was sometimes thought to be IgE. Now we know it to be a part of secretory IgA.

Allansmith and McClellan [2] reported

159

that the IgA content of tears was $\frac{1}{8}$ that of the serum IgA; the IgG in tears was $\frac{1}{70}$ that of the serum. The $\frac{1}{8}$ IgA included IgE. They indicated that in some cases the IgG content surpassed that of the IgA in the tears.

Sapse et al. [18] discovered IgA and IgG in the tears. Little et al. [14] found 21 mg % IgA in the tears of 10 persons. Bazzi et al. [5] reported 79 mg % IgA and 23 mg % IgG. IgM could only be found in traces. Centifanto et al. [8] found that in the tears of patients suffering from herpes simplex, the interferon level increased considerably in the first 5 weeks of poly I:C treatment.

According to Scalise et al. [19] the IgA immune globuline of the tears decreased considerably in $\frac{2}{3}$ of the patients with herpetic keratitis.

Based on investigations of 32 tear samples, Allansmith [2] stated in her monograph that normal human tears contained 16 mg % IgG and 18 mg % IgA. Changes are induced by diseases. She reported 18 mg % IgG and 22 mg % IgA in blepharoconjunctivitis, with 2 mg % of IgM; 26 mg % IgG and 23 mg % of IgA in herpetic keratitis. In acute conjunctivitis follicularis, IgG was 60 mg %, IgA 58 mg %, and IgM 46 mg %. In tears from healthy persons IgD could also be revealed, its level was less than 1 mg %; IgE was 200 µg %. In different diseases, IgG levels varied between 8 and 94 mg %, those of IgA between 9 and 82 mg %. IgM was not found in every disease. In case of pharyngoconjunctival fever, the specific antibody was found in the IgG fraction like in the serum. In the IgA fraction, an antibody against rhinovirus 15 was found. In the same monograph, Allansmith suggested that 5% of the tear globulins – which according to her make up 20% of the total proteins in tears – were immune globulins, while 20% of the serum globulins were immune globulins.

Kaneko [13] showed that by means of immunofluorescence techniques, the IgA level in tears decreased at the beginning of herpetic keratitis but later, in the course of recovery, increased; the tear IgG changed the other way.

In 1974 Muravieva et al. [16] examined 160 patients suffering from conjunctivitis, keratitis and uveitis by means of immundiffusion techniques. In inflammatory diseases, the IgA and IgG levels of the tears increased except in herpetic keratitis, where they decreased. The IgM level remained unchanged.

In the serum, the values of the three immune globulins varied between normal limits.

The immune chemistry of tears is a rather new branch of science. The results cited above, which are often contradictory, need to be examined and confirmed before they can be accepted.

**Materials and Methods**

In my immune electrophoretic tests, a plexi tub with platinum electrodes and a proper rectifier was used with 200 V and 4 h migration time. The 10 cm plates had a current intensity of 28–32 mA, the 12 cm plates 36 mA. A 10 V/cm voltage drop was observed. The tests were carried out in an ice chamber at + 4 °C.

A 0.5% agarose solution after Serva and Koch-Light was used. Agarose was diluted by the buffer solution just in use. The more the gel could be diluted the better the separation of fractions was.

Glass plates $10 \times 2.5$ cm and $12 \times 2.5$ cm made to order were used. Agarose gel was placed 2 mm thick on the smaller ones (2.5 ml) and on the larger ones (3 ml). The plates coated with agarose gel were connected by Macherey-Nagel 214 filter paper stripes with the buffer at the two ends of the plexi tub. Tris-EDTA-boric acid was used (pH 9.0 $I_c$ = 0.15 mol/l). Buffers were preserved by means of 1 ppm merthiolate or 10 ppm thymol solution.

In the agarose gel immuno-electrophoretic migrations, the following cutting pattern was used: cuttings to take up the antigen were made 38 mm from the negative pole on the 10 $\times$ 2.5 cm plates and 50 mm from the negative pole on the 12 $\times$ 2.5 cm plates. The circle to receive the antigen had a diameter of 1.8 mm on every plate type. In the middle there were troughs of different sizes for the immune serum: 80 mm $\times$ 1.5 mm on plates of 10 cm $\times$ 2.5 cm and 100 mm $\times$ 1.5 mm on those of 12 $\times$ 2.5 cm. The circular shaped cutting to receive the antigen was done at a 3 mm distance from the trough of the immune serum. The trough for immune serum was made 1 cm from each end of the plate.

For the electrophoretic migration 0.001 ml serum, and 0.002 or 0.003 ml tears were placed directly on the glass plate in the circular shaped cuttings of the antigen. After electrophoretic investigation the agarose was carefully removed by water pump from the pre-cut central trough, then 0.1 ml immune serum in 1:2 dilution was placed in the central trough directly on the glass plate. In the agarose-gel immuno-electrophoresis, the following immune serums were used:

Polyspecific immune serums precipitating human immune globulins:

1. antihuman IgG-IgM horse serum (IgGM)

2. antihuman IgG-IgA-IgM horse serum (IgGAM).

Monospecific immune serums precipitating human immune globulins:

1. antihuman IgG horse serum (IgG)

2. antihuman IgM horse serum (IgM)

3. antihuman IgA horse serum (IgA)

4. antihuman IgA goat serum (IgA)

5. antihuman IgA sheep serum (IgA).

Monospecific immune serums against some immunological structural units of human immune globulins:

1. antihuman kappa horse serum (anti-kappa)

2. antihuman lambda horse serum (anti-lambda)

3. antihuman IgG-Fc rabbit serum (IgG-Fc)

4. antihuman IgG-Fd rabbit serum (IgG-Fd)

5. antihuman IgG-Fab rabbit serum (IgG-Fab)

6. antihuman IgG-H rabbit serum (IgGH).

After placing the immune serum on glass plates they were put in moist chamber. Diffusion time was 24 h, followed by washing of plates with physiological common salt solution several times a day for 48 h to remove excess immune-serum. After drying and fixing of plates, proteins were stained with 1% amido-black 10B (Merck and Loba) or 2% acid fuchsin (Merck).

Sucked human tear samples were immediately investigated for quantitative changes by means of agarose gel immuno-electrophoresis of Backhausz. Tear samples taken from 31 patients suffering from herpetic eye diseases, 62 patients with conjunctivitis caused by adenovirus and 100 healthy persons were analysed.

## Results and Discussion

In each of the 100 healthy tear samples IgA and IgG could be revealed by specific antihuman immunoserum. Immune globulin IgM was found in three cases. Quantitative tests indicated an average level of 18 mg/100 ml IgA and 15 mg/100 ml IgG in the tears of healthy persons. When measurable, IgM was found at a concentration of 3 mg/100 ml.

In tears of the 62 patients suffering from adenovirus conjunctivitis, each sample contained IgA and IgG, but only six samples IgM. Quantitative analysis revealed 42 mg/100 ml IgA and 45 mg/100 ml IgG. IgM had a mean of 8 mg/100 ml.

Among the 31 patients suffering in herpetic eye diseases, 22 were diagnosed as suffering from keratitis dendritica herpetica, six from keratitis disciformis herpetica and three from iridocyclitis herpetica.

In the 22 cases of keratitis dendritica herpetica, IgA and IgG could be detected in each sample. IgM was not found. IgA averaged 12 mg/100 ml, IgG 28 mg/100 ml. In the six cases of keratitis disciformis herpetica 24 mg/100 ml IgA and 18 mg/100 ml IgG were measured. In the three patients suffering from iridocyclitis herpetica, 22 mg/100 ml IgA and 30 mg/100 ml IgG were found.

The following conclusions can be drawn:

1. Immune globulin IgA is more important in the human tears to control external eye diseases caused by bacteria or viruses than the other immune globulins.

2. In external herpetic eye diseases, the accumulation of immune globulins and their role in controlling the virus is less than in external inflammations caused by other viruses or bacteria.

3. IgA is of more importance in controlling herpetic conjunctivitis and superficial keratitis, while in deep herpetic diseases and iridocyclitis, IgG seems to be more important.

4. In herpetic eye diseases, the level of immune globulins only increases if the herpetic disease spreads to tissues with a good blood supply. Then herpes virus does not seem to mobilize the local or general immune system to such an extent as to induce production of an adequate quantity of antiserum.

To summarize we can say that the organism has little natural resistance against herpetic diseases and needs either a well proved vaccination or, what at present seems more promising, medicaments which reduce the activity of the herpetic virus.

# References

1. Adenis JP, Bonnet BJM, Queroy M, Rammaert B, Loubet A (1977) Etude immunopathologique dans un cas d'ulcere de Mooren. Résultats préliminaires. Bull Soc Ophthalmol Fr 77:719-721
2. Allansmith MR, McClellan B (1969) Immunoglobulin levels in human tears. Invest Ophthalmol Visual Sci 8:240-246
3. Allansmith MR (1973) Immunology of the tears. Int Ophthalmol Clin 13:47-72
4. Backhausz R (1967) Immunodiffusion and Immunoelektrophorese. Verlag der ungarischen Akademie der Wissenschaften, Budapest
5. Bazzi C, Cattaneo R, Migone V, Farine M (1970) Further observations on immunoglobulins of external secretions. Prog Immunobiol 4:333-335
6. Bluestone R, Easty DL, Goldberg LS, Jones BR, Pettit TH (1975) Lacrimal immunoglobulins and complement quantified by counterimmunoelectrophoresis. Br J Ophthalmol 59:279-281
7. Bonavide B, Sapse AT, Sercarz EE (1968) Rabbit tear proteins. I. Detection and quantitation of lysozyme in non-stimulated tears. Invest Ophthalmol Visual Sci 7:435-440
8. Centifanto YM, Goorha RM, Kaufman HE (1970) Interferon induction in rabbit and human tears. Am J Ophthalmol 70:1006-1009
9. Chodirker WB, Tomasi jr TB (1963) Gammaglobulins: quantitative relationship in humanserum and nonvascular fluids. Science 142:1080-1081
10. Ishizaka K, Ishizaka T, Bennich H, Johannson SGO (1970) Biologic activities of aggregated immunoglobulin-E. J Immunol 104:854-862
11. Jordano J, Ceres J, Pena J (1973) Estudio cuantitativo de la immunoglobulima a en lagrima humana. (Quantitative study of IgA in human tears.) Rev Clin Esp 130:481-486
12. Josephson AS, Weiner RS (1968) Studies of the proteins of lacrimal secretions. J Immunol 100:1080-1081
13. Kaneko M (1973) Studies on antibodies in serum and tears from patients with herpes simplex keratitis. Acta Soc Ophthalmol Jap 77:7-14
14. Little JM, Centifanto YM, Kaufman HE (1969) Immunoglobulins in human tears. Am J Ophthalmol 68:898-905
15. McClellan BH, Bettman jr JW, Allansmith MR (1974) Tear and serum immunoglobulin levels in Navajo children with trachoma. Am J Ophthalmol 78:106-109
16. Muravieva TV, Lyudogovskaya LA, Zaltseva NS (1974) Immunoglobulins in tears, anterior chamber humor and sera of patients with diverse eye diseases. Vestn Ophthalmol 3:40-43
17. Prause JU (1979) Immunoelectrophoretic determination of tear fluid proteins collected by the Schirmer test. Acta Ophthalmol 57:959-967
18. Sapse AT, Bonavida B, Stone jr W, Sercarz EE (1969) Proteins in human tears. I. Immunoelectrophoretic patterns. Arch Ophthalmol 81:815-819
19. Scalise G, Barca L, Sinicco A, Mura MS (1971) The behavior of immunoglobulins of the serum and of the lacrimal secretion in keratitis from herpes simplex. Boll Oculist 50:569-587
20. Sen DK, Sarin GS, Mani K, Saha K (1976) Immunoglobulins in tears of normal Indian people. Br J Ophthalmol 60:302-304
21. Sen DK, Sarin GS, Mathur GP, Saha K (1978) Biological variation of immunoglobulin concentrations in normal human tears related to age and sex. Acta Ophthalmol (Kbh) 56:439-444
22. Tapasztó I, Vass Z, Kiss L (1965) The agar immunoelectrophoresis of the protein fractions of the human tears. Acta Ophthalmol (Kbh) 43:802-807
23. Tapasztó I (1973) Pathophysiology of human tears. Int Ophthalmol Clin 13:119-147
24. Thompson RA, Asquith P, Cooke WT (1969) Secretory IgA in the serum. Lancet 2:517-519

Sundmacher, R. (Hrsg.):
Herpetische Augenerkrankungen
© J.F. Bergmann Verlag, München 1981

# Zur Klinik der granulomatösen Reaktion gegen die Descemetsche Membran

G.F. Kortüm, W. Seibel, H.E. Völcker, G.O.H. Naumann, Tübingen

**Key words.** Herpetic keratitis, granulomatous reaction against Descemet's

**Schlüsselwörter.** Herpeskeratitis, granulomatöse Reaktion gegen Descemet

**Summary.** In 1016 excised corneas after perforating keratoplasty between 1975 and 1979 we found histologically a granulomatous reaction against Descemet's membrane in 66 patients (6%). This granulomatous reaction against Descemet's membrane was seen only in those 99 corneas which had been excised in patients with a herpes cornea, that means in $^2/_3$ of all patients who had been operated because of this disease. The fragmentation of the Descemet's membrane is believed to be a precursor of corneal perforation.

The clinical correlation in 16 patients is characteristic:

1. On an average duration of disease 16 years
2. Deep circumscribed stromal infiltrate
3. Intensive edema of the cornea caused by endothelial decompensation
4. Folds in Descemet
5. Variable uveitis

In our opinion these findings are an indication to perform a curative perforating keratoplasty. Results in 16 patients are good.

**Zusammenfassung.** Unter 1016 Hornhaut-Exzisaten nach perforierender Keratoplastik zwischen 1975 und 1979 wurde histologisch eine granulomatöse Reaktion gegen die Descemet bei 66 Patienten (d.h. in 6%) beobachtet. Diese granulomatöse Reaktion gegen die Descemetsche Membran wurde ausschließlich unter den 99 Hornhaut-Exzisaten gesehen, die von Patienten mit einem Herpes corneae gewonnen wurden, d.h. in $^2/_3$ aller Patienten, die deswegen operiert wurden. Die Zerstörung und Fragmentierung der Descemetschen Membran wird als Vorstadium zur Hornhautperforation gedeutet.

Das klinische Korrelat bei 16 präoperativ fotografierten Patienten ist charakteristisch:

1. Durchschnittliche Erkrankungsdauer 16 Jahre.
2. Tiefes umschriebenes Hornhautinfiltrat.
3. Ausgeprägtes Hornhautoedem durch Endothel-Dekompensation.
4. Descemet-Falten.
5. Wechselnd ausgeprägte Begleituveitis.

Der genannte Befund stellt u.E. eine Indikation zur kurativen Keratoplastik dar. Die Ergebnisse bei 16 Patienten sind gut.

## Einleitung

Die granulomatöse Reaktion gegen die Descemetsche Membran in Verbindung mit einer ulzerierenden und häufig perforierenden herpetischen Keratitis ist ein seit langem bekannter histologischer Befund [1–6].

Im folgenden soll auf das charakteristische klinische Bild, den typischen Krankheitsverlauf und die folgerichtige Therapie hingewiesen werden.

## Patienten, Untersuchungsmaterial und Untersuchungsmethoden

Vom 1. 3. 75 bis 30. 11. 79 wurden im ophthalmo-pathologischen Labor der Univ. Augen-

**Tabelle 1.** Hornhaut-Exzisate nach Keratoplastik 1. 3. 75–30. 11. 79

| Diagnosen | |
|---|---|
| 1. Hornhautnarben | 359 = 34% |
| 2. Keratokonus | 208 = 20% |
| 3. Prim. + sek. Endothel-Dekompensation | 204 = 19% |
| 4. Chron. unspez. Keratitis | 103 = 10% |
| 5. Herpes corneae (anamn.) | 99 = 9% |
| 6. Dystrophie | 48 = 4% |
| 7. Verätzung | 48 = 4% |
| Gesamtzahl | 1061 = 100% |

klinik Tübingen 1061 Hornhautexzisate histologisch untersucht. Hierbei handelt es sich sowohl um Exzisate aus der eigenen Klinik als auch um Zusendung auswärtiger Kliniken (Tabelle 1).

16 Patienten, bei denen wir wegen einer histologisch gesicherten granulomatösen Reaktion gegen die Descemetsche Membran eine perforierende Keratoplastik an der Tübinger Augenklinik durchführten, wurden nachuntersucht.

## Ergebnisse

### Häufigkeiten

Klinisch wurde in dieser Serie die Diagnose eines Herpes corneae bei 99 Patienten = 9% angegeben (s. Tabelle 1). Eine virologische Absicherung lag in keinem Fall vor. Eine granulomatöse Reaktion gegen die Descemet wurde *ausschließlich* bei Patienten mit dieser klinischen Diagnose gesehen, und zwar bei 66 Exzisaten, d.h. bei $^2/_3$ aller wegen eines Herpes corneae operierten Patienten.

### Klinisch-histopathologische Korrelation

Anhand der 16 Patienten lassen sich folgende Aussagen über die Dauer der Erkrankung,

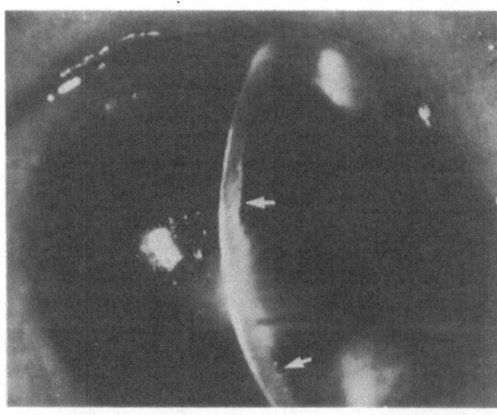

**Abb. 1.** A.B. ♀ 59 J. alt; granulomatöse Reaktion gegen die Descemetsche Membran; nach über 5 Jahren Rezidiv,

Herpetische Keratitis:
Spaltlampenmikroskopisch tiefes Stromainfiltrat mit Descemet-Falten und umschriebene Endothel-Epithel-Dekompensation (Pfeile)

über die biomikroskopischen präoperativen Befunde und den postoperativen Verlauf nach perforierender Keratoplastik machen:

### a) Anamnese

Die durchschnittliche Erkrankungsdauer vor Durchführung der Keratoplastik betrug 16 Jahre, längstens 33 Jahre und kürzestens 6 Wochen. Typisch in der Anamnese sind in unregelmäßigen Abständen auftretende Rezidive einer herpetischen Keratitis mit unterschiedlich stark ausgeprägter Begleituveitis, wobei beschwerdefreie Intervalle über mehrere Jahre hinweg nicht selten sind.

### b) Histopathologie

Die histologischen Kriterien sind geläufig. Zwischen nekrotischen Hornhautlamellen findet sich ein dichtes leukozytäres und lymphozytäres Infiltrat der tiefen Stromaschicht, um die Descemetsche Membran herum findet sich eine granulomatöse histiocytäre Infiltration mit Fremdkörperriesenzellen. Im Verlauf der Entzündung kommt es zur Faltenbildung, Aufsplitterung und zur Fragmentierung der Descemetschen Membran.

### c) Biomikroskopisches Bild

Das biomikroskopische Bild der granulomatösen Reaktion läßt sich aus einer Korrelation zum präoperativ fotografierten Befund ableiten:

1. Die entzündliche Infiltration konzentriert sich im *tiefen* Stroma nahe der Descemetschen Membran. Sie ist zwar unscharf begrenzt, aber zumindest anfangs *fokal betont.*
2. Vom Zentrum des Infiltrates gehen Descemet-Falten aus.
3. Als Folge der *Dekompensation des Hornhautendothels* fällt ein ausgeprägtes Oedem von Stroma und Hornhautepithel auf (Abb. 1).
4. Nur $^2/_3$ der Patienten (10 von 16) litten präoperativ an einem Hornhautulcus, welches bei 6 Patienten perforiert war (Abb. 2 und 3).
5. Augen mit einer granulomatösen Reaktion gegen die Descemet zeigten eine sehr wechselnd ausgeprägte Uveitis anterior, jedoch *kein* Hypopyon (Abb. 2a). Einige Augen erschienen äußerlich sogar reizfrei.

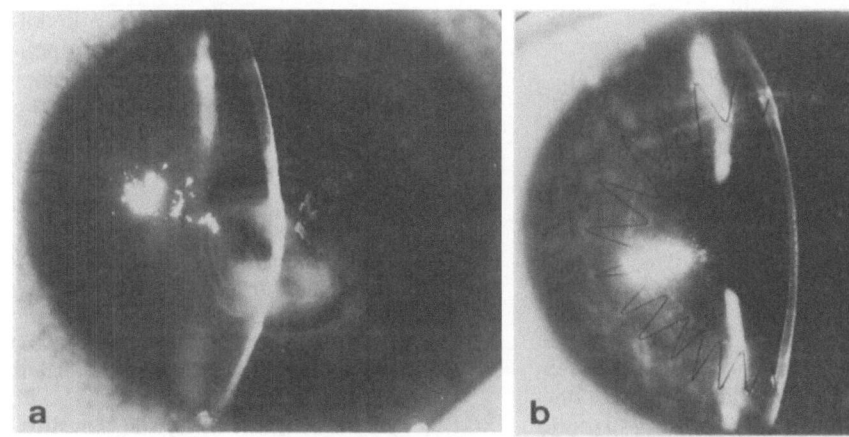

**Abb. 2.** K. Ch. ♀ 27 J.; nach über 4 Jahren Rezidiv.
**a** herpetische Keratitis; granulomatöse Reaktion mit therapieresistentem Ulkus und tiefer Stromainfiltration sowie Begleituveitis *ohne* Hypopyon; V = Handbewegung/30 cm
**b** 8 Mon. nach perf. Keratoplastik vor der Hornhautfadenentfernung; V = 0,6

d) Therapie

Der Durchmesser der perforierenden Keratoplastik variierte je nach klinischem Befund von 6,7 mm bis 10,5 mm (Abb. 2b und 3b).

Neben den sechs perforierten Hornhautulzera wurde die Keratoplastik nur einmal bei starker Begleituveitis (à chaud) durchgeführt. Die Nachbehandlung erfolgte bei allen Patienten mit lokaler Gabe von Corticosteroiden ohne Virustatika-Therapie. Eine immunologische Transplantatreaktion wurde bei keinem der sechs Patienten während des Nachbehandlungszeitraums von 1 Monat bis 4 Jahre gesehen. Durch die perforierende Keratoplastik ließ sich mit Ausnahme eines Patienten stets eine Visusbesserung erreichen (Tabelle 2).

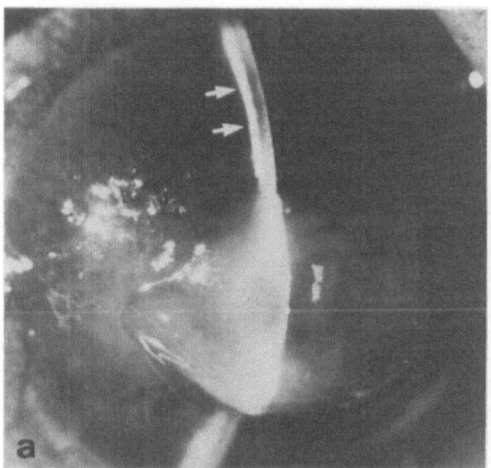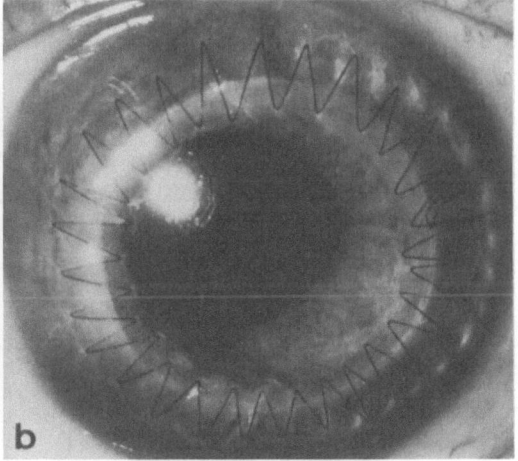

**Abb. 3.** LA. ♂ 37 J., 24 J. nach Rezidiv.
**a** herpetische Keratitis; granulomatöse Reaktion gegen die Descemetsche Membran mit Hornhautulkusperforation und aufgehobener Vorderkammer (Pfeile); V = Handbewegung/30 cm
**b** 3 Mon. nach perf. Keratoplastik à chaud kombiniert mit Cataract-Extraktion; V = 0,2

Tabelle 2.

| Präop. Visus | | Postop. Visus | |
|---|---|---|---|
| Lichtschein und | | bis 0,2⁻p | 4 Pat. |
| Projektion | 2 Pat. | 0,2–0,4 p | 6 Pat. |
| Handbewegungen | 6 Pat. | 0,4–0,8 p | 4 Pat. |
| Fingerzählen | 2 Pat. | 0,8 und besser | 2 Pat. |
| bis 0,1 | 6 Pat. | | |

## Diskussion

Die granulomatöse Reaktion gegen die Descemetsche Membran erklärt die typischerweise auch klinisch im tiefen Stroma sitzende und erkennbare entzündliche Infiltration.

Die dabei histologisch beobachteten Defekte in der Descemetschen Membran machen bei gleichzeitig ulzerierender Keratitis einmal die Gefahr der Ulkus-Perforation – und zwar ohne vorherige Descemetozele – verständlich und folgerichtigerweise eine *perforierende* Keratoplastik notwendig. Eine lamelläre Keratoplastik ist verständlicherweise kontraindiziert. Das gleichzeitig histologisch beobachtete Fehlen des Endothels in Nachbarschaft der granulomatösen Reaktion gegen die Descemetsche Membran ist Ursache für die klinisch zu beobachtende Endotheldekompensation. In der kleinen Fallserie traten bisher weder Rezidive noch eine immunologische Transplantatreaktion auf.

## Literatur

1. Green WR, Zimmermann LE (1967) Granulomatous reaction to Descemet's membrane. Am Ophthalmol 64:555–558
2. Hogan MJ, Kumura SJ, Tygeson P (1963) Pathology of herpes simplex keratoiritis Trans Ophthalmol Soc 61:75–99
3. Roll P, Hanselmayer H (1976) Die Ultrastruktur der granulomatösen Reaktion gegen die Descemetsche Membran. Klin Monatsbl Augenheilkd 168:819–824
4. Stock W (1939) Pathologische Anatomie des Auges. Enke, Stuttgart, S 41 ff
5. Vogel HM, Naumann GOH (1971) Die granulomatöse Reaktion gegen die Descemetsche Membran. Ber Dtsch Ophthalmol Ges 71:35–41
6. Zimmermann LE (1965) New concepts in pathology of the cornea. In: King RJ, McTigue JW (eds) The Cornea World Congress. Butterworths, London

Sundmacher, R. (Hrsg.):
Herpetische Augenerkrankungen
© J.F. Bergmann Verlag, München 1981

# Granulomatous Keratitis and its Relationship to Herpetic Disease

H. Witschel, J. Orsoni, Freiburg

**Key words.** Bowman's, Descemet's, giant cells, herpetic keratitis, granulomatous reaction

**Schlüsselwörter.** Bowman, Descemet, Riesenzellen, granulomatöse Reaktion

**Summary.** Among 141 specimens of corneal ulcers or chronic keratitis examined between 1969 and 1979, 19 cases of granulomatous inflammation with foreign body giant cell reaction to corneal structures were found. While herpes simplex infection was the prevalent underlying cause, granulomatous inflammation also occurred in other corneal diseases like rosacea keratitis, perforating injury, and after X-ray radiation. Besides the well-known reaction to Descemet's membrane, we also found giant cells around condensed and diseased stromal lamellae, fragments of Bowman's membrane, and around pieces of Descemet's from donor corneas used as "bio-patches". The significance of these findings is briefly discussed.

**Zusammenfassung.** Unter 141 Präparaten mit Hornhautulkus oder chronischer Keratitis, die zwischen 1968 und 1979 zur Untersuchung gelangten, fanden sich 19 Fälle von granulomatöser Entzündung mit Fremdkörperriesenzellen. Eine Herpes simplex-Infektion war zwar die häufigste Ursache der granulomatösen Entzündung, aber auch in Fällen von Rosacea-Keratitis, perforierender Verletzung und nach Röntgenbestrahlung traten gleichartige Veränderungen auf. Neben der bekannten Riesenzellenreaktion gegen Descemet fanden wir Riesenzellen auch an verdichteten Stromalamellen, an Bruchstücken der Bowmanschen Membran und an umwachsenen Stücken von Descemet aufgenähter Spenderhornhäute. Die Bedeutung dieser Befunde wird kurz diskutiert.

A granulomatous keratitis with giant cells, unrelated to a specific infection like tuberculosis or fungal disease, was first mentioned by Stock [4] and later described in more detail by Hogan and coworkers [2]. These authors found a foreign body giant cell reaction to Descemet's membrane in some cases of stromal herpetic keratitis and interpreted these findings as a probable result of necrosis of Descemet's membrane. Zimmerman [7] and Green and Zimmerman [1], however, after examining a larger series of cases, pointed to the fact that the pattern of this keratitis is very similar to that observed in phacoanaphylaxis and rheumatoid scleritis and thus speculated that the corneal disease could also be an autosensitivity reaction. While herpetic keratitis was also the prevalent disease in their series, they found the reaction to be rather non-specific, occurring in a number of different chronic corneal inflammatory and ulcerative diseases. Vogel and Naumann [5] reported on the clinical and histopathological picture of 12 cases. They observed that the giant cell reaction was exclusively centered around Descemet's membrane and stressed the importance of this disease for possible corneal perforation.

Our study was undertaken to find out whether the granulomatous giant cell reaction is actually exclusively directed to Descemet's membrane and whether it is most likely to be related to herpetic keratitis.

## Materials and Methods

141 corneal buttons and enucleated eyes, filed between 1968 and 1979 in the ophthalmic pathology laboratory of the University Eye Hospital in Freiburg and diagnosed as having chronic keratitis or corneal ulcers, were re-examined for the presence of granulomatous giant cell reaction in any of the corneal layers. Multiple sections, cut at 6 μ–8 μ from paraffin-embedded tissue, were available in each case. HE and PAS stainings were routinely done, while special staining techniques for bacteria and fungi were employed only when necessa-

ry. Cases were judged positively if clear-cut multi-nucleated giant cells were found. Corneas with giant cell reactions to sutures or other foreign body material were excluded, while a few cases of perforating corneal injury showing a giant cell reaction not related to foreign bodies were included. The available preoperative clinical pictures of the patients were studied, and an attempt to correlate the clinical and histopathological findings was made.

## Results

Among the 141 specimens examined, 19 cases of giant cell reaction were found. While herpes simplex was the prevalent underlying disease, the granulomatous reaction also occurred in a number of other corneal diseases such as rosacea-keratitis, mycotic ulcer, perforating injury, and after X-ray radiation for a malignant melanoma of the choroid. The incidence of the giant cell inflammation in the different diseases is given in Table 1.

The "classical" picture of giant cells centering around fragments or splinters of Descemet's or lining up against the intact membrane (Fig. 1b) was observed in 13 cases. However, there was also involvement of other corneal structures. Thus, we were able to find a giant cell granulomatous reaction around diseased or necrotic stromal lamellae (Fig. 1b) as well as to Bowman's membrane. In one case, the reaction to Bowman's membrane was in the donor button (Fig. 2), and in two cases, the giant cells were found around small fragments of Descemet's incorporated into the superficial stroma stemming from a donor button sown on as a "bio-patch" (Fig. 1c). The type and incidence of the corneal structures

**Table 1.** Incidence of the giant cell inflammation in the different diseases

| Herpetic Keratitis | |
| --- | --- |
| ulcerative | 7 |
| non-ulcerative | 4 |
| Other Inflammations | |
| Rosacea-Keratitis | 8 |
| Mycotic Ulcer | 1 |
| Bacterial(?) Ulcer | 1 |
| Trauma | |
| Perforating Injury | 3 |
| X-ray Radiation | 1 |

**Table 2.** Type and incidence of the corneal structures involved in the different diseases

| | Herpetic keratitis | Non-herpetic inflammations | Trauma |
| --- | --- | --- | --- |
| Descemet | 7 | 3 | 3 |
| Stroma | 4 | 1 | 2 |
| Bowman | 5 | – | – |
| Donor-Descemet | 2 | – | – |

involved in the different diseases is shown in Table 2.

The examination of the clinical pictures showed that in most cases of granulomatous giant cell reaction, there was a very severe corneal disease with deep ulceration and even perforation (Fig. 1). In some patients, however, a giant cell reaction could be found even with a rather inconspicuous clinical disease (Fig. 2).

## Discussion

The incidence of granulomatous giant cell reaction in our series of chronic and ulcerative keratitis was about 13%, thus slightly higher than that in the series of Green and Zimmerman [1], which was 9.4%. Our number would have been even higher if we included the granulomatous histiocytic reactions without giant cells. For reasons of clarity we excluded those cases, although Roll and Hanselmayer [3], in an electron microscopic study of granulomatous inflammation around Descemet's, were able to show that the histiocytic cells play the major role in the reaction, while the giant cells are not at all essential. We may therefore conclude that the granulomatous keratitis is more common than has been hitherto assumed.

Our series confirmed the findings by other authors [1, 5] that the granulomatous reaction is more frequently found in herpetic keratitis than in other forms of keratitis, although it is a rather non-specific reaction which occurs in a variety of corneal diseases. As yet it has only been reported in relation to Descemet's membrane, but we observed that it is not at all restricted to this membrane. It can also be found around diseased stromal lamellae and

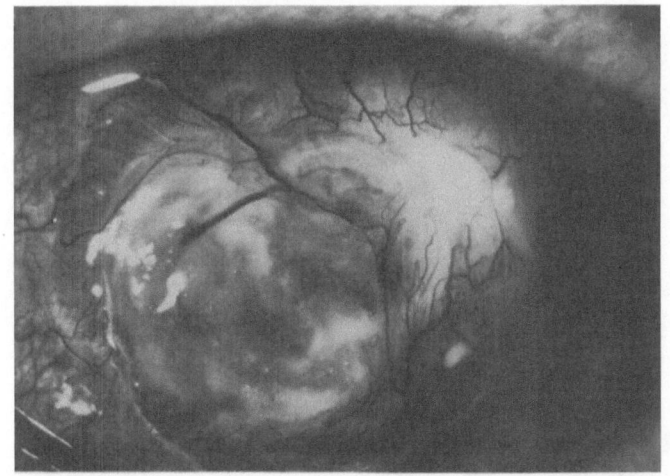

a

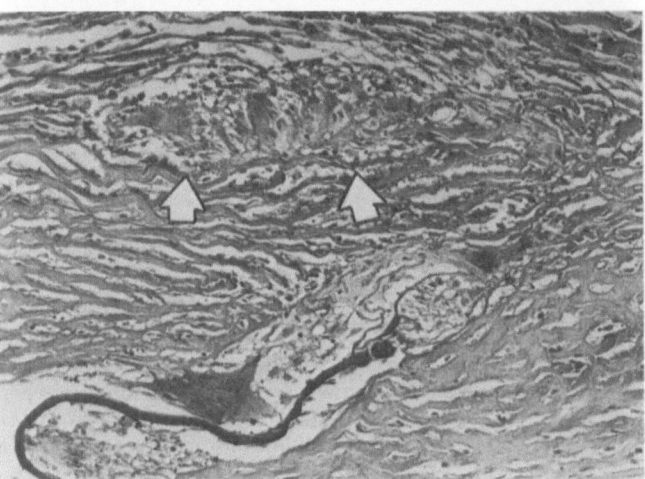

b

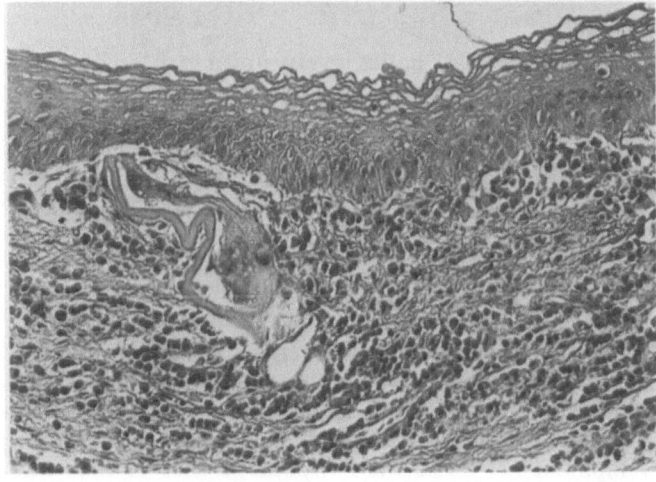

c

**Fig. 1.** Severe herpetic keratitis of more than 10 years duration. **a** Clinical picture, 8 months after "biopatching" with a sown-on donor cornea. **b** Giant cell reaction to Descemet's membrane and in the stroma (arrows). PAS, X 590. **c** Giant cells around a fragment of Descemet's membrane of the donor cornea. H and E, X 590

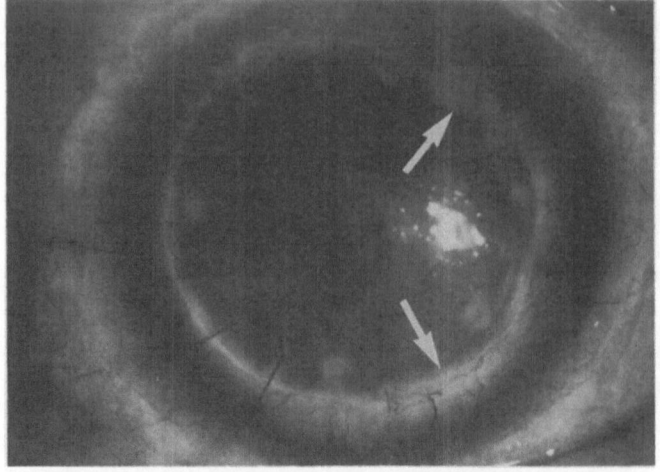

a

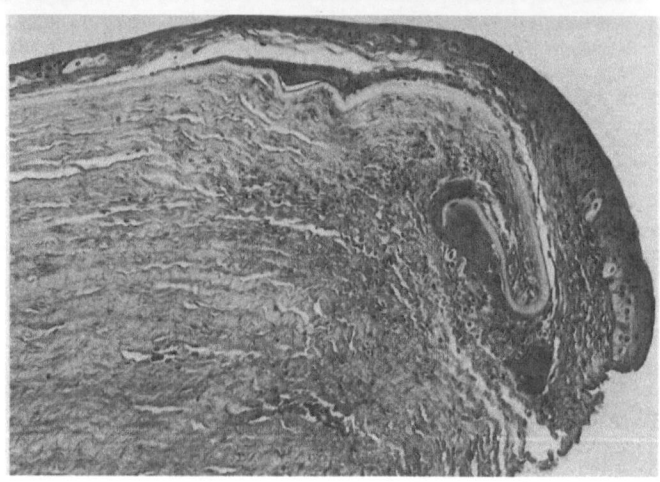

b

**Fig. 2.** Patient's eye 6 months after keratoplasty for severe herpetic keratitis. **a** Note the inflammatory infiltrates at the interface between host and donor tissues (arrows). **b** Giant cell reaction to donor Bowman near the edge of the button. PAS, X 230

around Bowman's membrane of host and donor tissue. These findings make an etiological explanation more difficult. Three hypotheses may nevertheless be considered in relation to etiology:

First, the physico-chemical nature of the corneal structures may be changed by the disease, giving them a "foreign body" nature.

Second, the reaction may be of the immunological type. This can be easily understood in cases where the granulomatous inflammation is directed against donor tissue. In cases of involvement of the host's own tissue, however, an altered antigenicity of the corneal structures with the consequent development of an autosensitivity reaction would be required. As mentioned earlier, Zimmerman [7] and Green and Zimmerman [1] emphasized that the histological picture of the granuloma-

tous keratitis is very similar to that of rheumatoid scleritis and phacoanaphylactic endophthalmitis, which are both considered to be autosensitivity reactions. This hypothesis is further supported by an observation of Wolter and co-workers [6] who described a patient with severe granulomatous keratitis in one eye and a consequent anterior uveitis in the other eye, presumably directed against Descemet's membrane. The uveitis immediately subsided after the enucleation of the first eye. This case was interpreted by the authors as an example of an acquired autosensitivity to Descemet's membrane.

The third hypothesis tries to take into account that the granulomatous reaction seems to be preferably centered around preformed "membranous" structures of the cornea. Though these "membranes" differ widely with respect to their histology and have quite different physico-chemical properties, they may well serve as a scaffold for easy adsorption of foreign antigen; viral, bacterial, or chemical.

Whatever the correct explanation may be, a better understanding of the nature of granulomatous giant cell keratitis is necessary for further therapeutic efforts.

## References

1. Green WR, Zimmerman LE (1967) Granulomatous reaction to Descemet's membrane. Am J Ophthalmol 64:555–558
2. Hogan MJ, Kimura SJ, Thygeson P (1963) Pathology of Herpes simplex kerato-iritis. Trans Am Ophthalmol Soc 61:75–99
3. Roll P, Hanselmayer H (1976) Die Ultrastruktur der granulomatösen Reaktion gegen die Descemetsche Membran. Klin Monatsbl Augenheilkd 168:819–824
4. Stock W (1939) Pathologische Anatomie des Auges. Enke, Stuttgart S 41
5. Vogel MH, Naumann G (1972) Die granulomatöse Reaktion gegen die Descemetsche Membran. Ber Dtsch Ophthalmol Ges 71:35–42
6. Wolter RJ, Johnson FD, Meyer RF, Watters JA (1971) Acquired autosensitivity to degenerating Descemet's membrane in a case with anterior uveitis in the other eye. Am J Ophthalmol 72:782–786
7. Zimmerman LE (1965) New concepts in pathology of the cornea. In: King RJ, McTigue JW (eds) Cornea World Congress. Butterworths, Washington D.C., pp 30–48

## Discussion on the Contributions pp. 163–171

J. Wollensak (Berlin)
In der allgemeinen Pathologie besteht die Auffassung, daß Riesenzellbildungen dann auftreten, wenn irgendwelches Fasermaterial abtransportiert werden soll. Und so vertreten zu meiner großen Überraschung die Pathologen die Auffassung, daß die Arteriitis temporalis eine Viruserkrankung sei und daß es bei dieser Viruserkrankung in der Arterie zum Untergang von Fasersubstanz kommt, und damit zur Riesenzellbildung. Meine Frage an die beiden Autoren: Was denken Sie darüber? Sind Reaktionen und Riesenzellen bei der Riesenzellarteriitis denen in der Cornea vergleichbar? Zweitens, haben Sie elektronenmikroskopische Befunde, denn mit deren Hilfe könnte man den Vergleich besser anstellen.

G.O.H. Naumann (Erlangen)
Das Anliegen war, die *klinischen* Kriterien zu diesem eigentümlichen histologischen Befund, der schon seit *Stocks* Zeiten bekannt ist (1939), herauszuarbeiten, weil wir ihn als eine Indikation zur kurativen Keratoplastik ansehen. Was die Ursache für den Befund angeht, müssen wir bekennen, daß wir im Spekulativen bleiben. Die Erklärungsmöglichkeiten wurden genannt, vom Fremdkörper bis zum autoimmunologischen Prozeß. Was im einzelnen zugrunde liegt, können wir nicht sagen.

Our basic thrust was to elaborate on the clinical criteria for this entity that has been well known to every ophthalmic pathologist because of the fact that this process is the precursor of a spontaneous perforation, and therefore, an indication for curative keratoplasty in our opinion. We have no etiologic proofs for this peculiar finding. We have no electron microscopic findings.

W. Böke (Kiel)
Ich möchte das etwas erweitern, was Herr Wollensak schon gesagt hat. Ihre Abschwächung, Herr Naumann, steht etwas im Gegensatz zu dem, was Herr Kortüm ziemlich deutlich angesprochen hat; nämlich, daß die Reaktion gegen die Descemet'sche Membran eine Autoaggressionsreaktion ist. Seit der ersten Mitteilung von Zimmermann, später von anderen und auch von Ihnen während Ihrer Hamburger Zeit, hat die Vorstellung einer Autoaggressionsreaktion eine Rolle gespielt. Wenn man sich mit der Immunologie und mit dem Vorgang der Autoaggression befaßt hat, muß man sich aber fragen, wo liegt der Beweis für diese Vermutung? Ich glaube, hier sollten wir vorsichtiger sein. Ich meine, man könnte die Reaktion, die Herr Wollensak soeben angedeutet und auch Herr Witschel ausgeführt hat, ebenso gut als eine sekundäre Reaktion gegen Läsionen verschiedener Art deuten. Daß Riesenzellen gefunden wurden, beweist noch nicht einmal einen immunopathologischen Vorgang geschweige denn Autoaggression. Vielleicht darf ich Sie, Herr Kortüm, auch darin korrigieren, daß der Wessely'sche Immunring keineswegs ein Zeichen eines Autoaggressionprozesses sein muß. Er kann auf vielerlei Weise und gegen vielerlei Antigene produziert werden und wird auch klinisch gesehen.

I would like to express the main points of my remarks in English: I objected to the idea that the granulomatous reaction against Descemet's membrane is to be taken for an auto-aggressive process. This may not necessarily be so, but various factors could induce such a response.

C. Kok van Alphen (Leyden)
I would like to ask what is the role of the endothelium.

G.O.H. Naumann (Erlangen)
It is probably destroyed. The signs of early corneal edema, that is endothelial decompensation, indicate that this crucial monocellular layer is affected in the initial phase.

R. Sundmacher (Freiburg)
This was also exactly the point I wanted to make because I think that deep corneal folds are mostly due to endothelial decompensation which, of course, may have different etiologies. In principal, I totally agree with your advice that these severely damaged eyes should undergo keratoplasty, because this will often eliminate recurrent inflammations and also restore vision. On the other hand, however, I do not follow you when you *generally* advise surgery in the *acute* stage already. One reason is that you may have unexpectedly good vision after conservative therapy. We happen to have treated a case from Tübingen which looked very similar to the last one you demonstrated. You ended up with a vision of 0.5 after keratoplasty, and we had a vision of 0.8 after conservative therapy. This does not say that we will not have to operate this patient sometime later in case of further recurring disease; I would prefer, however, to restrict immediate surgery to those cases with marked thinning and threatening perforation. In all other cases we would wait until the infiltrate has gone; but we too would certainly not wait for 1 or 2 years as has been recommended, but just for a couple of weeks or months.

G.O.H. Naumann (Erlangen)
It is not just an "infiltrate", it is a particular one. If it is the granulomatous reaction to Descemet's membrane, it is a frequent precursor of corneal perforation. To prevent that we believe a curative perforating corneal graft is indicated.

E. Kraus-Mackiw (Heidelberg)
Sometimes there is strong evidence, as Dr. Naumann pointed out, that there might be an autoimmune reaction to Descemet's. We saw a four-year-old girl who was hospitalized because of keratitis in both eyes. Three months after onset of the disease, keratoplasty à chaud was necessary in both eyes and histologically we found granulomatous reactions with macrophages and giant cells containing fragments of Descemet's, as demonstrated by Dr. Witschel. Since there has been no reaction to Descemet's of the donor grafts for 8 years now, it can be concluded that autoantibodies confined to the host tissue might be involved.

Furthermore, there was a recurrent herpes infection in the host corneas which stopped at the edge of the donor grafts: This observation may be attributed to the fact that corneal tissue varies in susceptibility to herpes virus infection depending on the differing genetic origin of receptor cornea and donor homograft.

G.O.H. Naumann (Erlangen)
Die Deutung dieses eigentümlichen klinischen und histopathologischen Phänomens ist bisher unklar. Wenn Herr Kortüm von autoaggressiven oder -immunologischen Prozessen sprach, so sind dies im Moment reine Vermutungen, wir wissen die Details nicht. Uns liegt es aber an was ganz anderem: Die Behandlung der Herpes corneae hängt, natürlich, entscheidend von der Virusisolation ab. Auch sind die Untersuchungen über die Serologie bzw. Immunologie, die wir heute nachmittag hörten, theoretisch sehr interessant und für das Verständnis der Krankheit wichtig. Was bisher kaum erwähnt wurde, waren die Veränderungen anderer Strukturen des Auges und speziell die handgreifliche granulomatöse Reaktion an der Descemet'schen Membran.

Zur Frage von Frau van Alphen über die Rolle des Endothels: Das Endothel ist bei dieser Reaktion zwangsläufig mitbetroffen. Selbstverständlich kommt es in Folge der entzündlichen Reaktion an der Descemet'schen Membran auch zu einer Endotheldekompensation und entsprechend dann zu dieser Faltenbildung, die wir klinisch als ein Kriterion für den Prozeß vor uns haben. Die Deutung des Wessely'schen Immunophänomens war nicht Anliegen unserer Demonstration. Es war aber unser Anliegen, die klinischen Kriterien der granulomatösen Reaktion an der Descemet'schen Membran, d.h. lange Anamnese, tiefes Infiltrat, Descemet-Falten, Begleituveitis, herauszuarbeiten und als eine definitive Indikation für ein aktives Vorgehen darzustellen. (Ich habe mich übrigens sehr gefreut, zu hören, daß die Freiburger uns als liebe Nachbarn genau so nett bei schwierigen Patienten aushelfen wie wir Ihnen!) Aber wir sind definitiv der Meinung, daß man beim Vorliegen einer Descemet-Ruptur − und die gehört zur granulomatösen Reaktion gegen die Descemet − allein aus tektonischen Gründen unbedingt zu einer kurativen perforierenden Keratoplastik raten sollte − auch dann, wenn das übrige Stroma noch nicht verdünnt ist. Wir haben mehrfach Patienten mit granulomatöser Reaktion gegen die Descemet beobachtet, die den Eingriff ablehnten, bei denen es innerhalb von Tagen zu einer spontanen Perforation kam. Deswegen möchte ich dezidiert den Vorschlag aufrecht erhalten, daß beim Vorliegen einer granulomatösen Reaktion gegen die Descemetsche Membran zur perforierenden Keratoplastik geraten werden sollte.

The idea was not to discuss the etiology, the

idea was to present the *clinical* features and to stress that our impression of this process as a precusor to corneal perforation represents a definite indication for a curative perforating keratoplasty. The role of the endothelium is that of an innocent, passive, suffering element that is damaged, which leads to endothelial decompensation. Frequently the peculiar granulomatous infiltration is visible only anterior to Descemet's membrane (away from the endothelium).

Sundmacher, R. (Hrsg.):
Herpetische Augenerkrankungen
© J.F. Bergmann Verlag, München 1981

# Scanning Electron Microscopic Investigations on the Development of the Dendritic Lesion in the Corneal Epithelium

J.-P. Harnisch, F. Hoffmann, Berlin

**Key words.** Dendritic lesion, SEM

**Schlüsselwörter.** Dendritikafigur, Rasterelektronenmikroskopie

**Summary.** The dendritic lesion in cases of HVH infection is provoked experimentally in the rabbit cornea and, based on scanning electron microscopic findings, a theory is formulated on the development of the dendritic lesion.

The dendritic lesion is typical for a herpes simplex infection of the cornea. Two developmental theories are known to us:
1. It is the result of the viruses spreading in the corneal nerves [1].
2. Resistent cell groups are responsible for a random course of infection pathways in the presence of viruses spreading from cell to cell [2].

**Zusammenfassung.** Die Dendriticafigur bei HVH-Infektion wird experimentell an der Kaninchen-hornhaut erzeugt und eine Theorie bezüglich ihrer Entstehung anhand rasterelektronenmikroskopischer Befunde entwickelt.

## Material and Method

1 drop of HVH type 1 ($10^4$–$10^5$ TCID$_{50}$/ml) is applied to the intact corneas of 18 rabbits. Three eyes are examined every 2nd day over a period of 12 days.

## Results

In ten rabbits epithelial alterations develop in

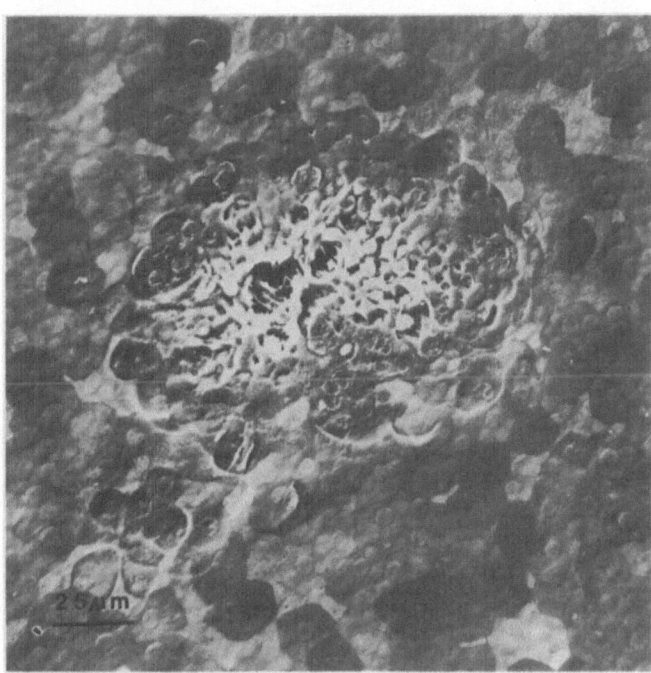

**Fig. 1.** Isolated focal lesion of the corneal epithelium

175

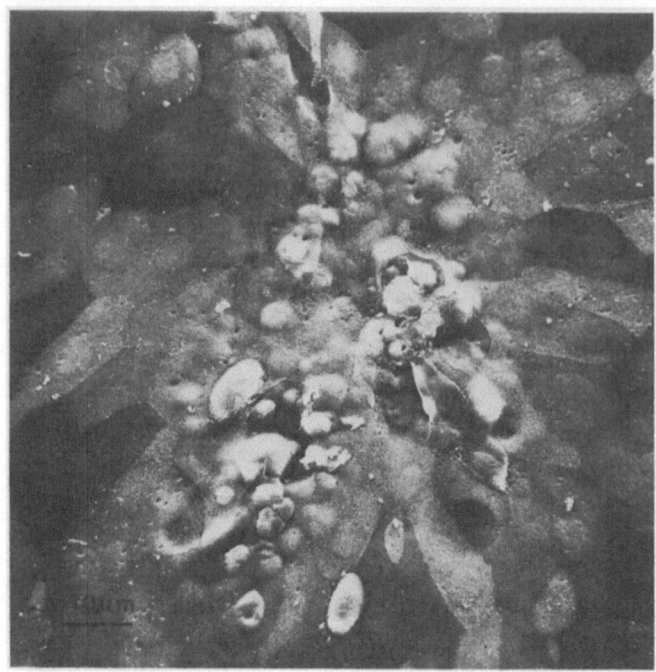

**Fig. 2.** Cellular movement of epithelial cells partly covering the epithelial defect

the form of isolated focal lesions (Fig. 1) and dendritic lesions. On the 4th day, there is no change in the epithelial cell pattern surrounding focal lesions. On the 6th day, the epithelial cells move towards the defect. On the 8th day, the surface cells are arranged in an asteroid alignment and may have partly covered the defect (Fig. 2).

The dendritic lesion from the 4th day on shows a more beaded configuration, i.e. the

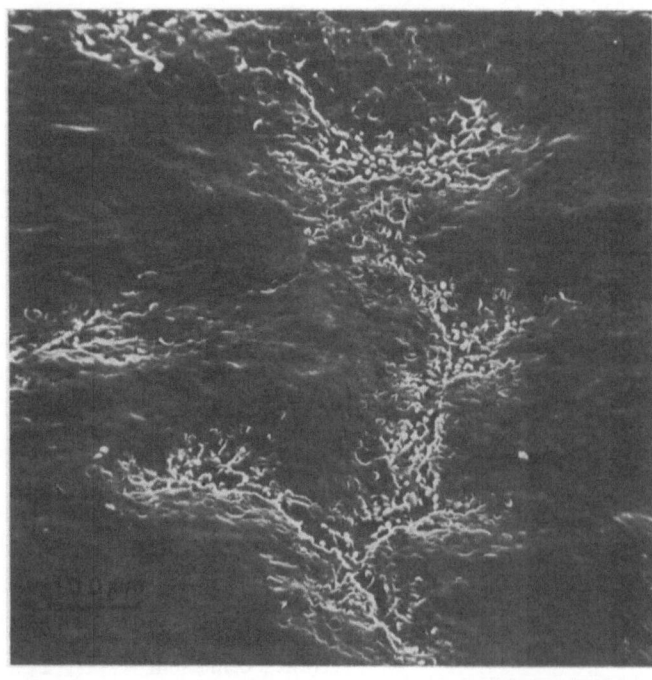

**Fig. 3.** Dendritic lesion on the 4th day, built up by connected focal defects

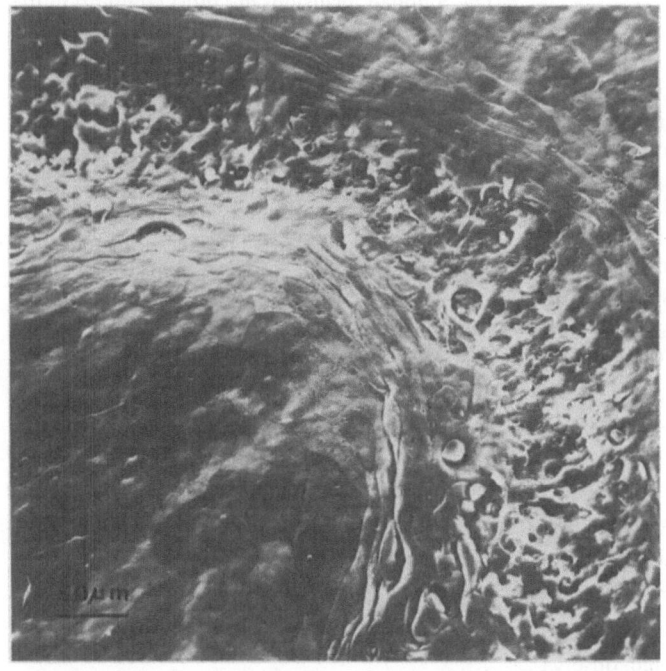

**Fig. 4.** Uniformly broad epithelial lesion on the 12th day

focal lesions are connected by string-like defects (Fig. 3). On the 6th day the connections are growing wider until, on the 12th day, a uniformly broad epithelial lesion has developed.

The original circular foci are no longer recognizable (Fig. 4). During the entire observation period, the diameter of isolated circular foci and dendritic lesions remained constant at 100 to 200 µm.

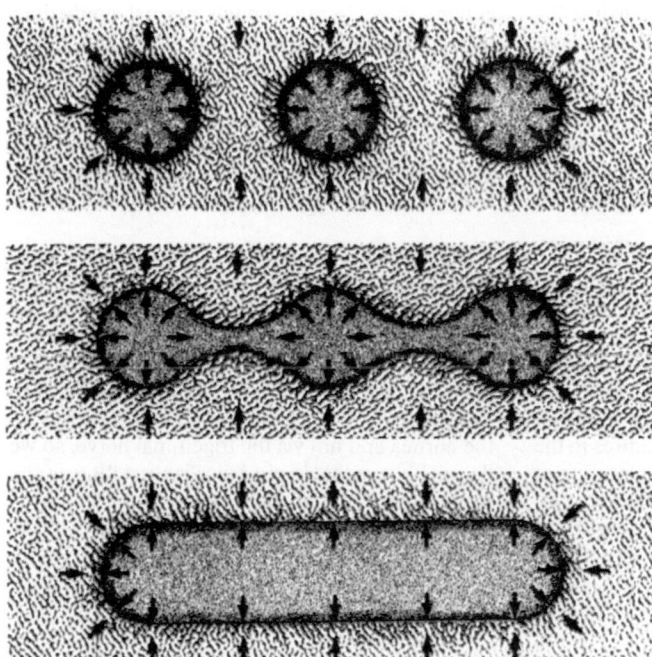

**Fig. 5.** Graphic presentation of the development of a dendritic lesion from adjacent focal defects

## Conclusion

We consider the focal lesion in the herpes simplex infection to be the primary epithelial defect. The reparative response to the defect demonstrated by SEM consists of epithelial movement. The balance between the cytopathic effect and the epithelial movement accounts for the constant size of the focal and dendritic lesion (Fig. 5). Between immediately adjacent defects there is too little epithelium capable of migration, so that the cytotoxic effect prevails and the dendritic lesion develops.

## References

1. Dawson CR, Togni B, Moore TE (1968) Structural changes in chronic herpetic keratitis studied by light and electron microscopy. Arch Ophthalmol 79:740–748
2. Spencer WH, Hayes TL (1970) Scanning and transmission electron microscopic observations of the topographic anatomy of dendritic lesions in the rabbit cornea. Invest Ophthalmol Visual Sci 2:183–195

## Discussion on the Contribution pp. 175–178

V. Victoria-Troncoso (Ghent)
As far as I see there is no opposition against the theory that the lesions confluence. In the same cornea, you can find focal lesions and dendritic lesions. Do they all confluence?

F. Hoffmann (Berlin)
Only those lesions confluence which are close together. If they are separated focal lesions, they normally disappear within a week.

P.C. Maudgal (Leuven)
I fully agree with what the authors of this poster have presented here, but I would like to discuss this poster in correlation to the histological findings. Histologically, there are also punctate epithelial lesions, as we see in the second photograph from the left. Herpes virus multiplies and matures in the infected cells and is released by the ballooning of the nuclear membrane. The released material reorganises into rounded inclusion bodies which can infect other cells to form more punctate lesions.

The rounded inclusions are most common in the 1st week of infection and were not seen in the late stages of experimental keratitis or dendritic ulcers of patients. Now, if we compare the dendritic lesion and the punctate lesion in this poster, the dendritic lesion shows elongated cells along the periphery which are absent in punctate lesions. What I am trying to emphasize is that there is a difference in the behaviour of cells in the early and late stages of infection. With the lapse of time, more and more cells become rounded and may fuse together to form syncytia. At the same time, the histochemical staining pattern changes. Pseudopodia-like processes extend from the rounded cells or syncytia to the peripheral cells. On coming in contact with these processes, the peripheral cells become rounded to form another lesion. I think the dendritic lesion is formed in this way. My question is if the authors of this paper saw any evidence of such pseudopodia processes in their scanning electron microscopic study.

F. Hoffmann (Berlin)
No, we did not. Four days after the infection you see normal epithelial cells in the area surrounding the focal lesions. Six days after the infection, you see the asteroid alignment of the epithelial cells in the area surrounding the focal lesion. While they are moving towards this defect in order to close it, the viruses are spreading and destroying the surrounding cells, so there is a balance between these forces; and, after a week or so, an immunity develops against the disease and the defect can be closed. But when focal lesions are very close together, there is not enough normal epithelium between lesions to outbalance the destructive force, and we have the dendritic lesion.

K. Lalau (Leyden)
I would like to ask whether you noticed any correlation between the corneal nerves in the epithelium and the development of the lesions.

F. Hoffmann (Berlin)
Of course, we also did transmission electron microscopy, but that does not enable us to answer this question. Ours is just a hypothesis that does not take into consideration infection via the trigeminal nerve. In our experimental set-up, the infection was induced by local application of the viruses on the cornea and not via the trigeminal nerve, so we do not believe that in our investigation there is any connection between the formation of a dendritic lesion and the arrangement of nerve fibers in the cornea.

Sundmacher, R. (Hrsg.):
Herpetische Augenerkrankungen
© J.F. Bergmann Verlag, München 1981

# Welcoming Address at the Wine Tasting Party

G. Mackensen, Freiburg

Dear Participants of our Herpes Symposium and especially, honored ladies,

I promised you this morning in my welcoming address that, outside of the scientific lectures and discussions, we would like to amuse you with those things which most typify the life style of this area.

Freiburg has experienced a great deal during the turbulence of European history. Since 1368, it belonged alternately to Austria and France. Only in the past 170 years had it been a part of the Baden region, and, hence, a part of what we now call Germany.

Accordingly, one is still able to clearly detect French and Austrian influences which complement the indigenous alemanian way of life. I cannot elaborate right now on how much the intelectual life and culinary pleasures of this region have been stamped by the harmony of these influences, but believe me, the life in this region, which – ignoring all borders – calls itself "Regio Basiliensis", is exceptionally charming.

Still, we are not concerned with getting you acquainted with the fine dining of our country. Tonight we would prefer to dine in the manner which comes to us from the peasant culture, and, here in Freiburg, wine plays an integral role. Therefore, we also offer you that which one drinks here in the country.

In Latin class we learned the phrase "in vino veritas" and probably didn't understand it at first. Now that we are older and wiser, we understand that it should be the motto for this evening. Wine makes us more friendly, it loosens our tongues and brings us closer to our partners in conversation. To this extent, it can play an important role in such a symposium as ours.

One could, however, attach a further meaning to the Latin proverb. The enormous variety of vintages demands that we compare these different wines. It is therefore not surprising that there is a science of wine tasting in which one is called upon again and again to compare the different types of grapes, their specific qualities and taste as dictated by the place in which they were grown and their year's vintage qualities.

Continuous testing to learn if it is more advisable to abide by one favorite wine or if one should remain open to new discoveries does have something in common with scientific developments. The wine tasting which we will now enjoy is, in this regard, a real component of our symposium.

In doing so let us not forget that we would like to use the harmonizing effect of the wine for being especially nice to the ladies. In vino veritas!

# Clinico-Serologic Correlations

Sundmacher, R. (Hrsg.):
Herpetische Augenerkrankungen
© J.F. Bergmann Verlag, München 1981

# A Micro-Immunofluorescence (IF) Test for Detecting Type-Specific Antibodies to Herpes Simplex Virus

S. Darougar, T. Forsey, London

**Key words.** HSV infections – diagnosis by micro-immunofluorescence (IF) test

**Schlüsselwörter.** HSV-Infektionen – Diagnose mit Mikroimmunfluoreszenztest

**Summary.** A rapid IF test capable of detecting and quantifying type specific IgG, IgM or IgA antibodies to Herpes simplex virus (HSV) type 1 and type 2 in blood or local discharges has been developed.

The antigens required for this test can be grown in bulk in tissue cultures and purified by a simple differential centrifugation. The amount of antigen required for each test is minimal since one ampoule containing 0.3 ml of purified virus can produce hundreds of slides.

Because of the small amounts of serum or whole blood or local discharge required for this test (0.1 ml) we found it feasible to collect these specimens by special cellulose sponges and transport them without requiring special arrangement for cold storage.

In our laboratory we found that the IF test is highly sensitive for detecting type-specific antibodies to HSV type 1 and type 2. Additionally, the test is also able to identify anti-herpes IgG, IgM or IgA classes of antibody in patients with ocular or genital HSV infection.

The results of studies on comparative sensitivity of IF test with that of the complement fixation test and cultural tests for the diagnosis of HSV infections of the eye and genital tract and the results of sero-epidemiological surveys of HSV ocular and genital infections using the IF test are discussed.

**Zusammenfassung.** Ein sehr schnell durchführbarer IF-Test, mit dem man Typ-spezifische IgG-, IgM- and IgA-Antikörper gegen Herpes simplex-Virus Typ 1 oder 2 im Blut oder in Absonderungen nachweisen kann, wurde von uns entwickelt.

Die für den Test benötigten Antigene kann man in großer Menge in Gewebekulturen erzeugen und dann durch einfache Differentialzentrifugierung reinigen. Die für den einzelnen Test benötigte Antigenmenge ist so gering, daß eine 0,3-ml-Ampulle mit gereinigtem Virus für die Herstellung von hunderten von Deckgläsern gebraucht werden kann.

Weil der Test auch mit sehr kleinen Serum- oder Vollblutmengen oder mit flüssigen Absonderungen durchgeführt werden kann (0,1 ml), haben wir die Gewinnung dieser Flüssigkeiten mit kleinen speziellen Zelluloseschwämmen als vorteilhaft empfunden. Sie können ohne spezielle Kühlvorrichtungen transportiert werden.

In unseren Laboratorien hat sich der IF-Test als äußerst empfindlich bei der Entdeckung Typ-spezifischer Antikörper gegen HSV Typ 1 und 2 erwiesen. Außerdem läßt sich dieser Test auch zur Identifizierung von Antiherpes-Antikörpern der Klassen IgG, IgM oder IgA bei Patienten mit okulärem oder genitalem Herpes anwenden. Wir werden über Studien zur Empfindlichkeit des IF-Testes im Vergleich mit der Komplementbindungsreaktion und virologischen Isolierungen bei der Diagnose von HSV-Augen- und Genitalinfektionen berichten sowie über die Ergebnisse von sero-epidemiologischen Studien mit dem IF-Test bei okulären und genitalen HSV-Infektionen.

## Discussion on the Contribution p. 183

J. Wollensak (Berlin)
I want to ask you why your blood donors have had such a very low ration of HSV antibodies, because, if I remember correctly, yours had only 20% and we think ours must have had 90% or more.

S. Darougar (London)
The low prevalence of HSV antibodies detected in blood donors (21% for HSV 1 and 7% for HSV 2) may be due partly to our starting dilution at $^1/_{16}$ (missing sera positive at levels of $^1/_8$ or lower) and

partly to the type of antigen (purified virus particles) used in the test. In our hands the sensitivity of microimmunofluorescence (IF) test appears to be slightly higher than that of the complement fixation test for detecting antibodies against herpes virus. Further work is in progress to compare the sensitivity of IF test with that of neutralization test and ELISA system. However, recent reports show a lower prevalence of antibody against HSV in the developed countries. Juel Jensen (1973) reported a 33% prevalence amongst a group of British students and Roome et al. (1975) reported a 50% (approximately) prevalence in a group of blood donors.

H.E. Kaufman (New Orleans)
It is a very interesting paper, but the real problem is what it all means. Some years ago, for example, we did a great deal of work on locally-produced IgA antibodies to herpes. We found that there were herpes-specific antibodies, more effective, in fact, than IgG. We found that putting dead antigen in one eye would selectively stimulate that eye to produce IgA, but we could never show that this prevented infection or prevented recurrence, or did anything at all. Although it's there, and the Lord must have had a purpose for it, we don't yet know what it is.

H. Moser (Marburg)
I just want to comment on your results concerning a supposed lower incidence of HSV infection due to a better hygiene standard in developed countries. In Marburg, West Germany, we recently examined a randomly selected group of 36 adult blood donors for anti HSV 1 immunity using complement fixation assays, microneutralization tests and the more sensitive enzyme immunoassays. In addition, the lymphocyte stimulation test was employed to detect specific cellular immunity. We found only three of the donors to be HSV negative in all the assays, while nine of them were negative in the less sensitive complement fixation and microneutralization test. This result indicates that detection of anti HSV antibodies depends largely on the sensitivity of the assays. Hence I would suggest that you would substantiate the validity of your results by employing a more sensitive method.

M. Zirm (Innsbruck)
I'd like to ask you about your last slide. If I understand it correctly, you find IgG antibodies more often than IgA. Could you explain this fact?

S. Darougar (London)
I am afraid in the present series we found only a few tears positive for IgA, whereas IgG was present in the tears of the majority of cases. I am sorry that at present we are unable to interpret this finding.

M. Zirm (Innsbruck)
You would expect IgA in tears in a much higher concentration.

S. Darougar (London)
In our experience the level of IgA in tears is very low if it is present at all.

D. Neumann-Haefelin (Freiburg)
I would like to ask you once more about the sensitivity of your test. Did you compare it with the sensitivity of an immunofluorescence test using infected cells as an antigen? Could you tell the actual titers in the sera tested, or at least the range of these titers?

S. Darougar (London)
I am afraid I am not able to answer your question regarding comparative sensitivities of these two tests as we have not yet compared them. In our test we have a standard end-point which can be followed without difficulty, whereas in using infected cells as antigen we have various responses including standard inclusions in the cytoplasm or in nucleus, whole stained cells or rings around the cells which causes variation in reading the results.

H. Shiota (Tokushima)
More than 90% of the adults have anti-HSV titers in their serum, usually type. 1. It is therefore possible that those who suffer from type 2 have the same titer. Have you ever seen a patient who showed the same titer against type 1 and type 2? In that case you may have difficulty in identifying which type the patient is suffering from.

S. Darougar (London)
In animals experimentally infected with HSV 2, sera react equally against HSV 1 and HSV 2, whereas sera from animals infected with HSV 1 react distinctively against HSV 1.

In examining positive sera from patients with genital herpes infection, we found that the level of antibody is raised against both serotypes equally in about 70% of patients (suggestive of an infection with HSV 2), whereas in 30% of patients we have a higher level of antibody against one or another serotype.

B.R. Jones (London)
Thank you very much. We should pass on to the next paper, but it would seem that there is a need for contemporary serological surveys concerning the epidemiology of herpes infections in various types of communities. I think it is not valid to apply to our communities today the doubt that arose in the earlier part of this century because of changing patterns of hygiene and interpersonal contact. It is a time now with new serological methods available which really lend themselves to sero-epidemiological studies; of course, these methods are also of value in the diagnosis of disease in individual patients, but, as Kaplan has pointed out, in this field there are much greater problems in interpretation.

Sundmacher, R. (Hrsg.):
Herpetische Augenerkrankungen
© J.F. Bergmann Verlag, München 1981

# Virologische Untersuchung bei endogenen Augenerkrankungen

G. Maass, B. Dieckhues, Münster

**Key words.** Antibody mediated immunity to HSV – correlation with endogenous eye diseases

**Schlüsselwörter.** Antikörpervermittelte Immunität gegenüber HSV – Korrelation mit endogenen Augenerkrankungen

**Summary.** In addition to presumed bacteriologic etiology for immunopathologic eye diseases (e.g. tuberculosis, toxoplasmosis, leptospirosis, streptococci etc.), a viral etiology for endogenous uveitis has been discussed recently. We investigated the titers of antibodies against the following viruses in patients with immunopathologic eye diseases and in normals: adeno-, mumps-, measles-, German measles-, herpes-, varizella-, hepatitis-B-, and cytomegalo-viruses.

**Zusammenfassung.** Neben bakteriologischen Ursachen immunpathologischer Augenerkrankungen, insbesondere Tbc, Toxoplasmose, Leptospirose, Streptokokken usw., wird in neuerer Zeit auch eine Virusätiologie der Uveitiden diskutiert. In der vorliegenden Arbeit wird über den Nachweis von Antikörpern gegen verschiedene Virusarten bei immunpathologischen Augenerkrankungen im Vergleich zu gesunden Versuchspersonen berichtet. Die zum Teil wiederholt durchgeführten serologischen Untersuchungen erstreckten sich auf folgende Viren:
Adeno-, Mumps-, Masern-, Röteln-, Herpes-, Varizellen-, Hepatitis-B- und Zytomegalie-Viren.

In der Pathogenese der endogenen Uveitis wird immunpathologischen Mechanismen eine bedeutende Rolle zugesprochen, wobei durch den Erstkontakt, z.B. mit einzelnen Bakterien oder ihren Toxinen, eine lokale Antikörpersynthese im Auge induziert werden soll, so daß bei einem erneuten Kontakt – z.B. auch durch eine hämatogene Aussaat der Mikroben – eine lokale Antigen-Antikörperreaktion ausgelöst wird, die sich als Entzündung des befallenen Auges äußert. Als Hinweis auf derartige immunologische Mechanismen bei der Entstehung der Uveitis kann die festgestellte Vermehrung von T-und B-Lymphocyten im Blut der Erkrankten gewertet werden [1].

Als auslösende Faktoren dieser immunologischen Reaktion bei endogenen Augenerkrankungen wurden bisher überwiegend Infektionen mit Bakterien oder Parasiten angeschuldigt, die sich jedoch nur bei einem kleinen Teil der Erkrankten nachweisen ließen. Wir interessierten uns für die Frage, wieweit akute oder chronische Virusinfektionen des Menschen eine Uveitis verursachen können. Ähnliche Untersuchungen wurden bereits u.a. von Witmer [5], Martenet [3] und anderen durchgeführt. Zur Beantwortung der Frage wurden bei etwa 190 Patienten im Alter zwischen 25 und 50 Jahren mit Uveitis und Neuritis im Vergleich zu einer Kontrollgruppe Antikörper mit unterschiedlichen Methoden gegen verschiedene Viren im Serum der Patienten nachgewiesen; die Untersuchungstechniken sind in Tabelle 1 zusammengestellt. KBR, HHT und RIT wurden in den jeweiligen Standardtechniken des US Public Health Service [2] durchgeführt, der Nachweis von Antikörpern gegen Zytomegalievirus erfolgte nach der Methode von Schmitz und Haas [4].

**Tabelle 1.** Methoden zum Nachweis von Antikörpern gegen verschiedene Virusarten bei Patienten mit Uveitis

| Virusart | Methode |
|---|---|
| Masern | HHT |
| Röteln | HHT |
| H. simplex | KBR |
| Varizellen | KBR |
| Adenovirus (Gruppenantigen) | KBR |
| CMV | IFT (IgM, IgG) |
| Hepatitis B | RIT |

**Tabelle 2.** Nachweis von Antikörpern (%) gegen verschiedene Virusarten bei Patienten mit Uveitis

| Virus | Perf. Verletzung n = 40 | Neuritis 41 | Vordere Uveitis 46 | Hintere Uveitis 61 | Uveitis 52 | Sonstige 14 |
|---|---|---|---|---|---|---|
| Masern | 93 | 95 | 98 | 95 | 87 | 93 |
| Röteln | 98 | 97 | 100 | 97 | 100 | 100 |
| H. simplex | 43 | 45 | 40 | 43 | 44 | 50 |
| Varizellen | 0 | 0 | 4 | 2 | 0 | 4 |
| Adenovirus-Gruppen-Antigen | 10 | 11 | 20 | 15 | 14 | 18 |

Die Häufigkeit von Antikörpern als Folge durchgemachter Infektionen mit den jeweiligen Viren in den verschiedenen Untersuchungsgruppen findet sich in Tabelle 2. Unterschiede zwischen den Patientengruppen mit verschiedenen Uveitisformen oder gegenüber der Kontrollgruppe, die aus Patienten mit perforierenden Hornhautverletzungen besteht, finden sich nicht. Die hohen Prävalenzraten der Antikörper gegen Masern- und Rötelnvirus entspricht der Durchseuchung der entsprechenden Altersgruppen mit diesen Viren. Die Angaben über die Infektionshäufigkeit mit Adenoviren geben – anders als bei den übrigen Viren – Auskunft über einen Kontakt mit mindestens einem Adenovirus, da für die KBR ein gruppenspezifisches Antigen verwendet wurde.

Untersucht man nicht die Häufigkeit von Antikörperträgern gegen die genannten Virusarten in den verschiedenen Gruppen, sondern die mittlere Antikörperkonzentration in den Gruppen, so ergibt sich das folgende Bild (Tabelle 3). Auf diesem Bild sind die geometrischen Mittelwerte der Antikörpertiter in den jeweiligen Gruppen – abgekürzt GMT – zusammen mit dem 95%-Vertrauensbereich dieser Werte angegeben. Es finden sich keine Unterschiede in den mittleren Antikörpertitern bei den Patienten mit verschiedenen Uveitisformen gegenüber der Kontrollgruppe.

Zu diesen Daten möchte ich ergänzen, daß wir bei drei von insgesamt 249 untersuchten Personen durch den Nachweis von HBsAg eine chronische, symptomlose Infektion mit Hepatitis-B-Virus ermitteln konnten, bei einer Kontrollperson und bei zwei Patienten mit Uveitis. Diese Häufigkeit von 1,2% für das asymptomatische Trägertum von Hepatitis-B-Virus entspricht dem Erwartungswert in der hiesigen Bevölkerung, der zwischen 0,7% und 1,2% liegt.

**Tabelle 3.** GMT (95% VB) gegen verschiedene Virusarten bei Patienten mit Uveitis

| Virus | Perf. Verletzung n = 40 | Neuritis 41 | Vordere Uveitis 46 | Hintere Uveitis 61 | Uveitis 52 | Sonstige 14 |
|---|---|---|---|---|---|---|
| Masern | 28.6 (28,3–28,7) | 47.5 (47,2–47,8) | 36.0 (35,7–36,3) | 34.3 (34,0–34,6) | 34.3 (34,0–34,6) | 47.5 (47,2–47,8) |
| Röteln | 75.1 (74,4–75,7) | 96.3 (96,0–96,7) | 84.6 (81,3–81,9) | 89.9 (89,5–90,2) | 91.8 (91,5–92,2) | 96.3 (96,0–96,7) |
| H. simplex | 4.9 ( 4,4– 5,4) | 4.4 ( 3,9– 4,9) | 4.4 ( 3,6– 4,6) | 4.6 ( 4,2– 5,0) | 4.9 ( 4,4– 5,4) | 4.0 |
| Varizellen | – | – | 6.0 | 4.0 | – | – |
| Adenovirus-Gruppen-Antigen | 5.0 ( 4,7– 5,3) | 4.0 | 5.0 ( 4,7– 5,3) | 5.9 ( 5,6– 6,2) | 4.9 ( 4,6– 5,2) | 4.0 |

**Tabelle 4.** Antikörper gegen CMV (IgM, IgG) bei Patienten mit Uveitis

| | Perf. Verletzung n = 44 | Neuritis 37 | Vordere Uveitis 55 | Hintere Uveitis 69 | Uveitis 57 | Sonstige 14 |
|---|---|---|---|---|---|---|
| CMV-IgM positiv | 15% | 32 | 33 | 32<br>p > 0,05 | 21 | 14 |
| CMV-IgG positiv | 62% | 62 | 68 | 55 | 54 | 36 |

Außer Antikörpern gegen die bisher genannten Virusarten wurde die Häufigkeit von Antikörpern gegen Zytomegalievirus sowohl in der IgG- als auch in der IgM-Fraktion der Immunglobuline der Patienten bestimmt; die Ergebnisse dieser Untersuchung sind in Tabelle 4 zusammengestellt.

Die Häufigkeit von Personen, die zumindest einmal mit Zytomegalievirus infiziert worden waren – kenntlich am Nachweis von Antikörpern in der IgG-Fraktion –, ist in den verschiedenen Untersuchungsgruppen praktisch gleich, wenn man einmal von der kleinen Gruppe „sonstige" absieht. Der Nachweis von IgM-Antikörpern gegen dieses Virus kann als Hinweis für eine floride Infektion mit dem Erreger angesehen werden, entweder als Primärinfektion oder als Folge einer Reaktivierung einer latenten Infektion oder – anders ausgedrückt – einer endogenen Reinfektion. Die Häufigkeit, mit der IgM-Antikörper gegen dieses Virus in den verschiedenen Untersuchungsgruppen nachgewiesen werden konnten, ist in der oberen Bildhälfte angegeben. Die Unterschiede zwischen den verschiedenen Gruppen mit Uveitis und der Kontrollgruppe sind – wie man nach entsprechender statistischer Prüfung mit Hilfe des $X^2$-Tests nachweisen kann – auf dem angegebenen Level nicht signifikant.

Zusammenfassend kann man also feststellen, daß die Häufigkeit von Infektionen mit Masern-, Röteln-, H. simplex-, Varizellen-Zoster-, Hepatitis-B-Virus und Adenoviren sowie die Nachweishäufigkeit von IgM-Antikörpern gegen Zytomegalievirus bei den verschiedenen Formen der Uveitis sich nicht von entsprechenden Daten in der Allgemeinbevölkerung unterscheidet. Diese Feststellung schließt nicht aus, daß im Einzelfall eine Uveitis im Gefolge einer Virusinfektion auftreten kann.

## Literatur

1. Dieckhues B, Jünemann G (1980) T- und B-Lymphocyten bei Augenerkrankungen. Ber Dtsch Ophthalmol Ges 77:889–890
2. Lennette EH, Schmidt NJ (1979) Diagnostic procedures for viral, rickettsial and chlamydial infections, 5th ed. Am Publ Health Ass, Washington DC
3. Martenet AC (1971) Virus et uvéites. Dois, Paris
4. Schmitz H, Haas R (1972) Determination of different cytomegalovirus immunoglobulins by immunfluorescence. Arch Virusforsch 37:332
5. Witmer R (1978) Clinical implications of aqueous humor studies in uveitis. Am J Ophthalmol 86:39

## Diskussion zum Beitrag S. 185–187

H. Neubauer (Köln)
Darf ich fragen, ob in der letzten Gruppe der Uveitis nur Pan-Uveitis-Fälle gemeint waren, oder waren da möglicherweise auch Augen mit vorderer Uveitis?

B. Dieckhues (Münster)
Es handelt sich bei dieser Gruppe nur um Pan-Uveitis-Fälle.

# Clinical Virology

Sundmacher, R. (Hrsg.):
Herpetische Augenerkrankungen
© J.F. Bergmann Verlag, München 1981

# Herpetic Chorioretinitis in Newborn Infants: An Experimental Study

J.O. Oh, P. Minasi, San Francisco

**Key words.** HSV-1, HSV-2, chorioretinitis, dermatotropism

**Schlüsselwörter.** HSV-1, HSV-2, Chorioretinitis, Dermatotropismus

**Summary.** Herpetic chorioretinitis in newborn infants has been associated exclusively with type 2 herpes simplex virus (HSV 2). The cause of this unique nature of the eye diseases is not clear at present. One possible cause is that the selective susceptibility of portal of entries of the virus may be a determining factor for the outcome of chorioretinal involvement in the newborn. This possibility was investigated in newborn rabbits.

One-day-old New Zealand white rabbits were inoculated with $10^3$ TCID$_{50}$ of type 1 HSV (HSV 1) and HSV 2 strains via intranasal and subcutaneous routes and ten-day-old rabbits were inoculated with the virus via corneal routes. Both HSV 1 and HSV 2 strains produced chorioretinal lesions in the eyes in an equal frequency following intranasal and corneal inoculation. Following subcutaneous inoculation, however, only HSV 2 strains were able to induce chorioretinal lesions. HSV 2 grew well in the skin and disseminated readily in many organs including the eye, while HSV 1 strains grew poorly in the skin, failed to disseminate and to induce ocular lesions. However, intracardiac injection of HSV 1 resulted in wide dissemination of the infection and chorioretinitis in the eye in a similar frequency as in the rabbits which received HSV 2 strains. These results appear to indicate that the dermatotropism of HSV 2 may be partly responsible for the unique association of herpetic chorioretinitis with HSV 2 in the herpetic infection of the newborns.

**Zusammenfassung.** Eine herpetische Chorioretinitis bei Neugeborenen hat man bislang ausschließlich durch die Infektion mit Herpes simplex-Virus Typ 2 (HSV 2) gefunden. Der Grund hierfür ist gegenwärtig noch nicht klar. Eine Erklärungsmöglichkeit könnte darin liegen, daß die Eintrittspforten, über die das Virus Zugang zum Körper erlangt und dann die Neugeborenen-Chorioretinitis erzeugt, eine gewisse selektive Empfänglichkeit haben. Dies haben wir bei neugeborenen Kaninchen untersucht. Einen Tag alte weiße Neuseeland-Kaninchen wurden mit $10^3$ TCID$_{50}$ eines HSV 1 und eines HSV 2 Stammes intranasal und subkutan infiziert; eine korneale Infektion mit den gleichen Stämmen erfolgte an zehn Tage alten Tieren. Sowohl HSV 1- als auch HSV 2-Stämme erzeugten nach intranasaler und kornealer Infektion in einer vergleichbaren Häufigkeit chorioretinale Entzündungen. Nach subkutaner Infektion gelang dies aber nur mit HSV 2. Dieser Stamm vermehrte sich gut in der Haut und streute leicht in viele Organe, das Auge eingeschlossen, während HSV 1 sich in der Haut nur schlecht vermehrte und von dort aus auch weder streute noch okuläre Entzündungen erzeugte. Injizierte man HSV 1 aber intrakardial, so war auch dieser Herpesvirustyp in der Lage, genauso wie Typ 2 zu disseminieren und eine Chorioretinitis zu erzeugen. Hieraus schließen wir, daß der Dermatotropismus der HSV 2-Stämme zumindest zum Teil dafür verantwortlich ist, daß die meisten herpetischen Chorioretinitiden bei Neugeborenen durch Typ 2 hervorgerufen werden.

## Introduction

A case of neonatal infection with herpes simplex virus (HSV) was first described by an Italian ophthalmologist, Betignani [3] in 1934. In this report of a newborn infant who developed conjunctivitis followed by keratitis, HSV was demonstrated by inoculation of material from the child's eye into rabbit corneas. Since then, over 150 cases of neonatal herpetic infections have been reported of which approximately 20% had some kind of ocular manifestations.

Herpetic chorioretinitis in newborn infants has been associated exclusively with type 2 HSV (HSV 2). As shown in Table 1, 27 patients have been described with chorioretinitis as a manifestation of neonatal herpetic

**Table 1.** Reported cases of neonatal herpetic chorioretinitis

| Authors | Year | No. of cases | HSV type |
|---------|------|--------------|----------|
| Smith et al. [32] | 1941 | 1 | NT |
| Florman et al. [11] | 1952 | 2 | NT |
| Mitchell et al. [17] | 1963 | 1 | NT |
| Cogan et al. [9] | 1964 | 1 | NT |
| Yen et al. [37] | 1965 | 1 | NT |
| Bahrani et al. [2] | 1966 | 1 | NT |
| Golden et al. [12] | 1969 | 1 | NT |
| Hagler et al. [13] | 1969 | 2 | HSV–2 |
| Cibis et al. [6] | 1971 | 1 | HSV–2 |
| Pettay et al. [28] | 1972 | 1 | NT |
| Cibis [7] | 1975 | 1 | HSV–2 |
| Nahmias et al. [22a] | 1976 | 6 | HSV–2 |
| Yanoff et al. [36] | 1977 | 1 | HSV–2 |
| Tarkkanen et al. [35] | 1977 | 4 | HSV–2 |
| Chalhub et al. [5] | 1977 | 1 | HSV–2 |
| Cibis et al. [8] | 1978 | 1 | NT |
| Mousel et al. [19] | 1979 | 1 | HSV–2 |
| Total | | 27 | 17 |

NT: not typed

infections, and HSV isolates from 17 cases were typed, and all were found to be HSV 2 [5, 8, 13, 19, 22a, 35, 36]. Why this should be so, is not clear. It has been postulated, however, that this unique association could be due to the predominance of HSV 2 in newborn herpetic infections or to the high susceptibility of chorioretinal tissues to HSV 2.

When neonates acquire herpes infection from the maternal genital tract, either in utero after its ascent from the cervix or during the course of delivery, the skin, eye and oronasal orifices are the most accessible sites and therefore the most likely areas of primary infection. The virus can spread locally and then invade the blood stream and various organs including the eye. Thus the selective susceptibility of the portal of entry for HSV may play an important role in determining the outcome of the viral infection of the eye. We investigated such a possibility in newborn rabbits.

This paper describes our comparative study of the eye lesions produced by type 1 HSV (HSV 1) and HSV 2 following ocular, oronasal or subcutaneous inoculation, and the role of dermatotropism of HSV 2 in the pathogenesis of ocular lesions in the newborn rabbits.

**Materials and Methods**

*Newborn Rabbits*

Mid-term New Zealand white pregnant rabbits were acquired from a local commercial vendor. Each rabbit was placed in a separate cage with a breeding box. The gestation period was 30 days, and the rabbits we used in the study were between 17 and 34 hours old, and 10 days old.

*Viruses*

We used four strains of HSV 1 (PH, Shealey, Tyler, W270#4) and four strains of HSV 2 (MS, Curtis, P124, P407). All but two (PH and MS) were recent isolates; PH and MS were laboratory strains with long histories of passages in various tissues. Their sources were all described in a previous paper [26]. Before using them in the study, we passed them once or twice in primary cultures of rabbit kidney cells grown in a medium consisting of 95% Medium 199, 5% rabbit serum, and antibiotics [23]. The final titers ranged between $10^6$ and $10^7$ TCID$_{50}$ per ml.

*Virus Inoculation*

a) Ocular Inoculation
Both eyes of the ten-day-old newborn rabbit received topical instillation of 0.01 ml of virus suspension containing $10^3$ TCID$_{50}$ of each strain of HSV 1 or HSV 2, then lids were closed for 10 s and the rabbits were returned to the cage. The rabbits were examined daily with slit lamp for any ocular changes, and on postinfection day 10, the rabbit was killed and histopathologic studies of the eye were carried out.
b) Oronasal Inoculation
The one-day-old newborn rabbit received 0.001 ml of each strain of virus containing $10^3$ TCID$_{50}$ to each nostril and into the mouth. The rabbit was examined daily for oronasal infection and systemic effects. On postinfection day 5, the rabbit was killed and eyes were fixed for histopathologic studies.
c) Subcutaneous Inoculation
With 26-gauge hypodermic needles, we made

subcutaneous injection of 0.01 ml of virus suspension containing $10^3$ $TCID_{50}$ of each strain of HSV 1 or HSV 2 into each of four sites on the back of the one-day-old newborn rabbit, two on each side of the midline, 2 cm apart. The rabbit was examined daily and killed on postinfection day 4 for histopathologic studies of the eyes.

d) Intracardiac Inoculation

With 26-gauge hypodermic needles 0.01 ml of virus suspension containing $10^3$ $TCID_{50}$ of each strain of HSV 1 or HSV 2 was injected intracardially to one-day-old rabbit, and the rabbit was killed for histopathologic and virologic studies on postinfection day 3.

In virus inoculation, litter mates received the same strain of HSV, and each strain of the virus was tested at least twice in different litters, totaling 10 to 16 rabbits.

## Collection of Blood and Tissue Specimens for Virus Assay and Histopathology

The rabbits were killed by intraperitoneal injection of sodium penobarbital, and the visceral organs were exposed by an aseptic technique. For virus isolation attempts, 2 ml of cardiac blood was collected immediately from each rabbit in a syringe containing 10 units of heparin. Various organs (lungs, liver, adrenal glands, skin, brain, and eyes) were then taken aseptically, and a piece of each organ (except one whole eye and one whole adrenal gland of each rabbit) was fixed in Bouin's fixative for histopathologic study. The remaining tissues, including the second adrenal gland and the second eye of each rabbit, were frozen at –60 °C until used for virus isolation attempts.

## Virus Isolation From Cardiac Blood

We added an equal volume of sterile physiological saline to the heparinized blood and separated the leukocytes in Ficoll-Hypaque gradient as described by Böyum [4]. The separated leukocytes were washed three times in 3 ml of phosphate buffered saline (PBS) at pH 7.3 and inoculated into two tubes of Vero cells. We also collected plasma layer and inoculated 0.5 ml of it into each of two tubes of Vero cells for virus isolation. The Vero-cell tubes were incubated in a stationary position at 36 °C, and the culture medium was completely changed 1 day later. We examined the

cells for cytopathic effects (CPE) daily for 7 days. The virus isolates were identified as HSV by a neutralization test in which we used anti-HSV 1 rabbit immune serum [25].

## Virus Isolation From Tissues

We ground a 1-cc piece of each tissue with a mortar and pestle, adding 1 ml of crystalline alumina (90 mish) to facilitate the grinding. Tissue homogenate, prepared by adding 2 ml of a medium consisting of 95% Eagle's minimum essential medium, 5% fetal calf serum, and antibiotics, was centrifuged at $800 \times g$ for 10 min at 4 °C. The resultant supernatent fluid was considered to be a $10^{-1}$ dilution of the specimen, and serial 10-fold dilutions were made with the medium. We inoculated Vero-cell tubes with 1 ml of each dilution, incubated the tubes in a stationary position at 36 °C, and examined them for CPE daily for 7 days. The reciprocal of the highest dilution showing CPE was considered to be the infectivity titer of the tissue homogenate per ml.

## Histopathologic Studies

All the tissues fixed in Bouin's solution were processed and embedded in paraffine, and 5-micron sections, stained with hematoxylin and eosin, were examined microscopically.

## Measurement of Skin Lesions

The lesions produced by the subcutaneous injection of HSV were examined daily, and their diameters were measured in millimeters. To calculate the average size of the lesions produced by a strain of HSV on a given day, we divided the sum of the diameters of all of the lesions on all of the rabbits on that day by the total number of skin sites injected.

## Experimental Results

### Production of Ocular Lesions by HSV Following Various Routes of Inoculation

To examine the role of various portal of entry for HSV in the production of herpetic ocular lesions in newborn rabbits, each strain of HSV 1 or HSV 2 ($10^3$ $TCID_{50}$) was inoculated

**Table 2.** Production of retinal lesions after various routes of inoculation of types 1 and 2 herpes simplex virus (HSV)

| HSV type | Strain | Eyes with retinal lesion (%) | | |
| --- | --- | --- | --- | --- |
| | | Ocular route | Oronasal route | Subcut. route |
| HSV 1 | Shealey | 33 | 25 | 0 |
| | Tyler | 27 | 10 | 0 |
| | W270 # 4 | 42 | 57 | 0 |
| | PH | 26 | 10 | 8 |
| HSV 2 | Curtis | 33 | 20 | 43 |
| | P124 | 15 | 12 | 50 |
| | P407 | 25 | 12 | 33 |
| | MS | 25 | 25 | 29 |

to rabbits via ocular, oronasal or subcutaneous route.

Both HSV 1 and HSV 2 strains produced retinal lesions in an equal frequency following ocular and oronasal inoculation of the virus as shown in Table 2. Following subcutaneous inoculation, however, only HSV 2 strains were able to induce retinal lesions in a significant number of eyes. All four strains of HSV 2 produced retinal lesions in 29 to 50% of

the eyes while only one strain (PH) of HSV 1 induced retinal lesions in only 8% of the eyes. The retinal lesions were characterized by the retinal folds with occasional foci of necrosis (Fig. 1). Such retinal changes were not observed in the eyes of normal newborn rabbits. A mild iritis, choroiditis and blepharitis were also seen in some rabbits following subcutaneous inoculation of HSV 2 and oronasal inoculation of HSV 1 or HSV 2. Severe keratitis, iritis, blepharitis and a moderate degree of choroiditis were seen in almost all eyes of rabbits which had received ocular inoculation of either HSV 1 or HSV 2 strains.

*Production of Skin Lesions by HSV 1 and HSV 2*

One day after subcutaneous injection of HSV ($10^3$ TCID$_{50}$), all four strains of HSV 2 produced slightly elevated erythematous lesions, ranging from 2 to 3 mm in diameter, on the skin at the injection sites (Table 3). The lesions steadily increased in size and had become vesicles by day 3. On day 4 their average size ranged from 7 mm for strain P124 to as much as 12 mm for strain P407. A crust was formed at the center of most of the lesions.

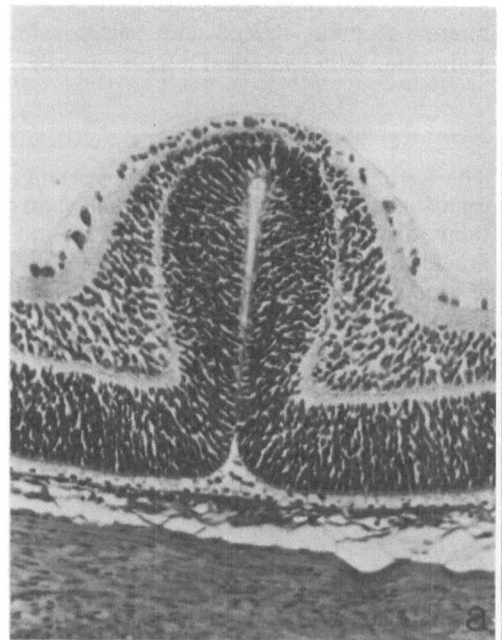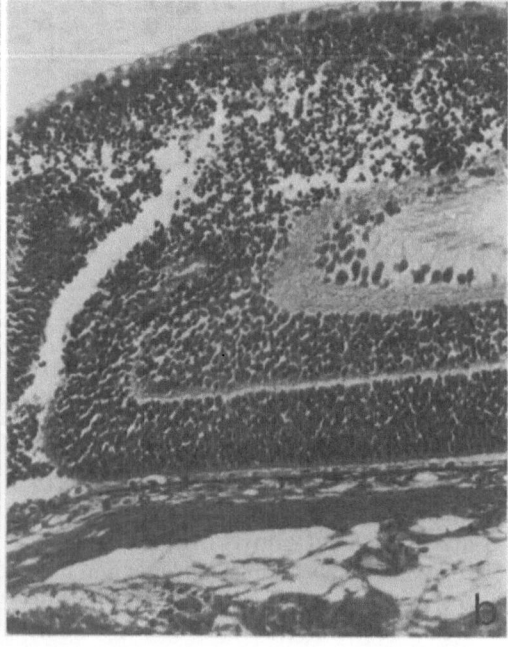

a          b

**Fig. 1.** Retinal lesions produced by herpes simplex virus in the eye of the newborn rabbit. Postinoculation day 4 (H & E stain, × 100). **a** A retinal fold, **b** A retinal fold with focal necrosis

**Table 3.** Production of skin lesions by types 1 and 2 herpes simplex virus (HSV)

| HSV type | Strain | Average size of skin lesions (mm) Postinoculation days | | | | |
|---|---|---|---|---|---|---|
| | | 1 | 2 | 3 | 4 | 5 |
| HSV 1 | Shealey | 0 | 0 | 0 | 0 | 0 |
| | Tyler | 0 | 1.0 | 0 | 0 | 0 |
| | W270 # 4 | 0 | 1.0 | 0.5 | 0.5 | 0.1 |
| | PH | 0 | 2.0 | 2.0 | 0 | 0 |
| HSV 2 | Curtis | 2.0 | 8.5 | 10.0 | 11.0 | |
| | P124 | 1.0 | 5.3 | 6.4 | 7.0 | |
| | P407 | 3.0 | 9.0 | 11.0 | 12.0 | |
| | MS | 1.0 | 5.0 | 9.5 | 11.0 | |

**Table 4.** Virus titers of skin lesions produced by types 1 and 2 herpes simplex virus (HSV)

| HSV type | Strain | No. of rabbit with skin infectivity | | | | | | |
|---|---|---|---|---|---|---|---|---|
| | | $Log_{10}$ TCID$_{50}$ | | | | | | |
| | | No virus | 1 | 2 | 3 | 4 | 5 | >5 |
| HSV 1 | Shealey | 4 | | 2 | | | | |
| | Tyler | 3 | | 1 | 1 | 1 | | |
| | W270 # 4 | 1 | 1 | 1 | 2 | 1 | | |
| | PH | 3 | | 1 | 2 | 1 | | |
| HSV 2 | Curtis | | | 1 | 1 | | 2 | 4 |
| | P124 | | | | | | | 6 |
| | P407 | | | | | 3 | 2 | 1 |
| | MS | | | | | 2 | 3 | 2 |

**Table 5.** Histopathologic lesions in various organs produced after subcutaneous inoculation of types 1 and 2 herpes simplex virus (HSV)

| HSV type | Strain | Histopathologic lesions | | | |
|---|---|---|---|---|---|
| | | Lung | Liver | Adrenal glands | Brain |
| HSV 1 | Shealey | 0/8[a] | 0/8 | 0/8 | 0/8 |
| | Tyler | 0/6 | 2/6 | 1/6 | 1/6 |
| | W270 # 4 | 0/6 | 4/6 | 0/6 | 0/6 |
| | PH | 4/7 | 2/7 | 0/7 | 0/7 |
| HSV 2 | Curtis | 2/7 | 4/7 | 3/7 | 5/7 |
| | P124 | 3/6 | 6/6 | 1/6 | 5/6 |
| | P407 | 6/6 | 4/6 | 3/6 | 6/6 |
| | MS | 4/7 | 5/7 | 0/7 | 2/7 |

[a] No. of organs with lesions/No. of organs examined on postinoculation day 4. (Reproduced by permission, see [25])

When we examined the histopathology of the HSV 2 lesions on day 4, we found extensive acute inflammatory reactions throughout the entire thickness of the skin, and scattered foci of necrosis. The infiltration of polymorphonuclear leukocytes was minimal, however. The epidermis was eroded over the area of necrosis, and the epithelium adjacent to the erosions contained multinucleated giant cells and typical Cowdry type A intranuclear inclusions.

In contrast, although all four strains of HSV 1 showed erythematous lesions on day 2, they were small in size, regressed rapidly (Table 3), and were completely healed by day 4. When we examined the histopathology of the lesions, we found a rather mild degree of inflammatory response in the papillary layer of the dermis and an epithelium that was for the most part intact.

*Virus Multiplication in the Skin*

On day 4 all the skin specimens inoculated with HSV 2 strains contained HSV in high titers ranging from $10^2$ to over $10^5$ TCID$_{50}$ (Table 4). In contrast, only half of the skin specimens inoculated with HSV 1 strains yielded virus, and the titers were lower than in the specimens inoculated with HSV 2.

*Dissemination of HSV*

As shown in Table 5, rabbits inoculated with HSV 2 strains showed widely disseminated lesions in their visceral organs much more frequently than those inoculated with HSV 1 strains. Liver and spleens were the sites of most of the lesions, which were multiple, well-circumscribed, and necrotic. The hepatic lesions were the same size, however, whether produced by HSV 1 or HSV 2. The adrenal glands showed microscopic foci of necrosis and hemorrhage in both cortex and medulla, pneumonitis was found in the lungs, and there was perivascular cuffing and encephalitis in the brain. All of these changes appeared for the most part in the HSV 2-inoculated animals.

A difference between the HSV 1 and HSV 2 strains was also seen in the frequency with which infectious HSV could be recovered from the affected organs. In general HSV could be recovered more often from HSV 2-infected rabbits than from HSV 1-infected

**Table 6.** Isolation of herpes simplex virus (HSV) from rabbit leukocytes and plasma after subcutaneous inoculation of types 1 and 2 HSV

| HSV type | Strain | Isolation of HSV from | |
|---|---|---|---|
| | | Leukocytes | Plasma |
| HSV 1 | Shealey | 0/7[a] | 0/7 |
| | Tyler | 0/6 | 0/6 |
| | W270 # 4 | 0/6 | 0/6 |
| | PH | 0/6 | 0/6 |
| HSV 2 | Curtis | 2/4 | 1/4 |
| | P124 | 3/6 | 0/6 |
| | P407 | 0/6 | 0/6 |
| | MS | 1/3 | 2/3 |

[a] No. of HSV isolation/No. of specimens tested on postinoculation day 4. (Reproduced by permission, see [25])

rabbits: twice as often from the liver, three times as often from the lung, adrenal glands, and brain, and ten times as often from the eye. The amounts of infectious HSV recovered, however, were not significantly different whether recovered from HSV 1- or HSV 2-infected organs.

## Isolation of HSV from Blood

None of the blood (leukocytes or plasma) obtained from rabbits inoculated with HSV 1 strains yielded HSV (Table 6). In contrast, the blood of animals inoculated with HSV 2 strains yielded virus, three of five strains from

**Table 7.** Effect of intracardiac inoculation of types 1 and 2 herpes simplex virus (HSV) on the eye and skin (Postinoculation day 3)

| HSV type | Strain | Eyes with retinal lesions (%) | Rabbits with skin lesions (%) | HSV in blood |
|---|---|---|---|---|
| HSV 1 | Shealey | 60 | 0 | + |
| | Tyler | 40 | 0 | + |
| | W270 # 4 | 60 | 0 | + |
| | PH | 17 | 10 | + |
| HSV 2 | Curtis | 26 | 33 | + |
| | P124 | 17 | 70 | + |
| | P407 | 20 | 50 | + |
| | MS | 17 | 66 | + |

leukocytes and two of five strains from plasma. Virus was recovered from the leukocytes of as many as 50% of rabbits infected with either Curtis or P124 strain of HSV 2.

## Production of Ocular Lesions Following Intracardiac Inoculation of HSV

We were uncertain whether the visceral organs also manifest the different degree of "tissue tropism" to HSV 1 and HSV 2 as observed in the skin, and it was thought possible that the high susceptibility of visceral organs to HSV 2 may also be responsible for the unique association of HSV 2 with the retinal lesions in the newborn rabbits following subcutaneous inoculation of the virus. To examine this possibility, one-day-old rabbits received an intracardiac inoculation of HSV 1 or HSV 2 ($10^3$ $TCID_{50}$), and eyes were examined for retinal lesions on postinfection day 3.

As shown in Table 7, all four strains of both HSV 1 and HSV 2 produced retinal lesions indicating that the retinal tissue is susceptible to HSV 1 as much as to HSV 2. It is interesting to note that both HSV 1 and HSV 2 strains caused viremia and widely disseminated visceral involvement, yet skin lesions were found almost exclusively in the rabbits inoculated with HSV 2 strains. The result is a further evidence for the dermatotropic nature of HSV 2 in the newborn rabbits.

## Discussion

Chorioretinitis in newborn infants has been associated almost exclusively with HSV 2 [5–7, 13, 19, 22a, 35, 36]. The cause of this unique relationship between chorioretinitis and HSV 2 is not clear at present. In our present study, both HSV 1 and HSV 2 strains produced retinal lesions in the eyes of the newborn rabbits in an equal frequency when they were inoculated with either oronasal, ocular or intracardiac route. Following subcutaneous inoculation, however, only HSV 2 strains were able to induce retinal lesions. The difference can be attributed to the fact that HSV 2 grows extensively in skin lesions and disseminates to various organs, including the eye, and that HSV 1 produces only insignificant skin lesions and no dissemination of virus to the eye. Thus dermatotropism of

HSV 2 may in part account for the chorioretinitis that occurs only in newborn infants infected with HSV 2 since the skin is a major portal of entry for HSV in newborns.

Similar differences in tissue and cell tropisms between HSV 1 and HSV 2 have been noted in other organs. In mouse and cell culture of human fetal brain, HSV 2 is more neurovirulent than HSV 1 [1, 20] and HSV 2 is also more paralytogenic for adult rabbits than HSV 1 [29]. HSV 2 produces larger pocks on the chorioallantoic membrane of embryonated eggs and affects the mesodermal, entodermal, and ectodermal layers, while HSV 1 almost exclusively the ectodermal layer [21]. In primary cultures of chick-embryo cells, HSV 2 produces plaques, whereas HSV 1 produces minute plaque or, more often, none at all [16]. In the rabbit eye, HSV 2 strains produce severe keratitis that affects an entire layer of the cornea, whereas HSV 1 strains produce only superficial lesions that affect the epithelium and the upper third of the corneal stroma [27, 33].

Dissemination of infection after the subcutaneous inoculation of newborn rabbits with HSV 2 was much more pronounced than after inoculation with HSV 1. In view of the fact that HSV could be isolated from the blood of HSV 2 infected animals but not from the blood of HSV 1-infected animals, viremia plays an important role in disseminating HSV 2 infections in this experimental model. In human infections, the route of HSV 2 dissemination to the central nervous system is also thought to be hematogenous [8, 10, 14, 31]; Craig and Nahmias [10] have recovered HSV 2 from the buffy coat of the blood of two adult patients suffering from aseptic meningitis. In contrast, the virus in cases of HSV 1 encephalitis is believed to travel into and through the nervous system by direct cell-to-cell infection. This theory is substantiated by the paucity of positive blood or buffy-coat cultures and the frequent focal nature of the encephalitis. Brain cultures in such patients often yield HSV 1, whereas cerebrospinal fluid cultures are sterile.

In hematogenous dissemination of HSV 2 in newborn rabbits, blood leukocytes, along with plasma, appear to play a significant role since the virus could often be recovered from leukocytes as well as plasma of the infected animals. It is not yet clear, however, which subgroups of leukocytes are associated with HSV 2, or whether or not the virus multiplies in the leukocytes. Future studies may provide answers to these questions. It should be noted, however, that in humans, HSV has been shown to multiply in both lymphocytes [2, 15, 29, 34] and monocytes [10, 29, 34]. Recently Morgensen [18] reported that macrophages of adult mice were more susceptible to HSV 2 than to HSV 1 and suggested that the differences in the hepatic lesions observed in mice after intraperitoneal injection of HSV 1 or HSV 2 could be explained by the differences in the susceptibility of the macrophages to these viruses.

**Acknowledgments.** This work was supported by research grants EY 00964 and EY 01578, and a core grant EY 01597 from the U.S. Public Health Service, National Institutes of Health. We would like to acknowledge the technical assistance provided by M. Kopal, H. Krasnobrod and C. Wilkey.

# References

1. Alford C, Snider M, Stubbs G (1967) Studies on virulence of herpes simplex viruses isolated from different clinical entities. Pediatr Res 1:209–210
2. Bahrani M, Bexerbaum B, Gilger A (1966) Generalized herpes simplex and hypoadrenocorticism. A case associated with adrenocortical insufficiency in a prematurely born male, clinical, virological, ophthalmological and metabolic studies. Am J Dis Child 111:437–445
3. Batignani A (1934) Conjunctivite da virus erpetico in neonato. Boll Ocul 13:1217–1220
4. Böyum A (1964) Separation of white blood cells. Nature 204:793–794
5. Chalhub EG, Baenziger J, Feigen RD, Middlekamp JN, Shackelford GD (1977) Congenital herpes simplex type II infection with extensive hepatic calcification, bone lesions and cataract: Complete postmortem examination. Dev Med Child Neurol 19:527–534
6. Cibis A, Burde RM (1971) Herpes simplex-virus-induced congenital cataracts. Arch Ophthalmol 85:220–223
7. Cibis GW (1975) Neonatal herpes simplex retinitis. Albrecht von Graefes Arch Klin Ophthalmol 196:39–47
8. Cibis GW, Flynn JT, David EB (1978) Herpes simplex retinitis. Arch Ophthalmol 96:299–302
9. Cogan DG, Kuwabara T, Young GF, Knox DL (1964) Herpes simplex retinopathy in an infant. Arch Ophthalmol 72:641–645

10. Craig CP, Nahmias AJ (1973) Different patterns of neurologic involvement with herpes simplex virus types 1 and 2: Isolation of herpes simplex virus type 2 from the buffy coat of two adults with meningitis. J Infect Dis 127:365–371
11. Florman AL, Mindlin RL (1952) Generalized herpes simplex in an 11-day-old premature infant. Am J Dis Child 83:481–486
12. Golden B, Ball WE, McKee AP (1969) Disseminated herpes simplex with encephalitis in a neonate. JAMA 209:1219–1221
13. Hagler WS, Walters PV, Nahmias AJ (1969) Ocular involvement in neonatal herpes simplex virus infections. Arch Ophthalmol 82: 169–176
14. Hevron JE (1977) Herpes simplex virus type 2 meningitis. Obstet Gynecol 49:622–624
15. Kirchner H, Kleinicke C, Northoff H (1977) Replication of herpes simplex virus in human peripheral T lymphocytes. J Gen Virol 37:647–649
16. Lowry SP, Melnick JL, Rawls WE (1971) Investigation of plaque formation in chick embryo cells as a biological marker for distinguishing herpes virus type 2 from type 1. J Gen Virol 10:1–9
17. Mitchell JE, McCall FC (1963) Transplacental infection by herpes simplex virus. Am J Dis Child 106:207–209
18. Morgensen S (1977) Role of macrophages in hepatitis induced by herpes simplex virus types 1 and 2 in mice. Infect Immun 15:686–691
19. Mousel DK, Missall SR (1979) Pan uveitis and retinitis in neonatal herpes simplex infection. J Ped Ophthalmol Strabismus 16:7–9
20. Nahmias AJ, Dowdle WR (1968) Antigenic and biologic differences in Herpesvirus hominis. Prog Med Virol 10:110–159
21. Nahmias AJ, Dowdle WR, Naib ZM, Highsmith A, Harwell RW, Josey WE (1968) Relation of pock size on chorioallantoic membrane to antigenic type of Herpesvirus hominis. Proc Soc Exp Biol Med 127:1022–1028
22. Nahmias A, Kibrick S, Rosan RC (1964) Viral-leukocyte interrelationships. I. Multiplication of a DNA virus-herpes simplex in human leukocyte cultures. J Immunol 93:69–74
22a. Nahmias AJ, Visintine AM, Caldwell DR, Wilson LA (1976) Eye infections with herpes simplex viruses in neonates. Surv Ophthalmol 21:100–105
23. Oh, JO (1976) Primary and secondary herpes simplex uveitis in rabbits. Surv Ophthalmol 21:178–184
24. Oh JO, Kimura S, Ostler HB (1975) Acute ocular infection by type 2 herpes simplex virus in adults. Arch Ophthalmol 93:1127–1129
25. Oh JO, Minasi P (1980) Different susceptibility of skin to type 1 and type 2 herpes simplex virus in newborn rabbits. Infect Immun 27: 168–174
26. Oh JO, Moschini GB, Okumoto M, Stevens T (1972) Ocular pathogenicity of types 1 and 2 Herpesvirus hominis in rabbits. Infect Immun 5:412–413
27. Oh JO, Stevens TR (1973) Comparison of types 1 and 2 Herpesvirus hominis infection of rabbit eyes: I. Clinical manifestations. Arch Ophthalmol 90:473–476
28. Pettay O, Leinikki P, Donner M, Lapinleimu K (1972) Herpes simplex virus infection in the newborn. Arch Dis Child 47:97–103
29. Plaeger-Marshall S, Smith JW (1978) Experimental infection of subpopulations of human peripheral blood leukocytes by herpes simplex virus. Proc Soc Exp Biol Med 158:263–268
30. Plummer G, Hackett S (1966) Herpes simplex virus and paralysis of animals. Br J Exp Pathol 47:82–85
31. Sköldenberg B, Jeansson S (1973) Herpes simplex virus type 2 in acute aseptic meningitis. Br Med J 2:611
32. Smith MC, Lennette EH, Reames HR (1941) Isolation of the virus of herpes simplex and the demonstration of intranuclear inclusions in a case of acute encephalitis. Am J Pathol 17: 55–68
33. Stevens TR, Oh JO (1973) Comparison of types 1 and 2 Herpesvirus hominis infection of rabbit eyes: II. Histopathologic and virologic studies. Arch Ophthalmol 90:477–480
34. Rinaldo jr CR, Richter BS, Black PH, Callery R, Chess L, Hirsch MS (1978) Replication of herpes simplex virus and cytomegalovirus in human leukocytes. J Immunol 120:130–136
35. Tarkkanen A, Laatikainen L (1977) Late ocular manifestations in neonatal herpes simplex infection. Br J Ophthalmol 61:608–616
36. Yanoff M, Allman MI, Fine BS (1977) Congenital herpes simplex virus, type 2, bilateral endophthalmitis. Trans Am Ophthalmol Soc 75:325–337
37. Yen SSC, Reagan JW, Rosenthal MS (1965) Herpes simplex infection in female genital tract. Obstet Gynecol 25:479–492

**Discussion on the Contribution pp. 191–198**

J. Wollensak (Berlin)
Did you get bilateral chorioretinitis in experiments and what was the cause of cases of human infection?

J. Oh (San Francisco):
Most of the chorioretinitis in human infants, quoted here, is bilateral. In our animal model, about

70% of chorioretinitis are bilateral, particularly following intracardiac inoculation of the virus; about 80% of the animals produced bilateral chorioretinitis.

G.O.H. Naumann (Erlangen)
I want to congratulate you on your beautiful study. You showed that you got a wide dissemination of virus in many organs, including the brain. How often did the virus actually produce lesions in the brain in your experiments and how often was there cerebral involvement in the patients quoted in the literature?

J. Oh (San Francisco)
As I indicated in the first slide, most of the earlier reports of chorioretinitis in newborns were found in non-ophthalmology journals, namely, pediatrics or gynecology journals, and all these patients had encephalitis. In the experimental model we used in this study, yes, the virus produced encephalitis, sometimes meningitis. I can't recall exactly what per cent of these animals had encephalitis.

Sundmacher, R. (Hrsg.):
Herpetische Augenerkrankungen
© J.F. Bergmann Verlag, München 1981

# Herpes Simplex Blepharitis of the Erosive-Ulcerative Type

I. Egerer, A. Stary, Wien

**Key words.** HSV blepharitis – erosive-ulcerative

**Schlüsselwörter.** HSV – erosiv ulzeröse Blepharitis

**Summary.** In contrast to the classical picture of herpes simplex infection involving the lids and lid margin characterized by the presence of a group of vesicles situated on a swollen erythematous base, the latter are usually lacking in the erosive-ulcerative type of herpes simplex blepharitis (Fig. 1, 2). Here the following features are encountered: single or multiple intermarginal erosions, single or multiple skin ulcers situated at the lid margin, or a combination of both. The affected lid portion usually exhibits slight swelling and tenderness upon palpation, moderate conjunctival injection especially adjacent to the lesion may be present, as well as ipsilateral palpable lymph nodes. A total of 42 cases has been observed within a period of 3 years. From the initial 28 patients smears were obtained for immunological proof of our diagnosis, which turned out to be positive in 26 cases, testifying to the reliability of the clinical features, which have been outlined in detail in our previous papers (Klin Monatsbl Augenheilkd 173:407–412 (1978), Arch Ophthalmol (in press)). In about 20% of the cases proven herpes simplex conjunctivitis has been encountered; therefore, local virustatics should be applied to the lesions as well as conjunctiva, especially in view of the fact that these drugs will find ready access to the viruses within the erosions and ulcers.

**Zusammenfassung.** Die Herpes simplex-Blepharitis vom erosiv-ulzerösen Typ äußert sich in Form von einzelnen oder multiplen Erosionen im Bereiche des intermarginalen Saumes oder Ulzera nahe dem Lidrand oder einer Kombination beider Formen (Abb. 1, 2). Nur ausnahmsweise können auch gleichzeitig charakteristische Herpesbläschen in unmittelbarer Umgebung registriert werden. Da die Ausbreitung der Viren auf die benachbarte Bindehaut ungehindert erfolgen kann, sollten hier unbedingt lokale Virustatika angewandt werden.

## Discussion on the Contribution p. 201

B.R. Jones (London)
Thank you very much for drawing our attention to this clinical picture. In a study of virologically proven primary herpes simplex conjunctivitis that we reported some time ago, about a quarter of the cases had lid lesions confined to the intermarginal strip, and as you pointed out they are erosive rather than vesicular. A very important diagnostic clinical sign.

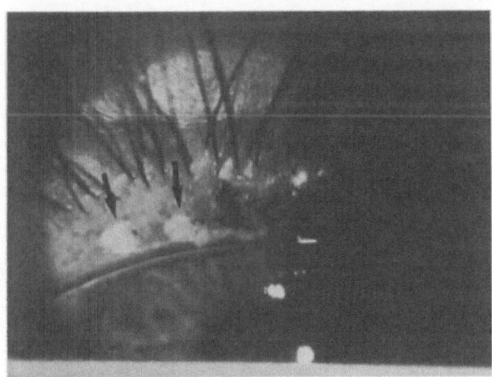

**Fig. 1.** Intermarginal erosions

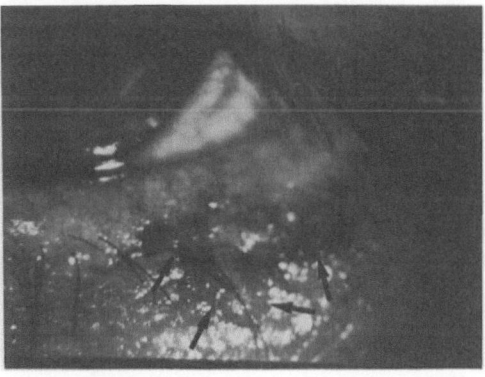

**Fig. 2.** Skin ulcer situated close to the lid margin

Sundmacher, R. (Hrsg.):
Herpetische Augenerkrankungen
© J.F. Bergmann Verlag, München 1981

# A Clinico-Virologic Classification of Herpetic Anterior Segment Diseases With Special Reference to Intraocular Herpes

R. Sundmacher, Freiburg

Key words. HSV – classification of anterior segment diseases, clinical diagnosis, intraocular herpes

Schlüsselwörter. HSV – Einteilung der Erkrankungen des vorderen Augenabschnittes, klinische Diagnose, intraokularer Herpes

Summary. Herpetic diseases of the eye may be classified differently depending on the various aspects which may be stressed. We suggest here a classification with only two major groups: I. viral diseases and II. nonviral (= metaherpetic) diseases. The division has mainly been made on the basis of clinico-virologic investigations. The very important immunologic aspects of various diseases do not explicitly show up in this classification. It is inferred, however, that immunology is always involved in the viral diseases and that only the importance of immunologic phenomena varies according to the structures which are attacked by the herpes simplex virus.

Zusammenfassung. Herpetische Augenerkrankungen kann man je nach dem Gesichtspunkt, den man betonen will, unterschiedlich klassifizieren. Hier soll eine Klassifikation vorgestellt werden, die mit zwei Hauptgruppen auskommt: I. Virale Erkrankungen und II. avirale (= metaherpetische) Erkrankungen. Die Einteilung der einzelnen Krankheitsformen in diese beiden Gruppen erfolgte – bis auf wenige Ausnahmen – auf der Grundlage unserer klinisch-virologischen Korrelationsstudien. Die für den Verlauf vieler Erkrankungsformen sehr wichtigen immunologischen Aspekte sind in dieser Einteilung nicht hervorgehoben. Es kann aber grundsätzlich davon ausgegangen werden, daß in der Gruppe I (virale Erkrankungen) immer auch Immunphänomene beteiligt sind. Diese werden sich unterschiedlich schwerwiegend auswirken, je nachdem, welche morphologische Struktur vom Herpesvirus angegriffen wird. So sind z.B. immunologische Phänomene für das Schicksal des Endothels bei der disciformen Keratitis sehr viel entscheidender

als für das Schicksal des Epithels bei der Keratitis dendritica.

Neben uncharakteristischen Entzündungszeichen bei herpetischen Augenerkrankungen gibt es biomikroskopisch eindeutig erkennbare Krankheitsbilder, die wie folgt klassifiziert werden:

*Virale Erkrankungen*
1. Herpesblepharitis
2. intermarginale Herpesblepharitis
3. limbäre Herpeskeratoconjunctivitis (primär)
4. epitheliale Herpeskeratitis (punctata, stellata, dendritica, geographica)
5. interstitielle Herpeskeratitis
6. ulzerierende interstitielle Herpeskeratitis
7. zentrale Endotheliitis (Keratitis disciformis)
8. periphere Endotheliitis (Trabeculitis)
9. fokale Herpesiritis
10. herpetische Episcleritis und Scleritis

*Metaherpetische (= avirale) Erkrankungen*
11. metaherpetische Erosio
12. metaherpetisches Ulcus
13. metaherpetische bullöse Keratopathie
14. chronisches Sekundärglaukom nach Trabeculitis

For some years we have been looking for culturable herpes simplex virus (HSV) in patients with herpetic anterior segment diseases. Two methods have been employed:

1. For identification of culturable HSV from lesions of the ocular surface, a drop of Eagle's minimal essential medium containing 0.5% human albumine was put into the conjunctival sac and recovered with an automatic micropipette after the eyelids had been gently rubbed. This procedure was repeated three times with every eye. Repeat attempts for isolation were made daily in every patient undergoing antiherpetic treatment. The specimens were stored either at 4 C for up to 6 hours or at –70 C for longer periods. Each sample was inoculated into human foreskin fibroblast cultures which were kept in glass tubes during the early years of our studies and on microplates later on. After 1 week,

negative cultures were passaged again and observed for another week. HSV was identified by its typical cytopathogenic effect (CPE). In the course of different studies, many isolates were further characterized by serological methods, e.g. neutralization tests with type-specific antisera.

2. For investigation of diseased ocular structures bordering the anterior chamber, acqeous taps were performed in selected patients after informed consent. In most of these patients, a local anesthesia with proxymetacaine plus cocaine 2% proved sufficient. The patients lay on the operating table and looked downward while a small *discision* needle entered the anterior chamber at the 12 o'clock position. A blunt anterior chamber canula was then cautiously inserted and as much of the acqeous aspirated as possible. The eye was bandaged after gentamycine ointment was applied and the chamber was left to restore spontaneously. The procedure had to be done with retrobulbar or with general anesthesia only in a couple of adults and children. The whole volume of the aspirate (up to 0.3 ml) was then put on a single culture of human foreskin fibroblasts, which had been growing for 12–24 hours in a 25–40 cm$^2$ bottle. Immediately before the paracentesis, keratokonjunctival washings, as described above, were obtained and processed identically to the acqeous humour as a control for a viral pick-up from the ocular surface. These controls have been consistently negative in all HSV-positive acqeous specimens reported here. Negative cultures were passaged two times and kept for a total of 4 weeks before definitely regarded as virus-negative.

## Results

In 1976 we reported on virological investigations of the ocular surface [1] which led us to differentiate between viral and aviral (=metaherpetic) types of diseases. The continuous study of many more patients since then has confirmed this basic concept. Other assumptions, however, had to be corrected. Whereas in 1976 we still classified disciform herpetic edema as an interstitial herpetic keratitis of mainly immunologic origin, the results of our acqeous humour studies, together with close clinical observations, have forced us to revise this view. Disciform

**Table 1.** Herpes simplex virus isolations from the acqeous humour. 77 taps in 70 patients; May 1976 – April 1980

| Diagnosis | No of Taps | Acqueous Humour HSV-Negative | HSV-Positive |
|---|---|---|---|
| Anterior uveitis of unknown etiology | 20 | 20 | – |
| Acute glaucoma with corneal edema mimicking endotheliitis | 1 | 1 | – |
| Zoster iritis, acute or chronic | 5 | 5* | – |
| *Patients with previous ocular herpes* | | | |
|   Clinically quiet scars | 3 | 3 | – |
|   Interstitial herpetic keratitis with "concomitant" uncharacteristic iritis | 10 | 10 | – |
| *Intraocular herpetic inflammation without significant stromal involvement* | | | |
|   Uncharacteristic anterior uveitis | 13 | 13 | – |
|   *Acute focal iritis* | 7 | 1 | 6 |
|   Peripheral or central *endotheliitis* (acute or subacute) | 18 | 12 | 6** |
| | 77 | 65 | 12** |

* Also, no varizella zoster virus could be isolated. ** In one patient with central plus peripheral endotheliitis (disciform edema plus trabeculitis) and longstanding severe secondary glaucoma, HSV could be isolated from the acqeous humour on two occasions at 14 day intervals. Thus, we have 12 positive isolations from 11 patients

**Table 2.** Correlation between acute secondary glaucoma in herpetic anterior segment diseases and culturable herpes simplex virus in the acqueous humour (n = 48 taps)

| | Virus-negative | Herpes simplex virus positive |
|---|---|---|
| No Glaucoma | 20 | 1 |
| *Glaucoma* | 16 | 11* |

* p < 0.01; Chi-square for 2 x 2 tables

edema is now classified as an HSV endotheliitis. Furthermore, we have added the somewhat new clinical entities of trabeculitis and focal herpetic iritis [2, 3].

Table 1 shows the actual state of our HSV isolation studies from the acqeous humour. The highest success rate was found in patients with focal herpetic iritis; whereas, in peripheral endotheliitis (= trabeculitis) or in central endotheliitis (= disciform edema) the success rate was lower, presumably because the amount of virus set free in these types of diseases is comparatively low. One factor correlating with a positive isolation was the presence of acute secondary glaucoma (Table 2). The important clinical aspect of this finding may be that with marked acute, secondary glaucoma, the chances of culturable HSV being present in the acqeous are quite high, and this of course has implications for the design of an appropriate therapy.

The bulk of "iritis" in herpes eyes, however, has turned out to be virus-negative − at least to the level of sensitivity of our methods (Table 1).

As it has turned out to be impossible to add a sufficient number of color photos for further illustration of the schematic classification in Figure 1, we give some short comment for each type of disease instead. Black and white photos of many of the clinical entities presented may be found in our respective publications [1–3].

*Viral Diseases*

1. *HSV blepharitis* may be recurrent (normally) or primary (rarely). If the lid margins are severely involved and the blisters relatively large and more watery than purulent for a prolonged time, a primary infection may be suspected, especially if an adenopathy together with some general illness is noted.

2. Except for primary infections where intermarginal blisters are quite common, there also exists an isolated *intermarginal HSV blepharitis* (see Chapter 32) in patients with an established anti-HSV immunity. This type of blepharitis is often overlooked because of its minuteness, but it is clinically quite characteristic.

3. A *limbal HSV keratokonjunctivitis* in its pure form has always been a sign of primary HSV infection in our patients. Most of these additionally have had severe HSV blepharitis (also intermarginal) so that the etiologic diagnosis could not be missed. Furthermore, these patients may develop stellate or dendritic corneal lesions. At that time, however, the limbal lesions have mostly resolved already without sequelae.

4. *Epithelial HSV keratitis* may take many forms from punctate via stellate via dendritic to geographic keratitis. Normally, the diagnosis of all of these lesions is easy as they all have a characteristic microstructure of their border when observed with a slit lamp before fluorescein staining. Patients with geographic keratitis have often been pretreated with steroids.

5. *Interstitial HSV keratitis* presents the most varying picture of all the types of HSV disease. This may be explained by varying degrees of virus multiplication and host response, resulting in infiltrates of subtle grey to dense white. A further subclassification may arise some day. At the moment, however, no results are available of virologic or immunologic studies of the stroma itself in herpes patients. Therefore, the classification of interstitial HSV keratitis as a viral disease has been done on the indirect evidence that virus may be obtained when these corneae ulcerate.

6. *Ulcerating interstitial herpetic keratitis* is a complicated form of # 5. HSV has been found in washings of the ocular surface and from corneal specimens obtained on the occasion of keratoplasty à chaud. The infiltrates represent the primary pathologic event and therefore, the ulcerated area in the beginning is small compared with the area of the infiltrates. Also, a significant inflammatory reaction in the ac-

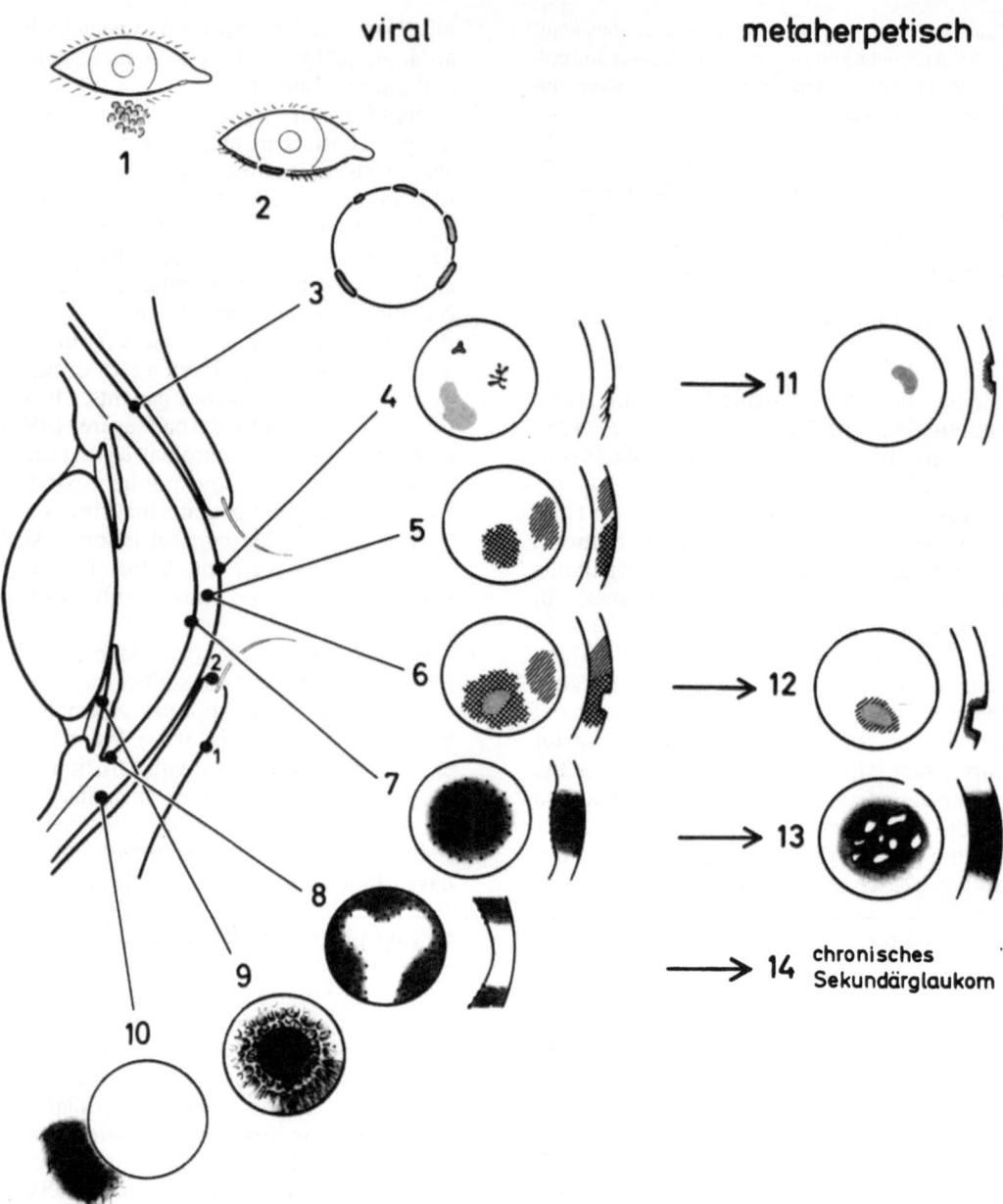

**viral**

**metaherpetisch**

**Fig. 1.** A clinico-virologic classification of herpetic anterior segment diseases. 1: HSV Blepharitis, 2: Inter-marginal HSV Blepharitis, 3: Limbal HSV Keratokonjunctivitis, 4: Epithelial HSV Keratitis, 5: Interstitial HSV Keratitis, 6: Ulcerating Interstitial HSV Keratitis, 7: Central HSV Endotheliitis (Disciform HSV Keratitis), 8: Peripheral HSV Endotheliitis (HSV Trabeculitis), 9: Focal HSV Iritis, 10: HSV-associated Scleritis and Episcleritis, 11: Metaherpetic Erosion, 12: Metaherpetic Ulcer, 13: Metaherpetic Bullous Keratopathy, 14: Chronic Secondary Glaucoma (after HSV Trabeculitis)

qeous is normally present. This makes a difference to metaherpetic ulcers (# 12).

7. *Central HSV endotheliitis* is the term which we suggest for herpetic disciform edema (Table 1). It is characterized by a focal disease of the corneal endothelium, which may or may not be disciform. Characteristically, localized precipitates with overlying corneal edema mark the area of the diseased endothelium. With the specular microscope, one may observe endothelial swelling and loss in the course of the disease (Sundmacher, unpublished). Disciform edema has been regarded as an immunologic disease, which usually responds well to steroids. As we have now found culturable virus in the acqeous humour of several patients with disciform edema, our hypothesis is that disciform edema primarily represents a viral disease of the corneal endothelium. In reaction to this, the endothelium is attacked by immunocompetent cells, and this attack is probably much more harmful to the cells than viral cytolysis alone. This calls for a combination of an effective antiviral together with steroids for the treatment of this type of disease.

8. *Peripheral HSV endotheliitis (trabeculitis)* has an etiopathology very similar to that of central endotheliitis. Trabeculitis, however, is much more dangerous in the long run, as it is often complicated by extremely severe forms of secondary glaucoma. For these cases, a potent antiviral therapy which acts in the trabecular meshwork is most urgently needed.

9. *Focal HSV iritis* is the third clinical entity which has evolved from our acqeous humour studies (Table 1). Characteristically, a limited area of the iris is slightly grey and swollen and somewhat hyperemic. The dilator in this region does not respond to mydriatics, which results in dysfiguration of the pupil. There is a marked augmentation of cells and flare in the acqeous humour (whereas in typical endotheliitis, cells and flare are comparatively sparse). Sometimes a limited corneal edema indicates a concomitant endotheliitis. In the course of the disease, which normally is benign, pigment epithelium defects in the iris evolve and serve as a permanent sign of a passed focal herpetic iritis. Recurrences of the disease are quite common and seem to have a predilection for parts of the iris which neighbour formerly diseased structures.

10. *HSV-associated scleritis* seems to occur rarely. Diagnosis is only possible in eyes with known herpetic history. No virologic evidence for the classification as a viral disease is as yet available.

*Aviral (=metaherpetic) Diseases*

11. Epithelial healing problems after HSV keratitis are quite common. They mostly present themselves as some kind of punctate epitheliopathy, but may cause many more kinds of epithelial disturbance. Sometimes they progress to recurring erosions and/or shallow epithelial defects with thick, grey borders which we classify as *metaherpetic erosions*. In most cases, the critical observation of the microstructure of the epithelial border, together with the shape of the defect, help in establishing the correct diagnosis. This is important as antivirals will not improve the condition but instead worsen it.

12. If the aviral destruction goes beyond Bowman's into the stroma, we call it a *metaherpetic ulcer*. It should be noted that in the classic European terminology a difference is made between an erosion (defect of the epithelium only) and an ulcer (all defects deeper than an erosion). The differential diagnosis of metaherpetic ulcers may be difficult, and sometimes it may even be impossible to judge on a clinical basis whether or not a herpetic ulcer is aviral or viral (# 6). We look and see how infiltrated the margins of the ulcer are, if this is comparatively little and if the underlying infiltrate − which may be considerable − is mostly confined to the ulcerated area. Then we feel that an aviral, metaherpetic process is more likely than a viral one, especially if the history of ulceration is long and refractiveness to multiple antiviral agents has been noted.

13. Central HSV endotheliitis may regress and leave functionally normal conditions if diagnosed early and treated properly. If, however, proper diagnosis or therapy do not take place, or if numerous attacks of endotheliitis have struck the cornea, a chronic bullous keratopathy is likely to develop. This *metaherpetic bullous kerato-*

207

*pathy* is differentiated from other conditions of this type by the patient's history and/or by acute HSV recurrences, which by themselves are diagnostic. If a metaherpetic bullosa is not complicated by glaucoma (# 14), such eyes are good candidates for a perforating keratoplasty, which we don't hesitate to perform if the patient is likely to benefit from a clear graft.

14. Peripheral endotheliitis (trabeculitis) may lead to permanent *chronic secondary glaucoma.* In the absence of acute inflammatory disease, these cases should be treated like chronic simple glaucoma. We avoid surgery as long as possible, as it has been our experience that filtering procedures don't have a very good prognosis. Apart from threatening loss of vision from glaucomatous atrophy of the optic nerve, this complication also obviates an otherwise promising keratoplasty if the intraocular pressure cannot be brought under control. In this respect it should be remembered that applanation or Schiötz tonometry often do not give consistent results in eyes with severely damaged anterior segments, and that therefore, in this special situation, digital estimation of the intraocular pressure should always be done in addition.

In designing this novel classification of herpetic anterior segment diseases, we have tried to rely mostly on facts gathered in clinico-virologic correlation studies. The very important immunologic aspects of various diseases do not explicitly show up in this classification, as no reliable information is available on the exact nature of immune reactions in herpes patients suffering from different types of diseases. It is inferred, however, that immunology is always involved in the viral diseases. The importance of immunologic reactions probably varies considerably according to the structures which are attacked by the herpes simplex virus. This deserves further studies, and the results of such studies will probably modify our current thinking on herpetic diseases. This may result in modifications of our classification which we do not expect to be a lasting one in every detail anyway. Also, it may be useful to point out that we did not intend to achieve a "complete" classification. The many different types of keratokonjunctivitis sicca after herpetic keratokonjunctivitis, e.g., were purposely left out in order not to overdo it. We wanted rather to present some main topics which we feel are important for pathophysiological thinking. For the application of this classification in the clinic, one should be aware that quite often herpetic anterior segment diseases present themselves in varying combinations of the pure types presented here. We would regard it as a success if this presentation would stimulate critical discussions and also lead to further investigations in the pathophysiologic nature of herpetic eye diseases in patients.

## References

1. Sundmacher R, Neumann-Haefelin D (1976) Keratitis metaherpetica, klinische und virologische Befunde. Klin Monatsbl Augenheilkd 169:728–737
2. Sundmacher R, Neumann-Haefelin D (1979) Herpes simplex virus-positive and -negative keratouveitis. In: Silverstein AM, O'Connor GR (eds) Immunology and immunopathology of the eye. Masson, New York, Paris, p 225–229
3. Sundmacher R, Neumann-Haefelin D (1979) Herpes simplex Virus Isolierung aus dem Kammerwasser bei fokaler Iritis, Endotheliitis und langdauernder Keratitis disciformis mit Sekundärglaukom. Klin Monatsbl Augenheilkd 175:488–501

A review of the literature may be found in [1] and [3].

## Discussion on the Contribution pp. 203–208

W. Böke (Kiel)
May I comment? I think we completely agree, Dr. Sundmacher, that there are some forms which are determined by the presence of the virus, and others in which the virus cannot be found. The latter fit into the term "metaherpetic keratitis".

However, I found this term not very appropriate because, particularly in Germany, it is mixed up with other forms; mainly with the stromal forms. This misunderstanding has its root in a textbook which was published about 30 years ago. In this book, the metaherpetic type was mixed up with the disciform type. I think it might be more appropriate to find any other name for the metaherpetic type. You yourself have pointed out its basically neurotrophic pathogenesis. Why not name this form neurotrophic herpetic keratitis?

R. Sundmacher (Freiburg)

Well, that is just a matter of nomenclature. You and others would, perhaps, prefer to apply the term "trophic" to the aviral group. Although this would often be a correct description, secondary glaucoma after trabeculitis, for example, would not really fit under this heading. "Metaherpetic" means simply something which occurs "after herpes", and as in the anglo-american literature authors have sometimes called aviral erosions after herpes "metaherpetic erosions", I have chosen this term for the whole aviral group of diseases. Of course, we could agree on some better term. Here, we only present our current terminology for discussion in order to stop the terrible confusion concerning disciform keratitis, metaherpetic keratitis, herpetic interstitial keratitis, and others which are certainly quite different entities as we have shown.

H.E. Kaufman (New Orleans)

Frankly, I don't know of any satisfactory nomenclature. However, one of the things that interests me is that we have done numerous aqueous taps also, and, although we've seen virus on electron microscopy, we have almost never cultured virus out of the anterior chamber. I know that you have cultured virus from the anterior chamber, and your method may be more sensitive than ours, but still, there is much more antigen than virus, and I wonder what the pathogenesis is. It is difficult to be sure by specular microscopy that virus is multiplying in the endothelium, even though we have reported such multiplication occurring in rabbits. This is central disciform edema, and you say that you can see the lesions disappear under therapy. I would like to ask, what kind of therapy?

R. Sundmacher (Freiburg)

I don't think that our virological methods are more sensitive than yours, but it is certainly the details which count. We do acqeous taps only in the very early and acute stages of the disease, we aspirate the maximum of fluid, and put it all together on an outgrowing culture of human foreskin fibroblasts immediately after the aspiration in the operating theater. The success rate in these selected cases is about 50% for endotheliitis and it approaches 100% for focal herpetic iritis. We cannot, of course, see the virus multiply in the endothelium; but what we see by specular microscopy is the development of "defects" and their disappearance in the course of amelioration of the disease. Our standard therapy would be five drops of trifluorothymidine per day plus mydriatics. Steroids are always added, the dosage depending on the activity of the disease. In case of secondary glaucoma we also give timolole.

W. Jaeger (Heidelberg)

In the past, we thought that the black precipitates on the endothelium were pathognomonic for zoster iritis. Do you also see such black precipitates in your cases of focal herpetic iritis and what can you say about the sensitivity of the cornea in these cases of isolated herpetic iritis?

R. Sundmacher (Freiburg)

Most of these have had some corneal herpetic disease before which has led to some reduction in sensitivity. If you deal, however, with the first manifestation of a focal herpetic iritis and there has been no prior herpes keratitis, I would suspect that you would find the sensitivity about normal.

Heavily pigmented precipitates, in my experience, are more often found in zoster patients than in herpes simplex patients and I think that this is simply due to the amount of destruction of the iris pigment epithelium which is certainly more often severe in zoster than in herpes; but we did find heavily pigmented precipitates in some of our patients with focal herpetic iritis.

M. Singh (Amritsar)

I have been interested in the peripheral type of endotheliitis that Dr. Sundmacher has just mentioned. I would like to know when these patients recover from herpetic endotheliitis, do they get any localised stromal defect at the back of their cornea, like what we usually call a localised posterior keratoconus?

R. Sundmacher (Freiburg)

In most cases, the endothelium slides over again, covers defects and keeps on working. If it decompensates, however, you get a chronic bullous keratopathy after herpes and no posterior keratoconus.

C. Kok van Alphen (Leyden)

I wanted to mention our findings because we did electron microscopical examinations of the discs which came from eyes which had keratoplasty: We found the virus in those pieces.

L.M.T. Collum (Dublin)

I'd just like to ask Dr. Sundmacher a question about his peripheral disease. I have seen a number of cases that go on to a moorenoid type lesion, that is a furrow lesion with sloping edges. They look like Mooren's ulcers and if you take conjunctival biopsies or treat them by conjunctivectomy, you can show immunoglobulin in large amounts in the epithelium and the subepithelial tissues, I wonder, in fact, if the use of current antiviral agents is changing the natural course of this disease and if you have any comment to make about this. I think that this is becoming more common as I see more of them. Perhaps you don't agree that they are moorenoid or perhaps this is the wrong expression to use, but I'd like to hear what you have got to say about that.

**B.R. Jones (London)**
Could I make a plea not to use the word moorenoid. What we see is a gutter and it's either acute or chronic, but to introduce the term moorenoid is another exercise of nomenclature which I feel is only going to confuse the issue.

**S. Darougar (London)**
May I add another group to Dr. Sundmacher's classification and that is acute conjunctivitis due to herpes simplex virus; it seems it is rather common.

**R. Sundmacher (Freiburg)**
I don't know whether a herpes conjunctivitis without concomitant keratitis or blepharitis is really common. We have tried to find such cases as they have been reported in the literature. In all the years we have not found more than a couple of them which means that we don't have experience with them. As to the peripheral "gutter" I can only say that we too have problems with this kind of herpetic disease which takes quite some time for healing. We almost never found virus in that type of chronic keratitis near the limbus.

A totally different story is the limbal erosions with some underlying infiltrates, which we have found only with primary herpes simplex infection proven by seroconversion. These "benign" limbal erosions in true primary infection heal very rapidly, and they certainly represent viral lesions.

**B.R. Jones, London**
It has also been my experience to see this latter type of lesion only in the primary infection.

Sundmacher, R. (Hrsg.):
Herpetische Augenerkrankungen
© J.F. Bergmann Verlag, München 1981

# Herpetic Keratitis Causing Lacrimal Hyposecretion and Xerosis

D. Singh, M. Singh, R. Singh, Amritsar

**Key words.** Herpetic keratitis – lacrimal hypose-cretion, xerosis, dry eyes

**Schlüsselwörter.** Herpeskeratitis – Tränenmangel, Xerose, trockene Augen

**Summary.** Lacrimal secretion has been found to be profoundly suppressed in cases of herpes simplex keratitis. Comparison with age matched control and statistical analysis has shown that the effect on the lacrimal secretion is highly significant.

The rate of recurrence is an important factor in the reduction of tear formation.

**Zusammenfassung.** Wir fanden nach Herpes sim-plex-Keratitis im Vergleich zu einer altersent-sprechenden Kontrollgruppe eine hochsigni-fikante Reduktion der Tränenproduktion. Das Ausmaß der Beeinträchtigung ist wesentlich von der Zahl der abgelaufenen Herpesrezidive ab-hängig.

Herpes simplex keratitis (HSK) is a very serious and common disease throughout the world. It remains an important cause of cor-neal opacification resulting in considerable visual disability.

The re-emergence of malaria on a large scale has greatly increased the incidence of herpes simplex keratitis (Chaddah MR, 1978, pers. Communications). Recurrence of HSK is common and a difficult problem in clinical practice. It very often leads to the formation of dense corneal opacities. Various patterns of HSK have been recognised for the purpose of clinical description but they all appear to be different expressions of a common patholog-ical process and are closely interrelated.

Extensive research is in progress throughout the world to understand the various mysterious aspects of HSK. It is sur-prising however that little attention has been paid so far to the effects of herpetic corneal disease on lacrimal secretion. The present study of lacrimal secretion in cases of HSK has shown a significant depression of tear production in a large number of patients.

## Materials and Methods

Lacrimal secretion has been studied in 250 eyes comprising of
1. Eyes suffering from HSK = 125
2. Normal eyes to serve as age matched con-trol for 1. = 125

The control group comprised of healthy medical students, nurses and attendants of the patients. Diagnosis of HSK was based on the following
1. Old record of the patient
2. Keratitis associated with febrile illness, particularly malaria
3. History of recurrence especially if asso-ciated with fevers
4. Presence of typical lesions on the cornea and skin
5. Thinning of the cornea
6. Hypoasthesia of the cornea
7. History of use of IDU

Lacrimal secretion was assessed by Schir-mer's test. The test was performed in a moderately lighted room. A $35 \times 5$ mm strip of Whatman No. 41 filter paper was used. A 5 mm tab was folded at one end and inserted over the lower lid margin into the lower con-junctival sac at the junction of the middle and temporal third of the lower lid. The strip is kept in place for 5 min and then removed. The reading is taken after waiting for a few sec-onds to allow final absorption of tears already on the paper.

This test however, also measures the tears already secreted before the paper is inserted and those already pooled in the fornix. This can be largely overcome by immediately re-peating the test and taking the second read-

**Table 1.** Age and sex distribution

| Age in years | Control group | | Herpetic keratitis group | |
|---|---|---|---|---|
| | Male | Female | Male | Female |
| 11–20 years | 13 | 12 | 15 | 6 |
| 21–30 years | 65 | 5 | 47 | 13 |
| 31–40 years | 0 | 11 | 19 | 9 |
| 41–50 years | 5 | 2 | 7 | 2 |
| 51–60 years | 5 | 0 | 5 | 0 |
| Above 60 years | 5 | 2 | 2 | 0 |
| Total | 93 | 32 | 95 | 30 |
| % | 74.4 | 25.6 | 76.0 | 24.0 |

ing. Measurements below 15 mm were considered abnormal.

## Results

The age and sex distribution is shown in Table 1. It will be noted that most of the cases of HSK belonged to the younger age group. 87.2% of the patients were below the age of 40 years. It will be further noted that HSK affected the males more frequently (76%) than the females (24%).

Table 2 shows the number of recurrent attacks of HSK suffered by the patients. There was no sex difference in the rate of recurrence and no specific correlation was found with any particular age pattern.

Table 3 shows the results of Schirmer's test in the control group. It will be seen that 22 cases (17.6%) showed hyposecretion. Most of

these cases (90%) having Schirmer's readings less than 10 mm were above 40 years of age. Secretion was reduced more in females (22%) than in males (16%).

Table 4 shows the results of Schirmer's test in the HSK group. Seventy-one cases (56.8%) of HSK showed reduced tear formation. Of the female patients 66.6% had hyposecretion as compared to 54% of the males. Most of the cases (81%) showing Schirmer's readings less than 10 mm were below 40 years of age.

Table 5 shows the relationship between the number of recurrent attacks and lacrimal secretion in HSK. It is evident that lacrimal secretion was adversely affected with the increased number of recurrent attacks. Forty-four patients (35.2%) visited the hospital during the first attack of HSK, and of these 21 cases (47.7%) showed hyposecretion. Twenty patients (16%) in this study had four or more recurrences and they all showed deficient tear production.

## Statistical Analysis

Mean value for rates of lacrimal secretion
Controls = 24 mm
Standard Deviation ±7.55
HSK = 17 mm.
SD ± 11.11
Chi square $x^2$ = 27.22
Degree of freedom DF = I
Probability value p = 0.00I
The conclusions drawn from the clinical data were found to be statistically highly significant.

**Table 2.** Number of attacks of herpetic keratitis suffered by the patients

| Age in years | Number of attacks of herpetic keratitis | | | | | | | | | |
|---|---|---|---|---|---|---|---|---|---|---|
| | One | | Two | | Three | | More than three | | Total | |
| | Male | Female | Male | Female | Male | Female | Male | Female | Male | Female |
| 11–20 years | 5 | 2 | 5 | 2 | 3 | 1 | 2 | 1 | 15 | 6 |
| 21–30 years | 21 | 6 | 10 | 2 | 11 | 3 | 5 | 2 | 47 | 13 |
| 31–40 years | 6 | 3 | 5 | 2 | 4 | 2 | 4 | 2 | 19 | 9 |
| 41–50 years | 1 | 0 | 2 | 1 | 2 | 1 | 2 | 0 | 7 | 2 |
| 51–60 years | 0 | 0 | 2 | 0 | 2 | 0 | 1 | 0 | 5 | 0 |
| Above 60 years | 0 | 0 | 0 | 0 | 1 | 0 | 1 | 0 | 2 | 0 |
| Total | 33 | 11 | 24 | 7 | 23 | 7 | 15 | 5 | 95 | 30 |
| % | 26.4 | 8.8 | 19.2 | 5.6 | 18.4 | 5.6 | 12.0 | 4.0 | 76.0 | 24.0 |

**Table 3.** Lacrimal secretion (mm of Schirmer's Test) in the control group

| Age in years | 0–5 mm Male | Female | 6–10 mm Male | Female | 11–15 mm Male | Female | 16–20 mm Male | Female | Above 20 mm Male | Female |
|---|---|---|---|---|---|---|---|---|---|---|
| 11–20 years | 0 | 0 | 0 | 0 | 1 | 1 | 1 | 2 | 11 | 9 |
| 21–30 years | 0 | 0 | 0 | 1 | 3 | 0 | 3 | 1 | 59 | 3 |
| 31–40 years | 0 | 0 | 0 | 0 | 0 | 3 | 0 | 2 | 0 | 6 |
| 41–50 years | 0 | 0 | 2 | 0 | 1 | 0 | 1 | 2 | 1 | 0 |
| 51–60 years | 1 | 0 | 1 | 0 | 1 | 0 | 2 | 0 | 0 | 6 |
| Above 60 years | 0 | 0 | 3 | 2 | 2 | 0 | 0 | 0 | 0 | 0 |
| Total | 1 | 0 | 6 | 3 | 8 | 4 | 7 | 7 | 71 | 18 |
| % | 0.8 | 0 | 4.8 | 2.4 | 6.4 | 3.2 | 5.6 | 5.6 | 56.8 | 14.4 |

**Table 4.** Lacrimal secretion (mm of Schirmer's Test) in herpetic keratitis group

| Age in years | 0–5 mm Male | Female | 6–10 mm Male | Female | 11–15 mm Male | Female | 16–20 mm Male | Female | Above 20 mm Male | Female |
|---|---|---|---|---|---|---|---|---|---|---|
| 11–20 years | 3 | 1 | 3 | 1 | 2 | 2 | 1 | 1 | 6 | 1 |
| 21–30 years | 7 | 2 | 6 | 2 | 7 | 3 | 2 | 1 | 25 | 5 |
| 31–40 years | 6 | 1 | 4 | 2 | 3 | 4 | 1 | 1 | 5 | 1 |
| 41–50 years | 2 | 1 | 1 | 1 | 2 | 0 | 1 | 0 | 1 | 0 |
| 51–60 years | 1 | 0 | 1 | 0 | 1 | 0 | 1 | 0 | 1 | 0 |
| Above 60 years | 1 | 0 | 1 | 0 | 0 | 0 | 0 | 0 | 0 | 0 |
| Total | 20 | 5 | 16 | 6 | 15 | 9 | 6 | 3 | 38 | 7 |
| % | 16.0 | 4.0 | 12.8 | 4.8 | 12.0 | 7.2 | 4.8 | 2.4 | 30.4 | 5.6 |

**Table 5.** Relationship between the number of attacks and lacrimal secretion in herpetic keratitis group

| No. of attacks | 0–5 mm Male | Female | 6–10 mm Male | Female | 11–15 mm Male | Female | 16–20 mm Male | Female | Above 20 Male | Female |
|---|---|---|---|---|---|---|---|---|---|---|
| One | 2 | 0 | 5 | 2 | 8 | 4 | 1 | 1 | 17 | 4 |
| Two | 5 | 1 | 4 | 1 | 4 | 3 | 0 | 0 | 11 | 2 |
| Three | 4 | 1 | 2 | 1 | 2 | 2 | 5 | 2 | 10 | 1 |
| More than three | 9 | 3 | 5 | 2 | 1 | 0 | 0 | 0 | 0 | 0 |
| Total | 20 | 5 | 16 | 6 | 15 | 9 | 6 | 3 | 38 | 7 |
| % | 16.0 | 4.0 | 12.8 | 4.8 | 12.0 | 7.2 | 4.8 | 2.4 | 30.4 | 5.6 |

## Discussion

Deficient tear secretion is a common observation in many patients with HSK [5]. The magnitude and pattern of this significant clinical observation has not been investigated. This study therefore is probably the first attempt in this direction. It is quite significant to note that whereas in the control group only 17.6% of the cases showed hyposecretion, 56.8% of the patients with HSK showed reduced tear production.

Roy [4] tabulated the various causes of paucity of tears into the following main groups:

*Xerosis – local tissue changes by*

a Cicatrical degeneration of the conjunctiva and the mucous tissue

b Exposure keratitis

*Keratoconjunctivitis Sicca (KCS)*

a Congenital

b Neurogenic

c Systemic Disease

d Toxic

We have tried to exclude all these causes as far as possible. The mechanism of deficient tear production in HSK is not very clear.

a Hypoasthesia of the cornea associated with the disease may be partly blamed.

b Direct invasion of the glandular tissue by the virus may cause structural damage.

c The immune response of the host might play some role.

How the lacrimal secretion is actually reduced needs further investigation.

The behaviour of herpetic ocular disease in the presence of hyposecretion is largely unknown and demands careful study. The role of tear film in corneal nutrition and metabolism is well established. A significant part of the $O_2$ requirements of the cornea is met from the precorneal tear film. It dissolves the atmospheric $O_2$ which diffuses into the corneal epithelium [1]. Similarly $CO_2$ is discharged into the atmosphere via the tear film [2]. Disturbances in these physiological processes might occur in cases of defective tear production and are likely to further aggravate the corneal pathology. Alterations in the quality of tears produced is another important aspect worthy of our future attention. Hyposecretion may be responsible for some of the slow healing herpetic corneal lesions.

It is believed that patients with defective tear secretion are more likely to develop toxic reactions to IDU [3]. Variations in the therapeutic role of other antiviral agents are also possible under these circumstances.

We have every reason to presume that in our country at least, herpes simplex infection plays a significant role independently in the causation of dry eyes (xerosis), as well as in combination with other factors like trachoma and malnutrition. Statistical analysis of our cases of HSK and their comparison with age matched controls has established that HSK causes suppression of tear formation in a high percentage of cases. The greater the number of attacks, the greater is the effect on secretion.

The study of lacrimal secretion in HSK thus assumes an importance in the management of initial active lesions and their subsequent sequalae.

**Acknowledgment.** Secretarial assistance of Miss Katy Smith is gratefully acknowledged by the authors.

## References

1. Farris RL, Takahashi GH, Donn A (1965) Oxygen flux across the in vivo rabbit cornea. Arch Ophthal 74:679
2. Fatt J, Hill RM, Takahashi GH (1964) Carbon dioxide efflux from the human cornea in vivo. Nature 203:738
3. McGill J, Williams H, McKinnon J, Holt-Wilson AD, Jones BR (1974) Idoxiuridine in herpetic keratitis. Trans Ophthal Soc UK 94:549
4. Roy FH (1975) Ocular differential diagnosis. Lea and Febinger, Philadelphia p 92
5. Watson PG (1973) In corneal graft failure. Discussion of NSC Rice and BR Jones p 221. Ciba Foundation Symposium 15:238

Sundmacher, R. (Hrsg.):
Herpetische Augenerkrankungen
© J.F. Bergmann Verlag, München 1981

# Impairment of Tear-Production in Corneal Herpetic Diseases

C.C. Kok van Alphen, H.J.M. Völker-Dieben, Leyden

**Key words.** Herpetic keratitis – tear production

**Schlüsselwörter.** Herpeskeratitis – Tränenproduktion

**Summary.** In the last 2 years 115 patients with a bad disciform herpes-keratitis were referred to our clinic for keratoplasty.

Of those patients 20 had a severe impairment of tear production. They had an insufficient tear production in reflectory lacrimation as well as in the continuous flow.

The consequences for the herpetic eye with insufficient lacrimation can be disastrous.

A corneal graft in such a case has little chance of success.

**Zusammenfassung.** Während der letzten zwei Jahre wurden uns 115 Patienten mit einer schweren herpetischen Keratitis disciformis zur Keratoplastik überwiesen. Bei 20 dieser Patienten fanden wir eine erhebliche Beeinträchtigung der Tränenproduktion, die sich sowohl bei der Prüfung der Basissekretion als auch der Reflexsekretion fand. Solch eine herabgesetzte, ungenügende Tränenproduktion kann für ein Herpesauge schlimme Folgen haben. So hat z.B. eine Keratoplastik in diesen Augen nur geringe Erfolgsaussichten.

In lacrimation we meet several types of tear-secretion. The most important types are:
1. continuous tears,
2. reflex tears.

Whitwell [1] has produced evidence that in humans sympathetic nerves do play a role in normal or continuous tear-flow.

Botelho et al. [2] have questioned Whitwell's conclusions. In the cat they demonstrated electric activity in the nerve when they stimulated the sphenopalatine ganglion but not when they stimulated the pre-ganglionic fibers of the cervical sympathetic chain. Thus the main lacrimal nerve of the cat contains only parasympathetic fibers.

Changes in membrane potential in the secretory lacrimal cell was associated with an increase in flow in the excretory duct. They also noted that vascular supply of the gland, pressure in the excretory ducts and perhaps humoral substances that influence metabolism of lacrimal cells can play a role in lacrimal secretion. Most reflex-lacrimation originates from stimulation of the first division of the trigeminal nerve. Any painful disease of the eye can produce extra reflex-lacrimation. The efferent innervation (brain → lacrimal gland) passes the geniculate ganglion and the sphenopalatine ganglion. Impaired tear production can be caused by obliteration of the excretory ducts of the lacrimal gland and the supplementary tear glands, by diseases of the tear gland itself or by disturbances in the nervous pathways.

From experimental investigations in animals we know that herpes virus can be found in the lacrimal gland and even in the sphenopalatine ganglion soon after the start of the infection [3, 4]. However, we don't know how much damage is caused there by the virus. It is not yet proven that it stays in those tissues in an inactive form to be triggered to new activity at the time of a re-infection [5, 6].

Guided by clinical facts we can construct a hypothesis of the cause of impaired lacrimation in chronic herpetic corneal disease. It was shown to us in our clinical material that some corneal grafts failed in severe herpetic disciform keratitis cases, and this failure was definitely not caused by rejection or re-infection (Fig. 1). To our astonishment we found an impaired tear production in those cases. Schirmer's test described in 1903 [7] is still the most simple and practical clinical test for evaluating tear production. Boberg-Ans [8] and MacMillan and Cone [9] described some modifications, but ultimately the Schirmer test proved to be the method of choice. The

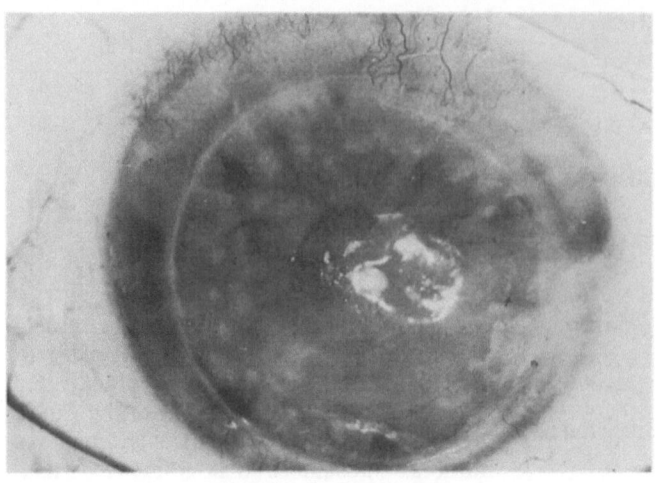

**Fig. 1.** Graft failure caused by impairment of tear production

quantitative values of Halberg and Berens were used in our investigation. Wetting of the filter-paper under 15 mm was considered pathological in patients under 40 years old. However, in older people a normal production may be 10–15 mm. The alterations with age show of course a gliding scale. The method has the disadvantage of not being exact. Ideally, tear secretion should be measured in the excretory ducts of the lacrimal gland, but these ducts are very small and are relatively inaccessible for practical clinical study.

In the last 2 years 115 patients with severe recurrent disciform herpes-keratitis were referred to our clinic for keratoplasty. Of those patients, 20 had a severe impairment of tear production. We always measured the reflex-tearing without giving anaesthetic drops before inserting the filterpaper-strip in the lower conjunctival fornix. When our attention was drawn to the tear production it struck us how many times before we had failed to examine the tear production. Inadequate lacrimation tends to have disastrous consequences for an eye with a herpes infection. It is not possible to create an adequate continuous tear-flow artificially. The best possibility is to transfer the excretory duct of the salivatory gland to the eye by an operation, provided the salivatory gland is still functioning.

However, it is important to institute palliative therapy as soon as the disturbance in lacrimation is known. Methylcellulose, artificial tears like Tears Naturale or Liquifilm Tears are very useful. When still a small tear production exists, we can improve the lacrimation by Dakryo-Biciron (Bromehexine-HCL), which stimulates the lacrimal gland. Sometimes a therapeutic soft-lens, combined with artificial tears can be a therapy.

In our clinical material 20 patients had a severe impairment of tear-production. They showed an insufficient Schirmer test and a significant difference in this test in the herpetic eye, compared with the normal eye. The average tear production was 4.0 mm in the diseased eye and 14.4 in the healthy eye.

In four patients an impaired tear production was measured on both eyes. Of those, three had a disciform herpes keratitis in both eyes. We only considered patients with herpes simplex, those with herpes zoster were excluded.

The number of years the patients suffered from recurrent herpes attacks was appallingly high. We found an average of 21.64 years in patients with insufficient lacrimation and of 20.12 years in the patients without pathology in lacrimation. We have to consider the handicap this must have been for these patients. An earlier keratoplasty would have possibly been much better for them.

When an eye with metaherpetic infection shows an insufficient tear production the chance to get an intercurrent bacterial or fungal infection is much higher. Those eyes are generally treated with antiviral as well as corticosteroid therapy. This intercurrent infection generally can lead to a descemetocele or even a perforation. Then we are forced to do a keratoplasty. However, this corneal

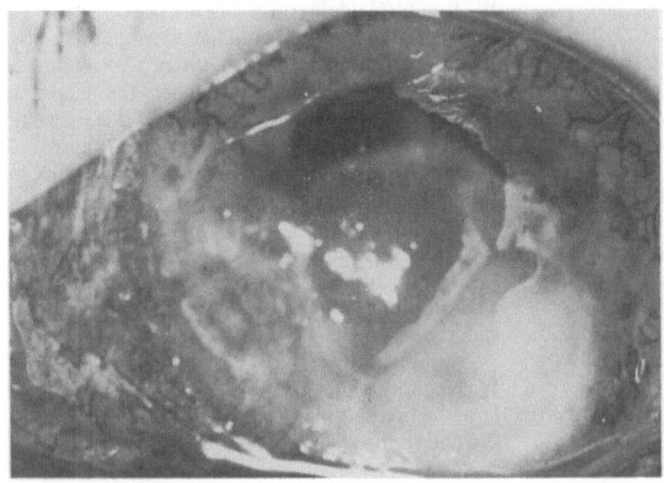

**Fig. 2.** Intercurrent infection in a herpetic eye with insufficient lacrimation

graft (Fig. 2) is rarely successful and shows clouding in due time. The lack of tears seems to be even more disastrous for the graft than for the pre-existing cornea itself.

We should like to postulate the hypothesis that the cause of the impairment of tear production is either due to obliteration of the excretory ducts or damage of the producing cells in the lacrimal gland. If the cause had to do with the supranuclear pathways or the sphenopalatine ganglion, the patients would also complain of a unilateral dry nose. This was not the case in the herpetic patients. However, we met this phenomenon in patients with pathological tear production caused by neurological diseases (Fig. 3).

We were amazed to find a poor or non-existing tear production change back to normal lacrimation. This phenomenon was accompanied by a striking improvement in either the cornea or the graft. In one of those cases a deterioration of the tear-production occurred again after 2 months and the beautiful graft, performed in the normal period, clouded in a few days.

It seems useful to start a qualitative investigation of the tear-fluid in chronic herpetic keratitis. In some cases with a normal Schirmer-test we found abnormalities in the graft, especially an abnormality of the epithelium, which pointed to disturbances in the composition of the tear fluid.

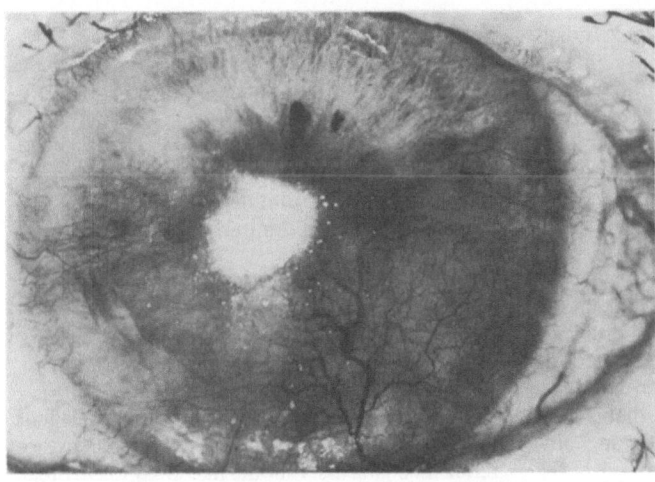

**Fig. 3.** Dry eye caused by neurological disease. This patient complained of a unilateral dry nose

## References

1. Whitewell J (1961) Role of sympathetic in lacrimal secretion. Br J Ophthalmol 45:439–445
2. Botelho SY, Hisada M, Fuenmayor N (1966) Functional innervation of the lacrimal gland in the cat. Origin of secretomotor fibers in the lacrimal nerve. Arch Ophthalmol 76:581–588
3. Brown DC, Kaufman HE (1969) Chronic herpes simplex infection of the ocular adnexa: persistence of virus in the rabbit after enucleation. Arch Ophthalmol 81:837–839
4. Nesburn AB, Cook ML, Stevens JG (1972) Latent herpes simplex virus. Arch Ophthalmol 88:412–417
5. Kaufman HE, Brown DC, Ellison EM (1968) Herpes virus in the lacrimal gland, conjunctiva and cornea of man. Am J Ophthalmol 65:32–35
6. Pavan Langston D, Nesburn AB (1968) The chronology of primary herpes infection of the eye and adnexa glands. Arch Ophthalmol 80: 258–264
7. Schirmer O (1903) Studien zur Physiologie and Pathologie der Tränenabsonderung und Tränenabfuhr. Albrecht von Graefes Arch Klin Ophthalmol 56:197–291
8. Boberg-Ans J (1955) Experience in clinical examination of corneal sensitivity. Corneal sensitivity and the naso-lacrimal reflex after retrobulbar anaesthesia. Br J Ophthalmol 39: 705–726
9. MacMillan JA, Cone W (1937) Prevention and treatment of keratitis neuroparalytica by closure of the lacrimal canaliculi. Arch Ophthalmol 18:352–355

## Discussion on the Contributions pp. 211–218

D. Epstein (Stockholm)
I'd like to address a question to Dr. Singh's Indian study. You mention in your last slide in point six what should be done and one of the things was, naturally, qualitative analysis because we know today that quantity probably is not the most important factor. Have you made any preliminary attempts to assess the quality, like the BUT and that sort of thing?

M. Singh (Amritsar)
We did not look into the quality of tears specifically. We were randomly selecting the patients and making a preliminary study just of the amount of lacrimal secretions. As I have mentioned earlier, as far as the quality is concerned, I think that is very important. I am afraid we have not done any qualitative study of that kind.

W. Jaeger (Heidelberg)
In terms of therapy, I would like to mention a substance derived from the octopus. It is named Eledoisin and strongly stimulates the lacrimal glands. It has two disadvantages, first it is very expensive, and second, it hasn't as yet been approved by our Drug Administration so that I, e.g., get it from Barcelona, Spain; but it is very helpful.

B.R. Jones (London)
Mr. Jaeger, this polypeptide from the octopus, does it cause allergic reactions from the continued application of it to the eye?

W. Jaeger (Heidelberg)
I got the first samples from Bietti some 5 or 6 years ago and have as yet not observed allergic reactions.

G. Smolin (San Francisco)
Frequently, in chronic inflammation, we observe decreased tears from the irritative phenomena and I was wondering if that effect may be occurring with the decreased tearing observed in herpes. Secondly, did you determine the lysozyme content of the tears? Thirdly, did you put ophthaine in the eyes to determine whether or not an anesthetic eye in a control group was identical to a herpetic anesthetic eye?

M. Singh (Amritsar)
No, we did not study the lysozyme at all in this series. We would in fact wish to do all the qualitative studies, but unfortunately we do not have the facilities for that at the moment in our hospital. As far as doing the Schirmer's test is concerned, the conditions were kept nearly the same in both study groups.

G. Sturrock (Basel)
Dr. Singh, did you instill local anaesthetic into the eye before you performed your Schirmer's test?

M. Singh (Amritsar)
No, we did not put any local anaesthetic into the eye, because these patients already had hypoaesthesia of their corneas.

G. Sturrock (Basel)
Is it possible that the diminished secretion was, to a large extent, due to diminished sensitivity in the herpetic eye?

M. Singh (Amritsar)
I think we can keep that as a possibility.

C. Kok van Alphen (Leyden)
We used both methods, but with the anaesthetic drops we found no tears at all. Then we went over to reflex mechanisms. I should like to say to Dr. Singh

that it is curious that we have such similar findings in such different countries.

**M. Singh (Amritsar)**
Yes, it is very interesting indeed. I was really amazed, because although we have slightly different types of set ups of Ophthalmology in two countries, we have come to have identical observations.

**J. Colin (Brest)**
Has somebody in the auditorium any experience with what else one could do with these dry eyes?

**H.E. Kaufman (New Orleans)**
In our experience, the problem is that a patient with herpes and an anesthetic cornea and dry eyes is in terrible trouble and is never discharged from the clinic as cured. As a result, studying herpes patients from the clinic results in a very high percentage of dry eyes also, and these are very hard to manage. What should be done is a prospective study, which would include both patients who get better as well as the ones who remain under medical supervision.

Also, the effects of anesthesia must be taken care of, and the dry eyes problem can also be helped with slow-release artifical tear inserts, a hydroxy-propylcellulose rod that dissolves continuously.

**H. Neubauer (Köln)**
Wilhelm Güter, whose picture was presented in the opening session by Wilhelm Böke, was a man who didn't like hasty publishing. Consequently, some of his knowledge was never published. His opinion was that dry eye in herpes only happens if the process is located in the peripheral parts of the cornea, especially if there is vascularization and a strong conjunctival process. He thought that even a recurrent herpes in the central part of the cornea will not lead to dry eyes. We did use Schirmer's test, but he always said that it's not a very sensitive test. We have seen pictures where the stripes were applied in the center of the lid. I think we have to expect strong irritation even in a cornea with hypoanesthesia.

# Antivirals

Sundmacher, R. (Hrsg.):
Herpetische Augenerkrankungen
© J.F. Bergmann Verlag, München 1981

# Development of Antiviral Drugs

W.H. Prusoff, New Haven

**Key words.** Nucleosides, thymidine kinase, DNA polymerase, antiviral drugs

**Schlüsselwörter.** Nukleoside, Thymidinkinase, DNA-Polymyerase, antivirale Medikamente

**Summary.** The development of antiviral drugs has progressed through several stages. We have witnessed within the past few years a major breakthrough in antiviral chemotherapy, because selectivity can now be based on a qualitative exploitation of unique virus enzymic activities. Thus, today we have several antiviral agents which have little or no host cell toxicity, because they are uniquely or preferentially activated (phosphorylated) by the herpesvirus encoded thymidine kinase which is present only in the infected cell. Examples include: 9-(2′ hydroxyethoxymethyl)guanine, 5-ethyl-2′-deoxyuridine, 5-propyl-2′-deoxyuridine, 5-iodo-5′-amino-2′, 5′-dideoxyuridine, 5-(2-bromovinyl)-2′-deoxyuridine, 5-methoxymethyl-2′-deoxyuridine and 2′-fluoro-5-iodo-arabinosyl cytosine.

A major problem which has not been solved is the availability of a reliable in vitro assay, biological or biochemical, that will predict efficacy of test compounds in animals or man.

**Zusammenfassung.** Die ersten antiviralen Substanzen wurden eigentlich mehr durch Zufall gefunden und dann durch breitgefächerte Suchmethoden weiter entwickelt. Inzwischen sind unsere Möglichkeiten zu einer rationaleren Entwicklung von Virustatika etwas besser geworden. Die meisten Bemühungen gehen heutzutage in Richtung einer strukturellen Modifizierung bekannter antiviraler Substanzen in der Hoffnung, hierdurch eine reduzierte Toxizität und eine verbesserte Wirkung zu erhalten. Mit unserer immer besser werdenden Kenntnis von der Biochemie der Virusreplikation und der Zwischenwirkungen von Wirtszelle und Virus lernen wir allmählich auch virusspezifische Angriffspunkte kennen. Die damit verbundene Hoffnung besteht natürlich darin, daß man hier-

durch in die Lage versetzt wird, Medikamente zu planen, die eine ganz spezifische antivirale Aktivität aufweisen. Obwohl wir eine ganze Reihe von Virustatika besitzen, die nur geringe oder gar keine Wirtszelltoxizität aufweisen, wie zum Beispiel 9-2′ Hydroxyethoxymethyl)Guanin, 5-Ethyl-2′-Deoxyuridine, 5-Propyl-2′-Deoxyuridine, 5-Iodo-5′-Amino-2′-Deoxyuridine, 5-(2-Bromovinyl)-2′-Deoxyuridine, 5-Methoxymethyl-2′-Deoxyuridine und 2′-Fluoro-5-Iodo-Arabinosyl Cytosine, so wurden diese doch alle entweder durch Modifikation schon bekannter Virustatika oder durch reine Zufallsbefunde entwickelt. Ob wir *neue* antivirale Moleküle dadurch planen und entwickeln können, daß wir die virusspezifischen biochemischen Angriffspunkte besser kennen lernen, muß sich in Zukunft erst noch erweisen. In vielen Laboratorien, u.a. auch bei uns, wird mit beträchtlichem Aufwand auf dieses Ziel hin gearbeitet.

Eines der Hauptprobleme bei der Entwicklung von neuen Virustatika ist die Entwicklung eines verläßlichen in vitro-Testsystemes, mit dem man die Wirkung von Virustatika in bestimmten klinischen Situationen richtig voraussagen kann.

My charge today is twofold − first, to present an overview of the development of antiviral drugs; second, to discuss the processes involved in the evaluation of the many compounds that are synthesized, as well as to discuss the decision making process involved in choosing compounds for study in animal systems. The significance of animal models will be discussed later by Dr. Kaufman. The development of antiviral drugs has passed through several stages of development (Table 1). During the first period it was generally accepted that a non-toxic antiviral agent could not be found, because a virus not only must replicate within a host cell, but in so doing, also utilizes much of the host cell's metabolic processes. Inhibition of viral replication was assumed to be a consequence of inhibition of the host cell, and hence any antiviral agent would be too toxic for practical use.

223

**Table 1.** Periods of antiviral drug development

---

*Discouragement*
*Enlightenment*
   Prophylactic: Amantadine; Marboran
   curative    : Idoxuridine (IdUrd);
              Vidarabine (ara-A);
              Trifluorothymidine ($F_3dThd$).
*Serendipitous Specificity*
   5'-Amino-IdUrd; ara-T; 5-Methoxymethyl-dUrd;
   5-Alkyl-dUrd; Acyclovir; FIAC.
*Directed Specificity*
   ? ? ? ?

---

The second period is termed "Enlightenment" since several compounds, such as Amantadine and Marboran, were found to be effective prophylactic agents: Amantadine for the prevention of respiratory infections caused by the influenza-A virus, and Marboran for prevention of smallpox.

A very significant advance in our thinking was made by Kaufman and his colleagues [8], with the remarkable discovery, that patients with an established virus infection, herpetic keratitis, could be cured. Thus, his use of Idoxuridine in the therapy of herpetic keratitis in man truly represented a milestone in the field of antiviral chemotherapy.

In addition to Kaufman, it is appropriate at this meeting to acknowledge the pioneering work of Wollensak, who as far back as 1959, was deeply involved in studies of the potential role of antimetabolites in the therapy of herpetic keratitis (references cited in [13]). Several others who also played a major part in establishing a role for antiviral drugs in Ophthalmology include Sundmacher in Germany, Jones in England and Pavan-Langston in the U.S.A. Obviously, there are others who also made important contributions.

Idoxuridine, although approved by the FDA for use in herpetic keratitis, is not the ideal agent, since it does have certain toxicities, and hence there is a need for compounds with more desirable properties. Thus today, in the United States, Vidarabine (ara-A) is also approved by the FDA for therapy of herpetic keratitis.

In Europe, Trifluorothymidine, first synthesized by Heidelberger, also represents a drug of the "Enlightenment" era, and in several respects it is a preferable drug to Idoxuridine or ara-A. However, all three of these drugs, Idoxuridine, ara-A and Trifluorothymidine, have certain undesirable toxicities.

The basis for the antiviral activity of both Idoxuridine and Trifluorothymidine is a consequence of the incorporation, of these metabolic analogues of thymidine, into the DNA of the herpes virus. Ara-A is also incorporated into viral DNA, and in addition inhibits herpes simplex virus DNA-polymerase to a greater extent than cellular DNA polymerases.

Unfortunately, these three compounds are also incorporated into the DNA of uninfected cells, that are in the S-phase of their cell cycle, and this is responsible for their cytotoxicity. Therefore, systemic use of Idoxuridine and Trifluorothymidine is limited because of bone marrow depression; and the use of ara-A in non-lethal infections should be limited because of its potential to be teratogenic and oncogenic.

The third state of antiviral drug development is where we are now, and this stage represents a major breakthrough in antiviral chemotherapy. This is because antiviral selectivity can now be based on a *qualitative* as well as a *quantitative* exploitation of viral associated enzymatic activities. The role of enzymes in antiviral chemotherapy will be developed more extensively by Cheng.

Within the past few years we have seen the development of a number of antiviral nucleosides that have little or no toxicity to the host cell (Fig. 1): 5-ethyl-, 5-propyl-, 5-methoxymethyl-, and 5-(2-bromovinyl)-2'-deoxyuridine; 5-iodo-5'-amino-2', 5'-dideoxyuridine, 5'-amino-5'-deoxythymidine, 2'-fluoro-5-iodo-arabinosylcytosine and acycloguanosine. The molecular basis for their decreased cytotoxicity is the *selective* or *preferential* phosphorylation of these agents by the herpesvirus encoded thymidine kinase.

Although there is great diversity in these structures, they are good substrates for the herpesvirus encoded thymidine kinase, but not for the cellular thymidine kinase. The question that we are trying to answer is "What are the common features of these compounds which enable the herpes enzyme, but not the cellular thymidine kinase, to either uniquely or preferentially phosphorylate these compounds". If we can solve this riddle, then we will be in a position to develop new antiviral agents which are *only* activated in the

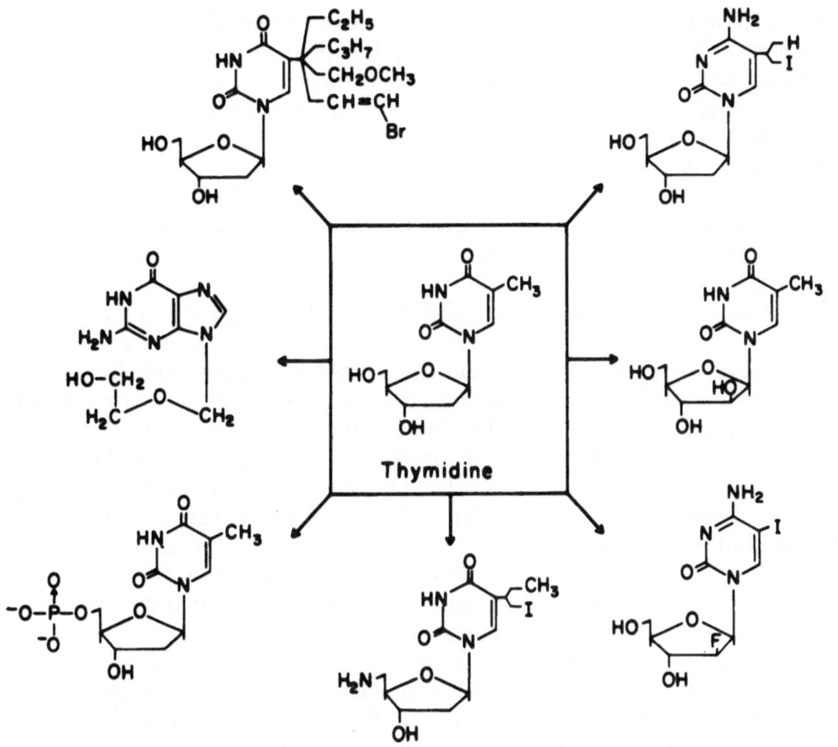

**Fig. 1.** Some compounds which act to a variable degree as specific substrates for herpesvirus induced Thymidine-kinase

virus infected cell, and are totally without toxicity to the uninfected cells.

There are several strategies that one can use to develop such compounds, and my laboratory as well as others are busily engaged in these directions. But this is a whole lecture by itself. What I have done so far is to indicate one approach to the development of potential antiviral agents.

The second part of my talk concerns the problem, that once a compound is synthesized, how do you determine whether it is worth pursuing in animal models, and more importantly in humans. There are two approaches to the in vitro evaluation, the most common being *biological* and the other *biochemical*.

Unfortunately there is *no* standard procedure to determine antiviral activity of a compound [7, 11, 12], and hence it is not surprising that varying results are produced, at times, in different laboratories. Sidwell [12] and also Schwöbel et al. [11] recently discussed the problems of in vitro evaluation.

**Biological Approach**

The host cell used to grow the virus is important. For example, if one evaluates the antiviral activity of 5-Iodo-2'-deoxycytidine (IdCyd) in cells which do *not* have cytidine deaminase activity, a very high therapeutic index is obtained. However, if one uses the same strain of virus in cells which do have this enzyme, then a low therapeutic index will result. IdCyd is rapidly deaminated to idoxuridine in the presence of cytidine deaminase, and therefore it is not surprising that a therapeutic index similar to idoxuridine is obtained. Also, reproducing cells are considerably more sensitive to the toxic effects of a compound, than are confluent cells, which are generally used when evaluating antiviral activity. Furthermore, the temperature of incubation and the pH of the media are also influential.

The strain of virus, the passage history of the virus, as well as the size of the inoculum is important. Thus we and others have seen

225

great variation, among prototype and clinical isolates, in their responsiveness to nucleoside antiviral agents. This may be a reflection, for example, of the relative amounts of cellular phosphorylase, which would inactivate a nucleoside drug and the kinase responsible for its activation. We know from the studies of Dundarov et al. [3], that there is great variation in the induction of thymidine kinase activity by different clinical isolates of HSV 1 and HSV 2. This will effect their sensitivity to certain antiviral agents.

In addition to variations in the host cell and virus, another major variation is the method of assay used. Studies by Griffith and Hsiung [5] found a marked variation in the extent of inhibition of HSV by 5-Iodo-5'-amino-2',5'-dideoxyuridine which was related not only to the strain of virus, but also the method of assay.

Several tests for in vitro susceptibility of HSV to drugs have been described, and there is disagreement as to which is the most reliable predictor. In an attempt to determine how to properly evaluate new compounds Collins and Bauer [2] compared three in vitro methods of assay:

Plaque Inhibition
Plaque Reduction
Yield Reduction

*Plaque Inhibition*

Vero cells in petri dishes were grown to confluency, and then infected with 100 pfu/ml of virus for 1 h. Paper discs impregnated with the drug were placed on each overlay, and the zones of plaque inhibition measured 96 h later.

*Plaque Reduction*

Vero cells in petri dishes were grown to confluency, and then infected with 100–200 pfu/ml of virus for 1 h. Varying concentrations of drug in an overlay medium were now added, and after an incubation period, the number of plaques were counted and compared to a control containing no drug.

*Yield Reduction*

Vero cells in petri dishes were grown to confluency and infected with 2–3 pfu/ml of virus for 1 h, followed by inclusion of varying amounts of drug. After 18 h incubation, the cells were disrupted and the virus yield determined by plaque assay, and the titers were compared with those of the untreated cultures.

Collins and Bauer [2] concluded that the plaque reduction test was the most reliable in vitro method for assaying drug activity against HSV.

Griffith and Hsiung [5] found the plaque reduction test to be of particular value for a *rapid* comparison of the susceptibility of different virus strains to drugs, since it obviated the time required for incubation and virus release which is required in the yield reduction method. However, with herpesvirus prototypes, the yield reduction assay proved to be more sensitive than the plaque reduction method, for testing compounds that are less potent then idoxuridine, such as 5'-amino-nucleosides (AIdUrd).

Schwöbel and coworkers [11] recently described procedures for standardization of in vitro tests for screening of antiviral drugs. First they used a plaque reduction assay, which was then followed by a Persistant Infection Cell Culture test, in which confluent cells were infected with HSV at a very low multiplicity of infection (0.1–0.001 PFU per cell). The test compound was added after adsorption of the virus, and at various intervals of time, new medium containing the drug was added. The extent of virus induced cell destruction was related to virus replication. This latter procedure was stated, to allow the determination as to whether the test compound can effect a cure, as well as to detect emergence of drug resistant virus.

Another complicating feature which may vary with drug, host cell, as well as strain of virus, relates to the effect on pool sizes of metabolites within the cell, with which the drug or its phosphorylated derivates may have to compete before the drug can get to the site of inhibition. Thus Cheng and Prusoff [1] found the 5'-amino analog of idoxuridine had a marked effect on the intracellular pool size of the various nucleoside triphosphates (dATP, dGTP, dCTP and dTTP) in the herpes simplex virus infected cell.

The picture is further complicated when one tries to correlate in vitro antiviral effects with responses in experimental animals. This is made evident by the study of North and

Pavan-Langston [9], in which they clearly found poor agreement between in vitro and in vivo results, in a comparison of the antiviral activity of vidarabine and idoxuridine. These data, as well as personal experience, would indicate that one should not discard a compound as being inactive based on in vitro data alone. The problem is that in vivo screening is long, laborious and expensive, and hence one is more likely to limit studies in experimental animals to those compounds that are active in vitro. However, such a decision may save time, effort and money, but the cost could be the failure to identify an antiviral agent that may be of value in animal systems and more importantly in man.

On the other hand a compound that is effective as an antiviral agent in vitro may be a complete failure when evaluated in animal systems for a variety of reasons. These have been tabulated by Sidwell [12]:

1. Enzymes may not be present in the host cell that is used in the in vitro assay, but if present in the animal or man, may either activate or inactivate the test compound.

2. Problems in solubility, adsorption, or distribution may not provide an adequate concentration in the infected tissues of animal or man.

3. The immune system often is critical for an effective antiviral effect, and suppression of immunity would not be detected in the in vitro assay.

4. The concentration of virus is critical, since if too high, then significant activity may not be seen.

5. Mycoplasma contamination, in the in vitro system, may inactivate an otherwise active compound.

6. In vitro activity may be expressed in only certain cells for unknown reasons.

## Biochemical Approach

The identification of enzymes that are encoded by the viral genome, not only affords a target for chemotherapy, but also can be used as a screen for evaluation of compounds for antiviral activity. Herpes simplex virus-DNA polymerase is an example of an appropriate target, provided cellular DNA polymerases ($\alpha$, $\beta$, $\gamma$) are used as the control.

Thus, Overby et al. [10] found phosphono-acetic acid to be a preferential inhibitor of HSV-DNA polymerase. Helgstrand and Oberg [6], used a cell-free polymerase model as a primary screen to find selective inhibitors of HSV-DNA biosynthesis, and they found phosphonoformate not only to be active in this system, but also to be effective in the therapy of cutaneous herpesvirus infection in guinea pigs.

Evaluation of nucleoside analogs in such a screen requires their conversion to the triphosphate derivative before testing as potential inhibitors of DNA polymerase. Thus, vidarabine (ara-A), after conversion to the triphosphate analog, inhibits HSV-DNA polymerase to about a 30–40-fold greater extent than cellular DNA polymerase.

Other nucleoside analogs, such as idoxuridine or the 5'-amino analog of idoxuridine have been shown by Fischer et al. [4] to exert their inhibitory effect after incorporation into the HSV-DNA, rather than by inhibition of DNA polymerase. In other words, the analogs, at the triphosphate level are alternate substrates for DNA polymerase. In fact, a direct correlation has been found between inhibition of the formation of infectious herpesvirus and incorporation into viral DNA. Since ara-A is also incorporated into HSV-DNA, this factor must also be considered in the screening procedure.

Another potential valuable procedure, at least for pyrimidine and possibly other nucleosides, is the use of HSV-encoded thymidine kinase to screen compounds for unique or preferential phosphorylation relative to cellular thymidine kinase. This will at least detect compounds that have little or no toxicity to the host cell, but does not necessarily imply antiviral activity.

*In conclusion*, we have made tremendous strides in the development of potent antiviral drugs that have little or no toxicity, but we are still in a primitive stage in finding a reliable in vitro assay that will predict efficacy in the animal model and more importantly in humans.

## References

1. Cheng YC, Prusoff WH Unpublished data
2. Collins P, Bauer DJ (1977) Relative potencies of antiherpes compounds. Ann NY Acad Sci 284:49–59
3. Dundarov S, Dundarova d, Todorov S, Kava-

klova L, Falke D (1978) Induction capacity and influence of dThdMP on thymidine kinase activity of type 1 and 2 strains of herpes simplex virus. Arch Virol 56:243–249

4. Fischer PH, Chen MS, Prusoff WH (1980) The incorporation of 5-Iodo-5′-amino-2′,5′-dideoxyuridine and 5-iodo-2′-deoxyuridine into herpes simplex virus DNA. Relationship between antiviral activity and effects on DNA structure. Biochim Biophys Acta 606:236–245

5. Griffith B, Hsiung E Unpublished data

6. Helgstrand E, Oberg B (1978) Antiviral screening based on cell-free polymerase models and a new selective inhibitor. Current Chemotherapy, Proceedings 10th Int Congr Chemother 1:329–330

7. Herrman jr EC (ed) (1965) Antiviral substances. Ann NY Acad Sci 130:1–483

8. Kaufman HE, Martola E, Dohlman C (1962) Use of 5-iodo-2′-deoxyuridine (IdU) in treatment of herpes simplex keratitis. Arch Ophthalmol 68:235–239

9. North RD, Pavan-Langston D (1976) Herpes simplex virus types 1 and 2: Therapeutic response to antiviral drugs. Arch Ophthalmol 94:1019–1021

10. Overby LR, Duff RG, Mao JC-H (1977) Antiviral potential of phosphonacetic acid. Ann NY Acad Sci 284:310–320

11. Schwöbel W, Streissle G, Kiefer G (1979) Attempts to standardize the screening for antiviral drugs by in vitro tests. Chemotherapy 25:268–278

12. Sidwell RW (1979) Test systems for evaluating the antiviral activity of nucleoside analogs. In: Walker RT, DeClercq E, Eckstein F (eds) Nucleoside analogues: Chemistry, biology and medical applications. Plenum, New York, pp 337–362

13. Wollensak J (1979) Herpes simplex of the eye and possibilities of its therapeutic control. Adv Ophthalmol 38:99–104

## Discussion on the Contribution pp. 223–228

G. Smolin (San Francisco)
The New York Academy of Science Symposium on antivirals devoted many articles to isoprinosine. Do you have any experience with the drug?

W.H. Prusoff (New Haven)
I have not had any direct experience with this drug. As I understand it, it's primary effect is at best on the immune system, but the data in support of antiviral activity is quite poor.

G. Streissle (Wuppertal)
Another disadvantage of many test models lies in the fact that one has to use a lethal infection to obtain reproducible results although the majority of natural virus diseases are not lethal.

W.H. Prusoff (New Haven)
I agree and probably Dr. Kaufman could go into this more.

J. Oh (San Francisco)
What is your own assessment of this new antiherpetic drug, Acyclovir?

W.H. Prusoff (New Haven)
I would say at this stage it looks like it's probably the most exciting drug which we've seen evaluated today. Acyclovir and the one that Dr. De Clercq is developing, 5-(2-Bromovinyl)-2′-deoxyuridine, are probably the two drugs which we will hear a great deal about within the next year or two. Exactly what their role will be clinically, obviously, we will have to wait and see how they perform during clinical evaluation.

B.R. Jones (London)
Just to point out that the laboratory test which is universally named plaque reduction test is really wrong named. It should have been named plaque inhibition test, because it measures the prophylactic effect. Interferon, for example, looks exceedingly good in such a system. We have endeavored to extrapolate from the laboratory model to an in vivo model on the rabbit cornea, and we first called our test the "corneal epithelial lesion reduction assay". Interferon, again, looks very good in this system. But then we realized that what we measured was not really lesion reduction or plaque reduction, it is lesion or plaque inhibition. Only when you delay the institution of treatment up to the time when lesions have already formed, you get a true lesion reduction assay. Shiota will, I hope, report on such a system later on. Of course, you can do the same thing in vitro; but I really wanted to ask you whether you feel that there is an additional dimension of information to be gained from a true plaque reduction test as distinct from a plaque inhibition test in the in vitro system?

W.H. Prusoff (New Haven)
I don't want to get into any semantic discussions. These were not my terms as applied to the tests. But I think any in vitro assay has certain limitations for the reasons which I gave. For example, you have no understanding of the immune response. You do not have the complication of the drug passing through the liver where it may either become inactivated or, possibly, converted into a toxic compound. There are a lot of complications with any in vitro assay. I agree with you completely that there may be better in vitro assays than the ones I've mentioned. I'm not critisizing but merely indicating that there are limitations.

Sundmacher, R. (Hrsg.):
Herpetische Augenerkrankungen
© J.F. Bergmann Verlag, München 1981

# Animal Models in the Development of Antiviral Therapy

H.E. Kaufman, New Orleans

**Key words.** Dendritic keratitis, stromal keratitis, iritis, interferon, acyclovir, trifluorothymidine, vidarabine

**Schlüsselwörter.** Keratitis dendritica, Stromaherpes, Iritis, Interferon, Acyclovir, Trifluorthymidin, Vidarabin

**Summary.** Virtually all medical laboratory experimentation involves the creation of models of human diseases which can be used in the preliminary evaluation of newly developed modes of therapy. The critical problem with such models is distinguishing between those models that are accurate representations of the human disease and its reaction to treatment and those models that are in some way separate or distinct from the human disease. This problem is clearly illustrated by the various animal models developed in the course of our search for a truly safe and effective treatment for herpesvirus ocular disease.

In the case of epithelial dendritic ulceration, antimetabolite therapy has been tested in the rabbit. The results seen in this animal model have proven highly predictive of actual therapeutic results obtained with antimetabolite drugs in man.

Epithelial disease can also be treated successfully with interferon and with interferon inducers, particularly for the prevention of recurrence of epithelial disease. However, interferon inducers are highly species-specific and, therefore, experimental results obtained in rabbits and rats cannot be usefully extrapolated to man. Thus, primates or even human subjects must be employed to provide relevant data. Actual interferon itself tends to be species-selective, and the quantitative determination of its efficacy in experimental animals, although possibly related to such results in man, may not prove reliable in human therapeutics.

Stromal disease can result from a primary host immune reaction either to viruses and antigen, or to extensive multiplication of virus that causes destructive stromal lesions. Each of these processes can be produced in an animal model on which drug evaluations can be performed; however, the exact relevance to man of these evaluations of immunosuppressive drugs or specific antiviral therapies remains uncertain because the role of each of the two processes in the production of the disease remains uncertain.

The chemical determination of drug penetration has been made more difficult by a lack of knowledge of essential drug concentrations. For example, a virus that multiplies rapidly in the epithelium may require a lower concentration of drug in the stroma where both cellular metabolism and viral multiplication may be different. Several topically administered drugs have been demonstrated to be active in the rabbit against stromal keratitis, but it is uncertain if they are equally active in man. Similar problems are involved in the interpretation of activity of systemically administered drugs on local ocular disease, even though the models for systemic effects such as prevention of death from encephalitis appear to be relevant to man.

**Zusammenfassung.** Im Prinzip besteht jegliche Laborforschung in der Entwicklung von Modellen und deren Prüfung. Das Kernproblem dabei ist, wie man klinisch relevante Modelle von solchen unterscheiden kann, die für menschliche Erkrankungen keine Bedeutung haben. Dies sei am Beispiel der Herpeserkrankungen gezeigt. Eine Keratitis dendritica kann man mit Antimetaboliten im Tierversuch behandeln und die Modelle sind sowohl hinsichtlich der Wirksamkeit als auch der relativen Wirkung solcher Substanzen in hohem Maße aussagekräftig.

Interferon-Induktoren vermögen einen epithelialen Herpes günstig zu beeinflussen und können Rezidive verhindern, sie sind aber hochgradig spezies-spezifisch, so daß Versuche mit Kaninchen oder anderen Nagetieren bei solchen Substanzen irrelevant sind. Hierfür muß man Primaten oder eben Menschen selbst benutzen.

Interferon selbst ist ebenfalls in gewissem Maße spezies-spezifisch und das bedeutet, daß eine Prüfung in Tiermodellen ebenfalls nicht sehr viel für die Klinik aussagt, obwohl in diesem Fall die Modelle schon mehr Bedeutung haben.

Ein Stroma-Herpes entwickelt sich entweder

durch eine Immunreaktion des Wirtes auf das Virus oder Virusantigene oder auf eine exzessive Virusvermehrung mit ausgedehnter Zellzerstörung im Stroma. Für beide Vorgänge kann man Tiermodelle entwickeln und die Medikamentenwirkung bei ihnen testen; es bleibt aber unklar, inwieweit man den Wert von Immunosuppressiva oder spezifischen Virustatika in solchen Tiermodellen auf die klinische Situation beim Menschen übertragen kann.

Bei der Bestimmung von Virustatikapenetrationen in die Hornhaut oder das Kammerwasser ist es bis jetzt nicht gut möglich gewesen, zu beurteilen, ob die gemessenen Konzentrationen am Ort noch wirksam sind oder nicht. So kann es zum Beispiel sein, daß man im Stroma, wo der Zellstoffwechsel ganz anders als im Epithel ist, sehr viel weniger Virustatikum braucht, um eine Virusvermehrung zu verhindern; auch geht vielleicht die Virusvermehrung im Stroma von Kaninchen anders vor sich als im Stroma von Menschen. So konnte man zum Beispiel zeigen, daß verschiedene lokal applizierte Virustatika bei der Stromakeratitis des Kaninchens wirksam sind; es ist aber völlig unklar, ob dies auch für den Menschen zutrifft. Ähnliche Einschränkungen treffen für die Beurteilung systemisch applizierter Medikamente bei Augenerkrankungen zu, obwohl solche Modelle für die Evaluierung systemischer Defekte gut sind, soweit sie den Schutz vor schweren systemischen Komplikationen wie einer Enzephalitis betreffen.

## Introduction

Diseases in animals that are similar to human disease provide models with which we can observe the effects of the disease, investigate the mechanisms by which the disease is produced, and most importantly for the clinician, evaluate various forms of therapy for the treatment of the disease in man.

In some cases, naturally-occurring analogues of human diseases have been found, and have proven to be of great value, particularly in the determination of the fundamental mechanisms underlying the disease processes, host resistance and immune protection. Artificially-produced animal models, however, have proven to be most effective in the evaluation of various modalities of therapy, and this is generally the case with the evaluation of therapeutic regimens for the treatment of herpes simplex virus infection. Using herpesvirus infection produced in the rabbit eye under laboratory conditions, it has been possible to determine many factors

involved in the pathogenesis of herpesvirus ocular disease, and from this information, to develop specific drugs for the treatment of this widespread and often damaging disease.

The use of such laboratory-produced models must provide parameters that are easily evaluated. For example, a very mild herpes infection will disappear so rapidly and be so transient that it is useless as an experimental model. A more severe infection may be mild enough to be successfully treated with any antiviral drug, so that rank order of potency cannot be determined. At the other end of the spectrum, some herpesviruses cause encephalitis, death and tissue destruction so rapidly that the effect of the drug cannot be quantitated. For these reasons, strains of herpesvirus that provide an intermediate level of infection are employed, so that rank order of potency and quantitation of various drugs can be assessed and compared.

Because infection with herpes simplex virus produces a number of types of disease, it has been necessary to attempt to develop more than one model in order to assure the accurate mimicry of the conditions of human herpes infection. It has been shown that some phases of herpes infection involve actively multiplying virus, some phases appear to be the result of immune damage to tissue that no longer contains virus, and some phases appear to be mainly the result of immune damage to residual viral antigen. In each case, understanding of these different processes and mechanisms of disease must be gained so that intelligent decisions concerning therapeutic approaches and sensibly-directed searches for future therapies can be carried out.

## Epithelial Herpes

Herpesvirus epithelial disease is easily mimicked in the rabbit. Rabbit eyes develop a typical epithelial herpes simplex infection with progressive superficial corneal ulceration. When treated with antimetabolite agents, the lesions respond almost exactly as do human infections, and the rank order of potency of drugs and their efficacy in the treatment of this disease have been reliably predicted in animal species [15].

The pathogenesis of active epithelial

herpes is cytodestruction by multiplying virus spreading from cell to cell. During the early stages of this infection, virus cultures are almost always positive, and viral antigen can be seen easily with fluorescent antibody staining as virus multiplies in the epithelial cells. Immunity does not seem to play a major part in the control of the infection, and there is little invasion seen histologically either in man or in the animal model. Although IgA antibody can be made locally, the application of antibody to the corneal surface of an already infected eye causes no significant changes in the progression of the disease [27].

In view of the nature of epithelial herpes, therapy must concern itself with stopping the spread of the multiplying virus. In the development of such antiviral drugs, we have found the rabbit keratitis model to be extremely valuable in predicting drug effects on epithelial herpesvirus infection in man. The efficacy of idoxuridine as an antiviral drug useful in the treatment of epithelial herpes was established in the rabbit model [14], and idoxuridine proved to be the first truly therapeutic antiviral drug for the treatment of human herpes ocular infection. Shortly thereafter, the rabbit model was used to demonstrate the toxicity of cytosine arabinoside, with the subsequent limitation of its use in man [16]. Adenine arabinoside (vidarabine) was also tested in this rabbit model, and was found to be effective as an antiviral and to have many characteristics in common with idoxuridine, such as similar solubility and acute toxicity; the therapeutic effect was later confirmed in human herpes simplex epithelial keratitis [1, 8, 20, 34].

A newer antiviral, trifluridine, was originally tested in the rabbit model, and was shown to be superior to the previously developed antiviral drugs [22]. When tested in man, trifluridine was shown to be clinically more effective than any drug now available [44]. Approximately 97% of ulcers treated with trifluridine are cured in about 2 weeks [24, 35]; dendritic epithelial keratitis is almost entirely cured; and large ameboid ulcers heal more rapidly with trifluridine treatment [7].

Interferon may play some role in the healing of epithelial ulcers, but this is not clear, and the mechanism by which the host controls the infection remains uncertain. It is clear that initial healing of ulcers can occur by epithelial sliding without much cell division.

The application of corticosteroids to animals infected with some types of herpesvirus prolongs the survival of the virus and renders the host animals unable to eradicate the virus normally. Although it may seem that corticosteroids are immunosuppressive, this becomes doubtful with the knowledge that this phenomenon also occurs in isolated tissue cultures [31].

## Stromal Disease

Stromal disease is a far more serious form of herpes simplex virus ocular infection because, although epithelial herpes infection does not normally produce permanent damage to the eye, stromal disease often does irreversible harm. Unfortunately, the development of animal models for the various forms of herpetic stromal disease, such as disciform edema, necrotizing stromal disease, and iritis, has been uncertain up to this time.

Although several strains of virus cause stromal keratitis in the laboratory [30, 39, 45], stromal disease can be produced either by suppression of the host immune response and active destruction of the stroma, or by minimal direct destruction of the stroma and a severe host immune response. Because the balance between these factors can be manipulated in either direction in the animal models of stromal disease, and because the real character of stromal disease in man is still uncertain, the testing of drug therapies for this disease and extrapolation to humans is much less reliable than in the case of epithelial herpes infection.

In disciform edema, the stroma usually is not scarred in the beginning, but the endothelium is damaged. Fluid can penetrate the endothelial cell layer, causing the central cornea to swell. If the edema persists, vascular invasion and scarring are frequent sequelae. The pathogenesis is not clear, but it is believed to be largely an immunological phenomenon. It has been shown that, in tissue culture of herpes infected cells, the herpetic antigens can be incorporated into the cell membranes [12]. When this occurs in vivo, the cell becomes antigenically foreign, creating a potential long-term focus for immunoreactivity [28]. The cornea is capable of a delayed hypersensitivity reaction [26], and disciform edema can be mimicked, albeit imperfectly, by injecting semi-purified herpes antigen into an immune animal [45]. In addition, virus antigen is easily demonstrated in the anterior chamber, but only occasionally cultured from the aqueous humor, even when virus particles are seen in the aqueous with the electromicroscope. This suggests that immune complexes may be involved. This phenomenon, more than any other, responds promptly and dramatically to corticosteroid therapy, which usually can be discontinued after about three months.

In necrotizing stromal disease, keratocyte death does not seem to be capable of causing the kind of scarring observed in the cornea. However, disruption of the collagen and ground substance must be responsible for most of the opacification and permanent blindness resulting from this disease. Since pathogenic viruses cause only cytodestruction, it seems improbable that direct virus invasion alone produces the necrotizing keratitis of destructive corneal herpes. More likely, the host immunological response is involved in some way.

Experimentally, it is possible to inject a strain of virus into the stroma and to produce a necrotizing keratitis at the same time that the virus disappears and becomes difficult or even impossible to culture [29]. Infection of the cells takes place, but disease is not apparent, and it is only with the gradual disappearance of the virus and the production of the host response that clinical disease is seen. There is, however, much evidence that the virus can multiply in the stroma, and similarly, that a wasting away of the stroma can occur in animals that are totally immunosuppressed. Although both the virus multiplication and the host response involved in the production of stromal disease can be reproduced in animal models, the precise relationship between the two in man is as yet unknown.

Acyclovir, a new topical drug, has some effect on stromal disease [9, 38], but is not a cure for the disease [43]. Vidarabine alone has no measurable effect on stromal disease in animals, but a combination of vidarabine and acyclovir produces an augmented therapeutic effect in both animal eyes [43] and tissue culture. In tissue culture, virus is eradicated more rapidly and completely with the combination of drugs than would be expected from increased concentrations of a single

drug [6]. In the rabbit eye, stromal disease can be essentially eliminated with this combination of drugs. It may be that the two components of stromal disease, viral multiplication and host response, can be more successfully attacked with this combination of antiviral agents.

Acyclovir differs from the normal metabolite only in that it has a deoxyribose analogue which is different from the normal deoxyribose of guanosine. The metabolite must be phosphorylated and enter into the metabolic chain to be useful to the cell, but normal cellular enzymes will not phosphorylate the abnormal acyclovir to a great degree. Therefore, the drug does not enter the metabolic processes of the normal cell [5, 11]. On the other hand, herpesvirus-induced enzymes do phosphorylate acyclovir, and once phosphorylated, the drug can enter the metabolic chain and kill the virus.

Acyclovir is a highly potent drug that is topically active in treating herpes simplex keratitis effectively [2, 10, 23, 40], with no apparent local toxicity [25]. Acyclovir also appears to be systemically active. We have shown that, if the drug is given at the time of initial ocular infection, it can prevent colonization of the trigeminal ganglion, possibly preventing later recurrent herpes disease. Using the mouse eye infected with herpes type 1, Pavan-Langston has reported that administering acyclovir chronically may reduce the incidence of ganglionic colonization [36], and may, either alone or in combination with other drugs, eradicate virus from the ganglion, but much more work will be required to confirm this, particularly the study of the ganglia for a longer period of time after cessation of drug therapy. This work suggests that virus in the ganglion may continue to multiply at a very slow rate [33, 42]; such multiplication, if it actually is taking place, could make the virus in the ganglion susceptible to antiviral drug therapy.

**Herpetic Iritis**

Herpesvirus infection of the deeper eye, herpetic iritis and anterior chamber inflammation may progress to necrosis of the iris and ciliary body, resulting in a hypopyon of purulent exudate in the anterior chamber, sometimes glaucoma and hemorrhage and a complete destruction of the anterior segment of the eye and cornea.

Therapeutically, there is very little that can be done for severe cases of this disease.

In animals, herpesvirus iritis has been produced primarily by direct injection of virus into the anterior chamber, with resulting inflammation [41]. Although this is not the perfect model for human iritis, it has permitted us to evaluate the effect on this disease of systemically active antiviral drugs and of topically applied antiviral drugs. Although epithelial disease may be graded in a roughly parametric form (percentage of the surface involved by ulceration), stromal disease and iritis are evaluated in a non-parametric way. For this reason, concurrent controls and masked studies are required for all animal experiments with ocular herpes, and non-parametric statistics must be used, especially in evaluating the deeper forms of the disease.

In the animal eye, trifluridine and acyclovir have been shown to enter the anterior chamber after topical application [32, 41] and to ameliorate iritis and stromal disease; however, these drugs have not been tested on this disease in humans. We have shown that intravenous vidarabine ameliorates herpetic iritis and stromal disease [1], but is seldom clinically useful because of the low solubility (requiring large volumes of fluids for administration) and the possible effects on the patient's cellular genetic material. Clinical results indicate that trifluridine and acyclovir are effective topically. Laboratory data suggest that combinations of the drugs may be additive or synergistic. There is some evidence that acyclovir penetrates the human anterior chamber [37], but these drugs do not act in cell-free aqueous humor and, whether acyclovir will prove therapeutically useful remains to be seen.

## Interferon

Information obtained concerning therapeutic effects of interferon in animal models has proven largely unreliable in human trials. Much work done with poly I:C, tilorone and other interferon inducers was eventually shown to involve major differences among species, and therefore, to be irrelevant to man until repeated in primate models [13, 17].

Interferon inducers such as poly I:C protected rabbits absolutely from herpes recurrences for 6 to 8 weeks [21]. No effect was seen in monkeys, and only a transient and not very effective interferon burst occurred in human subjects [4]. Not only does tilorone have very little interferon effect in man, but also it is stored in the corneal epithelium and perhaps in other organs. Both its long-term safety and its efficacy appear to be doubtful [3, 18].

In animals, the therapeutic effect of interferon seems weak compared with that of most antiviral drugs and even interferon inducers effective in these species produce only a modest therapeutic response. However, during the time that inducers are effective, both exogenous and spontaneously recurrent infections are almost wholly prevented [19]. With antiviral therapy, recurrences are minor and clear quickly, but some epithelial defects remain. Thus there seem to be both therapeutic and prophylactic effects, with the interferon system perhaps having major potential as a prophylactic agent.

Acknowledgment. Supported in part by USPHS grants EY02672 and EY02377 from the National Eye Institute, National Institutes of Health, Bethesda, Maryland.

## References

1. Abel jr R, Kaufman HE, Sugar J (1975) Intravenous adenine arabinoside against herpes simplex keratouveitis in humans. Am J Ophthalmol 79:659–664
2. Bauer DJ, Collins P, Tucker jr WE, Macklin AW (1979) Treatment of experimental herpes simplex keratitis with acycloguanosine. Br J Ophthalmol 63:429–435
3. Blanke RV, Saady JJ, Drummond DC, Weiss JN (1979) Tilorone determination in a corneal biopsy. J Analytical Toxicol 3:206–208
4. Centifanto YM, Goorha RM, Kaufman HE (1970) Interferon induction in rabbit and human tears. Am J Ophthalmol 70:1006–1009
5. Centifanto YM, Kaufman HE (1979) 9-(2-hydroxyethoxymethyl)guanine as an inhibitor of herpes simplex virus replication. Chemotherapy 25:279–281
6. Centifanto YM, Kaufman HE (in press) Sensitivity of HSV to antiviral therapy. Antimicrob Agents Chemother
7. Coster DJ, Jones BR, McGill JI (1979) Treatment of amoeboid herpetic ulcers with adenine arabinoside or trifluorothymidine. Br J Ophthalmol 63:418–421

8. Dresner AJ, Seamans ML (1975) Evidence of the safety and efficacy of adenine arabinoside in the treatment of herpes simplex epithelial keratitis. In: Pavan-Langston D, Alford CA (eds) Adenine arabinoside: an antiviral agent. Raven, New York, pp 381–392

9. Elion GB, Furman PA, Fyfe JA, Miranda P de, Beauchamp L, Schaeffer HJ (1977) Selectivity of action of an antiherpetic agent 9-(2-hydroxyethoxymethyl)guanine. Proc Natl Acad Sci USA 74:5716–5720

10. Falcon MG, Jones BR (1979) Acycloguanosine: antiviral activity in the rabbit cornea. Br J Ophthalmol 63:422–424

11. Fyfe JA, Keller PM, Furman PA, Miller RL, Elion GB (1978) Thymidine kinase from herpes simplex virus phosphorylates the new antiviral compound, 9-(2-hydroxyethoxymethyl)guanine. J Biol Chem 253:8721–8727

12. Henson D, Helmsen R, Becker KE, Strano AJ, Sullivan M, Harris D (1974) Ultrastructural localization of herpes simplex virus antigens on rabbit corneal cells using sheep antihuman IgG antihorse ferritin hybrid antibodies. Invest Ophthalmol 13:819–827

13. Hill DA, Baron S, Levy HB, Bellanti J, Buckler CE, Cannellos P, Carbone P (1971) Clinical studies of induction of interferon by polyinosinicpolycytidylic acid. Perspectives in virology, vol VII. Academic, New York, pp 198–222

14. Kaufman HE (1962) Clinical cure of herpes simplex keratitis by 5-iodo-2'-deoxyuridine. Proc Soc Exp Biol Med 109:251–252

15. Kaufman HE (1965) In vivo studies with antiviral agents. Ann NY Acad Sci 130:68–180

16. Kaufman HE, Capella JA, Maloney ED, Robbins JE, Cooper GN, Uotila MH (1964) Corneal toxicity of cytosine arabinoside. Arch Ophthalmol 72:535–540

17. Kaufman HE, Centifanto YM (1971) Species differences in interferon response in primates and man as compared to rodents. J Clin Invest 50:53a

18. Kaufman HE, Centifanto YM, Ellison ED, Brown DC (1971) Tilorone hydrochloride: human toxicity and interferon stimulation. Proc Soc Exp Biol Med 137:357–360

19. Kaufman HE, Ellison ED, Centifanto YM (1972) Difference in interferon response and protection from virus infection in rabbits and monkeys. Am J Ophthalmol 74:89–92

20. Kaufman HE, Ellison ED, Townsend WM (1970) The chemotherapy of herpes iritis with adenine arabinoside and cytarabine. Arch Ophthalmol 84:783–787

21. Kaufman HE, Goorha R (1970) Interferon and ocular virus disease. Surv Ophthalmol 15:169–178

22. Kaufman HE, Heidelberger C (1964) Therapeutic antiviral activity of 5-trifluoromethyl-2'-deoxyuridine. Science 145:585–586

23. Kaufman HE, Varnell ED, Centifanto YM, Rheinstrom SD (1978) Effect of 9-(2-hydroxyethoxymethyl)guanine on herpesvirus-induced keratitis and iritis in rabbits. Antimicrob Agents Chemother 14:842–845

24. Laibson PR, Arentsen JJ, Mazzanti WD, Eiferman RA (1977) Double controlled comparison of IDU and trifluorothymidine in 33 patients with superficial herpetic keratitis. Trans Am Ophthalmol Soc 75:316–324

25. Lass JH, Pavan-Langston D, Park NH (1979) Acycloguanosine and corneal wound healing. Invest Ophthalmol Visual Sci (Suppl) 18:57

26. Lausch RN, Swyers JS, Kaufman HE (1966) Delayed hypersensitivity to herpes simplex virus in the guinea pig. J Immunol 96:981–987

27. Little JM, Centifanto YM, Kaufman HE (1969) Immunoglobulins in human tears. Am J Ophthalmol 68:898–905

28. Metcalf JF, Helmsen R (1977) Immunoelectron microscopic localization of herpes simplex virus antigens in rabbit cornea with antihuman IgG-antiferritin hybrid antibodies. Invest Ophthalmol Visual Sci 16:779–786

29. Metcalf JF, Kaufman HE (1976) Herpetic keratitis – evidence for cell-mediated immunopathogenesis. Am J Ophthalmol 82:827–834

30. Metcalf JF, McNeill JI, Kaufman HE (1976) Experimental disciform edema and necrotizing keratitis in the rabbit. Invest Ophthalmol 15:979–985

31. Nishiyama Y, Rapp F (1979) Regulation of persistent infection with herpes simplex virus in vitro by hydrocortisone. J Virol 31:841–844

32. O'Brien WJ, Edelhauser HF (1977) The corneal penetration of trifluorothymidine, adenine arabinoside and idoxuridine: a comparative study. Invest Ophthalmol Visual Sci 16:1093–1103

33. Park N, Pavan-Langston D, McLean SL, Albert DM (1979) Therapy of experimental herpes simplex encephalitis with aciclovir in mice. Antimicrob Agents Chemother 15:775–779

34. Pavan-Langston D, Dohlman CH (1972) A double blind clinical study of adenine arabinoside therapy of viral keratoconjunctivitis. Am J Ophthalmol 74:81–88

35. Pavan-Langston D, Foster CS (1977) Trifluorothymidine and idoxuridine therapy of ocular herpes. Am J Ophthalmol 84:818–825

36. Pavan-Langston D, Park NH, Lass JH (1979) Herpetic ganglionic latency: acyclovir and vidarabine therapy. Arch Ophthalmol 97:1508–1510

37. Poirier RH (1979) Aqueous penetration characteristics of three antiviral compounds, trifluridine, Ara-AMP, and acycloguanosine.

Presented at Ocular Microbiology Group Annual Meeting, San Francisco, Nov 3, 1979
38. Schaeffer HJ, Beauchamp L, Miranda P de, Elion GB (1978) 9-(2-hydroxyethoxymethyl) guanine activity against viruses of the herpes group. Nature 272:583–585
39. Sery TW, Nagy RM, Nazario R (1972/3) Experimental disciform keratitis. II. Local corneal hypersensitivity to a highly virulent strain of herpes simplex. Ophthalmic Res 4:99–109
40. Shiota H, Inoue S, Yamone S (1979) Efficacy of acycloguanosine against herpetic ulcers in rabbit cornea. Br J Ophthalmol 63:425–428
41. Sugar J, Varnell ED, Centifanto YM, Kaufman HE (1973) Trifluorothymidine treatment of herpetic iritis in rabbits and ocular penetration. Invest Ophthalmol 12:532–534
42. Trousdale MD, Dunkel ED, Nesburn AB (1979) The effect of 9-(2-hydroxyethoxymethyl)guanine on CNS spread of ocular herpes virus infection in rabbits. Invest Ophthalmol Visual Sci (Suppl) 18:234
43. Varnell ED, Kaufman HE (1980) Antiviral agents in experimental herpetic stromal disease. This vol.
44. Wellings PC, Awdry PN, Bors PH, Jones BR, Brown DC, Kaufman HE (1972) Clinical evaluation of trifluorothymidine in the treatment of herpes simplex corneal ulcers. Am J Ophthalmol 73:932–942
45. Williams LE, Nesburn AB, Kaufman HE (1965) Experimental induction of disciform keratitis. Arch Ophthalmol 73:112–114

## Discussion on the Contribution pp. 229–235

H. Shiota (Tokushima)
I'd like to ask you about your in vitro study using IDU and other agents. There were several lines. Some of the lines are different, I mean, sharp lines or slow lines. Could you tell me what it means? Is it due to different permeability or different mechanisms of the agent?

H.E. Kaufman (New Orleans)
I don't know the reason for the slope of the dose-response curve. In fact, the oculopharmacology of these agents has not been thoroughly and carefully investigated.

D. Easty (Bristol)
We have evidence that previous experience of virus disease in the skin does seem to protect the cornea; how do you explain the effect of topical steroid if immunity has no protective effect?

H.E. Kaufman (New Orleans)
There is evidence that primary infection is worse

than an infection in a pre-immunized animal. Our results in similar studies have been very much like yours. In the primary infection, I think there is infection not only of the cornea, but also of the ocular adnexa. Originally, it was found that treating an animal with a primary infection until the cornea is well and then stopping treatment results in a recurrence of the disease. One reason is that the cornea is living in a sea of virus which is coming from the conjunctiva and from the rest of the adnexa. This happens in a primary infection, but is much reduced in the pre-immunized animal. I think this is the major factor here.

As far as I know, nobody knows why corticosteroids make virus persist. There are, however, tissue culture studies in which a slowly-reproducing virus is eliminated, but the addition of corticosteroids to the cultures allows the virus to persist and to multiply actively, even to the point of destroying the culture. This is not a function of cellular synthesis or cellular rate of multiplication. The mechanism by which the corticosteroids produce this effect is not at all understood.

B. Öberg (Södertälje)
Do you think that immunized rabbits are better models than nonimmunized for the recurrent infection?

H.E. Kaufman (New Orleans)
I think that the only thing that is important is whether the model is predictive of the treatment of human disease. It seems to be clear that non-immunized rabbits with primary infections show a reliable predictive therapeutic effect that correlates with the effect of treating dendritic ulcers in man. With other diseases, however, this predictive effect is not so clear.

R. Delgadillo (Antwerpen)
I would like to ask whether you know the titer of virus released into the conjunctival fluid in primary herpetic keratitis in man, and experimentally in rabbits.

H.E. Kaufman (New Orleans)
We have titered rabbits, but I don't remember the precise data, and I don't know the comparable figures in man.

H. Moser (Marburg)
You reported negative results trying to induce interferon by application of poly I:C. Did you also administer the more stable complex poly ICLC for interferon induction?

H.E. Kaufman (New Orleans)
I've worked with Hilton Levy, who has shown that there is an enzyme in the blood that hydrolyzes

poly I:C. RNA, which is normally double-stranded, can be made triple stranded by adding a polylysine. This three-stranded RNA is more resistant to the hydrolyzing enzyme and may actually be active in man and in the monkey. We studied interferon production in both man and monkeys using poly I:C-lysine as the inducer, and found it to be variable. This was some time ago, and there may have been manufacturing problems with the batches of poly I:C-lysine, but we did find some interferon produced, although not a tremendous amount.

One problem with the interferon inducers is that there is a hyporesponse period, i.e., you can't stimulate the interferon system continuously for a long period of time. Because interferon is not a very good therapeutic agent, a constant level must be produced to prevent recurrences, and the hyporesponse effect disrupts this. I think poly I:C-lysine needs further study.

G.O.H. Naumann (Erlangen)
You showed beautifully that a satisfactory model for stromal herpes disease of the cornea doesn't exist yet and that it is very unreliable. To a clinical ophthalmologist it is almost intimidating to hear about all the virologic-immunologic-pharmacologic aspects that we know of in this disease. Have you tried to correlate the disease's variable stromal manifestation, which really make up a large spectrum, to some of these aspects? I think it is not without significance whether we have a stromal disease with an intact Bowman's membrane, or whether we have, for example, a deep granuloma around Descemet's membrane? Clean morphologic criteria are of value in a clinical situation – and they should not be neglected in the experimental model.

H.E. Kaufman (New Orleans)
I agree. I used to think that disciform edema was largely an immunological phenomenon, partly because it responds so rapidly to corticosteroid therapy, sometimes in as little as 2 or 3 days. Certainly, necrotizing keratitis with granulomas responds less well to corticosteroids, but how it will respond to drugs that stop virus multiplication isn't known. Our studies with intravenous adenine arabinoside suggest some response, but at this time, we know only that there is some host immune response and some virus multiplication and that we probably need to work on stopping both.

Sundmacher, R. (Hrsg.):
Herpetische Augenerkrankungen
© J.F. Bergmann Verlag, München 1981

# Molecular Basis and Pharmacological Consideration of Selective Antiherpetic Agents

Y.C. Cheng, Chapel Hill

**Key words.** Nucleosides, thymidine kinase, DNA polymerase, antiviral drugs

**Schlüsselwörter.** Nukleoside Thymidinkinase, DNA-Polymerase, antivirale Medikamente

**Summary.** Selective antiherpes agents exert their action by taking advantage of the biochemical differences between virus infected and uninfected cells. In order to use these drugs effectively as antiherpes agents, it is important to understand their mode of action, their mechanism of selectivity, and their metabolism. The increasing knowledge of molecular biology and biochemistry of herpes viruses will facilitate new drug development.

In general, those discovered selective antiherpes virus agents which do not exert their action by inactivation or interfering with the uptake of the virus particle have one or several of following properties.
*1. They can be selectively activated by virus specific enzymes.* Herpes virus thymidine kinase dependent agents have this property.
*2. They can selectively inhibit the synthesis or the activity of virus specific enzymes which are required for virus replication.* Phosphonoformate and phosphonoacetate have this property. They can inhibit the synthesis and the activity of virus specific DNA polymerase which are required for virus replication. Some of the phosphorylated derivates of herpes thymidine kinase dependent agents such as 5-propyl deoxyuridine and acycloguanosine also have this property. 5-propyl deoxyuridine could inhibit the synthesis of herpes virus specific DNA polymerase and acycloguanosine triphosphate could preferentially inhibit the activity of herpes virus specific DNA polymerase.
*3. They can be inactivated by normal cellular enzymes to the metabolites which still retain antivirus activity and loss of anti-cell activity of the agents.* The reason for the selective antiherpes virus action of adenine arabinoside may be due to this reason. Adenine arabinoside could be deaminated by cellular adenosine deaminase to Ara-H which still has antivirus activity but loses the anti-cell activity possessed by adenine arabinoside. Thus, the combination of adenine arabinoside with adenosine deaminase inhibitor such as deoxycoformycin is not beneficial for the selective antivirus activity of adenine arabinoside. Ara-H or monophosphate of Ara-H will be worthwhile for further clinic trials.
*4. They can reversibly suppress both normal cell metabolism and virus replication or maturation processes.* This could lead to the irreversible damage of virus replication due to be unstable nature of virus genome in infected cells. The virus genomes presented in virus infected cells may not be stable enough to sustain long term suppression of its replication and thus become disintegrated by cellular enzyme or even virus induced DNase whereas the normal cells could sustain longer term of the suppression of their replication without disintegrating their replication machine. The end result is that the virus replication will be damaged irreversibly but the normal cell replication is only temporarily inhibited by the agent and can be reversed once the drug is not presented. Certain aspects of the antivirus action of phosphonoformate or even 2-deoxyglucose may be related to this.

**Zusammenfassung.** Die Wirkung von selektiven antiherpetischen Substanzen beruht auf dem biochemischen Unterschied zwischen einer infizierten und einer nicht-infizierten Zelle. Um diese Stoffe wirkungsvoll nutzen zu können, sollte man möglichst viel über ihren Wirkungsmechanismus, über die Grundlagen ihrer Selektivität sowie über ihren Stoffwechsel wissen. Auf der Basis zunehmender Kenntnisse von der Molekularbiologie und Biochemie der Herpesviren wird es dann auch leichter möglich sein, neue Wirkstoffe zu entwickeln. Sieht man von den Stoffen ab, die mit der Virusaufnahme in die Zeile interferieren oder das Virus direkt inaktivieren, gibt es folgende Wirkmöglichkeiten für bereits bekannte Virustatika:
*1. Selektive Aktivierung des Wirkstoffes durch virusspezifische Enzyme.* Diese Eigenschaften haben z.B. die Herpesvirus-Thymidinkinase-abhängigen Substanzen.

2. *Selektive Synthesehemmung oder Blockierung von virusspezifischen Enzymen, die für die Virusreplikation unerläßlich sind.* Hierzu gehören Phosphonoformat und Phosphonoacetat. Sie blockieren die Synthese und die Wirkung von virusspezifischer DNA-Polymerase, die für die Virusvermehrung benötigt wird. Einige der Thymidinkinase-abhängigen Substanzen (s. 1) haben zusätzlich diese Wirkung, sobald sie phosphoryliert sind, z.B. 5-Propyldesoxyuridin und Acycloguanosin. Dabei wird die Synthese der DNA-Polymerase von 5-Propyldesoxyuridin und die Aktivität des Enzyms vor allem von Acycloguanosin-Triphosphat gehemmt.

3. *Aktivierung durch normale Zellenzyme zu Metaboliten, die eine Virusspezifität bei relativ geringerer Zelltoxizität aufweisen.* Auf diesem Mechanismus beruht vielleicht die selektive antivirale Wirkung von ara-A. Ara-A wird durch zelluläre Adenosindeaminasen zu ara-H deaminiert, das immer noch antivirale Wirkung aufweist, dessen antizelluläre Potenz aber relativ geringer ist. Aus diesem Grunde ist auch eine Kombination eines Deaminase-Hemmstoffes (z.B. Deoxycoformicin) zusammen mit ara-A in Hinblick auf die Selektivität der Substanz gar nicht günstig. Man sollte statt dessen lieber Ara-H oder das Ara-H-Monophosphat intensiver in der Klinik austesten.

4. *Reversible Hemmung sowohl des zellulären als auch des Virusstoffwechsels mit der Möglichkeit, daß das Virusgenom dank seiner relativen Instabilität in den infizierten Zellen irreversibel geschädigt wird.* Dabei geht man davon aus, daß die Virusgenome in infizierten Zellen möglicherweise dann nicht sehr lange stabil sind, wenn ihre Replikation dauernd unterdrückt wird. Sie unterliegen dann der Zerstörung durch Zellenzyme und möglicherweise sogar durch ihre eigene Virus-DNAse, während normale, nicht mit Virus befallene Zellen wahrscheinlich längere Zeit eine Unterdrückung ihrer Replikationsmechanismen überleben, bevor sie irreversiblen Schaden nehmen. Das könnte dazu führen, daß die Virusvermehrung irreversibel, die Zellvermehrung aber nur reversibel gestört wird und wieder aufgenommen wird, sobald das Virustatikum nicht mehr einwirkt. Einige Besonderheiten der Wirkung von Phosphonoformat und vielleicht auch 2-Deoxyglucose kann man vielleicht mit einem solchen Mechanismus erklären.

Herpes viruses are DNA viruses. Once they infect cells, they can induce many biochemical changes which are virus specific [1, 2]. Thus, it is obvious that a rational approach for developing specific antiherpes virus agents is to take advantage of the biochemical differences between virus infected and uninfected normal cells. Among the protein induced by herpes simplex virus type 1 (HSV 1) and type 2 (HSV 2), three enzyme activities – Thymidine kinase (TK), DNA polymerase (DP), and Alkaline DNase (DS), are clearly identified as virus specific. All three activities from either HSV 1 or HSV 2 infected cells were highly purified and demonstrated to have unique properties which are not shared by their counterparts in host human cells [3–16]. On the basis of their unique behaviors, different strategies were proposed for developing antiherpes agents [17–19, 46].

Recently, several antiherpes simplex agents have been developed which have potent antiherpes virus activity with low toxicity. On the basis of their selective antiherpes virus effects, they can be classified into two groups:

1. Herpes Virus thymidine kinase dependent agents.

2. Herpes Virus thymidine kinase independent agents.

## Herpes Virus Thymidine Kinase Dependent Agents

This group of agents exert their selective antiherpes virus effects by being able to act as "selective alternative substrates" of virus TK. It includes those compounds such as 5-ethyl deoxyuridine, 5-propyl deoxyuridine, 5-mercaptomethyl deoxyuridine, 5'-amino 5-Iodo deoxyuridine E-5-(2-bromovinyl) deoxyuridine, 5-bromodeoxycytidine, thymine arabinoside, 2'-Fluoro-5-Iodo cytosine arabinoside, and acycloguanosine as shown in Fig. 1 [20–36]. All these nucleosides must be phosphorylated in cells to exert their antivirus or anticell activity. HSV 1, HSV 2, or VZV type specific thymidine kinase have much higher affinity for these nucleosides and can utilize these nucleosides more efficiently as substrates than the host cellular thymidine kinases [6, 7, 30, 33, 37]. Thus, they can be preferentially phosphorylated in those cells which have virus thymidine kinase. Uninfected normal cells can not phosphorylate these agents well since their thymidine kinase can not efficiently utilize these compounds as substrates [30, 33, 38]. Once these agents are phosphorylated to monophosphate nucleotides by TK, they can either stay as monophosphate nucleotides or be further phosphorylated to diphosphate or triphosphate nucleotides by the host mono-or diphosphate nucleotide kinases [30, 33, 38].

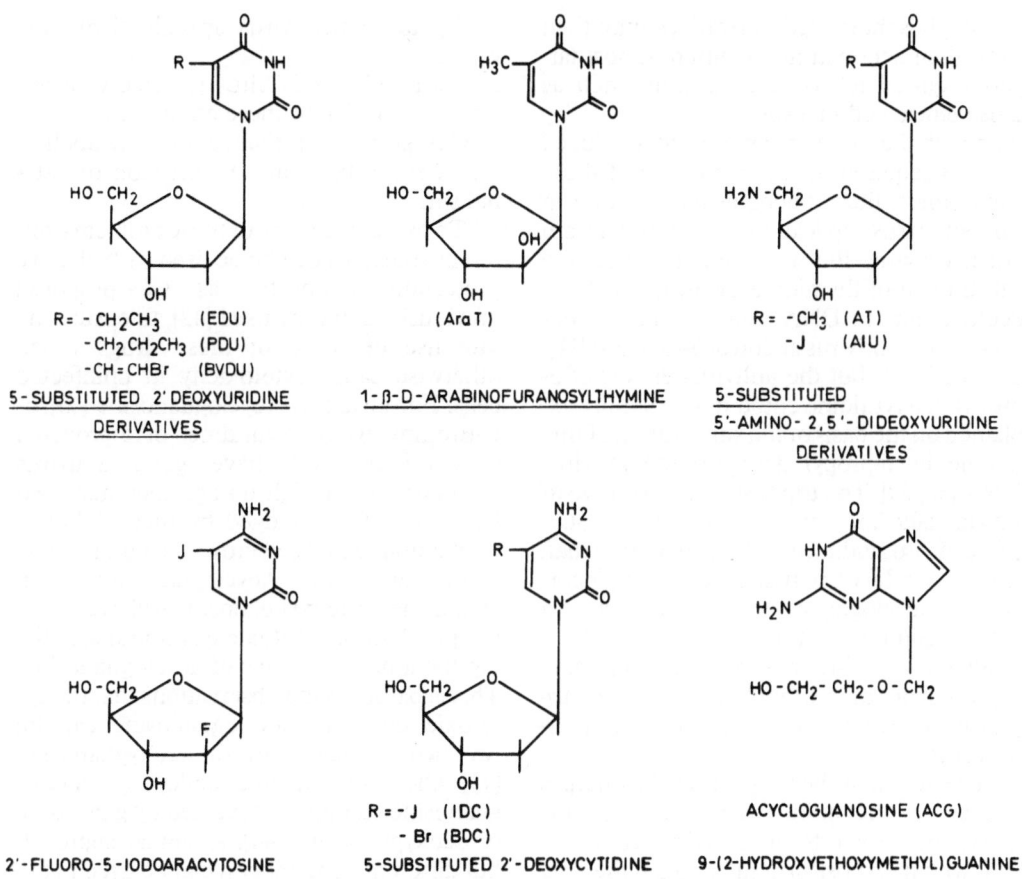

**Fig. 1.** Herpes virus thymidine kinase dependent agents

**Table 1.** Metabolism and action of the phosphorylated derivatives of virus thymidine kinase alternative substrates

| Metabolism | Potential Targets | Consequences |
|---|---|---|
| X MP ↓ X DP ↓ X TP ↓ X in DNA or RNA | NMP Kinase (e.g. TMP kinase) Synthesis of NMP (e.g. TMP synthetase) Ribonucleotide Reductase DNA polymerase RNA polymerase | dNDP or NDP ↓ dNMP or NMP ↓ dNTP ↓ DNA synthesis ↓ RNA synthesis ↓ DNA damage ↓ RNA damage ↓ Protein synthesis ↓ |

X = nucleoside

These phosphorylated derivatives may then exert their action at many different host targets required for virus replication such as those elucidated in Table 1.

Although the same enzyme – virus induced TK – is required for the activation of these compounds, their mechanisms of action in stopping virus replication or cell growth are not necessarily the same. For instance, the substitution of thymidine by 5-Iodo 5'-NH$_2$- deoxyuridine in DNA seems to be responsible for the antivirus action of 5-Iodo 5'-NH$_2$- deoxyuridine, but the antivirus effects of 5-propyl deoxyuridine could not be simply explained on the basis of the substitution of thymidine by 5-propyl deoxyuridine in virus DNA [38, 39]. The triphosphate derivative of acycloguanosine can serve as a better substrate of virus induced DNA polymerase than that of host DNA polymerase and the incorporated acycloguanosine can then act as a DNA chain terminator to stop further DNA synthesis [40]. 5-Iodo-5'-NH$_2$ deoxyuridine triphosphate or 5-propyl deoxyuridine triphosphate can not serve as DNA chain terminators.

The action of these agents against herpes viruses can be quite irreversible. 5-propyl deoxyuridine exerts its antivirus effects in cells within 9 h post virus infection. If the drug is removed 9 h post infection, the virus will not be able to regrow in those infected cells [41].

Since the selective antivirus effects of this group of agents relies on the ability of a herpes virus to induce a thymidine kinase which can recognize them as substrates in infected cells and the different types of herpes virus have different abilities to induce virus TK (CMV and EBV can not induce virus type specific TK) and furthermore the virus induced TK's of HSV 1, HSV 2, and VZV are different in substrate specificity [7, 17, 18, 37], it is anticipated that these agents will have different effects on different types of herpes virus.

There are several other considerations in the utilization of these types of agents against herpes infection. This is summarized in the following:

1. Compounds may not be totally inert toward the human nucleoside kinase. Therefore, at high concentrations, they may exert cytotoxic effects.
2. Compounds may induce the development of virus mutants which are deficient in their ability to induce virus specific thymidine kinase.
3. Not all phases of virus infected cells are equally sensitive to these compounds.
4. Compounds or their active metabolites may have a fast rate of excretion or catabolism.

To overcome some of these problems, different strategies can be devised. A "selective protection approach", as we proposed previously, could be used [42], to ensure the safe use of some of these drugs which otherwise cause cytotoxicity in uninfected cells. For instance, Acycloguanosine [43], 5-E-Bromovinyl deoxyuridine, or 5-propenyl deoxyuridine [42], have good antivirus activities, but at high dosage they may also have side effects judged by their ability to inhibit uninfected cell growth in culture. The combination of Acycloguanosine with guanosine or deoxyguanosine will overcome the problem of cytotoxicity without sacrificing the antivirus effects of acycloguanosine. This is based on the observations that the cytotoxic effect of acycloguanosine can be reversed by guanosine or deoxyguanosine [43] and the antivirus action of acycloguanosine can not be reversed by guanosine or deoxyguanosine [44]. A similar approach but different combination can be used in the case of 5-E-bromovinyl deoxyuridine or 5-propenyl deoxyuridine; the combination of either drug with a low dosage of thymidine could protect cells against the cytotoxic effects of the two compounds without decreasing their anti-HSV 1 effects. In addition, thymidine could also decrease catabolism of 5-E-bromovinyl deoxyuridine or 5-propenyl deoxyuridine by thymidine phosphorylase [45]. Recently, a "specific inhibitor approach", as discussed previously by us [46], was elegantly demonstrated by Dr. Prusoff et al. [47], the cytotoxicity of Iododeoxyuridine could be selectively prevented by 5'-NH$_2$ thymidine, which is an inhibitor of host cellular TK [48] and a substrate of virus induced TK, without sacrificing its antivirus activity. The concern of selecting TK$^-$ virus mutants in the clinic after treatment of virus diseases with this group of agents needs to be looked at. It should be pointed out that at present it is unclear whether a TK$^-$ virus mutant could reside in nerve terminals as does the latent virus and be reactivated when a proper stimulus is given. It is conceivable that the ability of virus to induce virus TK is essential for its reactivation in neurons due to: (1) nerve terminals have no efficient mechanism to make thymidine nucleotide available for virus DNA synthesis, (2) Only herpes virus, which has the ability to induce virus TK, is found at the nerve terminals, namely HSV 1, HSV 2, and VZV but not CMV or EBV, (3) Virus induced TK is more efficient than host TK in securing thymidine for DNA synthesis. Thus, the concern of selecting TK⁻ mutants, which cause the same type of virus infectious diseases currently seen in the clinic, due to the use of this group of virus TK dependent compound may not be a problem; but the potential problem that these TK⁻ virus mutants, if they arise, may cause a different spectrum of diseases similar to CMV or EBV and not yet seen in the clinic, still exists. In order to overcome the possibility of having TK⁻ virus mutants arised, two approaches could be taken: (1) a combination of antivirus compounds which have independent modes of activation and action such as adenine arabinoside and these virus thymidine kinase dependent agents, (2) the use of high dosages of compounds in combination with protective agents.

In general, these agents have a relatively short half-life in plasma and are only active in certain phases of cells post virus infection. In order to suppress virus replication completely, the effective level in plasma or at disease sites should be kept longer than one generation of virus replication. Therefore, the pharmacokinetics of these agents in humans should be considered in order to use them effectively as antivirus drugs. Patients with kidney or sometimes liver problems may retain these compounds longer, thus, these agents should be cautiously used on patients with kidney or liver problems.

### Herpes Virus Thymidine Kinase Independent Agents

Compounds included in this group are those compounds which exert their antiherpes virus action without the requirement of the participation of virus induced thymidine kinase. Pyrophosphate analogs such as phosphonoacetate and phosphonoformate, deoxyadenosine analogs such as adenine arabinoside, and glucose analogs such as 2-deoxyglucose [49–56] are in this category as shown in Fig. 2.

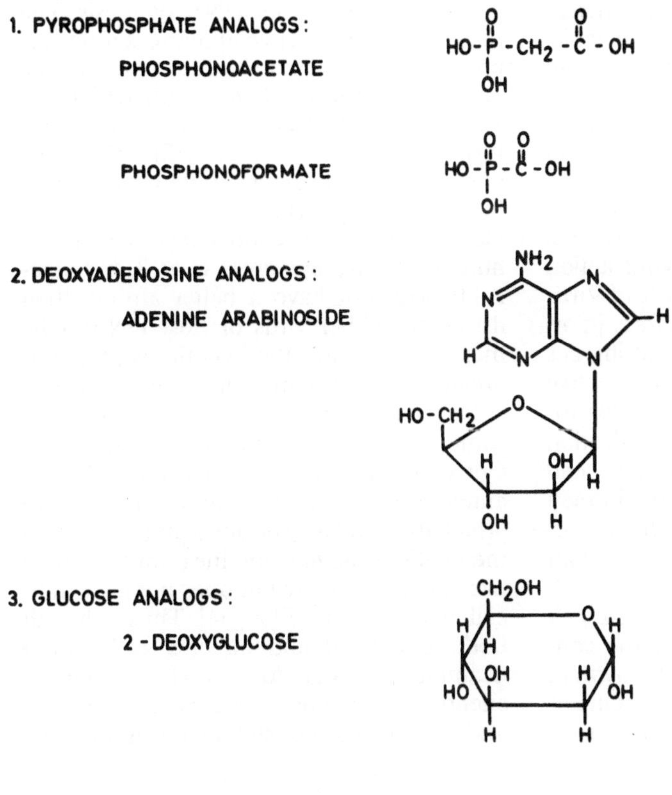

Fig. 2. Virus thymidine kinase antiherpes agents

Pyrophosphate is the product of DNA polymerase action. Analoges such as phosphonoacetate and phosphonoformate are more inhibitory to HSV 1 and HSV 2 induced DNA polymerase than to host DNA polymerases, and they behave as noncompetitive inhibitors with respect to deoxynucleoside triphosphate and noncompetitive inhibitors with respect to DNA [57–59]. All five types of herpes virus can induce their type specific DNA polymerase which is required for their DNA replication [19, 49], these virus induced DNA polymerases have similar sensitivity toward phosphonoacetate and phosphonoformate. Both agents were shown to have a broad spectrum suppressing all five types of herpes virus replication [49]. At the same concentration, phosphonoformate is more potent than phosphonoacetate as an anti-HSV 1 agent. The concentration of these compounds required to exert antivirus action in cell culture is higher than that required to inhibit virus DNA polymerase in vitro [55, 57]. This may be related to the poor permeability of these agents through cell membranes. The most sensitive period of the infected cells is 3 to 9 h post infection, which coincides with the period of virus DNA synthesis. Since the compounds are reversible inhibitors of virus DNA synthesis, the reversibility of antivirus effects exerted by these agents is predictable. The reversibility of antivirus action of both agents was found to depend on the time of exposure of infected cells to the compounds. When the infected cells were exposed to phosphonoformate for more than one generation of virus replication, irreversible inhibition of virus growth could be observed. This partial irreversibility of antivirus action may be related to the unstable nature of Virus DNA in infected cells [55]. Therefore, in order to obtain the most effective antiherpes virus effect in vivo, maintaining an effective dosage in serum or of diseased tissues for more than one generation of virus replication is recommended. Phosphonoformate and phosphonoacetate can also inhibit human cell growth in culture; the concentration required to inhibit cell growth is higher than that which shows strong anti-HSV 1 or HSV 2 effects. The inhibitory effect against cell growth is reversible [55], therefore the consideration of inhibiting normal cell growth in vivo by these agents is not necessary. One of the side effects of phosphonoacetate is its

ability to cause skin irritation when applied topically; phosphonoformate does not share this side effect [60]. Both agents deposit in bone when they are used in vivo; whether the deposition of these agents in bone is harmful to bone metabolism is still unclear. Recently, it was shown that the deposition of these agents in bone is reversible [60]; thus if the deposition in bone is not harmful to bone metabolism, this slow release of compound from bone could be an advantage to keep an effective dosage in serum for a longer period of time. Another potential problem of utilizing phosphonoformate in treating herpes virus infectious diseases is the development of virus mutants which are resistant to these pyrophosphate analogs [60, 61].

Adenosine arabinoside, a deoxyadenosine analog has antiherpes virus activity in vitro as well as in the clinic. Its mode of selective antivirus action is still unclear, the current thought is that Ara-A is phosphorylated to Ara-ATP by cellular kinases (which kinase are not clear), the activities for the phosphorylation of Ara-A in infected or uninfected cells are about the same [50, 51], Ara-ATP could then compete with dATP for incorporation into DNA [57, 62]. The incorporated Ara-A may then serve as a DNA chain terminator which prevents further DNA synthesis. The reason for the selective antivirus action was previously suggested to be due to the fact that Ara-ATP competes better with dATP for Virus induced DNA polymerase than that for host DNA polymerases [62]. Recently, observation made in this laboratory indicated that Ara-ATP has a higher affinity to HSV 1 or HSV 2 induced DNA polymerase than that to human DNA polymerase $\alpha$ or $\beta$, but Ara-ATP does not have a better affinity than dATP for either virus or host DNA polymerase [57]. Thus, the hypothesis proposed previously [62] concerning the selective antivirus action of Ara-A is questionable, and some other mechanisms may be involved. Currently, we propose that the selective antivirus action of Ara-A may not be due to Ara-A itself and may be due to its deaminated metabolite Arahypoxanthine (Ara-H), which has antivirus activity but does not have anticell activity by itself [50, 54]. Thus although both uninfected and infected cells could deaminate Ara-A to Ara-H by cellular adenosine deaminase, Ara-H is no longer toxic to the cells but still retains its antivirus activity. The use of Ara-H for clinic trials as antivirus agent should be further explored.

A glucose analog, 2-deoxyglucose, was shown to have antivirus activity in vitro. Recently, its antivirus activity was also demonstrated in vivo. Its mode of action is attributed to the inhibition of the synthesis of glycoproteins, which are required for virus maturation. The antivirus action of this agent is readily reversible. This could hinder the clinical use of this agent. Whether this agent has selective action against virus replication vs. normal cell metabolism must be further investigated.

**Dedication.** This is dedicated to Dr. William H. Prusoff under whom I did my postdoctoral training a few years back and for whom I hold a great admiration for and the person who I consider to be a cherished friend and advisor.

**Acknowledgment.** Supported by Grant CH-29-C From the American Cancer Society.

# References

1. Roizman B, Furlong D (1974) "The Replication of Herpesvirus" In: Compr Virology 3: 229
2. Cheng Y-C, Goz B, Prusoff WH (1975) "Deoxyribonucleotide Metabolism in Herpes Simplex Virus infected HeLa Cells," Biochim Biophys Acta 390:253
3. Cheng Y-C, Ostrander M (1976) "Herpes Simplex Type I and Type II Specific Thymidine Kinase I. Induction, Purification and General Properties". J Biol Chem 251:2605
4. Hoffman PJ, Cheng Y-C (1978) "The Deoxyribonuclease Induced after Infection of KB Cells by Herpes Simplex Virus Type I or Type 2 Purification and Characterization of the Enzyme". J Biol Chem 253:3557
5. Lee L-A, Cheng Y-C (1976) "Human Thymidine Kinase I. Purification and General Properties of the Cytosol and Mitochondria Thymidine Kinase Derived from Human Acute Myelocytic Blast Cells". J Biol Chem 251:2600
6. Lee L-S, Cheng Y-C (1976) "Human Deoxythymidine Kinase 2. Substrate Specificity and Kinetic Behaviors of the Cytoplasmic and Mitochondria Isozymes Derived from the Blast Cells of the Acute Myelocytic Leukemia"
7. Cheng Y-C (1976) "Deoxythymidine Kinase Induced in HeLa TK⁻ Cells by Herpes Simplex Virus Type I and Type II 2. Substrate Specificity and Kinetic Behaviors" Biochim Biophys Acta 452:370
8. Purifoy DJM, Powel KL (1977) "Nonstructural Proteins of Herpes Simplex Virus I. Purification of the Induced DNA Polymerase". J Virol 24:618
9. Ostrander M, Cheng Y-C (1980) "Properties of Herpes Simplex Virus Type 1 and Type 2 DNA Polymerase". Biochim Biophys Acta 609:232
10. Ostrander M, Cheng Y-C (1977) "Purification and Characterization of DNA Polymerase Induced by Herpes Simplex Virus Type 1 and Type II". The Pharmacologist 19:166
11. Hoffman PJ, Cheng Y-C (1979) "The DNase Induced after Infection of KB Cells by Herpes Simplex Virus Type 1 and Type 2: Characterization of Associated Endonuclease Activity". J Virol 32:449
12. Ogino T, Shiman R, Rapp F (1973) "Deoxythymidine Kinase From Rabbit Kidney Cells Infected with Herpes Simplex Virus Types 1 and 2". Intervirology 1:80
13. Jamieson AT, Subak-Sharpe JH (1974) "Biochemical Studies on the Herpes Simplex Virus-specified Deoxypyrimidine Kinase Activity". J Gen Virol 24:481
14. Thonless MC (1972) "Serological Properties of Thymidine Kinase Produced in Cells Infected with Type 1 and Type 2 Herpes Simplex". J Gen Virol 17:307
15. Kit D, Leung WC, Jorgeson GN, Dubbs DR (1974) "Distinctive Properties of Thymidine Kinase Isozymes Induced by Human and Avian Herpesviruses". Int J Cancer 14:598
16. Kit D, Dubbs DR (1965) Properties of Deoxythymidine Kinase Partially Purified from Noninfected and Virus Infected Mouse Fibroblast Cells". Virology 26:16
17. Cheng Y-C (1977) "A Rational Approach to the Development of Antiviral Chemotherapy: Alternative Substrates of Herpes Simplex Virus Type 1 and Type II Thymidine Kinase". Ann Rev N Y Acad Sci 284:594
18. Cheng Y-C, Hoffman PJ et al (1979) "Properties of Herpes Virus Specific Thymidine Kinase DNA Polymerase and DNAase and Their Implications in the Development of Specific Antiherpes Agents". Adv Opthalmol 38:173
19. Cheng Y-C, Ostrander M et al (1979) "Development of Antiherpes Agents on the Bases of Virus Induced Enzymes". Nucleoside Analogues Plenum, p 249
20. Gauri KK, Maloney G (1967) "Chemotherapie der Herpesinfektion mit neuen 5-Alkyluraaldesoxyribosiden". Arch Pharmakol 257:21
21. Walter RD, Gauri KK (1975) "5-Ethyl-2'-Deoxyuridine-5'-Monophosphate Inhibition of the Thymidylate Synthetase from Escherichia Coli". Biochem Pharmacol 24:1025
22. DeClercq E, Shugar D (1975) "Antiviral Activity of 5-Ethyl Pyrimidine Deoxynucleosides". Biochem Pharmacol 24:1073

23. Davis ED, Oakes JE, Taylor JA (1978) "Effect of Treatment with 5-Ethyl-2'-Deoxyuridine on Herpes Simplex Virus Encephalitis in Normal and Immunosuppressed Mice". Antimicrob Agents and Chemother 14:743

24. Cheng Y-C, Domin B, Sharma R, Bobek N (1976) "Studies on the Antiviral Action and Cellular Toxicity of Four Thymidine Analogs − 5-Ethyl-, 5-Vinyl-, 5-Propyl-, and 5-Allyl Deoxyuridine". Antimicrob Agents Chemotherapy 10:119

25. DeClercq E, Decamps J et al (1979) "(E)-5-(2-Bromovinyl)-2'-deoxyuridine: A Potent and Selective Anti-Herpes Agent". Proc Natl Acad Sci USA 76:2947

26. Gentry GA, Aswell JF (1975) "Inhibition of Herpes Simplex Virus Replication by araT". Virology 65:294

27. Aswell JF, Gentry AG (1977) "Cell Dependent Antiherpesviral Activity of 5-Methylarabinosylcytosine, and Intracellular Ara-T Donor". Ann N Y Acad Sci 284:342

28. Hardi R, Hughes RG, Ho YK et al (1976) "Differential Effects of 5-Methylmercapto-2'-Deoxyuridine on the Replication of Herpes Simplex Virus Type 1 in Two Cell Systems". Antimicrob Agents Chemother 10:682

29. Cheng Y-C, Goz B, Neenan JP, Ward DC, Prusoff WH (1975) "The Selective Inhibition of Herpes Simplex Virus by 5'-Amino-2'-Dideoxy-5-Iodouridine, a Novel Thymidine Analogue with Antiviral Activity". J Virol 15:1284

30. Chen MS, Ward DC, Prusoff WH (1976) "Specific Herpes Simplex Virus Induced Incorporation of 5-Iodo-5'-Amino-2', 5'-dideoxyuridine into Deoxyribonucleic Acid". J Biol Chem 251:4833

31. Cooper GN (1973) Phosphorylation of 5-Bromodeoxycytidine in Cells Infected with Herpes Simplex Virus". Natl Acad Sci USA 70: 3788

32. Greer S, Schildkraut I, Zimmerman T, Kaufman H (1975) 5-Halogenated Analogs of Deoxycytidine as Selective Inhibitors of the Replication of Herpes Simplex Viruses in Cell Culture and Related Studies of Intracranial Herpes Simplex Virus Infections in mice". Ann N Y Acad Sci 255:359

33. Elion GB, Furman PA, Fyfe JA, Miranda PD, Beachamp L, Schaeffer HJ (1977) "Selectivity of Action of an Antiherpetic Agent, 9-(2-hydroxyethoxymethyl) guanine". Proc Natl Acad Sci 74:5716

34. Schaeffer HK, Beachamp L, Miranda P, Elion GB, Baner PJ, Collins P (1978) "9-(2-Hydroxyethoxymethyl) guanine activity against viruses of the Herpes Group". Nature 272:583

35. Wantanabe KA, Reichman U et al (1979) "Synthesis and Antiherpes Virus Activity of Some 2'-Fluoro-2'-deoxyarabinofuranosylpyrimidine Nucleosides". J Med Chem 22:21

36. Lopex C, Livelli T et al (1979) 2'-Fluoro-5 Iodo-Aracytosine: A Potent Anti-Herpesvirus Nucleoside With Minimal Toxicity To Normal Cells". Proc Am Assoc Cancer Res 20:183

37. Cheng YC, Tsou R, Hackstat T, Mallavia LK (1979) "Induction of Thymidine Kinase and DNase in Varicella Zoster Virus Infected Cells and Kinetic Properties of the Virus Induced Thymidine Kinase". J Virol 31:172

38. Chen J-Y, Cheng YC (1979) "Mode of Action of 5-Propyldeoxyuridine as a Selective Antiherpes Simplex Virus Agent." The Pharmacologist 21:20

39. Fischer PH, Chen MS, Prusoff WH (1980) "The Incorporation of 5-Iodo-5'-Amino-2', 5'-dideoxyuridine and 5-Iodo-2'-Deoxyuridine into Herpes Simplex Virus DNA Relationship Between Antiviral Activity and Effects on DNA Structure". Biochim Biophys Acta 606: 236

40. Keller PM, Fyfe JA (1980) "A Detailed Examination of the Thymidine Kinase Induced By A Strain of Herpes Simplex Virus Resistant to Acyclovir". International Conference on Human Herpesviruses, March 17, 1980 Atlanta Ga USA Y 18

41. Cheng Y-C, Grill S, Dutschman G (1979) "Time Dependent Action of 5-Propyl Deoxyuridine as Antiherpes Simplex Virus Type 1 and Type 2 Agents". Biochem Pharmacol 28: 3529

42. Cheng Y-C, Grill S, Ruth J, Bergstrom D (1980) "Antiherpes Simplex Virus/Antihuman Cell Growth Activity of E-5-Propenyl-2'-Deoxyuridine and the Concept of "Selective Protection" in Antivirus Chemotherapy". Fed Proc Abstract 3118

43. Schnipper LZ, Kaufman ER, Davidson RL, Crumpacker CS (1980) "Resistance of HSV Intertypic Recombinants Both to Acycloguanosine (ACG) and to Phosphonoacetic Acid (PAA) Is Due to Altered Viral DNA Polymerases". International Conference on Human Herpesviruses, March 17, 1980 Abstract Y30

44. Furman P, Elion G Unpublished Results

45. Cheng YC Unpublished Results.

46. Cheng YC (1979) "Strategy for the Development of Selective Antiherpes Virus Agents Based on the Unique Properties of Viral Induced Enzymes − Thymidine Kinase, DNase and DNA Polymerase". In: Proc Antimetabolites in Biochemistry, Biology and Medicine, Pergamon p. 263

47. Fischer PH, Lee JJ, Chen MS, Lin TS, Prusoff WH (1979) "Synergistic Effect of 5'-Amino-5'-Deoxythymidine and 5-Iodo-2'-Deoxyuridine

Against Herpes Simplex Virus Infections in Vitro". Biochem Pharmacol 28:3483

48. Cheng YC, Prusoff WH (1974) "Mouse Ascites Sarcoma 180 Deoxythymidine (dThd) Kinnase". Biochemistry 13:1179

49. Boezi JA (1979) "The Antiherpesvirus Action of Phosphonoacetate". Pharmacol Ther 4:231

50. Shipman Jr. C, Smith SH, Carlson RH, Drach JC (1976) "Antiviral Activity of Arabinosyladenine and Arabinosylhypoxanthine in Herpes Simplex Virus Infected KB Cells: Selective Inhibition of Viral Deoxyribonucleic Acid Synthesis in Synchronized Suspension Cultures". Antimicrob Agents Chemotherp 9:120

51. Schwartz PM, Shipman Jr C, Smith SJ, Sandbag JN, Drach JC (1976) "Antiviral Activity of Arabinosyladenine and Arabinosylhypoxanthine in Herpes Simplex Virus-Infected KB Cells: Selective Inhibition of Viral Deoxyribonucleic Acid Synthesis in the Presence of an Adenosine Deaminase Inhibitor". Antimicrob Agents Chemotherp 10:64

52. Courtney RJ, Sloan SM, Benyesh-Molnick M (1976) "Effects of 2-deoxy-D-glucose on Herpes Simplex Virus Replication". Virol 52:447

53. Gallaher WR, Levitan DB, Blough HA (1977) "Effect of 2-Deoxy-D-Glucose on Cell Fusion Induced by Newcastle Disease and Herpes Simplex Viruses". Virology 55:193

54. Schabel Jr. FM (1968) "The Antiviral Activity of 9-β-D-Arabinofuranosyl Adenine (AraA)". Chemotherapy 13:321

55. Cheng YC, Grill S, Chen JY, Derse D, Caradonna SJ, Connor K (1980) "Mode of Action of Phosphonoformate as Antiherpes Simplex Agent". International Conference on Human Herpesviruses, March 17, 1980 Atlanta Ga USA Abstract Y25

56. Helgstrand E, Eriksson B, Johansson NG, Lanuero B, Larsson A, Misiorny A, Noren JO, Sjoberg B, Stenberg K, Stening G, Stridh S, Oberg B, Alenius S, Philipson L (1978) "Trisodium Phosphonoformate, A New Antiviral Compound". Science 201:819

57. Derse D, Cheng YC (1980) "Inhibition of Purified Host and HSV Induced DNA Polymerase by Substrate and Product Analysis". International Conference on Human Herpes Viruses, Atlanta GA USA March 17, 1980, Abstract Y24

58. Eriksson B, Larsson A, Helgstrand C, Johansson N-G, Oberg B (1980) "Pyrophosphate Analogues as Inhibitors of Herpes Simplex Virus Type 1 DNA Polymerase". Biochim Biophys Acta 607:53

59. Leinbach SS, Reno JM, Lee IF et al (1976) "Mechanism of Phosphonoacetate Inhibition of Herpesvirus-Induced DNA Polymerase". Biochem 15:426

60. Oberg B, Eriksson B, Helgstrand E, Flodh

Lundstrom J (1980) "Trisodium Phosphonoformate Antiviral Activities, Pharmacokinetics and Safety Evaluation". International Conference on Human Herpes Viruses, Atlanta Ga USA March 17, 1980, Abstract Y 26

61. Eriksson B, Oberg B (1979) „Characteristics of Herpesvirus Mutants Resistant to Phosphonoformate and phosphonoacetate". Antimicrob Agents Chemotherp 15:758

## Discussion on the Contribution pp. 237–245

E. De Clercq (Leuven)
Dr. Cheng, could you please elaborate: for EB virus you mentioned that the induction of thymidine kinase was ±. What do you mean by "plus-minus"?

Y.C. Cheng (Chapel Hill)
EBV could not induce thymidine kinase. This is based on the observation made in my laboratory and in several other laboratories, but there is one report indicating EBV could induce TK, therefore, I said the induction was ±. My personal belief at present is that EBV could not induce virus specific TK.

E. De Clercq (Leuven)
So, I guess we should assume that EBV does not induce thymidine kinase.

Y.C. Cheng (Chapel Hill)
I felt that we should leave room for some doubt and respect our other colleagues' different observations at this point.

E. De Clercq (Leuven)
My second question was: did you evaluate whether 5-propyl and 5-propenyl 2′-deoxyuridine are incorporated into DNA, either viral or cellular DNA?

Y.C. Cheng (Chapel Hill)
In the case of 5-propyl deoxyuridine in viral infected cells, the drug could incorporate into the viral DNA, but that incorporation did not directly correlate to the antiviral action of the drug. Thus the incorporation of 5-propyl dUrd does not explain its antiviral action.

E. De Clercq (Leuven)
And propenyl?

Y.C. Cheng (Chapel Hill)
This we haven't pursued yet because of lack of radioactive compounds.

E. De Clercq (Leuven)
Then I'll turn to my last question. You mentioned that by adding thymidine you could reverse the cy-

totoxic but not the antiviral activity of 5-propenyl 2'-deoxyuridine. Did I understand this correctly? If so, we must conclude that the cytotoxicity and antiviral activity are based on different modes of action. I would postulate that the cytotoxicity is due to an inhibition of thymidylate synthesis, which could be circumvented readily by the salvage pathway of thymidine, whereas the antiviral activity may be due to an inhibition of DNA synthesis, which would be much less reversible with the addition of thymidine. Do you share these points of view?

Y.C. Cheng (Chapel Hill)

Yes, thymidine at low concentration could reverse the cytotoxic but not the antiviral activity of 5-propenyl-2'-deoxyuridine. The rational for this selective protection approach is that 5-propenyl-2'-deoxyuridine is a poor substrate relative to thymidine for host cytosol TK. Therefore, thymidine could easily prevent the phosphorylation of 5-propenyl-2'-deoxyuridine in uninfected cells, which will prevent the cytotoxicity of 5-propenyl-2'-deoxyuridine in uninfected cells. In contrast, 5-propenyl-2'-deoxyuridine is as good a substrate relative to thymidine for virus specific TK. Thus, thymidine could not easily prevent 5-propenyl-2'-

deoxyuridine-phosphorylation by virus thymidine kinase. In virus infected cells the phosphorylated derivative will be able to exert its antiviral activity. It is too early to make the conclusion as you suggested.

H.J. Field (Cambridge)

I'd just like to comment about the TK⁻ mutants. There seem to be many different kinds of these and the one you mentioned (MDK) is unusual in that it is completely TK negative. Mutants selected in vitro often do induce small amounts of the enzyme and this could confer sensitivity to different drugs which are also mediated by the thymidine kinase.

Y.C. Cheng (Chapel Hill)

The MDK mutant we used is TK⁻. In other words, it could not include virus specific TK in virus infected cells.

H.J. Field (Cambridge)

The majority of mutants we have studied which have acquired resistance in the presence of acyclovir do have the polypeptide and do usually express a small amount of TK activity.

Y.C. Cheng (Chapel Hill)

Yes, in that case it will be a different story.

Sundmacher, R. (Hrsg.):
Herpetische Augenerkrankungen
© J.F. Bergmann Verlag, München 1981

# Systemic Application of Antivirals for Herpes Infections

T.C. Merigan, Stanford

**Key words.** Herpetic infections, antiviral drugs – systemic application

**Schlüsselwörter.** Herpesinfektionen, antivirale Medikamente – systemische Therapie

**Summary.** This review has attempted to synthesize work on antiviral chemotherapy, particularly pointing up the possibility of immunosuppression by drugs and the importance for antivirals of cooperative effects with immune and nonspecific recovery mechanisms. With the current successes and crucial need for antiviral chemotherapy, it is likely present efforts will be superseded by future work. A particularly attractive possibility which has only just begun to be investigated is the combination of chemo- and immunotherapy.

**Zusammenfassung.** Trotz der Entwicklung wirksamer Impfmethoden und hygienischer Maßnahmen gibt es doch noch eine ganze Reihe von Problemen mit Virusinfektionen beim Menschen, und deshalb bemüht man sich auch seit langem intensiv um die Entwicklung einer parenteralen Virustatikatherapie. In den letzten Jahren wurden zwei Substanzen entdeckt, die sich ganz besonders gegen virusinfizierte Zellen und weniger gegen normale Zellen richten und die sich bei akuten Viruserkrankungen als nützlich erwiesen haben. Beide Substanzen werden weiterhin gründlich untersucht, um ihr Anwendungsgebiet besser kennenzulernen. Wir haben uns hauptsächlich mit einer dieser Substanzen, dem menschlichen Leukozyten-Interferon, befaßt und dabei besonders seinen Wert bei der Behandlung akuter Herpesinfektionen bei immunosupprimierten Patienten untersucht, zum Beispiel bei Krebspatienten, bei denen solche Infektionen die schwersten Erkrankungen hervorrufen. Bei dem Versuch, auch chronische Viruserkrankungen, wie die Hepatitis B, mit Interferon zu behandeln, fanden wir, daß es von Vorteil ist, es mit Adenin-Arabinosid zu kombinieren, Ara-A ist das andere zur Zeit erhältliche systemisch wirksame Virustatikum. In neuester Zeit lernen wir aufgrund der großen Fortschritte in den Grundlagen-Wissenschaften nicht nur immer mehr über die Struktur des Interferons, sondern auch über seine Wirkmechanismen und sein Wirkungsspektrum, so daß sich neue pharmakologische Applikations-Verbesserungen und neue Möglichkeiten für die klinische Anwendung andeuten. Interferon verstärkt eine ganze Anzahl von Immun-Funktionen und wirkt auch unmittelbar hemmend auf das Wachstum von Tumorzellen, so daß man es auch bei verschiedenen Malignomen des Menschen erprobt. Untersuchungen in Stanford haben die günstige Wirkung des Interferons gegen gewisse Lymphome erwiesen. Gegenwärtig arbeiten wir daran, die Applikation des Interferons so zu optimieren, daß das Leben solcher Patienten bei uns und andernorts solange wie möglich erhalten werden kann.

## Introduction

Systemic antiviral therapy has had much appeal because of the persistent difficulties of viral infection in human populations despite developments in vaccination and public health disease control measures. Yet, progress in this area has been slow and the agents which have been developed appear to have only very specialized usages rather than broad spectrum application as desired by some. However, at least two appropriately selective agents have been shown to have systemic antiviral activity in man and these and others are under continued investigation to determine the full range of diseases and hosts in which they will be active.

In this review I will attempt to not only present new data as to the usefulness of these agents, but also bring out their limitations and what we might expect in the future from efforts at clinical application.

## Immunosuppression and Viral Chemotherapy

Because of the close coupling of the replication of animal viruses and host cell functions, successful antiviral therapy has demanded agents specifically directed against virus infected cells. In addition, the spread of virus within an infected individual involved a wide variety of cells in which antiviral drugs may or may not act with similar efficacy. Recent studies [40] have demonstrated that host defense to viral infection involves a multititered series of interrelated, but yet independent reponses, which act on virus infected cells as well as on extracellular virus to diminish spread of the agent within the host. The proper function of all of these events obviously depends on a complex series of host biosynthetic and differentiation steps.

The systemic use of antivirals in such a setting is hazardous if they do not have specificity for the virus infected cell. A number of studies have demonstrated that the host may be relatively immunosuppressed in a variety of cellular and humoral immune responses during systemic virus infections [62]. It is even possible that the pathogenicity of certain agents depends upon their having evolved such immunosuppressive abilities. In the absence of certain host defenses, others may be called upon for more efficient function and thus spread somewhat more thinly, making those remaining functions quite vulnerable to the action of metabolic inhibitors. Thus, skillful use of antiviral agents which are specific is particularly important when they are to be used therapeutically in order to avoid adding to immunosuppression. It seems quite likely that if we could measure specific host defenses to tumors with accuracy in man we would find that they also must function in close concert with antitumor agents for their most efficient therapeutic action.

This situation with viruses should be contrasted with chemotherapeutics active against more complicated microorganisms such as bacteria and fungi. Here, the site of action of the antimicrobial can be so selected as to minimize any effect on the cells of the host. For example, penicillin and amphotericin B are directed against components of the parasite's cell wall which are not present in the host cells [45] and immunosuppression is not reported with their use. With other agents the selectivity is based on an action on enzymes unique to the parasite. For example, the antifolates, pyrimethemine and trimethoprin, which are used against protozoa and bacteria, are much more active against the dihydrofolate reductase of the parasite than that of the host [6]. In the case of the antifungal, 5-fluorocytosine, its selective toxicity for the parasite depends upon the organism but not the host cell possessing cytosine deaminase which will degrade the drug to the toxic metabolite, 5-fluorouracil [33]. On the other hand, chloramphenicol and rifamycin have been demonstrated under certain conditions to inhibit host humoral and cellular immune functions [17, 48] as well as having potent antimicrobial properties. The antihelminthic, niridazole, also inhibits cell mediated immune responses in man and animals [57]. However, neither in the case of this agent nor the two previously mentioned is there any direct evidence for the immunosuppressive capacity leading to increased susceptibility to infection. However, it has been observed that prompt treatment of tularemia with tetracycline or streptomycin not only impaired the patient's production of precipitin antibody [56] but also produced increased frequency of relapse and susceptibility to reinfection.

## Present Status of Antivirals

Initially the focus for development of human antivirals was either 1) on local therapy to sites which could be exposed to high concentration of antiviral agents without systemic absorption or 2) on systemic prophylaxis. For example, the success of iododeoxyuridine [30] and cytosine arabinoside [29] in herpetic keratitis depended on their local application to the cornea, a site where quite high concentrations could be built up without effects on lymphatic or bone marrow cells which would have been manifest if the agents were given systemically. Furthermore, the use of amantadine in influenza [28] and isatin in smallpox [3] prophylaxis during the incubation period has prevented or diminished infection. As this action occurs quite early in the infectious process, the need for cooperation with host defenses is minimized. In fact, with the effective use of both these latter agents, antibody responses are inhibited in contrast to untreated controls. This is most likely because the therapy prevents development of an antigenic mass sufficient for immune sensitization. The net result was that the drug protected host not only did not have symptomatic disease but did not develop immunity and was susceptible on rechallenge. In controlled trials with volunteers locally applied interferon has also been effective in preventing respiratory tract infection [38] as well as vaccinial skin lesions [50], and here again immunity did not develop – most likely because of the restricted development of antigenic mass.

Amantadine's activity in preventing influenza was reaffirmed in a recently published field trial [39]. At present it is licensed for use with virtually all influenza A strains and a recent NIH sponsored consensus conference strongly advocated its increased usage given the limitations in our current vaccine stragegy.

Cytosine arabinoside was utilized systemically for varicella or zoster in a number of immunosuppressed patients on the basis of apparent success in single anecdotal cases. Carefully controlled trials revealed no evidence that the course of zoster was improved by this agent [4, 14, 49, 55]. In fact, in a randomized placebo controlled double blind trial [55] in patients with lymphoma at Stanford, it was observed that parenteral cytosine arabinoside actually prolonged the course of disseminated zoster concomitantly with its delay of host defenses. Specifically, it delayed the appearance of varicella zoster complement-fixing antibody in the serum and the local vesicle fluid interferon responses in the treated patients who had received recent chemotherapy and irradiation when their responses were compared to similar placebo treated controls.

In the last 3 years beneficial results have been reported with systemic administration of agents which seem to inhibit virus replication when given after symptoms have appeared. Specifically, we have found [37] intramuscular leukocyte interferon appears to shorten the course of zoster in immunosuppressed individuals as others have also observed in similar studies with intravenously administered adenine arabinoside [58]. Adenine arabinoside also decreased mortality in the encephalitis produced by type 1 herpes simplex [59]. Beneficial effects of adenine arabinoside will also soon be reported in neonatal encephalitis due to type 2

herpes simplex [60] which on cell culture testing is generally more resistant to antivirals than the other strain. Both these agents [1, 9, 20] as well as iododeoxyuridine [2] and cytosine arabinoside [36], can decrease urinary excretion of cytomegalovirus, although the response it somewhat variable and only a transient suppression is observed in most treated individuals. This latter result may be due to the lack of specific host immune responses available to cooperate with these antivirals in the neonates and transplant recipients who were treated. This latter point was also underscored by results in a recent double blind placebo controlled trial of human leukocyte interferon in renal transplant recipients [7]. Three million units, given prophylactically, twice weekly for 6 weeks resulted in a decreased incidence of CMV viremia and a delayed onset of CMV shedding. Interferon's effects were greater in patients not receiving antithymocyte globulin suggesting that the agent was most active in the setting of at least partially intact host defenses.

Optimal usage and demonstration of therapeutic efficacy of interferon and adenine arabinoside has depended upon early utilization of these antiviral agents. It has been important to carefully follow the effect of these agents on the development of the immune responses in the treated individuals because they were given in the midst of critical events in host response to the antigens of the infecting agents. Although large doses of mouse interferon have been demonstrated to suppress antibody production [8] and cellular immunity [18], these are greater than those which are required to limit acute viral infection. Adenine arabinoside has been observed to be not as toxic in vivo as cytosine arabinoside or iododeoxyuridine [34] and actually was selected as an antiviral agent for widespread trials because of its lack of immune suppression [54, 66]. Furthermore, in contrast to iododeoxyuridine and cytosine arabinoside, it was able to produce a therapeutic effect, even when given as late as 7 days after vaccinia or herpes simplex infection of immunosuppressed mice [63, 64]. The leukocyte interferon trials in zoster were conducted primarily in lymphoma patients. No impairment was observed in the antibody production of the interferon recipients as compared to that of the placebo recipients, even at a level of 35 million reference units per day [37]. It is possible that this occurs because this antibody response is an amnestic one to an agent with which the host is persistently infected. In a smaller uncontrolled and unconfirmed trial, it was suggested that lower doses, that is 3 million references units daily, would terminate new lesion formation in the primary dermatome in normal individuals with zoster [21]. Normal individuals may require less of this or other antiviral agents because of their intact immune responses.

## Future Perspectives for Acute and Chronic Infections

There is now evidence that it takes 1 or more days of antivirals to begin to act and many herpesviral diseases in which they are to be used only last a few days. Hence, there is a strong rationale for the use of antiviral agents in such infections as early as possible in the infection, if maximum prevention of pathology in the treated individuals is to be achieved. Yet it is also clear that in many this is one of the most sensitive times for possible interference with the immune responses and thus immunological parameters should be measured in all such trials to determine whether certain patients — rather than being helped — may be further immunocompromised by such agents. Assays of specific cellular immunity to viruses in man are being developed and will be particularly useful to monitor during trials considering the apparent importance of thymus derived lymphocytes in recovery. Both prolonged herpes simplex [46] and herpes zoster [23] have both observed to be paralleled with depressed specific T lymphocyte reactivity to the specific viral agent in transplant or cancer patients in whom immunosuppressive agents were continued after infection had developed. Most recently our group has observed that Dane particle levels are heightened by use of the immunosuppressive regimen commonly utilized for treatment of chronic hepatitis and cessation of such therapy is consistently associated with a fall in Dane particle number [51].

The neonate is at special risk for persistent herpesviral infections, and significant pathological sequelae are present in children who have been born infected with HSV, CMV, rubella and varicella-zoster virus.

Evidence is presently emerging that specific deficiencies associated with the immunological immaturity of the newborn [24] may be associated with the establishment of such neonatal disease which is often quite prolonged as compared to that in more mature individuals. Numerically, chronic CMV infection is probably the most important of these four and the long term neurological sequelae of such infections are of significant economic importance in our society. Yet, as mentioned previously, adenine arabinoside and interferon have only transiently suppressed CMV viruria [1, 9, 20], and the effect of interferon on cells chronically infected with rubella [19] suggests it also will be resistant to such therapy. It is possible that some carefully planned combination of chemo- and immunotherapy will be required to clear such persistent infections. For example, prevention of herpes simplex encephalitis in mice with adenine arabinoside was improved by the concomitant administration of specific immune globin [11]. The use of such combined therapy was particularly beneficial in infections of newborn of immunodeficient nude mice [10]. Whether such effects can be obtained with Cornynebacterium parvum, BCG, levamisole, or other agents [22, 25, 31, 35, 53] requires further study.

Recently our group has observed both leukocyte interferon and adenine arabinoside will favorably influence chronic hepatitis B virus infection [26, 44]. This persistent infection appears suppressible by both treatment modalities. Utilizing a 50-fold range of interferon dosage and a 6-fold range of adenine arabinoside, we find some patients appear much more responsive to this therapy than others, although all demonstrate a progressively increasing effect with increased dosage. The most responsive appear to have the most prolonged responses, and in 13 followed over a year Dane particles have not returned [52]. If Dane particles can be fully cleared from the blood by either agent, the effect persists and $HB_sAg$ titers fall as well. In fact, in three of our patients, all virologic markers of hepatitis B virus infection have disappeared. It appears to us that as yet undefined host factors condition the outcome of such therapy. We are currently trying to determine the optimum dosing regimen for these agents in combination. Combination therapy regimen apparently

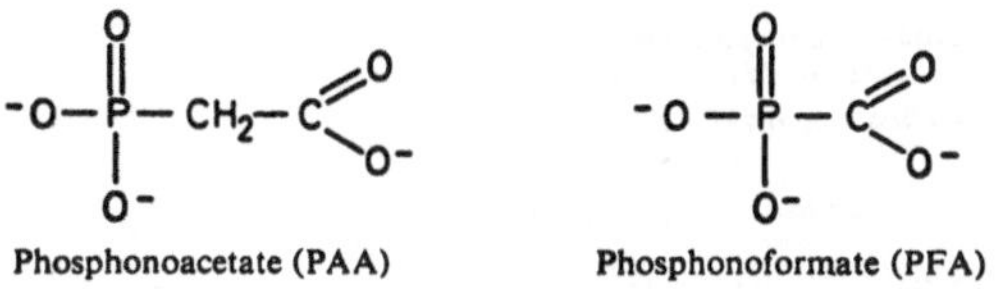

Phosphonoacetate (PAA)    Phosphonoformate (PFA)

**Fig. 1.** Phosphonoacetate and phosphonoformate

produces a greater immediate suppressive effect and likelihood of long term Dane particle eradication [52]. With Dane particle infectious for chimpanzees and liver function parameters are stabilized or improved. However, this last point can only be rigorously tested in randomized controlled trials. We are encouraged by present results that, by determining the extent of Dane particle suppression in the first weeks of therapy, we might be able to predict the outcome of the several month course of therapy which is required to eradicate the infection. Patients with high titers of Dane particles pretreatment are proving to be more difficult to treat in both obtaining 1) complete suppression during therapy and 2) enduring erradication of Dane particles on cessation of therapy.

Development of an optimum combination therapy to evaluate in a controlled trial has been delayed because of an increased incidence of adenine arabinoside neurotoxicity seen in the interferon treated hepatitis patients compared to other patients treated with the same dosage of drug. Pharmacokinetic studies [47] have revealed approximately 2-fold higher adenine ara-

binoside levels in the interferon treated hepatitis patients compared to others and neurotoxicity appears at lower adenine arabinoside dosages during combination therapy than if it is given alone.

It is apparent that greater sophistication in selecting agents which are less likely to be immunosuppressive has been crucial in producing a second generation of systemically administered antiviral agents, specifically adenine arabinoside and leukocyte interferon. Hopefully, better insights into the natural history and the nature of the host defenses will allow the development of more and better agents. Particularly interesting classes of agents at present appear to fall into two categories [12]. The first, which includes phosphonoacetic acid (Fig. 1) are agents which have a greater affinity for the viral DNA polymerase than for the host DNA polymerases. Secondly, novel nucleotides have been found which are phosphorylated by the virus pyrimidine kinase but not by the host cell thymidine kinase. Hence, these nucleoside analogues can only be incorporated into the DNA of virus infected cells but not of normal cells. Such agents as acycloguanosine (Fig. 2) and certain 5' substituted pyrimidines (Fig. 3) fall into this latter category. If such agents can be discovered which have appropriate pharmacologic distribution properties and lack significant side effects, it is anticipated their specificity will restrict their action to antiviral effects. Thus, one would avoid significantly effecting lymphoid cells or bone marrow, two of the most

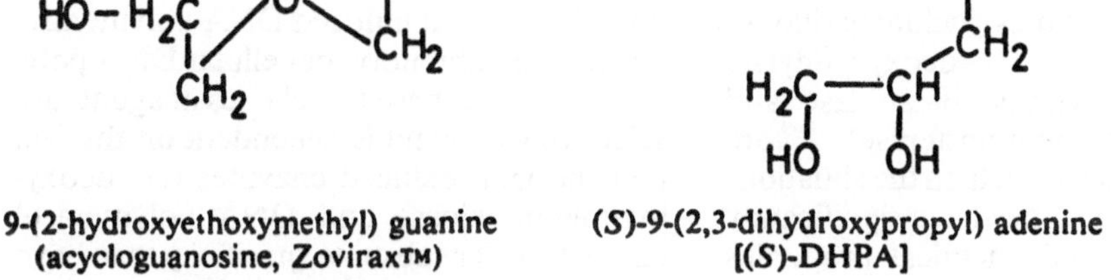

9-(2-hydroxyethoxymethyl) guanine
(acycloguanosine, Zovirax™)

(S)-9-(2,3-dihydroxypropyl) adenine
[(S)-DHPA]

**Fig. 2.** Acyclic nucleoside analogues

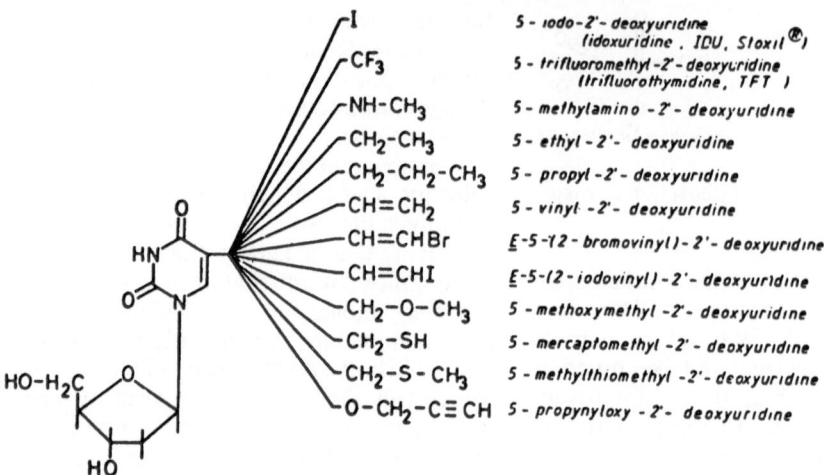

| | |
|---|---|
| I | 5 - iodo-2'- deoxyuridine (idoxuridine, IDU, Stoxil®) |
| CF₃ | 5 - trifluoromethyl -2'- deoxyuridine (trifluorothymidine, TFT ) |
| NH-CH₃ | 5 - methylamino - 2' - deoxyuridine |
| CH₂-CH₃ | 5 - ethyl - 2' - deoxyuridine |
| CH₂-CH₂-CH₃ | 5 - propyl -2'- deoxyuridine |
| CH=CH₂ | 5 - vinyl - 2'- deoxyuridine |
| CH=CHBr | E -5 -(2 - bromovinyl) - 2'- deoxyuridine |
| CH=CHI | E -5- (2 - iodovinyl ) - 2'- deoxyuridine |
| CH₂-O-CH₃ | 5 - methoxymethyl -2'- deoxyuridine |
| CH₂-SH | 5 - mercaptomethyl -2' - deoxyuridine |
| CH₂-S - CH₃ | 5 - methylthiomethyl -2'- deoxyuridine |
| O-CH₂-C≡CH | 5 - propynyloxy - 2'- deoxyuridine |

**Fig. 3.** 5′Substituted 2′deoxyuridines

critical and easily compromised rapidly dividing cell populations in the whole animal. Acycloguanosine is theoretically a particularly appealing compound as it appears to have a dual basis for its specificity in that the drug is active after only being initially phosphorylated by the viral induced kinase and also has a greater affinity for the viral rather than cellular DNA polymerases.

One additional acyclic compound with significant anti-viral activity has been identified by De Clercq [15] in his screening of 60 newly synthesized nucleoside compounds of this type. Surprisingly, this agent, (5)-9-(2, 3-dihydroxyprophyl) adenine, has been active against both RNA and DNA viruses and its mechanism of action has not yet been clarified (Fig. 2).

Herpesviral infection results in the intracellular appearance of many new proteins coded for by the viral genome. Some of these are structural proteins associated with the mature virus particle, while others are enzymes involved in the synthesis of viral DNA. In addition to the induction of deoxypyrimidine kinase and DNA polymerase, the activities of other enzymes (including ribonucleotide reductase, deoxycytidylate deaminase, deoxycytidine deaminase and nucleoside phosphotransferase) are increased in the infected cell. In the situations studied, the viral enzymes have significantly different physical and chemical properties (including substrate specificity and regulation by nucleotides) thereby providing candidate targets for potentially selective anti-herpes agents. As mentioned above, several recently described antiherpes agents, eg. 5-N-propyl-2-deoxyuridine, 5-amino-5-iododeoxyuridine, Ara-T and acycloguanosine all appear to be specific for the virus infected cell by virtue of being selectively phosphorylated by the virus induced deoxypyrimidine kinase but not the kinase of the non-infected cell. Because of particularly promising animal and tissue culture model infection findings, Phase I and II testing of acycloguanosine has been completed recently and large scale controlled trials are underway both in the U.S. and U.K. to assay its effects on HSV and VZ infection in several specific clinical settings. Another newly described 5′ substituted deoxyuridine (dU) (E-5(2′-bromovinyl)-2′dU) [16] has such a high level of activity in tissue culture and wide therapeutic ratio in animal herpes infections that it also deserved early clinical evaluation (Fig. 3).

The other currently interesting agents such as phosphonoacetate, phosphonoformate and zinc ion appear selectively inhibitory for the viral induced DNA polymerase, and are not inhibitory for cellular DNA polymerases. That these two classes of agents are selectively antiviral is dependent on the fact that the viral induced enzymes (i.e. deoxypyrimidine kinase and DNA polymerase) have a broader substrate specificity than have the enzymes from the non-infected cells. Obviously, the development of agents which are inhibitors of other enzymes (or proteins) involved in the replication of herpesviruses would be of great interest. One recently reported trial of deoxyglucose, an antiviral agent which is thought to inhibit glucosylation of viral glycoproteins or glycolipids has been interpreted to demonstrate a beneficial effect on local application to herpes genitalis lesions [5]. However, clinicians have raised doubts about the study as very prolonged viral shedding has been seen in the placebo treated group, perhaps related to a disease enhancing effect of the cream vehicle utilized for the study [13].

Of course, there are other characteristics that are important in an ideal antiviral. In the long run, the fact that interferon, like antibody, is part of normal host defenses, also may be of special advantage in its potential lack of the two most difficult to assess long term toxicities – that is, mutagenicity and teratogenicity. Iododeoxyuridine and cytosine arabinoside have been observed to be teratogenic in rodents [42], and the latter also has been noted to increase the number of chromosome breaks in herpes simplex infected cells [41]. The propensity of phosphoacetic and phosphoformic acid to deposit in bone make their systemic administration an unknown risk, for the long term and has slowed and may prevent their clinical study. The recently described mutagenic and teratogenic effects of adenine arabinoside must be taken into consideration in its use [43]. Finally, the long exposure of pathogens to interferon as a normal host defense without development of resistance also might be a special advantage in its clinical application. Resistance to acycloguanosine has developed under prolonged tissue culture exposure and can be due to mutations in either the kinase and polymerase genes in HSV. Combination antiviral therapy may be a useful means to prevent emergence of resistant mutants as has been the case with combination antibiotic therapy particularly in tuberculosis.

The greatest challenge to antiviral chemotherapy is the eradication of persistent infection in ganglia where it is already known that potent antivirals such as adenine arabinoside, phosphonoacetic acid [32, 61] and acycloguanosine can not inhibit or depress the extent of ganglia involvement in mice once the herpes simplex has reached that site. It is possible that virus replication is not in a productive phase at that site and thus is even less susceptible to selective chemotherapeutic action. On the other hand, it is also possible that certain antigens may be expressed in such persistently infected cells which might make them susceptible to selective immunotherapy. Alternatively, if viral enzymes are produced in the latently infected cells as has been suggested by certain recent observations [65], then it is possible they may provide the key to selective kill of those cells as mentioned above. Finally, it may be possible that use of antivirals may abort clinical manifestations of recurrent HSV disease even though ganglia are still chronically infected as the recent work of Hill and Blyth [27] has suggested can be accomplished with acycloguanosine in their recurrent mouse ear infection model. Obviously work will be continuing on such questions in years to come.

**Acknowledgments.** This work was kindly presented by R.B. Pollard, M.D., Galveston, as Dr. Merigan was prevented from attending. The work described in this manuscript was supported in part by U.S. Public Health Service grant AI-05629 and contract NIH-73-2501. The figures were taken with permission from a review article entitled, "New Trends in Antiviral Chemotherapy" by Eric DeClercq (1979) Archives Internationales de Physiologie et de Biochemie 87:353–395.

References

1. Arvin AM, Yeager AS, Merigan TC (1976) In: Merigan TC (ed) Antivirals with clinical potential. University of Chicago Press, Chicago, pp 205–210
2. Barton BW, Tobin JO (1970) Ann NY Acad Sci 173:90
3. Bauer DJ, St Vincent L, Kempe CH, et al (1969) Am J Epidemiol 90:130
4. Betts RF, Zaky DA, Douglas jr RG, et al. (1975) Ann Int Med 82:778
5. Blough HA, Giuntoli RL (1979) JAMA 241:2798
6. Burchall JJ, Hitchings GH (1965) Mol Pharmacol 1:126
7. Cheeseman SH, Rubin RH, Stewart JA, et al. (1979) N Engl J Med 300:1345
8. Chester TJ, Paucker K, Merigan TC (1973) Nature 246:92
9. Ch'ien LT, Whitley RJ, Dismukes WE, et al. (1974) J Infect Dis 130:32
10. Cho CT, Feng KK (1977) J Infect Dis 135:168
11. Cho CT, Feng KK, Brahmacupta (1976) J Infect Dis 133:157

12. Cohen SS (1977) Cancer 40:509
13. Corey L, Homes KK (1980) JAMA 243:29
14. Davis CM, VanDersarl JV, Coltman jr CA (1973) JAMA 224:122
15. DeClercq E, Holy A (1979) J Med Chem :
16. DeClercq E, Descamps J, DeSomer P, et al. (1979) Proc Natl Acad Sci 76:2947
17. Della Bella D, Petrescu D, Marca G, et al. (1973) Chemotherapy 18:99
18. Maeyer-Guignard J de, Cachard A, Maeyer E de (1975) Science 190:574
19. Desmyter J, Rawls WE, Melnick JJ, et al. (1967) J Immunol 99:771
20. Emodi G, O'Reilly R, Muller A (1976) In: Merigan TC (ed) Antivirals with clinical potential. University of Chicago Press, Chicago, pp 199–204
21. Emodi G, Rufli T, Just M, et al. (1975) Scand J Infect Dis 7:1
22. Fischer GW, Podgore JK, Bass JW, et al. (1975) J Infect Dis 132:578
23. Gallagher JG, Merigan TC (1979) Annals of Internal Medicine 91:842–846
24. Gehrz RC, Knorr SO, Marker SC, et al. (1977) Lancet p 844
25. Glasgow LA, Fischbach J, Bryant SM, et al. (1977) J Infect Dis 135:763
26. Greenberg HB, Pollard RB, Lutwick LI, et al. (1976) N Engl J Med 295:517
27. Hill TJ, Blyth WA (in preparation)
28. Jackson GG (1971) Hospital Practice Nov:75
29. Kaufman HE, Maloney ED (1963) Arch Ophthalmol 69:626
30. Kaufman HE, Martola EL, Dohlman CH (1962) Arch Ophthalmol 68:235
31. Kirchner H, Hirt HM, Munk K (1977) Infect Immun 16:9
32. Klein RJ, Friedman-Kien AE (1977) Antimicrob Agents Chemother 12:577
33. Koechlin BA, Robio F, Palmer S, et al. (1966) Biochem Pharmacol 15:435
34. Kurtz SM, Fisken RA, Kaump DH, et al. (1969) Antimicrob Agents Chemother 1968:180
35. McCord RS, Breinig MK, Morahan PS (1976) Antimicrob Agents Chemother 10:28
36. McCracken GH, Luby JP (1972) J Pediatr 80:488
37. Merigan TC, Rand KH, Pollard RB, et al. (1978) N Engl J Med 298:981
38. Merigan TC, Reed SE, Hall TS, et al. (1973) Lancet 1:563
39. Monto AS, Gunn RA, Bandyk MG, et al. (1979) JAMA 241
40. Notkins AL (ed) (1975) Viral immunology and immunopathology. Academic, New York
41. O'Neill FJ, Rapp R (1971) J Virology 7:692
42. Percy DH (1975) Teratology 11:103
43. Petrick T (1977) Discussion at Adenine Arabinoside Collaborative Study Group, Bethesda, MD., Nov. 17
44. Pollard RB, Smith JL, Neal EA, et al. (1978) JAMA 239:1648
45. Pratt WB (1977) Chemotherapy of infection Oxford University Press, New York
46. Rand KH, Rasmussen LE, Pollard RB, et al. (1977) N Engl J Med 296:1372
47. Sacks S (1980) Submitted for publication
48. Sanders jr WE (1976) Ann Int Med 85:82
49. Schimpff SC, Fortner CL, Greene WH, et al. (1974) J Infect Dis 130:673
50. Scientific Committee on Interferon (1962) Lancet 1:872
51. Scullard G (1980) Submitted for publication
52. Scullard G (1980) Submitted for publication
53. Starr SE, Visintine AM, Tomeh MO, et al. (1976) Proc Soc Exp Biol Med 152:57
54. Steele RW, Keeney RE, Brown III J, et al. (1977) J Infect Dis 135:593
55. Stevens DA, Jordan GW, Waddell TF, et al. (1973) N Engl J Med 289:873
56. Vosti RL, Ward MK, Tigertt WD (1962) J Clin Invest 41:1436
57. Webster LT, Butterworth AE, Mahmoud AAF, et al. (1975) N Engl J Med 292:1144
58. Whitley RJ, Ch'ien LT, Dolin R, et al. (1976) N Engl J Med 294:1193
59. Whitley RJ, Soong SJ, Dolin R, et al. (1977) N Engl J Med 297:289
60. Whitley RJ (1980) Submitted for publication
61. Wohlenberg CR, Walz MA, Notkins AL (1976) Infect Immun 13:1519
62. Woodruff JF, Woodruff JJ (1975) In: Notkins AL (ed) Viral immunology and immunopathology. Academic, New York, pp 393–418
63. Worthington M, Conliffe M (1977) J Gen Virol 36:329
64. Worthington MG, Conliffe M, Williams J (1977) Proc Soc Exp Biol Med 156:168
65. Yamamoto H, Wale MA, Notkins AL (1977) Virology 76:866–869
66. Zam ZS, Centifanto YM, Kaufman HE (1974) Interscience conference. Antimicrob Agents Chemother Am Soc Microbiol (abstr) 4:139

Sundmacher, R. (Hrsg.):
Herpetische Augenerkrankungen
© J.F. Bergmann Verlag, München 1981

# The Chemotherapy of Herpetic Keratitis in Rabbits

W.J. O'Brien, J.L. Taylor, J.D. DeCarlo, D.W. Clough, R.O. Schultz, Milwaukee

**Key words.** Antiviral antiherpetic drugs, herpetic keratitis

**Schlüsselwörter.** Antivirale antiherpetische Medikamente, Herpeskeratitis

**Summary.** Several antiviral agents were compared for efficacy in treatment of herpetic keratitis in rabbits. The compounds studied include: three nucleoside analogues; 1-β-D-arabinofuranosylthymine (ARA-T), 9-(2-hydroxyethoxymethyl) guanine (ACG), and 5-trifluoromethyl-2'-deoxyuridine ($F_3$TdR); the interferon inducer, 10-carboxymethyl-9-acridanone (CMA); and the retinoid; retinoic acid. The relative antiviral activity of these compounds in vitro was ARA-T > $F_3$TdR > ACG >> retinoic acid >> CMA. In the rabbit keratitis model 1% $F_3$TdR, 1% ARA-T, and 3% ACG were all about equally effective when given topically. Given intravenously ARA-T increased the frequency of disciform keratitis, and CMA was effective only when treatment was begun the same day as virus infection. Retinoic acid possessed antiviral activity in cell cultures, however, topical administration of 0.1% retinoic acid in a sesame oil vehicle resulted in reduced lesion scores which were not significantly different from the vehicle alone.

**Zusammenfassung.** Zur Behandlung der epithelialen Herpeskeratitis durch HSV Typ 1 bei Kaninchen benutzten wir antivirale Substanzen aus drei verschiedenen Gruppen: 1. Nucleosidanaloge, 2. einen Interferoninductor, 3. eine viruzide Substanz. Eine 1%ige Lösung des Nucleosidvirustatikums 1-β-D-Arabinofuranosylthymin (ARA-T) war weniger wirksam als eine 1%ige Lösung des 5-Trifluoromethyl-2'-Deoxyuridin ($F_3$TdR); sie war aber genauso wirksam wie eine 1%ige $F_3$TdR- und eine 3%ige 9-(2-Hydroxyethoxymethyl)-Guanin(Acyclo-G)-Salbe bei der Reduktion des epithelialen Herpes. ARA-T war zwar gegenüber den Serum-Nucleosid-Phosphorylasen bei systemischer Gabe stabil; eine systemische ARA-T-Therapie führte aber bei allen Tieren zu einer disziformen Keratitis. Der Interferoninduktor 9-Carboxymethyl-2-Acridanon (CMA) war bei der epithelialen Herpeskeratitis lokal gegeben unwirksam. Nach intraperitonealer Injektion induzierte CMA geringe Interferon-Titer in den Kaninchen. Die viruzide Substanz Retinol-Säure, die sich in vitro als Hemmer der Herpes simplex-Virusreplikationen erwiesen hat, zeigte als 0,1%ige Lösung nach lokaler Applikation keine Wirkung bei den Tieren.

Die Infektion der Kaninchenhornhäute (weiße Neuseelandkaninchen, 2–3 kg Gewicht) mit $10^6$ p.f.u. des HSV-Typ 1-Stammes McKrae erfolgte nach geringer epithelialer Skarifikation. Die Lokalbehandlung begann dann jeweils erst nach 72 Std, wenn sich die Effloreszenzen entwickelt hatten. Die Epitheldefekte wurden täglich mit Fluoreszein angefärbt und ihr Ausmaß bewertet. Die statistische Bewertung der dabei ermittelten Schweregradsziffern erfolgte mit dem Wilcoxon-Rank-Summentest.

Unsere Ergebnisse zeigen, daß 1. das Nucleosidanalog ARA-T nach lokaler Gabe wirksam ist, bei systemischer Gabe aber toxisch oder immunsuppressiv wirkt, daß 2. der niedermolekulare Interferoninduktor CMA bei der Lokaltherapie der Keratitis dendritica bei Kaninchen wirkungslos ist und daß 3. lokal gegebene Retinolsäure in vivo kein wirksames Virrustatikum darstellt.

## Introduction

Chemotherapy of herpetic keratitis has been one of the most successful antiviral chemotherapy treatment programs. Nucleoside analogues such as 5-iodo-2'-deoxyuridine (IUdR) were the first compounds used to inhibit herpes simplex type 1 (HSV) replication in the corneal epithelium of rabbits and man [13, 14]. In recent years nucleoside analogues which are more selectively metabolized by virus infected cells have been developed. The analogues 9-(2-hydroxyethoxymethyl)guanine (ACG), 5-amino-2'-5'-dideoxy-5-iodouridine (AIU) and 1-β-D-arabinofuranosylthymine (ARA-T) serve as excellent substrates for the HSV pyrimidine kinase while being low affinity substrates for cellular kinases [1, 7, 9].

Antimetabolites such as nucleoside antivirals are only one form of antiviral chemotherapy. The induction of host factors such as interferon which regulate the antiviral state of the host have met with mixed success in the treatment of herpetic keratitis. Treatment with preparations of interferon have been shown to be effective in preventing herpetic keratitis when used prophylactically but interferon was neither effective in reducing the severity nor in altering the healing rates of established disease [16, 17]. The induction of interferon by large molecular weight polyanionic molecules, such as poly IC, have also met with little success in the treatment of keratitis in monkeys and man but slight therapeutic and prophylactic effects were observed in rabbits [5, 11, 12]. Low molecular weight interferon inducers such as 10-carboxymethyl-9-acridanone (CMA) and substituted arylpyrimidines have been shown to be effective in reducing the severity of other viral infections when given therapeutically [15, 18, 23]. In these cases the levels of interferon induced appear to be dependent upon the route of administration and the species of animal receiving the drug.

Virucidal/antiviral effects have recently been attributed to a third class of compounds, retinoids. Retinal acid has been reported to be an effective virucidal agent in vitro [2]. In vivo, retinoic acid given intraperitoneally reduced the severity of keratitis in a chronic herpes model [21]. In other in vitro studies, retinoic acid was shown to inhibit the induction of Epstein-Barr virus from the latent state [24]. Such properties of retinoids which apparently suppress the expression of latent virus as well as the inhibition of viral growth make retinoic acid a good prospect for use as a chemotherapeutic agent. The mechanism by which retinoids express antiviral activity is presently unknown, however, it is possible that the mechanism may involve the regulation of gene expression as well as virucidal properties [4].

The purpose of our experiments was to investigate the relative antiviral activity of ACG, F$_3$TdR, ARA-T, CMA, and retinoic acid in conjunctival epithelial cells in vitro and to test the relative therapeutic efficacy of these compounds in treating herpetic keratitis.

**Materials and Methods**

*Infection and Treatment of Rabbits*

New Zealand white rabbits (2 to 3 kg) were infected with 10$^6$ plaque forming units (pfu) of either the McKrae strain or RE strain of herpes simplex virus type 1 (HSV 1) after lightly scarifying the corneal epithelium with a trephine. Lesions were allowed to develop for three days prior to initiation of treatment unless otherwise stated. Both eyes of each rabbit were infected and treated identically. Epithelial lesion sizes were graded daily after fluorescein staining by examination using a slit lamp. Epithelial lesions involving 100% of the corneal area were given a score of 4, 75% = 3, 50% = 2, and 25% = 1. Scores were evaluated daily by two observers and averaged to give the daily lesion score. Treatments with all drugs were initiated on the 3rd day after infection and administered five times per day at 2 hour intervals unless otherwise specified. Lesion scores were evaluated statistically for significant difference by one way analysis of variance and the Waller Duncan Adapted t Test.

*In Vitro Antiviral Tests*

The in vitro antiviral activity of each compound against the McKrae strain of HSV 1 was quantitated by yield reduction assays in Chang conjunctival cells. Chang cells, derived from normal human conjunctival epithelium [6], were planted at 1.5 × 10$^5$ cells/tube (16 × 125 mm) in medium 199 (M 199) containing 10% heat inactivated calf serum and organic buffers (10 mM BES, 10 mM TES and 15 mM HEPES) pH 7.1. Two days later, the medium was removed and the cells were infected with 10$^6$ pfu/tube (MOI ≅ 5) of the McKrae strain of HSV 1. After 1 h of adsorption, the unabsorbed virus was removed, and cells washed one time with Earle's Balanced Salts, and cells overlayed with M 199 containing the antivirals at various concentrations. Twenty-four hours after infection, the cells were frozen and thawed three times and the virus titered in Chang cells with the same medium described above containing 1.5% methyl cellulose. The concentration of drug required to reduce the viral yield by 99% ($ED_{99}$) was calculated from computer fit curves showing the relationship of drug concentration to virus titers. The effect of each drug on the viability of the Chang cells was determined by the change in colony forming ability after 24 h of drug exposure [8].

### Stability of ARA-T in Rabbit Serum

The resistance of ARA-T to metabolism was assayed by incubating varying concentrations of ARA-T in rabbit serum and monitoring the changes in optical density at 268 nm and 290 nm as described by Aswell et al. [1].

### Materials

5-Trifluoromethyl-2'-deoxyuridine ($F_3TdR$), 9-(2-hydroxyethoxymethyl)guanine (ACG), solution vehicle, and ointment placebo were a gift of the Burroughs Wellcome Company, Research Triangle Park, North Carolina; 1-β-D-arabinofuranosylthymine (ARA-T) from Raylow Chemicals Ltd, Alberta, Canada; 10-carboxymethyl-9-acridanone (CMA), a gift from Hoffmann-LaRoche Laboratories, Nutley, New Jersey; retinoic acid from Sigma Chemical Company, St. Louis, Missouri; and sesame oil (U.S.P.) from Humco Laboratory, Texarkana, Texas.

### Results

#### In Vitro Antiviral Activity

Each of the antiviral compounds to be tested in vivo were evaluated in vitro to determine their antiviral potency against the McKrae strain of HSV 1 in epithelial cells of ocular origin. The concentration of drug required to reduce viral yield by 99% ($ED_{99}$) was determined for each drug (Table 1). Of the compounds to be tested in vivo, the antiviral activity of ARA-T > $F_3TdR$ > ACG >> retinoic acid >> CMA. The order of toxicity established in vitro was CMA ≤ ACG ≤ retinoic acid < ARA-T ≪ $F_3TdR$ (Table 1).

#### In Vivo Antiviral Activity

The effect of ARA-T and $F_3TdR$ treatment

**Table 1.** The antiviral activity ($ED_{99}$) against the McKrae strain of HSV 1 and cytotoxicity ($LD_{50}$) in Chang conjunctival cells

| Antiviral | $ED_{99}$ (µM) | $LD_{50}$ (µM) |
|---|---|---|
| ARA-T | 4.4 | 32.6 |
| $F_3TdR$ | 6.3 | 8.3 |
| ACG | 8.1 | > 100 |
| IUdR | 44.0 | 27.6 |
| AIU | 86.3 | > 100 |
| ARA-A+ | 94.4 | 55.0 |
| ARA-AMP | 130.0 | 63.3 |
| Retinoic Acid | 190.0 | > 100 |
| CMA | | > 1000 |

+ Indicates the presence of adenosine deaminase inhibitor R-3 (2 deoxy-β-D-erythro-pentofuranosyl) – 3, 6, 7, 8 – tetrahydroimidazo [4,5d] [1,3] diazepin-8-ol at 1 µg/ml

on corneal lesion scores is shown in Fig. 1. One percent solutions of ARA-T and $F_3TdR$ significantly reduced the lesion scores and increased the healing rates of corneal lesions as compared to nontreated and placebo treated controls. On the 6th and 7th day after infection, the $F_3TdR$ lesions were significantly better than those treated with ARA-T. A comparison of 1% $F_3TdR$ ointment, 3% ACG ointment, and 1% ARA-T drops all given five times per day at 2 hour intervals indicated that all three compounds were equally effective (Fig. 2). The administration of ARA-T intravenously at a concentration of 5 mg/kg four times per day did not result in a significant decrease in corneal lesion scores (Fig. 3). Epithelial lesions of the intravenously treated rabbits healed to the same degree as the controls after 10 days; however, nine of ten eyes examined had severe disciform keratitis. In vitro incubations of rabbit serum with $10^{-4}M$ ARA-T did not result in significant cleavage of ARA-T to thymine and arabinose (Fig. 4).

CMA, a low molecular weight inducer of interferon was effective in reducing the lesion scores in rabbits as compared to saline treated controls (Fig. 5a, b) only if treatment was begun soon after infection. CMA administration begun within 2 h after infection with either the McKrae or RE strain of HSV 1 showed a moderate but significant reduction of lesion scores. CMA treatment of established corneal lesions produced by the McKrae strain of virus, did not result in

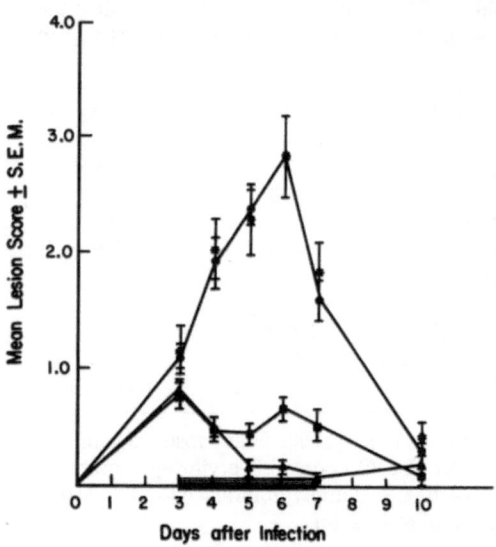

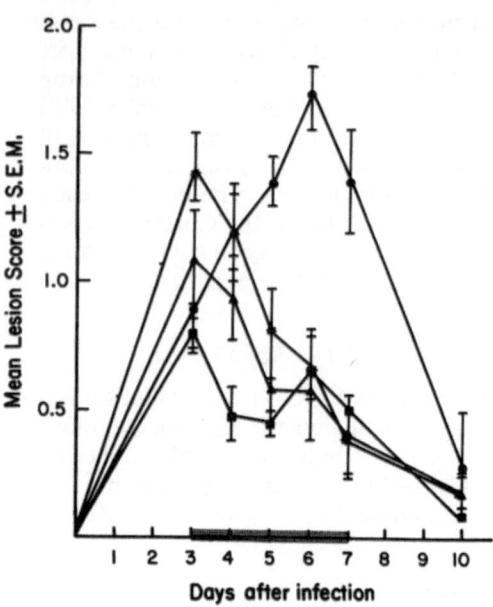

**Fig. 1.** The effect of topically applied solutions of ARA-T and $F_3$TdR on corneal lesion scores. Rabbit corneas were infected on day 0 with $10^6$ pfu of the McKrae strain of HSV 1. Treatment was initiated on the 3rd day after infection and continued for 4 days as indicated by the shaded area on the abscissa. Two drops were given to each eye five times per day at 2 h intervals. Each point represents the mean lesion score ± the standard error of the mean (N = 20). (*) No treatment, (●) vehicle, (■) 1% ARA-T, (▲) 1% $F_3$TdR

**Fig. 2.** The effect of topically applied ointments of ACG and $F_3$TdR on corneal lesion scores as compared to ARA-T solutions. Rabbit corneas were infected with $10^6$ pfu of the McKrae strain of HSV 1 and treatment was initiated 3 days later. Each drug was administered five times per day at 2 h intervals. Treatment was continued for 5 days as indicated by the shaded area on the abscissa. Each point represents the mean lesion score ± the standard error of the mean (N = 10). (●) Placebo ointment, (▲) 1% $F_3$TdR, (*) 3% ACG, (■) 1% ARA-T

significant reduction of lesion scores (Fig. 6). The treatment groups in which CMA therapy was initiated 3 days after infection were found to have significantly worse scores than saline treated controls by the 10th day after infection. The corneas of CMA treated animals had stromal edema and 360° pannus formation. Rabbits which were not infected but received one drop of 10% CMA hourly, nine times per day for 7 days, showed no obvious signs of ocular toxicity.

Treatment of established corneal lesions topically 0.1% retinoic acid in a sesame oil with vehicle resulted in a significant reduction in mean lesion scores as compared to saline treated group (Fig. 7). The reduction in lesion scores of the retinoic acid treated groups were not significantly better than those treated with sesame oil alone. The eyes of the animals receiving 0.1% retinoic acid in sesame oil showed no signs of ocular toxicity.

## Discussion

The relative antiviral activity of the three nucleoside analogues examined in these studies varied over a two-fold range in vitro and was nearly equal in vivo. None of the three compounds produced gross signs of ocular toxicity when applied topically. In cell culture, however, our studies have shown that ACG is clearly the least toxic of the three compounds while $F_3$TdR is the most toxic. The cell culture system used in these studies was designed to measure toxicity in rapidly growing cultures in which anabolic processes are high. Therefore, one would anticipate maximal toxicity. The role of anabolic enzymes such as cellular thymidine kinase in $F_3$TdR toxicity was examined by Wigdahl [25]. His studies indicated that nongrowing mouse L cells were at least 1000-fold less sensitive to $F_3$TdR than actively growing cells.

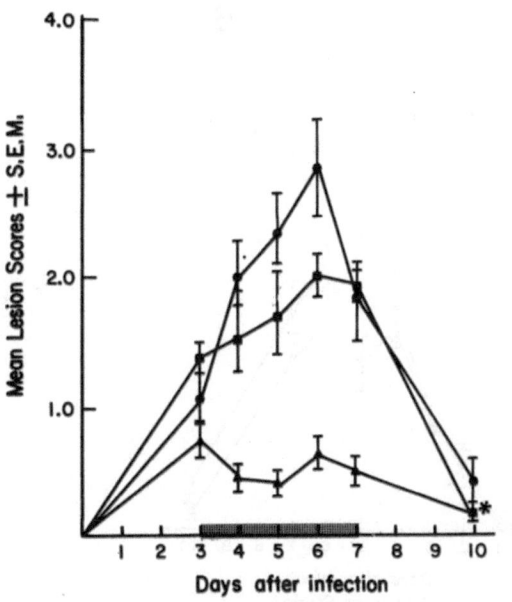

Fig. 3. Comparison of corneal lesion scores in rabbits treated topically with 1% ARA-T versus intravenous ARA-T. Rabbit corneas were infected with $10^6$ pfu of the McKrae strain of HSV 1. Both topical and intravenous treatment was initiated 3 days after infection and continued for 5 days as indicated by the shaded area of the abscissa. Each point represents the mean lesion score ± the standard error of the mean (N = 10). (●) No treatment (▲) 1% ARA-T topical, (■) 5 mg/kg I.V. ARA-T

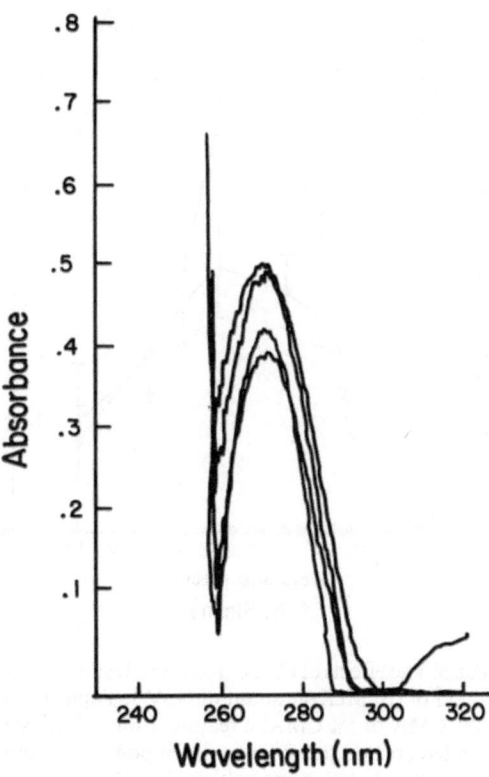

Fig. 4. The ultraviolet absorbance spectra of ARA-T in rabbit serum. ARA-T was incubated in rabbit serum at 37 °C. At time intervals of 0, 1, 2, 4, 8, 12 h aliquots were taken and adjusted to pH 12.0 for spectral analysis. All spectra indicate a λ max of 268 nm

The differences in toxicity were most likely due to the fact that $F_3TdR$ is poorly anabolized by nongrowing cells while it is actively metabolized by rapidly growing corneal and conjunctival epithelial tissues [19]. ARA-T unlike $F_3TdR$ has been reported to be resistant to metabolism in noninfected animals and cells [1]. The resistance of ARA-T to catabolism by pyrimidine nucleoside phosphorylase suggested that it may be useful for systemic therapy to reduce the establishment of trigeminal ganglia infections which may result from herpetic keratitis. Our data indicate that intravenous treatment with ARA-T resulted in severe disciform keratitis and corneal edema. Presently it is unclear whether the ocular complications were caused by systemic toxicity or suppression of the host immune response. Studies by Aswell et al. [1] indicate that larger systemic doses

than used in these studies were not toxic to mice. Recently, however, ARA-T was shown to reduce the ability of lymphocytes to respond to mitogen stimulation thereby suggesting that it was immunosuppressive [3].

Chemotherapy of herpetic keratitis with the low molecular weight interferon inducer, CMA, produced statistically significantly lower lesion scores than saline treated controls. Clinically the small degree of reduction and the need for treatment before appearance of lesions limit its value. Other interferon inducers and interferon itself have also been shown to be effective only if given prophylactically or very soon after virus infection. CMA has been shown to be an extremely potent interferon inducer in mice [23], however, only very low levels of interferon can be detected in rabbits (data not shown). These results

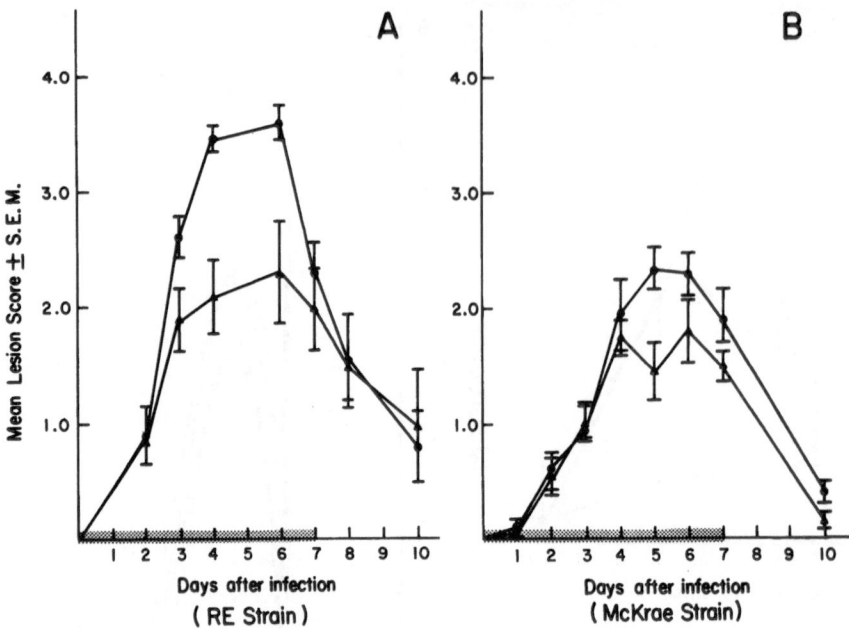

**Fig. 5.** The effects of CMA on corneal lesion scores. Rabbits were infected with $10^6$ pfu of either the (A) RE strain of (B) McKrae strain of HSV 1. Topical treatment was initiated 2 hours after infection with either 10% CMA or 5% CMA. Treatment was administered five times per day for the 7 days as shown by the shaded area on the abscissa. Each point represents the mean lesion score ± standard error of the mean (N = 10). (A) [●] saline vehicle, [▲] 10% CMA (B) [●] saline vehicle, [▲] 5% CMA

suggest that low molecular inferferon inducers have potential as antiviral agents, however, they must be evaluated in many animal species.

The data presented here suggest that retinoic acid may be of potential value in treating herpetic keratitis. Our data suggest that the virucidal effects of the long chain length fatty acids contained in the sesame oil are equally as effective in reducing corneal lesion scores as oil supplemented with 0.1% retinoic acid. Our in vitro studies, however, clearly show the virucidal activity of retinoic acid. Studies are currently in progress to evaluate the efficacy of higher concentrations of retinoic acid on lesion scores and ganglia latency. Retinoic acid (≈ 40,000 IU/kg) administered intraperitoneally has been observed to produce milder, more rapidly healing epithelial lesions, with minimal stromal complications in a chronic herpetic keratitis model [21]. The mechanism responsible for the virucidal or antiviral properties are presently speculative at best. The numerous biological properties associated with retinoids such as immunological penetration, inhibition of interferon production, stimulation of cell division, and antineoplastic properties yield a very complex mechanistic picture [4, 10, 21, 22, 24].

Currently nucleoside analogues provide the most effective means of reducing the severity of a corneal lesion produced by HSV 1. No compounds are currently available to reduce the frequency of recurrence. In experimental models, prolonged treatment with ACG has been shown to reduce the frequency with which virus can be cultured from ganglionic tissue [20], however, no evidence exists for a reduction of recurrence in patients. Other forms of therapy may hold the potential to solve the critical problems of acute, chronic, and recurrent infections, however, substantial work remains to be done.

**Acknowledgment.** Supported in part by grants EY-02834 and EY 01931 from the National Eye Institute (UPHS) and an unrestricted grant from Research to Prevent Blindness, Inc.

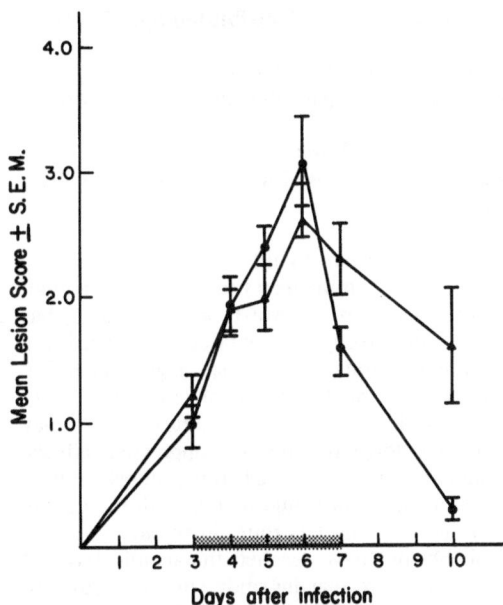

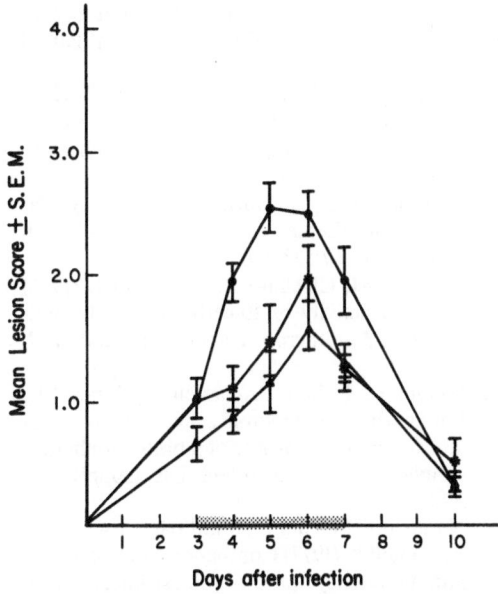

**Fig. 6.** Effects of CMA on established HSV corneal lesions. Rabbits were infected with $10^6$ pfu of the McKrae strain of HSV 1 and topical treatment with 5% CMA was initiated three days after infection. Therapy was continued for 4 days as shown by the shaded area on the abscissa. Each point represents the mean lesion score ± standard error of the mean (N = 10), (●) Saline vehicle, (▲) 5% CMA

**Fig. 7.** The therapeutic effect of retinoic acid on herpetic keratitis. Corneas were infected with $10^6$ pfu of the McKrae strain of HSV 1 and topical treatment with 0.1% retinoic acid was initiated 3 days after infection. Treatment was given five times per day for 5 days as indicated by the shaded area on the abscissa. Each point represents the mean (N = 10). (●) Saline, (*) sesame oil vehicle, (▲) sesame oil containing 0.1% retinoic acid

## References

1. Aswell JF, Allen GP, Jamieson AT, Campbell DE, Gentry GA (1977) Antiviral activity of arabinosylthymine in herpes viral replication: mechanism of action in vivo and in vitro. Antimicrob Agents Chemother 12:243–254
2. Auperin D, Reinhardt A, Sands J, Snipes W (1980) Characterization of virucidal activities of retinoids. In: Nelsen JD, Grass C (eds) Current chemotherapy and infectious disease, vol 2. American Society for Microbiology Press, Washington DC, pp 1368–1369
3. Barnett JM, McGowan JJ, Gentry GA (1979) Arabinosylthymidine: inhibitor of splenic lymphocyte macromolecular synthesis in vitro. Infect Immun 26:294–297
4. Blalock JE, Gifford GE (1977) Retinoic acid (vitamin A acid) induced transcriptional control of interferon production. Proc Natl Acad Sci USA 74:5382–5386
5. Centifanto YM, Goorha RM, Kaufman HE (1970) Interferon induction after poly I:C in rabbit and human tears. Am J Ophthalmol 70:1006–1009
6. Chang RS (1954) Continuous subcultivation of epithelial-like cells from normal human tissues. Proc Soc Exp Biol Med 87:440–443
7. Cheng YC, Goz B, Neenan JP, Ward DC, Prusoff WH (1975) Selective inhibition of herpes simplex virus by 5-amino-2, 5-dideoxy-5-iodouridine. J Virol 15:1284–1285
8. Drewinko B, Roper RP, Barlogie B (1979) Patterns of cell survival following treatment with antitumor agents in vitro. Eur J Cancer 15:93–99
9. Elion GB, Furman PA, Fyfe JA, Miranda P de, Beauchamp L, Schaeffer HJ (1977) Selectivity of action of an antiherpetic agent, 9-(2-hydroxyethoxymethyl) guanine. Proc Natl Acad Sci USA 74:5716–5720
10. Felix EL, Loyd B, Cohen MH (1975) Inhibition of growth and development of transplantable murine melanoma by vitamin A. Science 189:886–888
11. Kaufman HE, Ellison ED, Centifanto YM (1972) Difference in interferon response and protection from virus infection in rabbits and monkeys. Am J Ophthalmol 74:89–92
12. Kaufman HE, Ellison ED, Waltman SR (1969)

Doublestranded RNA, interferon inducer, in herpes simplex keratitis. Am J Ophthalmol 68:486–491

13. Kaufman HE, Martola E, Dohlman C (1962) Use of 5-iodo-2'-deoxyuridine (IDU) in treatment of herpes simplex keratitis. Arch Ophthalmol 68:235–239
14. Kaufman HE, Nesburn AB, Maloney DE (1962) IDU therapy of herpes simplex. Arch Ophthalmol 67:583–591
15. Kramer MJ, Cleeland R, Grunberg E (1976) Antiviral activity of 10-carboxymethyl-9-acridanone. Antimicrob Agents Chemother 9: 233–238
16. McGill JI, Collins P, Cantell K, Jones BR, Finter NB (1976) Optimal schedules for use of interferon in the corneas of rabbits with herpes simplex keratitis. J Infect Dis (suppl) 133: A13–A17
17. Neumann-Haefelin D, Sundmacher R, Skoda R, Cantell K (1977) Comparative evaluation of human leucocyte and fibroblast interferon in prevention of herpes simplex virus keratitis in a monkey model. Infect Immun 17:468–470
18. Nichol FR, Weed SD, Underwood GE (1976) Stimulation of murine interferon by a substituted pyrimidine. Antimicrob Agents Chemother 9:433–439
19. O'Brien WJ (1979) The metabolism of trifluorothymidine by cells of the rabbit cornea. Exp Eye Res 29:619–624
20. Pavan-Langston D, Park NH, Lass JH (1979) Herpetic ganglionic latency. Arch Ophthalmol 97:1508–1510
21. Smolin G, Okumoto M, Friedlaender M, Kwok S (1979) Herpes simplex keratitis treatment with vitamin A. Arch Ophthalmol 97: 2181–2183
22. Sporn MB, Clamon GH, Dunlop NM, Newton DL, Smith JM, Saffiotti U (1975) Activity of vitamin A analogues in cell cultures of mouse epidermis and organ cultures of hamster trachea. Nature 253:47–50
23. Taylor JL, Schoenherr C, Grossberg SE (1980) Carboxymethylacridanone, a potent interferon inducer and antiviral agent. In: Nelsen JD, Grass C (eds) Current chemotherapy and infectious disease, vol 2. American Society for Microbiology Press, Washington DC, pp 1604–1605
24. Yamemoto V, Bister K, Hausen H zur (1979) Retinoic acid inhibition of Epstein-Barr virus induction. Nature 278:553–554
25. Wigdahl BL (1979) Inhibition of HEp-2 cell, mouse L cell, and herpes simplex virus type 1 replication by 5-trifluoromethyl-2'-deoxyuridine: role of cellular and HSV-1-induced deoxythymidine kinases. PhD Thesis. The Medical College of Wisconsin, Milwaukee WI

## Discussion on the Contribution pp. 255–262

R. Wigand (Homburg/Saar)
From which company did you get your Ara-T?

W.J. O'Brien (Milwaukee)
Raylow Chemicals Ltd., Edmonton, Alberta Canada

Y.C. Cheng (Chapel Hill)
I just want to comment on your systemic treatment of keratitis by using Ara-T, which, indeed, has some immuno-suppressive effect when used in a high concentration in guinea pigs. These are observations which were recently made by Gentry and coworkers; but at a therapeutic dosage, it may not have longterm immunosuppressive effects. That is one point to be taken into consideration. The second point would be that with the dosage you used (5 mg/kg; four times/day) you will probably not have reached therapeutic levels. I think, therefore, that this study, concerning the systemic use of Ara-T for treatment of herpes keratitis, is too premature at the moment to draw valid conclusions.

B.R. Jones (London)
Could I ask what concentration of retinoic acid you applied topically and whether, if you continued such applications, you get into a range of toxic effects on the corneal epithelium?

W.J. O'Brien (Milwaukee)
We applied 0,1% retinoic acid in a sesame oil vehicle. This concentration didn't produce any gross signs of ocular toxicity. We haven't looked to see if DNA or protein synthesis are altered in the epithelial cells of treated animals.

G. Smolin (San Francisco)
I was wondering which form you used. The 13 Cis or all-trans form. Secondly, since the retinoic acid enhances epidermal cell DNA synthesis was the effect you observed due to cell turnover or a direct effect on the virus?

W.J. O'Brien (Milwaukee)
We used all trans-retinoic acid made in sesame oil. It was stored in a dark bottle under nitrogen. We continually checked the absorption spectra in order to determine if the compound retained its proper λ max.

As far as the mechanism of action of retinoic acid, I'm really not sure. The effects of retinoic acid on DNA synthesis are very concentration dependent. It's hard to say what is happening at the molecular level, the mechanism of the antiviral activity of retinoic acid certainly is something worth investigating.

Sundmacher, R. (Hrsg.):
Herpetische Augenerkrankungen
© J.F. Bergmann Verlag, München 1981

# Adverse Reactions in the Eye From Topical Therapy With Idoxuridine, Adenine Arabinoside and Trifluorothymidine

M.G. Falcon, B.R. Jones, H.P. Williams, K. Wilhelmus, D.J. Coster, London

**Key words.** Antiviral drugs, toxicity, hypersensitivity

**Schlüsselwörter.** Antivirale Medikamente, Toxizität, Überempfindlichkeit

**Summary.** In this paper we describe the incidence and the factors associated with the development of hypersensitivity and toxicity to IDU, AraA and $F_3T$. We review the clinical features of antiviral toxicity, which included an ischaemic reaction in the conjunctiva which was associated with $F_3T$ therapy. We conclude with a discussion of the mechanisms of antiviral toxicity.

**Zusammenfassung.** Auf der Basis von über tausend Krankengeschichten von Patienten, die bei uns während der letzten zehn Jahre Virustatika lokal erhielten, berichten wir über die Häufigkeit einer Toxizität von oder einer Überempfindlichkeit gegen IDU, Ara-A sowie TFT und gehen dabei auch auf die Faktoren ein, die eine solche Entwicklung fördern. Zu den Formen der antiviralen Toxizität gehört auch eine ischämische Bindehautreaktion bei TFT-Therapie. Die verschiedenen Mechanismen einer Virustatika-Toxizität werden diskutiert.

## Introduction

Although it is widely known that local hypersensitivity reactions, and a variety of local toxic reactions may occur as a result of topical therapy with Idoxuridine (IDU), Adenine Arabinoside (AraA) and Trifluorothymidine ($F_3T$) [1–5], there has been no detailed enquiry to assess these considerable problems in man in full. Their clinical features have been described, but their incidence, and the factors which may lead to their development, and their outcome, have not been fully investigated.

This paper presents our experience in treating over 1000 patients during recent years who have suffered from herpes simplex eye disease, and who have been treated with one or more antiviral compound. We indicate the incidence and clinical features of hypersensitivity reactions to IDU, AraA and $F_3T$. We assess the incidence of toxic reactions to these three antivirals, and describe their clinical features, which include a serious and unexpected manifestation of toxicity of $F_3T$.

## Methods

We used our Herpes Simplex Coding System [6], to obtain details of patients in our care who had suffered from hypersensitivity or toxic reactions to antiviral; where possible we compared the records of other patients who had not suffered from these adverse reactions. Unless indicated otherwise, all these patients received at least a full therapeutic course of antiviral, which consisted of the administration of one or other antiviral compound five times daily for at least 10 days.

IDU was used in a 0.5% ointment of BPC ointment base (liquid paraffin 10%, woolfat 10%, yellow soft paraffin 80%), which was prepared by Moorfields Eye Hospital Pharmacy. IDU drops have been used only briefly in a few of our patients, and have not been associated with hypersensitivity or toxic reactions. AraA was used in a 3% ointment as now marketed by Parke-Davis under the name ViraA. $F_3T$ was used as a 1% solution containing 1% $F_3T$, 0.9% sodium chloride, 0.005% Thiomersal and water to 100, with a pH between 4 and 6.5. It was prepared by Moorfields Eye Hospital Pharmacy.

## Results

### Local Hypersensitivity Reactions

The local hypersensitivity reactions to antiviral did not differ in their clinical features from contact dermatitis due to other topical therapy, and there were occasional difficulties in determining the sensitising agent when several drugs were being applied. In our patients there was typically an acute onset of a moist itchy erythematous reaction on the lids and adjacent skin, with subsequent scaling during resolution. These reactions did not occur in less than 8 days of antiviral therapy, except in previously sensitised individuals, and resolved in 3 to 8 weeks (often aided by the application of steroid cream to the skin). Of 550 patients using one or more courses of IDU, 45 developed local hypersensitivity (8%). For AraA the figures were 270 and 2 (0.4%), and for $F_3T$ they were 400 and 18 (4.6%). These comparisons should be viewed with caution, however, since in general IDU was used for longer than was AraA or $F_3T$, and it is to be expected that hypersensitivity reactions become more likely in an individual as the duration of the treatment is extended. Two patients were sensitive to both IDU and $F_3T$. In two patients there was a sensitivity to ointment base, but in none was there clear evidence that preservative was to blame.

### Toxic Reactions

#### IDU

Of the 550 patients receiving 710 courses of treatment with IDU, toxic reactions developed in 66 (12% of patients). These reactions have become less common and less severe in recent years because of the availability of alternative antivirals, which obviate the need for prolonged therapy with IDU. Apart from one patient who had had treatment with $F_3T$ thrice daily for 7 weeks immediately preceding the commencement of IDU therapy, all patients had had IDU treatment only. The earliest toxic reaction occurred $3\frac{1}{2}$ weeks after the initiation of IDU treatment five times a day and the latest occurred 11 months after IDU treatment had begun. The mean interval between commencement of therapy and development of toxicity was 4 months. There was no clear relationship between the frequency and duration of IDU treatment and the development of toxicity, but in general early toxicity resulted from intensive IDU therapy and affected principally the conjunctival and corneal epithelium, whereas protracted and usually less intensive treatment led in addition to changes in the lids and puncta. All but 8 of 66 patients required their IDU treatment to cover steroid therapy which was given for inflammatory herpetic disease.

A punctate epitheliopathy of the conjunctiva and cornea was the first sign of IDU toxicity in all our cases, and was manifest in several patients by the failure of an ulcer to heal, in spite of the absence of signs of continuing viral activity in the ulcer edge or the presence of stromal disease. Indeed, IDU toxicity was sometimes implicated as an important factor in the development of indolent (metaherpetic) ulceration. The punctate epitheliopathy was reversible in all of our patients, clearing generally within 6 to 8 weeks, in spite of the substitution of AraA or $F_3T$ therapy for IDU therapy. The signs of more chronic toxicity, namely conjunctival infiltration, follicular reaction and lid margin keratinisation, were reversible, whereas punctal occlusion was permanent in 7 of 14 patients who developed it.

#### AraA

Of the 270 patients who had 310 courses of AraA therapy, nine developed a toxic reaction (3%). Three other patients experienced discomfort in the eye following the administration of AraA ointment, which was severe enough in one to prevent the continuation of this treatment. Three patients had had treatment with another antiviral before commencing AraA therapy: one had had $F_3T$ for the previous 3 months (without toxicity), and developed AraA toxicity 10 weeks later. The second patient, who had a reduced tear film, had had IDU toxicity and $F_3T$ toxicity previously. She developed AraA toxicity on two occasions 3 weeks after using AraA five times daily. The third patient had had a brief course of IDU, to which there was no therapeutic response. When AraA was substituted, toxicity occurred 3 weeks later. The earliest toxic reaction occurred 2 weeks after the initiation of AraA therapy five times a day; the latest toxic reaction occurred after 17 weeks' AraA therapy. The mean interval between commencement of therapy and development of toxicity was 7 weeks. Many other patients have received more AraA treatment over a longer period of time without showing any sign of toxicity.

The clinical features of AraA toxicity in our patients were as follows: A punctate epitheliopathy of conjunctiva and cornea was present in all nine patients, and cleared in each case within 6 weeks, in spite of the use of an alternative antiviral in five patients. The epitheliopathy was considered to contribute to metaherpetic ulceration in three patients including one in whom a deposit of ointment collected in the ulcer base. We did not find punctal occlusion or lid changes in any of the nine patients.

## $F_3T$

Of the 400 patients who received 560 courses of $F_3T$ therapy, toxic reactions occurred in 18 (4.5%), and three patients suffered a neuralgia-like discomfort in and around the eye after instillation of $F_3T$, which caused them to stop treatment. Ten patients had received IDU prior to using $F_3T$: the interval between the end of IDU treatment and the start of $F_3T$ treatment varied between 8 and 0 months, and the duration of prior IDU treatment was 1 to 6 months. One patient was suffering from IDU toxicity (punctate epitheliopathy) at the time of starting $F_3T$, and this improved for the first 3 weeks, before an increase in the signs of toxicity was observed, attributable to $F_3T$.

There were two principle types of toxic response to $F_3T$: a marked corneal epitheliopathy, sometimes with diffuse epithelial oedema, occurring in a total of six patients within 4–25 days of starting intensive $F_3T$ treatment (ie. two-hourly); and a response to longer-term treatment, occurring in the remaining 12 patients who had received one to four daily drops of $F_3T$ for between 1 and 12 months (mean $4\frac{1}{2}$ months), who developed punctate lesions in the conjunctival and corneal epithelium (seven patients) or punctal occlusion (seven patients). These changes occurred together in two patients. The epitheliopathy, whether of the acute or chronic form, cleared in all patients in 3–10 weeks, but punctal occlusion was permanent in four patients. $F_3T$ was implicated in the production of metaherpetic changes in one of

the patients, who also had a diffuse toxic epitheliopathy.

The substitution of AraA for $F_3T$ allowed the toxic signs to improve (but not always the punctal occlusion), with the exception of one patient, who developed AraA toxicity on two occasions 3 weeks after the change of treatment.

One patient, who had previously suffered from $F_3T$-induced punctal stenosis, developed an acute ischaemic reaction in the conjunctiva. Prior to the development of this response, she had been receiving two or three drops of $F_3T$ daily for 4 months (as antiviral cover for steroid therapy for refractory herpetic keratouveitis). During the ensuing week the conjunctiva was noted to be swollen and oedematous, with extensive vessel closure mainly the lower bulbar and lower tarsal conjunctiva. These conjunctival changes were suggestive more of extrinsic toxicity than of intrinsic disease, and the diagnosis rested between $F_3T$ toxicity and artefacta; the latter was initially considered to be more likely, but was later excluded. On withdrawal of all topical therapy of 10 days, the conjunctival appearances began to improve. A vigorous neovascularisation of the ischaemic tissue followed, and there was the expected rebound of keratouveitis. Topical steroids and AraA were commenced, which brought this, and the exuberant neovascularisation, under control.

Two conjunctival biopsies were performed 20 days after the onset of the ischaemic response. The specimens were reported by Professor Alec Garner as follows:

"Sections of the clinically avascular bulbar conjunctiva show an epithelial layer which is marginally hyperplastic with an absence of goblet cells: there is also a hint of keratinisation of the most superficial cells. The supporting connective tissue includes several thin-walled vascular channels, many of which are devoid of blood cells but there is no sign of tissue infarction. Only a few leucocytes are seen. The appearances are those of incipient epidermalisation.

Sections of the (clinically) relatively healthy conjunctiva show generalised infiltration of the subepithelial stroma by lymphocytes and plasma cells. There is a moderate degree of vascular congestion and the overlying epithelium is markedly atrophic, being reduced to an incomplete unicellular layer in places. None of the few arterioles show evidence of vasculitis and the picture is one of non-specific chronic inflammation with nothing to indicate a 'collagen disease'. No pathogen is detectable in the sections but the possibility of a response to external irritation cannot be ruled out."

There was a continued clinical improvement during the following 3 months, and a further conjunctival biopsy at the end of that time was reported by Professor Alec Garner as follows:

"Histology of the conjunctiva now shows a loose vascularised connective tissue stroma covered by epithelium which in most places is a little acanthotic. Goblet cells are present in apparently normal numbers. There is a mild infiltration of the stroma with diffusely scattered lymphocytes and plasma cells, and in one small focus co-existent polymorphs have invaded the overlying epithelium.

Overall, however, the appearances represent a return to normality, there being much less inflammatory reaction and epithelial damage compared with the earlier specimen."

Two other patients have been brought to our attention independently who have had highly similar manifestations of $F_3T$ toxicity following a prolonged and relatively intensive regimen of $F_3T$.

**Discussion**

This study shows that even in this large series of patients, it was rarely possible to detect a clear relationship between the intensity and duration of treatment, and the development of antiviral toxicity. Probable exceptions are the toxicities from long-term IDU or $F_3T$ therapy, and the early $F_3T$ epitheliopathy. Otherwise, local and individual factors exert more influence; these include factors associated with the use of treatment (ie. the regularity and enthusiasm with which it is applied); local physical factors such as the tear film and the rate of turnover of the epithelial cells; and finally the considerable variability, between individuals, of the rate of drug metabolism − which, if comparable to the known variability in the metabolism of some systemic medication, may be very important.

The mechanism of IDU toxicity is assumed to be through its blocking of thymidine metabolism and incorporation into host DNA, although changes identical to those caused by IDU can be associated with the prolonged administration of preservative [7]. IDU toxicity is now rarer than hitherto, because of the availability of alternative antivirals.

AraA toxicity has been an infrequent and minor problem, which is outweighed in most patients by the severity of their herpetic disease. It may be argued that a low incidence of toxicity to AraA would be expected because of its more specific mode of action in blocking virally-directed DNA polymerase, and thus being only minimally incorporated into host DNA. This may well be the case, but the possibility of unexpected (and inexplicable) drug reactions should be borne in mind − such as were seen with Practolol [8], or in experimental studies with AraAMP [9, 10].

In certain circumstances $F_3T$ is superior to AraA [11] and these considerations may override the slightly greater problems of $F_3T$ toxicity compared with AraA. The early toxic reaction, which can result from intensive $F_3T$ treatment, and which is more common in those who have received IDU before commencing $F_3T$, could be explained on the basis that the metabolic pathways of IDU and $F_3T$ are similar: both block thymidine metabolism, but $F_3T$ has greater solubilities. The clinical features of toxicity from long-term $F_3T$ therapy also differ very little from those caused by IDU, and the figures for the speed of onset and regression are strikingly similar for the two antivirals (Table 1). We have not seen extreme examples of $F_3T$ toxicity, such as were earlier seen with IDU; this may indicate an increasing awareness among ophthalmologists of the possible risks of long-term therapy with one antiviral.

The conjunctival ischaemic response which we have described is difficult to explain. It could have been caused by degradation products of $F_3T$ if the preparation was not fresh, although $F_3T$ solution stored at 2 °C still retains 95% of its $F_3T$ unchanged after 3 months (Watkins R, personal communication). In our patient's case the solutions were freshly made up. It is of interest that an ointment preparation, with the $F_3T$ in particulate form, would have greater stability, although on the other hand there might be greater problems of toxicity from the more prolonged ocular contact time.

**Table 1.** Comparison between certain aspects of toxicity to IDU and F$_3$T. NB. This excludes the acute F$_3$T epitheliopathy

|  | IDU (66 patients) | F$_3$T (12 patients) |
|---|---|---|
| Interval between start of therapy and onset of toxic signs: | | |
| range | 3½ weeks – 11 months | 1 month – 12 months |
| mean | 4 months | 4½ months |
| Time for reversal of signs of toxicty (excluding punctal occlusion) | 3–8 weeks | 3–10 weeks |
| Punctal occlusion: reversed in | 7/14 patients | 3/7 patients |

This unexpected toxic reaction from F$_3$T reminds us that adverse drug reactions can be predicted only to a limited degree by extrapolation from experimental and pharmacological data, and a continued awareness of the possibility of toxicity is required. It is encouraging that our increasing topical ocular use of Acyclovir has so far been associated only with a mild and rapidly reversible punctate epitheliopathy in a small proportion of patients.

**Acknowledgment.** We are grateful to Mr. R. Watkins, Chief Pharmacist, Moorfields Eye Hospital, for advice.

**References**

1. Patterson A, Jones BR (1967) The management of ocular herpes. Trans Ophthalmol Soc UK 87:59–84
2. McGill J, Williams HP, McKinnon JR, Holt-Wilson AD, Jones BR (1974) A reassessment of idoxuridine therapy of herpetic keratitis. Trans Ophthalmol Soc UK 94:542–551
3. Jones BR, McGill JI, McKinnon JR, Holt-Wilson AD, Williams HP (1975) Preliminary experience with Adenine Arabinoside in comparison with Idoxuridine and Trifluorothymidine in the management of Herpetic Keratitis. In: Pavan Langston D, Buchanan RA, Alford jr CA (eds) Adenine Arabinoside; an antiviral agent. Raven, New York, p 411–416
4. McGill J, Holt-Wilson AD, McKinnon JR, Williams HP, Jones BR (1974) Some aspects of the clinical use of Trifluorothymidine in the treatment of herpetic ulceration of the cornea. Trans Ophthalmol Soc UK 94:342–352
5. Falcon MG, Jones BR, Williams HP, Coster DJ (1977) Management of herpetic eye disease. Trans Ophthalmol Soc UK 97:345–349
6. McKinnon J, McGill J, Jones BR (1975) Summary Code for Ocular Herpes Simplex. Br J Ophthalmol 59:539–544
7. Wright P (in press) Squamous metaplasia of the conjunctiva as an adverse reaction to topical medication.
8. Wright P (1975) Untoward effects associated with Practolol administration: oculomuco cutaneous syndrome. Br Med J 1:595
9. Falcon MG, Jones BR (1977) Antivirals for therapy of herpetic eye disease. Trans Ophthalmol Soc UK 97:330–332
10. Foster CS, Pavan Langston D (1977) Corneal wound healing and antiviral medication. Arch Ophthalmol 95:2062
11. Coster DJ, Jones BR, McGill JI (1979) Treatment of Amoeboid Herpetic Ulcers with adenine arabinoside or trifluorothymidine. Br J Ophthalmol 63:418–421

**Discussion on the Contribution pp. 263–267**

O.P. van Bijsterveld (Utrecht)
I want to ask you if the dryness you observed in the eyes that were treated with virostatic drugs could, in fact, be due to the herpes infection itself, as was discussed this morning?

M.G. Falcon (London)
Certainly. We did not wish to imply that it was due to the treatment.

J. Wollensak (Berlin)
Why were the antivirals used for such a long time?

M.G. Falcon (London)
Almost invariably, it was for antiviral cover for patients receiving steroid therapy.

R. Sundmacher (Freiburg)

I feel that dry eyes are a major contributing cause for the development of antiviral toxicity. We, therefore, very often combine artificial tears with antivirals.

There are, of course, other reasons for reaching the threshold of toxicity. I have been treating, for instance, a patient whose epithelium just fell off, and then we detected that the pH of the commercially available TFT was only 3.3. In another case which looked quite similar, the pH was 4.8, which is much better; but this patient had severe diabetes with resultant metabolic disturbance in the epithelium. There are certainly lots of other reasons why antivirals in certain patients may turn out to be toxic and we will not always be able to suspect the cause or causes.

M.G. Falcon (London)

Could I add that the stability of $F_3T$ is certainly a problem – at least when it's in solution. After 3 months, even if it's kept at 2 °C, 5% of the $F_3T$ has been broken down into potentially toxic products.

J. McGill (Southampton)

Have you seen dry eyes produced by AraA or $F_3T$? I've noticed that with IDU-induced dry eyes you can tell when the toxicity is going because the patients complain of watering eyes. Have you found that?

M.G. Falcon (London)

Occasionally. Of course it can be due to punctal problems too.

W.H. Prusoff (New Haven)

I guess I'm concerned with the fact that 5-trifluoro-methyl-2'-deoxyuridine (Trifluorothymidine) even at neutral pH will breakdown to 5-carboxy-2'-deoxyuridine which now can give you a low pH.

M.G. Falcon (London)

The Moorfields $F_3T$ is made up at pH 4–6.5, because it tends to be more stable in acid solution. Some patients find it very uncomfortable (even if it's quite fresh) and were unable to continue with it.

W.H. Prusoff (New Haven)

It's hard to keep sterile too.

D. Easty (Bristol)

Do you have any comments to make about differences between the use of ointment and drops. IDU as drops I found were less toxic. Your comparison when you use ointment and drops might have less validity based on the difference in formulation. Do you think that drops are less toxic?

M.G. Falcon (London)

We used IDU ointment because it seems to be easier for patients to use that five times a day rather than using drops every hour or two. In view of other comments I wonder if we should be using $F_3T$ ointment rather than drops.

D. Easty (Bristol)

Our experience with $F_3T$ ointment was that it seemed to be less effective than the drops.

Sundmacher, R. (Hrsg.):
Herpetische Augenerkrankungen
© J.F. Bergmann Verlag, München 1981

# The Cytotoxicity of Nucleoside Antivirals to Epithelial Cells of Ocular Origin

J.L. Taylor, W.J. O'Brien, Milwaukee

**Key words.** Nucleosides, antiviral drugs, cytotoxicity, epithelial cells

**Schlüsselwörter.** Nukleoside, antivirale Medikamente, Zytotoxizität, Epithelzellen

**Summary.** The toxicity of several antiviral agents was tested in Chang conjunctival cells, an epithelial cell line originating from normal human conjunctiva. The antivirals tested were the nucleoside analogues: 9-β-D-arabinofuranosyladenine (ARA-A), 9-β-D-arabinofuranosyladenine-5'-monophosphate (ARA-AMP), 1-β-D-arabinofuranosylthymine (ARA-T), 5-iodo-2'-deoxyuridine (IUdR), 5'-amino-2', 5' dideoxy-5-iodouridine (AIU) 5-trifluoromethyl-2'-deoxyuridine (F$_3$TdR) and 9-(2-hydroxyethoxymethyl) guanine (ACG).

The relative toxicity of these compounds was measured by inhibition of growth in the presence of the nucleoside analogues and reduced viability as measured by plating efficiency after drug exposure. These studies established the relative order of toxicity as follows: ACG $\leq$ AIU $\ll$ ARA-A $\leq$ ARA-T $\leq$ ARA-AMP $<$ IUdR $<$ F$_3$TdR. The toxicity of ARA-A and ARA-AMP were enhanced by the addition of adenosine deaminase inhibitors. Several major catabolic products of IUdR, F$_3$TdR, and ARA-A were found to have no toxicity for Chang conjunctival cells.

**Zusammenfassung.** Die Toxizität von Nucleosid-Analoga, die sich bei der Therapie einer Herpeskeratitis als wirksam erwiesen haben, wurde in vitro an Hand der Wachstumshemmung und der Auswachsrate von Chang-Bindehautzellen ermittelt. Es handelt sich hierbei um eine kontinuierliche Zellinie vom Menschen. Die Toxizitätsspanne reichte von fehlender Toxizität des 9-(2-Hydroxethoxymethyl)Guanin (Acyclo-G) in einer Konzentration von 10$^{-4}$ M bis zu totalem Zelluntergang durch 5-Trifluoromethyl-2'-Deoxyuridin (F$_3$TdR) in einer Konzentration von 10$^{-5}$ M. Mit 10$^{-4}$ M 5'-Amino-2'-5'-, Dideoxy-5-Iodo-

uridin (AIU) konnte keine Toxizität beobachtet werden, wohingegen 10$^{-5}$ M 5-Iodo-2'-deoxyuridin (IDU) nach dreitägiger Einwirkung die Auswachs-Effizienz um 70% reduzierte. Die Zytotoxizität des 1-β-D-Arabinofuranosylthymin (ARA-T) war geringer als die des IDU, aber größer als die des 9-β-D Arabinofuranosyladenin (ARA-A). ARA-A war weniger toxisch als ARA-AMP, aber toxischer als Acyclo-G. Die Zugabe eines Adenin-Deaminasen-Inhibitor zum Kulturmedium führte zu einem totalen Zelluntergang der Kulturen sowohl mit 10$^{-4}$ M ARA-A oder ARA-AMP. Dies ist eine Konzentration, bei der ohne Inhibitor nur eine geringe Toxizität erreicht wird.

Die Pathomechanismen, über die Nucleosid-Analoga eine Zytotoxizität induzieren, stehen oft in unmittelbarem Zusammenhang mit dem Zustand des Wirtszellstoffwechsels. Unsere Untersuchungen zeigen, daß F$_3$TdR von normalen Hornhautepithelzellen verstoffwechselt und auch in die DNA mit einer Frequenz eingebaut wird, die etwa 30% derjenigen exogenen Thymidins entspricht. Auch Abbauprodukte muß man bei der Entwicklung einer Toxizität in Erwägung ziehen. Zwei solcher F$_3$TdR Abbauprodukte, 5-Carboxy-2'-Deoxyuridin und 5 Carboxyuracil waren aber bei Konzentrationen bis zu 10$^{-4}$ M nicht toxisch. Iodouracil, ein Metabolit des IDU war ebenfalls für Chang-Conjunctivalzellen in Kultur atoxisch. Das gleiche trifft für 10$^{-4}$ M Arabinofuranosylhypoxanthin (ARA-Hx) zu, ein Metabolit des ARA-A.

Aufgrund dieser Daten läßt sich eine Zytotoxizitäts-Rangordnung von Nucleosidvirustatika bzgl. wachsender epithelialer Zellen okulären Ursprungs aufstellen: ACG $\leq$ AIU $\ll$ ARA-A $\leq$ ARA-T $\leq$ ARA-AMP $<$ IUdR $<$ F$_3$TdR. Die Ergebnisse zeigten weiterhin, daß die Auswachseffizienz von virustatikabehandelten Zellen verglichen mit der von Kontrollzellen das beste Toxizitätskriterium für schädliche Medikamenten-Konzentrationen darstellt.

## Introduction

Nucleoside analogues possessing antiviral

269

activity have been shown to be effective in treating the epithelial stages of herpetic keratitis in man and animals [1, 14–16, 22, 26, 29]. The efficacy and toxicity of such analogues depend on the properties of both the virus and the host. For example, the degree of toxicity of the nucleoside antivirals can often be related to the extent of metabolism of the drug by host-cells. In general, the inability of host tissues to anabolize nucleoside analogues results in increased efficacy and decreased toxicity as demonstrated by recent studies on 9-(2-hydroxyethoxymethyl) guanine (ACG) and 5'-amino-2', 5'dideoxy-5-iodouridine (AIU) [4, 9].

Complete evaluation of cytotoxicity, however, should include both in vivo and in vitro studies. The toxicity of nucleoside antivirals to ocular tissues has been extensively evaluated in vivo in animal systems. The thymidine analogue, 5-iodo-2'-deoxyuridine (IUdR) has been shown to produce punctate keratitis and impaired wound healing in experimental animals [17, 20]. Studies of Hana [12] indicate that IUdR or a metabolite of IUdR is incorporated into the DNA of both corneal and stromal cells in situ, thereby inducing lethal effects. Toxic effects of 5-trifluoromethyl-2'-deoxyuridine ($F_3$-TdR) such as punctate keratitis, impaired re-epithelialization and wound healing have also been reported [13, 18, 19]. Studies in our laboratory indicate that $F_3$TdR is incorporated into the DNA of rapidly corneal growing conjunctival epithelium at about 30% of the rate of exogenous thymidine [21]. The adenine analogue, 9-β-D-arabinofuranosyladenine (ARA-A) has been reported to be less toxic than IUdR and $F_3$TdR to corneal tissue in situ, however, the extent of anabolism of this compound by ocular tissues has not been established [23]. Catabolism of ARA-A in vivo by adenine deaminase present in ocular tissue clearly decreased efficacy and toxicity [24].

In cell culture systems, the metabolism of nucleoside antivirals is a function of the many cell characteristics such as cell type, cultural conditions, growth phase, and nature of the assay system. For example, cell culture studies indicate that adenosine deaminase inhibitors increase the efficiency of ARA-A in HeLa cell systems by fortyfold while having no effect on the activity in Vero cells [32]. These results suggest that cellular adenosine deaminase levels are not the same in these two cell types. Umeda and Heidelberger [31] examined the toxicity of $F_3$TdR and IUdR in cells of human, rat and mouse origin in culture, and detected a 100-fold variation in the toxic levels among the cell lines studied. Similar studies have indicated variations in the $ED_{50}$ of ACG on different indicator cell lines such as LM and Vero [9, 10].

In ocular toxicity studies conducted in vivo, it is often difficult to evaluate the mechanisms responsible for the observed toxic reaction. Often there can be no correlation between in vitro antiviral activities and clinical usefulness unless there is careful design and understanding of the in vitro model [7]. We have sought ocular cell systems in which to study the mechanisms of toxicity of nucleoside antivirals. Currently we are striving to culture corneal and conjunctival epithelial cells. Pure populations of passable epithelial cells which are suitable for cytotoxicity studies have not been obtained. We have been able to evaluate the metabolism and toxicity of nucleoside antivirals by cornea organ culture and with a continuous line of human conjunctival epithelial cells. In these studies we report the comparative toxicity of numerous nucleoside antivirals as measured in cell culture using Chang conjunctival cells (clone 1-5c-4), originally isolated from normal human conjunctiva.

## Materials and Methods

### Cells

Clone 1-5c-4 of Chang conjunctival cells were obtained from Dr. E. Kilborne. These cells were originally isolated from normal human conjunctiva [3]. Cells were grown in Medium 199 containing 10% calf serum and organic buffers, 10 mM BES, 10 mM TES and 15 mM HEPES adjusted to pH 7.1. It should be noted that this cell line is continuous, polypoid, and possesses some HeLa cell marker chromosomes. The cells do grow in D-valine medium, a characteristic of epithelial cell strains [11].

### Measurement of Toxicity

Cells were planted at $10^4$ cells/16 × 125 mm glass tube. After 1 day, medium was replaced with fresh medium with or without drug. Cytotoxicity was monitored daily by three methods.

Cells were washed once and removed from the glass with 0.02% ethylenediamine tetraacetic acid (EDTA) in phosphate buffered saline (PBS). Following centrifugation at 350 xg, the pelleted cells were resuspended in saline and counted using a Coulter counter. The same cultures were assayed for cell viability by staining with Erythrosin B and counting in a hemocytometer [27]. In addition, a portion of the sample was plated in medium without drug to determine plating efficiency and cell viability based on colony formation [8]. Colonies of 30 or more cells as visualized by staining with crystal violet were counted after approximately 14 days. All analyses were done in duplicate.

Growth curves were constructed by plotting cell number as determined by each method vs. time. Individual growth curves were constructed by computerized exponential curve fits in order to calculate generation times. Generation time $\alpha = \dfrac{\log N_1 - \log N_2}{0.301 \,(t_1 - t_2)}$ where: $N_1$ and $N_2$ equal the cell number as determined Coulter counts, hemocytometer counts, or colony counts, while: $t_1$ and $t_2$ represent the time of sampling (hours) of $N_1$ and $N_2$ respectively. Throughout the duration of these experiments, the mean generation time of the Chang cells was 34.2 hr $\pm$ 2.1 ($\overline{X} \pm$ S.E.M.) n = 18.

Reduced viability was measured by the change in colony forming ability as compared to untreated controls. The decrease in viability after exposure of cells to various concentrations of drug for a time equal to three generation times was used as a measure of drug induced toxicity. The percent reduction in viability after the equivalent of three generations times of control was calculated for each drug concentration from computer fit curves constructed by plotting colony forming units vs. time of exposure. $LD_{50}$ was calculated for dose response curves generated by plotting viable cell number after three generations versus drug concentration. $ED_{99}$, the dose required to reduce the yield of infectious virus by 99%, was calculated from curve fits obtained by plotting drug concentration versus virus yield [22].

*High Performance Liquid Chromatography (HPLC)*

HPLC analyses of the tissue culture medium were routinely run in order to analyze the breakdown of the nucleoside antivirals. Analyses were conducted on a Perkin-Elmer Series 3, Model 65 HPLC system equipped with a variable wavelength UV detector. Media samples were deproteinated by perchloric acid percipitation before analysis. Metabolites were chromatographed on either of two systems; 1) Whatman Partsil 10SAX eluted isocratically with butanol: glacial acetic acid: water (2:1:1), 2) Aminex A-10 eluted isocratically with 5 mM $NH_4 HPO_4$ acetonitrile (13/87).

*Compounds*

5-iodo-2'-deoxyuridine (IUdR) was obtained from P·L Biochemicals, Milwaukee, Wisconsin; 5-iodouracil and 2,4-dihydroxy-pyrimidine-5 carboxylic acid (5-carboxyuracil) were from Aldrich Chemical Company, Inc., Milwaukee, Wisconsin; 9-β-D-arabinofuranosyladenine (ARA-A), 9-β-D-arabinofuranosyladenine-5'-monophosphate (ARA-AMP), 9-β-D-arabinofuranosylhypoxanthine (ARA-Hx) and R-3-(2-deoxy-β-D-erythro-pentofuranosyl)-3, 6, 7, 8-tetrahydroimidazo [4, 5d] [1, 3] diazepin-8-ol an adenosine deaminase inhibitor were obtained from Parke-Davis and Company, Ann Arbor, Michigan; 1-β-D-arabino-furanosylthymine (ARA-T) from Raylow Chemicals, Ltd., Edmonton, Alberta, Canada; 5'-amino-2'-5'dideoxy-5-iodouridine (AIU) from Calbiochem-Behring Corporation, LaJolla, California; 9-(2-hydroxyethoxymethyl) guanine (ACG) and 5-trifluoromethyl-2'-deoxyuridine ($F_3$TdR) from Burroughs-Wellcome Company, Research Triangle Park, North Carolina; and 5-carboxy-2'-deoxyuridine (5-COOH-UdR) was prepared in our laboratory by case catalyzed hydrolysis of $F_3$TdR [28] and purified by thin-layer chromatography on MN cellulose developed in butanol: glacial acetic acid: water (2:1:1).

**Results**

*Evaluation of Methods*

All of the cell growth rate data presented in this manuscript was obtained from growth curves constructed by plotting cell numbers determined by colony forming units vs. time. The plating efficiency of untreated Chang conjunctival cells was $100.0 \pm 9.3\%$ (N = 17). The mean correlation coefficient of the exponential curve fits of growth curves for nontreated cells was $0.8588 \pm 0.0303$ (N = 15).

Growth curves and estimates of viability based upon hemocytometer counts and Erythrosin B staining produced highly variable data which defied statistical or any other sort of analysis. Coulter counts were reproducible; however, they could not be used to distinguish between nonviable intact cells and nongrowing cell populations of viable cells. Toxicity in our system can be regarded as any property of a drug which limits a cell's ability to replicate and form a colony.

*Effect of Nucleoside Analogues on Cell Growth and Viability*

Chang conjunctival cells were plated at a low density ($\simeq 10^4$ cells/ml) and allowed to grow in medium containing various concentrations of the nucleoside antivirals. Growth curves were constructed and the generation times calculated from computer fit data. The data indicate that all of the concentrations of ACG tested did not produced no significant alterations in the growth rate when compared to the growth rates of cells grown in the absence of drug (Table 1). The highest nontoxic concen-

tration of ACG examined, 100 µM, was therefore at least twelve times greater than $ED_{99}$ of ACG against the McKrae strain of herpes simplex virus in the Chang cell system. Cell viability, as measured by the ability of the cells to replicate and form colonies after ACG exposure for a time equal to three generation times, was not significantly altered by ACG concentration as high as 100 µM (Table 2).

Similarly AIU at 100 µM caused no increase in the generation time or viability of the cells (Table 1 and 2). The concentration of AIU, which produced a 99% reduction in virus yield, was at least 1.2 times less than the concentration required to show any significant decrease in cell viability.

ARA-A in the presence of adenosine deaminase inhibitor was lethal to Chang cells at 100 µM while having no effect on cell growth or viability at 10 µM (Table 1 and 2). Adenosine deaminase inhibitor (1.0 µg/ml) alone had no detectable effect on cell growth rate or viability. HPLC analysis indicated that in the Chang cell system no detectable ($< 0.05$ µg/ml) ARA-A remained in the culture media after 72 hrs if adenosine deaminase inhibitor was omitted. The addition of the deaminase inhibitor to cell culture media prior to the addition of ARA-A totally inhibited the conversion of ARA-A to ARA-Hx. In the presence of the deaminase inhibitor, the concentration of ARA-A re-

**Table 1.** Effects of nucleoside antivirals on cell generation time

| | % Change in generation time Drug Concentration (µM) | | | |
|---|---|---|---|---|
| Drug | 100 | 10 | 1 | 0.1 |
| ACG | + 23.5 | + 19.0 | − 5.4 | − 3.7 |
| AIU | 13.6 | + 31.7 | | |
| ARA-A† | ∞ * | + 18.2 | | |
| ARA-T | ∞ *C | + 25.6 | + 1.9 | |
| ARA-AMP | ∞ *C | + 36.6 | + 15.0 | + 28 |
| IUdR | ∞ *L | + 74.7* | + 22.7 | + 14.4 |
| F$_3$TdR | ∞ *L | ∞ *L | ∞ *L | − 7.1 |

* Indicates a change in generation time equal to or greater than two standard deviations from that of control cells grown in the absence of drug. Generation time for control cells was 34.2 hr $\pm$ 2.1 ($\overline{X} \pm$ S.E.M.)

+ Indicates increase in generation time and – indicates a decrease in generation time

L Cell lysis and death

C Cytostatic – no change in cell number with time

† Indicates presence of adenosine deaminase inhibitor 1.0 µg/ml R-3 (2-deoxy-β-D-erythro-pentofuranosyl)-3,6,7,8-tetrahydroimidazo [4,5d] [1,3] diazepin-8-01

∞ Indicates no cell growth

**Table 2.** Effects of nucleoside antivirals on cell viability

| | % Viable Drug concentration (µM) | | | |
|---|---|---|---|---|
| Drug | 100 | 10 | 1 | 0.1 |
| ACG | 110 | 107 | 121 | 114 |
| AIU | 120 | 98 | | |
| ARA-A† | 9* | 103 | | |
| ARA-T | 28* | 62 | 97 | |
| ARA-AMP | 0* | 94 | 107 | 95 |
| IUdR | 0* | 29* | 91 | 96 |
| F$_3$TdR | 0* | 4* | 10* | 62 |

\* Indicates a 50% or greater change in cell viability as measured by plating efficiency compared to untreated controls

† Indicates the presence of adenosine deaminase inhibitor R-3(2deoxy-β-D-erythro-pentofuranosyl)-3,6,7,8-tetrahydroimidazo [4,5d] [1,3] diazepin-8-o1

quired to reduce the viral yield by 99% was 1.7 times greater than that required to reduce cell viability 50%.

ARA-T did not cause gross cell death or lysis at 100 µM concentrations, however, no net increase in cell number was observed after three generations of drug exposure (Table 1). As indicated in Table 2, after exposure for three generation times, viable cell number was 28% of control value. HPLC analysis of the culture media indicated that ARA-T remained unchanged during 3 days in the culture medium. The concentration of ARA-T required to reduce viral yields by 99% was 8.8 times less than the concentration required to reduce cell viability by 50%.

ARA-AMP was cytostatic at 100 µM (Table 1). No increase in the number of viable cells occurred during a time equal to three cell generations when Chang cells were cultured in the presence of 100 µM ARA-AMP (Table 2). The concentration of ARA-AMP required to kill 50% of the cells was 63.3 µM while the concentration required to inhibit viral yield by 99% was 130.0 µM. In our system, adenosine deaminase inhibitor increased both the cytotoxicity and efficacy of ARA-AMP. This later observation is currently under investigation.

IUdR produced significant decreases in growth rate and viability of Chang cells at 10 µM concentrations (Table 1 and 2). The LD$_{50}$ of IUdR in the Chang conjunctival cells was 27.6 µM while the concentration of IUdR required to reduce viral production by 99% was 44.0 µM.

F$_3$TdR was clearly the most toxic of the nucleoside analogues which we have screened. Our data indicate that 1 µM F$_3$TdR produced cell lysis and nearly 100% loss in viability after exposure to cells for a time equal to three generation times (Table 1 and 2). The

**Table 3.** Effect of catabolites formed from nucleoside antivirals on cell generation time and viability

| Compound | Parent drug | % Change in generation time Drug concentration (µM) | | | | % Viable Drug concentration (µM) | | | |
|---|---|---|---|---|---|---|---|---|---|
| | | 100 | 10 | 1 | 0.1 | 100 | 10 | 1 | 01 |
| Fluoride ion | F$_3$TdR | + 6.0 | + 7.3 | − 1.0 | + 1.0 | 97.8 | 98.6 | 119.1 | 87.2 |
| 5 carboxyuracil | F$_3$TdR | + 17.5 | + 8.0 | + 17.5 | + 23.6 | 121.0 | 113.7 | 117.3 | 105.4 |
| 5 carboxy-2'-deoxyuridine | F$_3$TdR | − 9.9 | − 4.7 | − 3.5 | + 4.6 | 119.6 | 95.3 | 107.7 | |
| Iodouracil | IDU | + 8.3 | + 6.9 | − 1.3 | + 5.1 | 115.6 | 92.3 | 103.9 | 125.7 |
| Hypoxanthine arabinoside | ARA-A | − 9.3 | | | | 110.4 | | | |

$LD_{50}$ of $F_3TdR$ in the Chang cell system was 8.3 µM while the dose required to reduce viral production by 99% was 6.3 µM.

## Effect of Catabolites of Nucleoside Analogues on Cell Growth and Viability

ARA-A, IUdR, and $F_3TdR$ are all catabolized and/or hydrolyzed in our system. The primary catabolites of each compound are listed in Table 3. None of these compounds had any effect on cell growth rates or viability of Chang conjunctival cells at concentrations equivalent to toxic levels of the parent compound.

## Discussion

Our data establish the relative toxicity of the nucleoside antivirals in the following order: $ACG \lesssim AIU \ll ARA\text{-}A \lesssim ARA\text{-}T \lesssim ARA\text{-}AMP < IUdR \ll F_3TdR$. Surprisingly, principal catabolites produced by metabolism of ARA-A, IUdR and $F_3TdR$ were not toxic to Chang cells when added individually to the culture medium in concentrations as high as 100 µM. It is difficult to relate the antiviral concentration used in these cell culture studies to the actual concentration of antivirals attained at the corneal or conjunctival surface because little information is available regarding the actual concentration of antiviral drugs after topical application. Aqueous humor concentrations as high as 44 µM may be attained in humans after intensive topical therapy, therefore, we feel that the drug concentrations used in these studies are in a range comparable to that sustained in vivo [25].

ACG is reported in the literature to have an $ED_{50}$ for Vero cells of 300 µM while LM cells have an $ED_{50}$ of 26 µM [9, 10]. Our data indicate that Chang conjunctival cells have an $LD_{50}$ of greater than 100 µM and an $ED_{99}$ of 8.1 µM. The large difference between $ED_{99}$ and $LD_{50}$ reflect the lack of cytotoxicity, as has been observed by others.

AIU has been reported to have no cytotoxicity at concentrations up to 400 µM. Numerous tumor cell lines, nontumor lines, L cells and secondary chick embryo fibroblasts were included in the study [4]. Our data indicate that Chang cell viability, as measured by the ability to replicate and form colonies was unaffected by concentrations of AIU as high

as 100 µM. Although the growth rate of Chang cells is unchanged by 100 µM AIU, changes in cell size were not measured to determine if an imbalance of growth exists in these cells.

Cheng et al. [4] reported that ARA-A produced "moderate" toxicity in Vero cells at 20 µM in the absence of adenosine deaminase inhibitors. Plunkett and Cohen [28] reported that the same concentration caused a 75% loss of viability in mouse L cell cultures. In our system, 100 µM ARA-A completely inhibit cell growth during the first 72 h of exposure. The amount of catabolism of ARA-A was so great that after 72 h no ARA-A remained and the surviving cells then grew at a normal rate. In the presence of adenosine deaminase inhibitor, the $LD_{50}$ in Chang cells was 55 µM. In mouse L cell systems, 10 µM ARA-A in the presence of a deaminase inhibitor was lethal [28]. The apparent increase in activity observed in the presence of deaminase inhibitor is consistent with observations made in other systems [30]. ARA-Hx, the deaminated catabolite of ARA-A, was not toxic to Chang cells in culture.

Under the conditions of our assay system, ARA-AMP was cytostatic to Chang cells at 100 µM. These observations are consistent with those of Plunkett and Cohen [28] who observed that 200 µM ARA-AMP caused a loss of both viability and growth in mouse L fibroblasts. Our preliminary data indicate that the toxicity and efficacy of ARA-AMP is potentiated by adenine deaminase inhibitor such that 100 µM ARA-AMP was lethal to Chang cells. These observations are in direct conflict with those of Plunkett and Cohen [28] who used a Vero cell system in their studies. The difference probably reflects variances in phosphorylase levels between the two systems. Studies are in progress to resolve these differences.

ARA-T at 100 µM concentrations completely inhibited growth and resulted in a 70% loss of viability. These data indicate that ARA-T is more toxic to Chang cells than to LM, BHK and HEp-2 cells as reported by Aswell et al. [2]. They observed a 17% inhibition of cell growth with 100 µM ARA-T. ARA-T appeared not to be catabolized in our system and therefore ARA-T may be of potential value for systemic delivery. The great antiviral potency and moderate toxicity of ARA-T make it appear to have therapeutic potential. It should be noted, however, that like other thymidine analogues, resistant mutants may arise by mutation in the HSV thymidine kinase gene [2].

IUdR produced measurable toxicity at 10 μM and a complete loss of cell viability at 100 μM ($LD_{50}$ = 28 μM). Cheng et al. [4] reported complete inhibition of Vero cell growth at 50 μM IUdR. Other cell lines were subject to growth inhibition in concentration ranges between 1000 μM and 0.01 μM depending on their origin [31]. The metabolite 5-iodouracil showed no growth inhibition at concentrations as great as 100 μM.

$F_3$TdR was clearly the most toxic of all the drugs examined. Our data indicate that 8.3 μM produced a 50% reduction in cell viability. Wigdahl [33] reported that LM cells treated with 5 μM $F_3$TdR had a 42% plating efficiency as compared to untreated controls. HEp2 cells were shown to have a 50% inhibition of plating efficiency at 0.1 μM. Studies clearly indicate that under conditions in which cells express high cellular thymidine kinase activities, there is an increase in the cytotoxicity of $F_3$TdR [6]. Studies in our laboratory have shown actively growing epithelial cells of both corneal and conjunctival origin can incorporate $F_3$TdR into their DNA at significant rates [21]. These observations may account for the poor quality of the regenerating corneal epithelium observed during $F_3$TdR treatment [13].

The metabolites of $F_3$TdR, $F^-$ ion, 5 carboxyuracil and 5-carboxy-2'-deoxyuridine (5-COOH-UdR) had no effect on cell growth at the concentrations examined. Clough et al. [5] reported a 91% inhibition of HEp2 cell growth by 100 μM 5-COOH-UdR. Our studies indicate that although 5-COOH-UdR may be present in the media, corneal and conjunctival cells do not accumulate the compound in cellular pools [21].

The data reported here establish ranges of cytotoxic drug concentrations for many commonly used nucleoside antivirals. These data provide a quantitative assessment of toxicity in epithelial cells of ocular origin. A better assessment of toxicity as it relates to the in vivo situation requires the assessment of toxicity in normal diploid epithelial cells grown on a collagen matrix. Studies are currently in progress in an attempt to achieve such a system.

**Acknowledgment.** Supported in part by Grants EY 02834 and EY 01931 from the National Eye Institute (USPHS) and an unrestricted grant from Research to Prevent Blindness, Inc.

## References

1. Albert DM, Lahav M, Bhatt PN, Reid TW, Ward RE, Cykiert RC, Lin TS, Ward DC, Prusoff WH (1976) Successful therapy of herpes hominis keratitis in rabbits by 5-iodo-5'-amino-2'-5'-dideoxyuridine (AIU): A novel analog of thymidine. Invest Ophthalmol 15: 470–478
2. Aswell JF, Allen GP, Jamieson AT, Campbell DE, Gentry GA (1977) Antiviral activity of arabinosylthymine in herpesviral replication: mechanism of action in vivo and in vitro. Antimicrob Agents Chemother 12:243–254
3. Chang RS (1954) Continuous subcultivation of epithelial-like cells from normal human tissues. Proc Soc Exp Biol Med 87:440–443
4. Cheng YC, Goz B, Neehan JP, Ward DC, Prusoff WH (1975) Selective inhibition of herpes simplex virus by 5'-amino-2', 5'dideoxy-5-iodouridine. J Virol 15:1284–1285
5. Clough DW, Wigdahl BL, Parkhurst JR (1978) Biological effects of 5-carboxy-2'-deoxyuridine: Hydrolysis product of 5-trifluoromethyl-2'-deoxyuridine. Antimicrob Agents Chemother 14:126–131
6. DeClerq E, Drajewska E, Descamps J, Torrence PF (1977) Anti-herpes activity of deoxythymidine analogues: specific dependence on virus-induced deoxythymidine kinase. Mol Pharmacol 13:980–984
7. Drach VC, Shipman C (1977) The selective inhibition of viral DNA synthesis by chemotherapeutic agents: an indicator of clinical usefulness. Ann NY Acad Sci 284:396–409
8. Drewinko B, Roper PR, Barlogie B (1979) Patterns of cell survival following treatment with anti-tumor agents in vitro. Eur J Cancer 15:93–99
9. Elion GB, Furman PA, Fyfe JA, DeMiranda P, Beauchamp L, Schaeffer HJ (1977) Selectivity of action of an antiherpetic agent, 9-(2-hydroxyethoxymethyl) guanine. Proc Natl Acad Sci USA 74:5716–5720
10. Furman PA, McGuirt PV, Keller PM, Fyfe JA, Elion GB (1980) Inhibition by acyclovir of cell growth and DNA synthesis of cells biochemically transformed with herpesvirus genetic information. Virol 102:420–430
11. Gilbert SF, Migeon BR (1975) D-valine as a selective agent for normal human and rodent epithelial cells in culture. Cell 5:11–17

12. Hana C (1970) On the mechanism of the antiherpetic action of iodoxuridine. Ann Ophthalmol 2:345–353

13. Hyndiuk RA, Charlin RE, Alpren TVP, Schultz RO (1978) Trifluridine in resistant human herpetic keratitis. Arch Ophthalmol 96:1839–1841

14. Kaufman HE (1978) Herpetic keratitis. Invest Ophthalmol 17:941–957

15. Kaufman HE, Heidelberger C (1964) Therapeutic antiviral action of 5-trifluoromethyl-2'-deoxyuridine in herpes simplex keratitis. Science 145:585–586

16. Kaufman HE, Nesburn AB, Maloney ED (1962) IDU therapy of herpes simplex. Arch Ophthalmol 67:583–591

17. Langston RHS, Pavan-Langston D, Dohlman CH (1974) Antivirals and corneal wound healing. Arch Ophthalmol 92:509–513

18. Lerche W, Domarus DV, Hanhe C, Maass C, Gauri KK (1979) Electron microscopic studies following treatment with 5-ethyl-2'-deoxyuridine. Adv Ophthalmol 38:49–59

19. McGill J, Fraunfelder FT, Jones BR (1976) Current and proposed management of ocular herpes simplex. Surv Ophthalmol 20:358–365

20. McGill J, Williams H, McKinnon J, Holt-Wilson AD, Jones BR (1974) Reassessment of idoxuridine therapy of herpetic keratitis. Trans Ophthalmol Soc UK 94:542–551

21. O'Brien WJ (1979) The metabolism of trifluorothymidine by cells of the rabbit cornea. Exp Eye Res 29:619–624

22. O'Brien WJ, Taylor JL, DeCarlo JC, Clough DW, Schultz RO (1980) The chemotherapy of herpetic keratitis in rabbits. This vol

23. Pavan-Langston D, Buchanan RA, Alford C (1975) Adenine Arabinoside: A new antiviral. Raven, New York

24. Pavan-Langston D, Buchanan RA (1976) Vidarabine therapy of simple and IDU-complicated herpetic keratitis. Trans Am Acad Ophthalmol Otolaryngol 81:OP-813-825

25. Pavan-Langston D, Nelson DJ (1979) Intraocular penetration of trifluridine. Am J Ophthalmol 87:814–818

26. Pavan-Langston D, North RD, Geary PA (1976) ARA-AMP-A new highly soluble antiviral drug. Ann Ophthalmol 8:571–579

27. Phillip HJ, Terryberry JE (1957) Counting actively metabolizing tissue culture cells. Exp Cell Res 13:341–347

28. Plunkett W, Cohen SS (1975) Two approaches that increase the activity of analogues of adenine nucleosides in animal cells. Cancer Res 35:1547–1554

29. Sidwell RW, Dixon GJ, Schabel FM, Kaump DH (1968) Antiviral activity of 9-β-D-arabinofuranosyladenine. II. Activity against herpes simplex keratitis in hamsters. Antimicrob Agents Chemother 8:148–154

30. Sloan BJ, Kielty JK, Miller FA (1977) Effect of a novel adenosine deaminase inhibitor (covidarabine, Co-V) upon the antiviral activity in vitro and in vivo of vidarabine (Vira-A$^{TM}$) for DNA virus replication. Ann NY Acad Sci 284:60–80

31. Umeda M, Heidelberger C (1968) Fluorinated pyrimidines. XXX. Comparative studies with various cell lines. Cancer Res 28:2529–2538

32. Wigand R (1979) Adenine arabinoside inhibition of adenovirus replication enhanced by an adenosine deaminase inhibitor. J Med Virol 4:59–65

33. Wigdahl BL (1979) Inhibition of HEP-2 cell, mouse L cells, and herpes simplex type 1 replication by 5-trifluoromethyl-2'-deoxyuridine: Role of cellular and HSV-1 induced deoxythymidine kinases. PhD Thesis. The Medical College of Wisconsin, Milwaukee WI

Sundmacher, R. (Hrsg.):
Herpetische Augenerkrankungen
© J.F. Bergmann Verlag, München 1981

# The Effect of Trifluorothymidine on Epithelial Wound Healing in Rabbit Cornea. A Scanning Electron Microscopic Study

H. Brewitt, C. Feuerhake, Hannover

**Key words.** Corneal epithelium, wound healing trifluorothymidine, SEM

**Schlüsselwörter.** Hornhautepithel, Wundheilung, Trifluorthymidin, Rasterelektronenmikroskop

**Summary.** A scanning electron microscopic study with rabbits was made on the influence of tri-fluorothymidine ($F_3T$) on regeneration of the corneal epithelium following epithelial abrasion. With $F_3T$ medication, a dose-dependent delay in epithelial wound healing occurred. After six applications per day of $F_3T$, there was no apparent retardation of wound healing; in contrast, twelve applications per day clearly resulted in delayed epithelization. In addition to the uniformity in the morphological appearance of the migrating corneal epithelial cells after the twelve applications of $F_3T$, damage in the region of the migrated epithelial cells was clearly evident (i.e., reduction of the microstructure of the cell surface, break-up of the plasma membrane, eventual cell desquamation). The results are discussed and considered in relation to the literature.

**Zusammenfassung.** Es wurde das morphologische Bild des Hornhautepithels in der Regeneration nach Hornhautabrasio unter dem Einfluß von Trifluorthymidin beim Kaninchen mit Hilfe des Rasterelektronenmikroskopes untersucht. Unter der Medikation von Trifluorthymidin ($F_3T$) kam es zu einer dosisabhängigen Verzögerung der epithelialen Wundheilung. Nach 6maliger Applikation von $F_3T$ pro Tag kam es zu keiner faßbaren Verzögerung der Wundheilung, dagegen führte eine 12-malige Applikation von $F_3T$ pro Tag zu einer deutlich verzögerten Epithelisierung. Neben einer Uniformität des morphologischen Erscheinungsbildes der migrierenden Epithelzellen finden sich vor allem nach 12maliger Applikation von $F_3T$ Schäden im Bereich der migrierten Epithelzellen, wie Reduzierung der Mikrostruktur der Zelloberfläche, Aufbrüche der Plasmamembran bis hin zu Zelldesquamation. Die Ergebnisse werden diskutiert und mit der Literatur verglichen.

## Introduction

The treatment of herpetic keratitis with antimetabolites was first suggested in 1960 by Wollensak. Idoxuridine (IDU) was the first useful local antiviral agent [13]. Little information concerning tolerance of the medication was available and reports soon appeared about the side effects of this antiviral compound. Some side effects of IDU were delayed healing of epithelial erosion and disturbance of the regeneration of the stroma corneae. The influence of IDU on wound healing in the cornea serves as an index for the toxicity of this antiviral agent and is even today an important topic in clinical and experimental research (see 7, 9, 14–16, 18, 20, 22–24, 29]).

Recently, trifluorothymidine ($F_3T$) has been used for treating the herpetic corneal diseases. Like IDU, this substance is incorporated into the DNA-molecule of the virus [5]. $F_3T$ is more soluble and should be about twice as effective as IDU [11, 12, 19, 25, 27].

With the usual clinical dose ($5 \times F_3T$/ die) there have been no apparent side effects; however, with higher doses, pointlike erosion of the corneal epithelium has been observed [17]. For this reason Sundmacher [26] has warned against administering higher doses.

Foster and Pavan-Langston [4] as well as Gasset and Katzin [6] have described disturbances of the epithelium and delayed wound healing of the stroma due to the application of $F_3T$. In contrast, Holtmann and Stein [10] showed that no delay in regeneration of the corneal epithelium occurred.

The delayed wound healing of the cornea indicates the toxicity of the antiviral agent. To further elucidate this property of the antiviral compound F3T, the present scanning electron microscopic study was undertaken to examine the morphological changes in the corneal epithelium during regeneration under the influence of F₃T.

## Materials and Methods

Twenty fully grown rabbits of 2–3 kg weight and with normal eyes were used. Anesthesia was administered, and under microscopical observation a central lesion was made using a 2.5 mm-trephine. The epithelium within this area was then removed using a hockey knife, taking care that the basement membrane remained undamaged. Finally, three test groups were formed:

Group 1 (8 animals): Each animal received 6 drops of F₃T per day (application every 2 hours)[a],

Group 2 (8 animals): Each animal received 12 drops of F₃T per day (application every hour)[a],

Group 3 (4 animals): Each animal received 12 drops of the vehicle without the antiviral agent F3T per day (application every hour)[a].

After 0, 6, 15 and 48 hours, the animals were killed and the corneas was continuously irrigated for 5 min with 4% glutaraldehyde in Sörensens phosphate buffer (pH 7.2). Finally

the corneas were excised and fixed in the same solution. After rinsing in Sörensens phosphate buffer, the specimens were further fixed in osmium tetroxide. They were then dehydrated in increasing acetone concentrations and dried at the critical point. All preparations were coated with a 20 nm gold layer and examined in a "Stereoscan 600" [1].

## Results

*Group 1: 6 × F₃T/die, Application Every 2 Hours*

### Zero Time After Epithelial Lesion

In the surveying magnification, the basement membrane which had been stripped of epithelium appeared as a homogeneous grey area. The cells at the wound edge were rounded off. The intracellular spaces of the epithelial cells were disrupted in the area of the wound edge (Fig. 1a).

### 6 Hours After Epithelial Lesion

Leukocytes were found at the edge of the epithelial defect (Fig. 1b). The original wound edge was rounded off. The superficial epithelial cells were sloping markedly. They had migrated over the wound edge and were connected with the basement membrane. Very flat cells with microvilli-free zones on their free edges were characteristic at this point in time (Fig. 1c).

### 15 Hours After Epithelial Lesion

Leukocytes were no longer found (Fig. 1d). For the first time, basal epithelial cells with

a 1% Trifluorthymidin Augentropfen (5-Trifluoromethyl-2′-Deoxyuridine) and the vehicle were kindly supplied to us by Fa. Dr. Mann, Berlin

**Fig. 1.** Group 1 (6 applications of F₃T per day)

**a** Zero time after epithelial lesion: View of a portion of the epithelial lesion. Basement membrane (B) recognizable as homogeneous gray surface. Rounded-off epithelial cells (arrow) on the wound edge. Epithelium (E). 145×

**b** 6 hours after epithelial lesion: Rounded wound edge. In the wound bed cell-rich leukocytes (L) are found. Basement membrane (B), epithelium (E). 190×

**c** Enlargement of a portion of Fig. 1b.: Superficial epithelial cells (E) have closed the wound edge and reached the basement membrane (B) (arrow). Desquamated epithelial cells (*), Leukocytes (L). 2035×

**d** 15 hours after epithelial lesion: View of a portion of the wound; no leukocytes in the wound bed. Basement membrane (B), epithelium (E). 130×

**e** Enlargement of a section of Fig. 1d: Migrating basal-lying epithelial cell with folded microvilli-free edges. Basement membrane (B). 7250×

**f** 48 hours after epithelial lesion: Wound epithelized, cell desquamation indicative of vulnerability of migrated epithelium. 145×

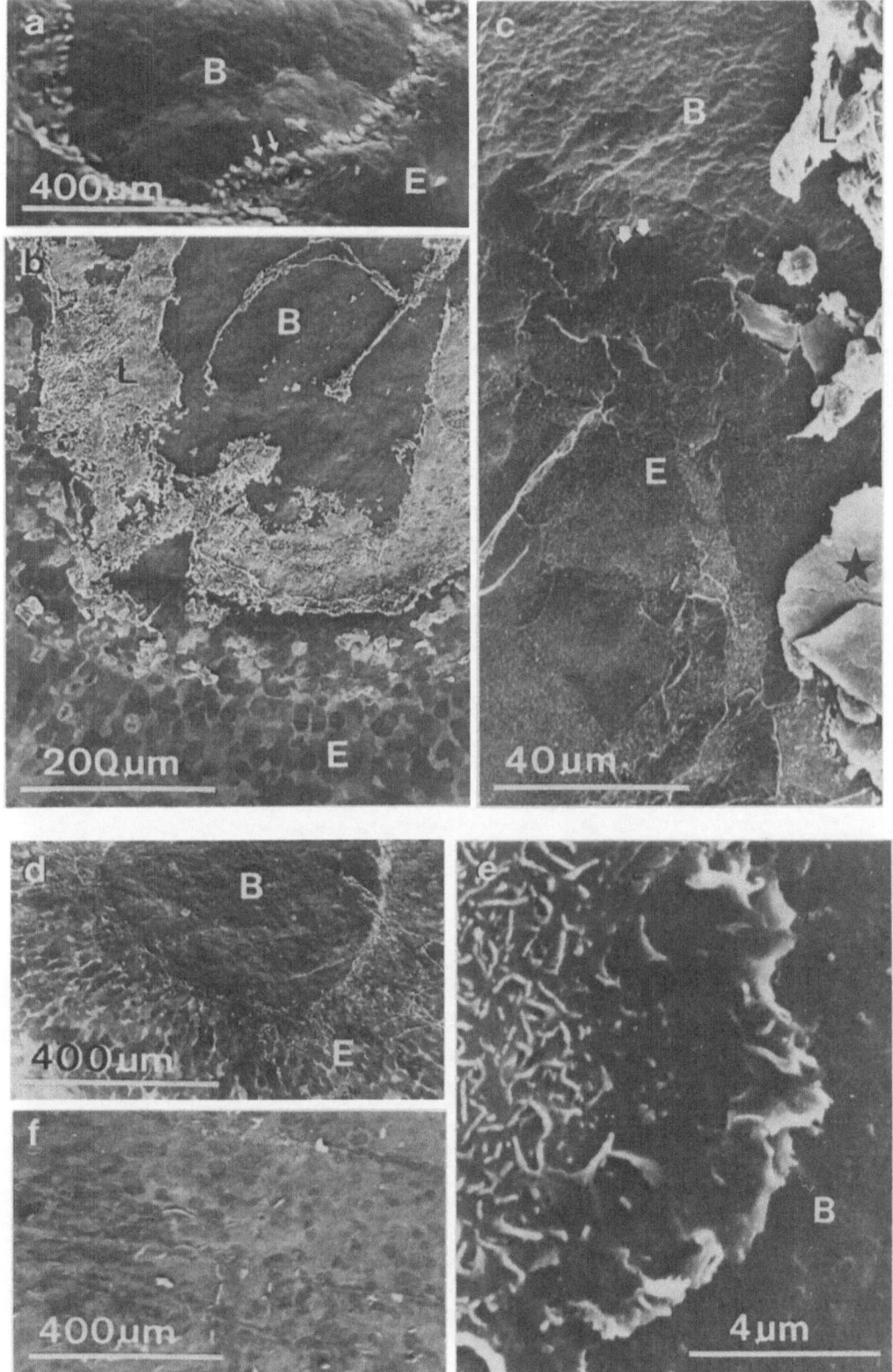

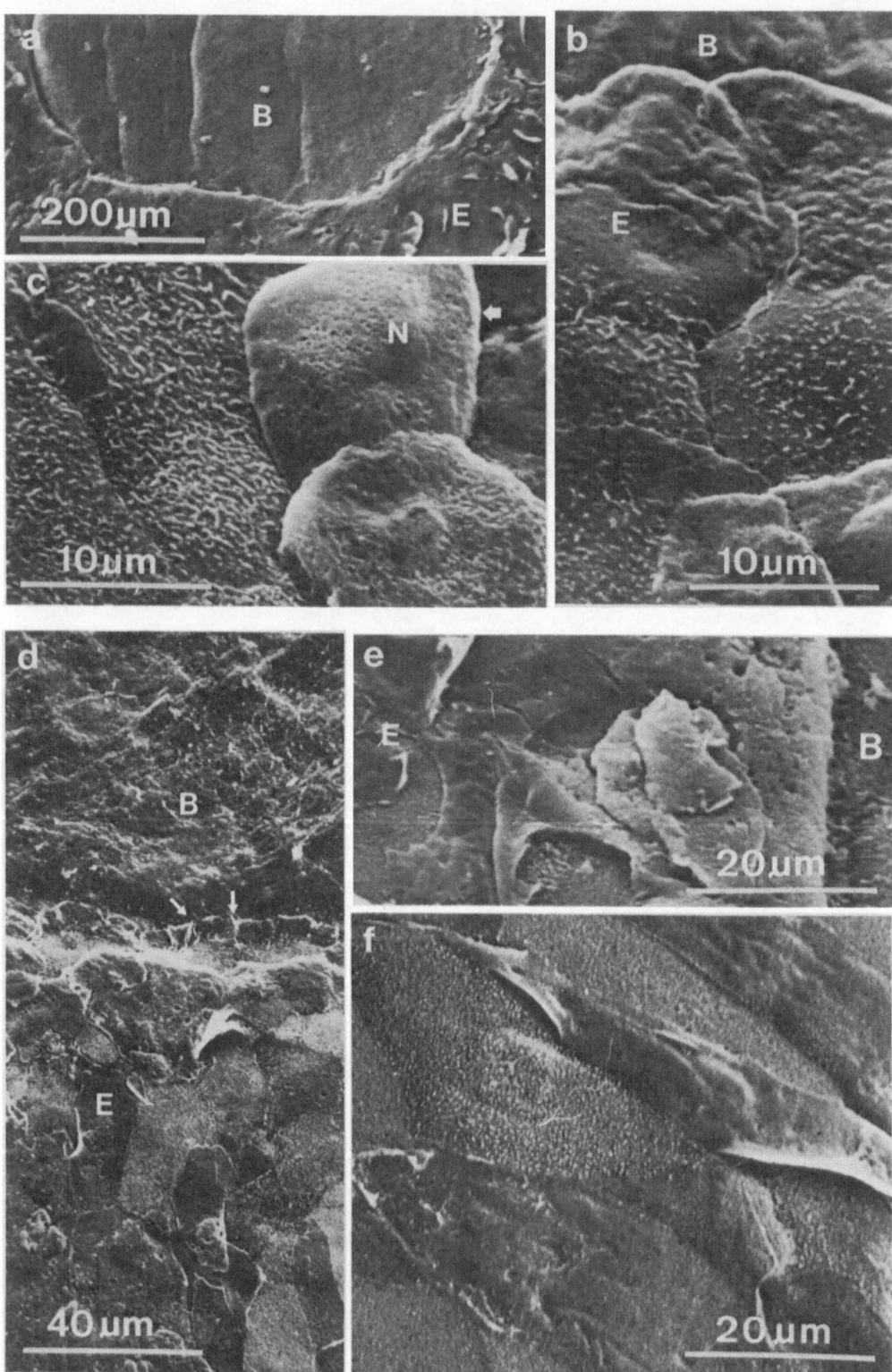

folded migratory edges followed by a further cell layer were observed (Fig. 1e). Occasionally, flat cells with smooth cell edges and microvilli-free zones could still be found at this stage of wound healing.

## 48 Hours After Epithelial Lesion

The whole wound area was epithelized; however, large numbers of detached cells were seen as the visible evidence of the vulnerability of the migrated epithelium (Fig. 1f). In contrast to the epithelium in untreated wound healing, the number of detached cells was increased and there were large areas of desquamated cells on whose surface no regular microstructure could be detected.

## Group 2: 12 × F₃T/die, Applications Hourly

*Group 2: 12 × F$_3$T/die, Applications Hourly*

Zero time after epithelial lesion: see comments for group 1.

## 6 Hours After Epithelial Lesion

No leukocytes were seen in the wound bed (Fig. 2a). The superficial epithelial cells had already migrated over the wound edge onto the basement membrane and showed the typical form of cell movement. The cells were very flat and possessed no microvilli on their migratory edges (Fig. 2b). Outside the area of the wound edge, marked changes of the epithelial cells, such as outlining of the cell nucleus, loss of microstructure on the surfaces and disruption of the intercellular spaces, had taken place (Fig. 2c).

## 15 Hours After Epithelial Lesion

The basal epithelial cells with serrated cell

edges led the migration (Fig. 2d). The migrating superficial epithelial cells at the wound edge showed marked damage to their cell surfaces. The intercellular spaces were disrupted and a regular structure was only occasionally found (Fig. 2e). Outside the actual migration zone typically extended cells with visible nuclei and short, sparce microvilli populations on their surfaces were found. Also in these areas the intercellular spaces were frequently open (Fig. 2f).

## 48 Hours After Epithelial Lesion

At this time, although the basement membrane was covered with epithelium, complete epithelization was not achieved. Radially directed epithelial projections interlocked with one another, indicating the still existing migrating activity (Fig. 3a). Migrating epithelial cells with pseudopodia-like projections were found (Fig. 3b). The superficial corneal epithelial cells of the already covered wound area possessed only a sparce population of microprocesses and their cell nuclei were recognizable. The intercellular spaces were open as a sign of damage.

## Group 3: 12 × vehicle/die, Application Hourly

*Group 3: 12 × vehicle/die, Application Hourly*

The vehicle without the agent F$_3$T effected no significant delay in epithelization of the corneal wound and the morphological appearance of migrating corneal epithelial cells.

## Discussion

The morphological appearance and the time course of the regeneration of the corneal

---

**Fig. 2.** Group 2 (12 applications of F$_3$T per day)

**a** 6 h after epithelial lesion: View of a portion of the wound; no leukocytes in wound bed; desquamated epithelial cells on wound edge. Basement membrane (B), epithelium (E). 145×

**b** Enlargement of a section of Fig. 2a: Flat epithelial cells with rare microvilli have reached the basement membrane (B), epithelium (E). 2900×

**c** Enlargement of a section of Fig. 2a: Migrated epithelial cells are again withdrawing from the cell bond (arrow); more visible cell nucleus (N); no regular microstructure on the surface 2900×

**d** 15 h after epithelial lesion: View of a portion of the wound; basal epithelial cells are leading the migration (arrow); basement membrane (B), epithelium (E). 825×

**e** Enlargement of Fig. 2d: Migrated superficial cells are detached and show no regular microstructure on their surface. 1450×

**f** Enlargement of Fig. 2d: Beyond the migration zone itself, desquamation occurs in longer, further migrated epithelial cells. Indicative of their cell damage, these cells exhibit no microstructure on their surface. 1450×

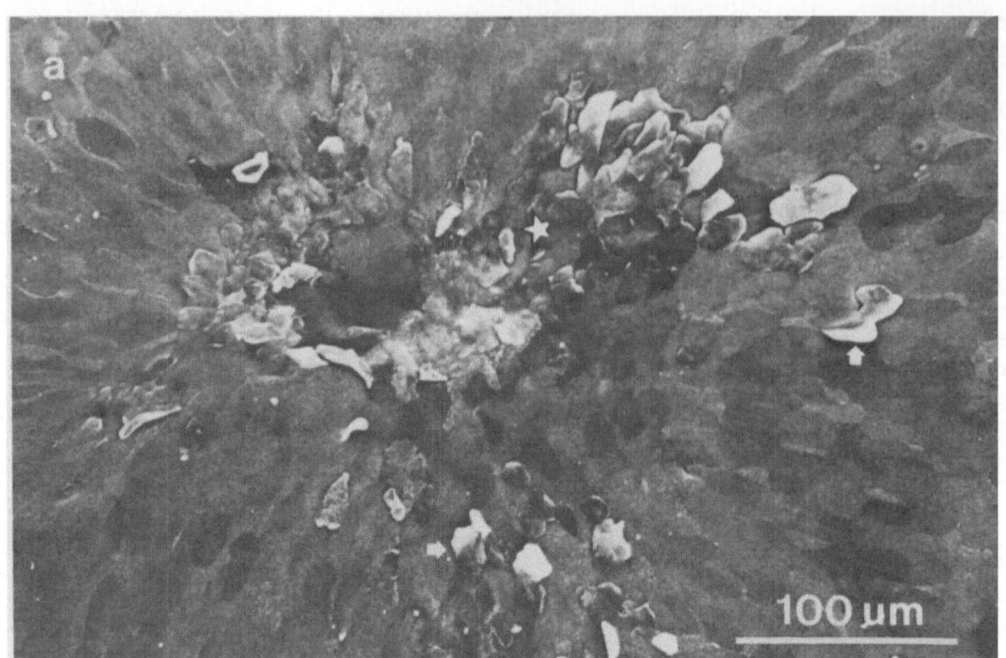

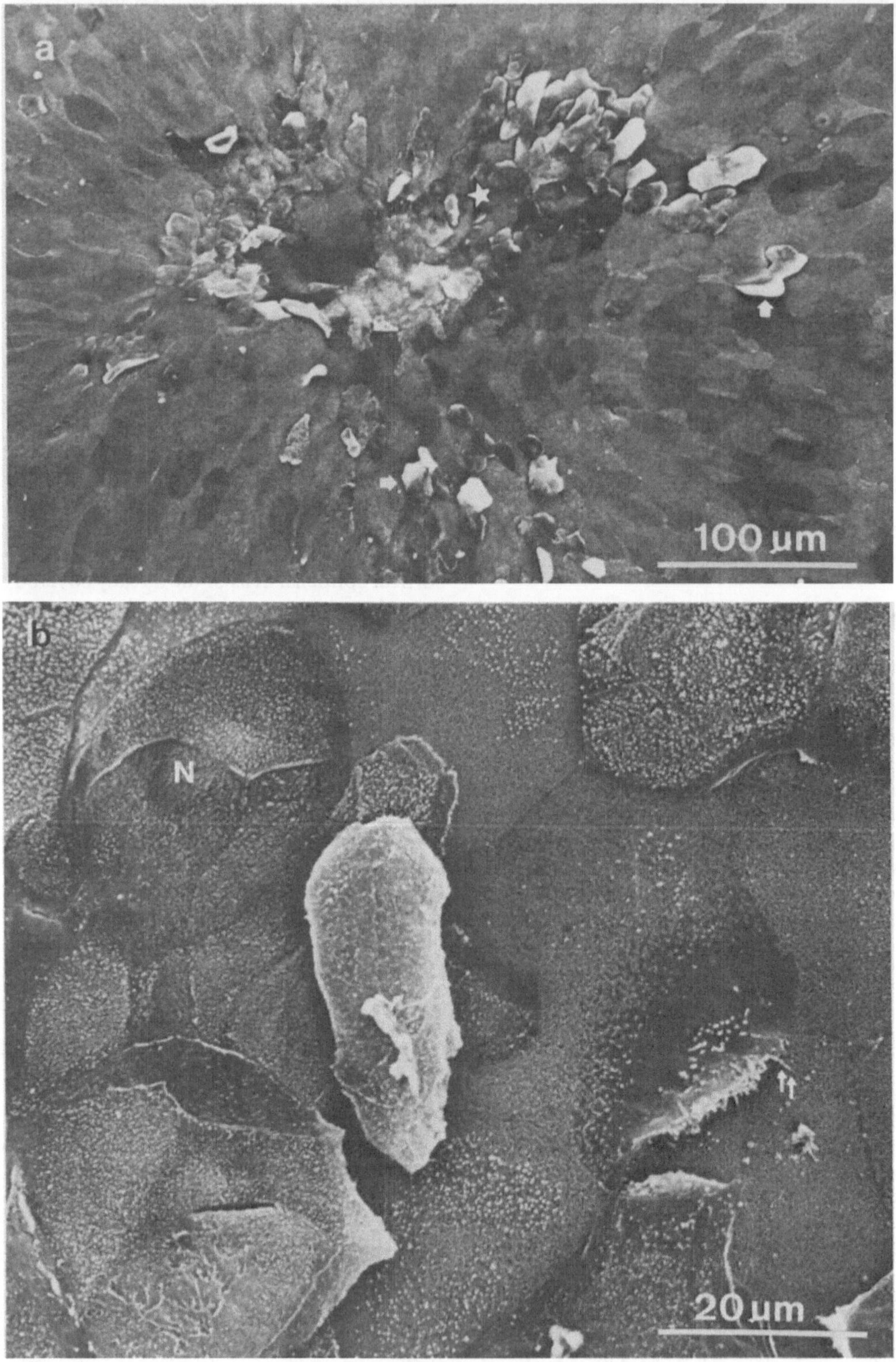

epithelium have been studied by several investigators using the scanning electron microscope [2, 3, 8, 21]. It has previously been shown [2], that after retraction of the wound edge, the superficial epithelial cells cross the free wound edge. These cells are very flat and possess a microvilli-free zone on their free cell edge. The basallying epithelial cells initiate the covering of the defect. During the cell movement, besides the very flat cells with wide cell borders, cells which have pronounced marginal folding at their edges and which send filopodia or claw-like projections over the basement membrane are found. A central epithelial lesion of 2.5 mm diameter is closed within a period of 48 hours. The average migration rate is 0.025 mm per h. The greatest activity in epithelial cell migration is observed after 6 and 15 h.

The present investigation, in which these particular times were studied, indicates that changes occurred during the migration of the corneal epithelial cells when Trifluorothymidine was used. With six applications of $F_3T$ per day, the speed of epithelization compared to that in untreated wound healing differs only slightly and is hardly measurable. However, the absence of leukocytes 15 hours after corneal epithelial lesion and the uniformity in the appearance of the migrating epithelial cells are noteworthy. The presence of the very flat cells with serrated edges is also significant.

Here, pseudopodia on the migrating cell border are only infrequently present, as are the claw-like processes which creep over the basement membrane. The number of damaged cells in the freshly epithelized area is particularly noticeable and must be due to the $F_3T$, even though these migrating cells are clearly more vulnerable than the old epithelial cells in an intact cell cover.

With 12 applications of $F_3T$ per day, the leukocytes are missing 6 hours after corneal epithelial lesion. At each point in time, the surface structure of the migrating epithelial cells changes. Microprocesses are either completely lacking or are only rarely found. Intercellular connections are almost routinely open. In contrast with untreated epithelization of epithelial wounds of similar size [2], the migration is not complete even after 48 hours when 12 x $F_3T$ per day is applied.

In summary, the application of $F_3T$ six times daily in the usual clinical procedure does not lengthen the time required for epithelization. However, the integrity of the epithelized area is very susceptible to even the smallest noxious substances, so that especially after application of $F_3T$, renewed disruptions of the epithelium can be expected. A 12-fold application of $F_3T$ leads to a significant delay in corneal epithelial wound healing and marked damage to the migrating epithelial cells; thus, higher doses of the antiviral agent are not recommended. These findings emphasize the previously described toxic effects of antiviral agents [4, 6]. In contrast to the untreated epithelial migration [2, 3, 21], the morphological picture of the migrating epithelial cells after application of $F_3T$ is very uniform; it is a visible expression of the influence of the antiviral agent on the cell movement. Furthermore, since this investigation involves the regeneration of epithelium in healthy rabbit corneas, it must be assumed that the capacity for regeneration of an herpetically affected human cornea will be limited by additional trophic disturbances.

**Acknowledgment.** This investigation was made possible with the cooperation of the Institut für Elektronenmikroskopie der Medizinischen Hochschule Hannover. The authors are greatly indebted to Prof. Dr. E. Reale for advice.

## References

1. Brewitt H (1979) Sliding of epithelium in experimental corneal wounds. A scanning electron microscopic study. Acta Ophthalmol (Kbh) 57:945–958
2. Brewitt H (1980) Rasterelektronenmikroskopische Untersuchungen über das Hornhaut-

**Fig. 3.** Group 2: 48 h after epithelial lesion

**a** View of a portion of the same wound: Radially-directed epithelial projections in the center; desquamation of migrated epithelial cells (arrow). Section of Fig. 3b (*). 290×

**b** Enlargement of a section of Fig. 3a: Further epithelization and development of pseudopodia (arrow) indicative of still-existing migration activity. Cells with scarce microvilli on the surface; visible cell nuclei (N). 1450×

epithel in der Regeneration nach mechanischer Schädigung. In: Naumann OHG, Gloor B. (eds) Wundheilung des Auges und ihre Komplikationen. Springer, Berlin, Heidelberg, New York, 175–178

3. Buck RC (1979) Cell migration in repair of mouse corneal epithelium. Invest Ophthalmol Visual Sci 18:767–784
4. Foster CS, Pavan-Langston D (1977) Corneal wound healing and antiviral medication. Arch Ophthalmol 95:2062–2067
5. Fujiwara Y, Oki T, Heidelberger C (1970) XXXVII. Effects of 5-Trifluoromethyl-2'-deoxyuridine on the synthesis of Deoxyribonucleic acid of mammalian cells in culture. Mol Pharmacol 6:273–280
6. Gasset AR, Katzin D (1975) Antiviral drugs and corneal wound healing. Invest Ophthalmol Visual Sci 14:628–630
7. Graeber W (1964) Tierexperimentelle und klinische Erfahrungen mit der IUDR-Behandlung des Herpes Corneae. Klin Monatsbl Augenheilkd 144:75–81
8. Haik BG, Zimny ML (1977) Scanning electron microscopy of corneal wound healing in rabbit. Invest Ophthalmol Visual Sci 16:787–796
9. Hanna C (1966) Effect of IDU on DNA synthesis during corneal wound healing. Am J Ophthalmol 61:279–282
10. Holtmann HW, Stein HJ (1977) Zur Frage der Epithelregenerationshemmung bei Trifluorothymidin-Behandlung. Klin Monatsbl Augenheilkd 171:576–579
11. Kaufman HE (1975) Therapy and prophylaxis of herpetic eye disease. Vortrag, Universitätsaugenklinik Freiburg
12. Kaufman HE (1979) Antiviral update. Ophthalmology 86:131–136
13. Kaufman HE, Heidelberger C (1964) Therapeutic antiviral action of 5-trifluoromethyl-2'-deoxyuridine in herpes simplex keratitis. Science 145:585–586
14. Kilp H, Walzer P, Hardke W (1976) Beeinflussung der Epithelisierungsgeschwindigkeit beim Kaninchenauge durch IDU- und tromantadinhaltige Augensalben. Klin Monatsbl Augenheilkd 168:354–361
15. Küchle HJ (1963) Zur Frage unerwünschter Nebenwirkungen von IDU auf die Hornhaut. Ber Dtsch Ophthalmol Ges 65:409–413
16. Laibson PR, Sery TW, Leopold IH (1963) The treatment of herpetic keratitis with 5-iodo-2'-deoxyuridine (IDU). Arch Ophthalmol 70:52–58
17. McGill J, Holt-Wilson AD, McKinnon JR, Williams HP, Jones BR Some aspects of the clinical use of trifluorothymidine in the treatment of herpetic ulceration of the cornea. Trans Ophthalmol Soc UK 94:342–352

18. Neubauer H, Severin M (1974) Die herpetischen Hornhauterkrankungen. In: Meyer-Schwickerath G, Ullerich K (Hrsg) Probleme entzündlicher Augenaffektionen. Enke, Stuttgart, S 32–53
19. Pavan-Langston D, Foster CS (1977) Trifluorothymidine and idoxuridine therapy of ocular herpes. Am J Ophthalmol 84:818–825
20. Payrau P, Dohlman CH (1964) IDU in corneal wound healing. Am J Ophthalmol 57:999–1002
21. Pfister RR (1975) The healing of corneal epithelial abrasions in the rabbit: a scanning electron microscope study. Invest Ophthalmol Visual Sci 14:648–661
22. Polack FM, Rose J (1964) The effect of 5-Iodo-2-Deoxyuridine (IDU) in corneal healing. Arch Ophthalmol 71:520–527
23. Pülhorn G, Sosath G, Thiel H-J (1978) The effect of 5-Iodo-2' deoxyuridine (IDU) and dexamethasone on corneal wound healing in the rabbit. Acta Ophthalmol (Kbh) 56:40–52
24. Reim M (1965) Beobachtungen bei der Behandlung der Keratitis dendritica mit 5-Joduracil-2-desoxy-ribosid (JUDR). Klin Monatsbl Augenheilkd 147:760–767
25. Sundmacher R (1976) Herpestherapie und -prophylaxe. I. Versuch einer kritischen Wertung. Klin Monatsbl Augenheilkd 169:308–325
26. Sundmacher R (1978) Trifluorthymidinprophylaxe bei der Steroidtherapie herpetischer Keratouveitiden. Klin Monatsbl Augenheilkd 173:516–519
27. Wellings PC, Awdry PN, Bors FH, Jones BR, Brown DC, Kaufman HE (1972) Clinical evaluation of trifluorothymidine in the treatment of herpes simplex corneal ulcers. Am J Ophthalmol 73:932–942
28. Wollensak J (1960) Neuere Gesichtspunkte zur Therapie des Herpes corneae. Tagung der Bay. Augenärzte, München
29. Wollensak J, Kypke W (1965) Hemmung von Epithelregeneration und cornealer Wundheilung beim Kaninchen durch Antimetaboliten. Albrecht von Graefes Arch Klin Ophthalmol 168:102–115

## Discussion on the Contribution pp. 277–284

H.E. Kaufman (New Orleans)
Did you use a control, such as frequent application of the vehicle without the trifluorothymidine?

H. Brewitt (Hannover)
Yes, we made a control; the vehicle, applied six times per day effected no delay in the epithelial regeneration.

H.E. Kaufman (New Orleans)
What about 12 times?

H. Brewitt (Hannover)
With 12 applications of the vehicle per day, the speed of epithelialization compared to that in untreated wound healing as neither significantly nor measurably changed. However, reduction of surface microprojections of migrated cells can be seen and intercellular spaces are sporadically open.

B.R. Jones (London)
What was the pH of the vehicle?

H. Brewitt (Hannover)
The pH was 5.1.

Sundmacher, R. (Hrsg.):
Herpetische Augenerkrankungen
© J.F. Bergmann Verlag, München 1981

# Der Einfluß von Virustatika und Steroiden auf die stromale Wundheilung

K.K. Gauri, H. Miestereck, Sauerlach

**Key words.** Antiviral drugs, corticosteroids, wound healing

**Schlüsselwörter.** Antivirale Medikamente, Kortikosteroide, Wundheilung

**Summary.** In view of the frequent clinical application of virostatic drugs in combination with steroids, it appeared important to re-evaluate their effect in stromal wound healing by adapting an efficient and quantitative animal model. Thus, the influence of Trifluorothymidine, Vidarabine, Triamcinolonacetonide, Dexamethasonsulfobenzoate-Na and Hydrocortisonacetate in combination and as single drugs has been investigated on extensive stromal wounds of 50 mm$^2$ in rabbits. Guidelines for designing useful combinations are also discussed.

**Zusammenfassung.** Da Virustatika klinisch sehr häufig in Verbindung mit Steroiden angewandt werden, erschien es uns wichtig, ihren Einfluß auf die stromale Wundheilung an Hand eines aussagekräftigen und quantifizierbaren Tiermodelles nachzuuntersuchen. Wir benutzten hierzu Trifluorthymidin, Vidarabin, Triamcinolonacetonid, Dexamethasonsulfobenzoat-Na und Hydrocortisonacetat sowohl in Kombination als auch als Einzelsubstanzen. Die Stromawunden der Kaninchen maßen 50 mm$^2$. Wir geben auch Anhaltspunkte dafür, welche Kombinationen vorteilhaft sein könnten.

Die Zahl der Virustatika, die topisch am Auge bei HSV-Infektionen eingesetzt werden können, nimmt ständig zu, so daß die Frage der Arzneimittelinteraktionen an Bedeutung gewinnt. Häufig werden diese Virustatika klinisch in Kombination mit Steroiden eingesetzt.

Da sowohl Virustatika wie auch Steroide konzentrationsabhängig einen negativen Einfluß auf die Wundheilung haben können, erschien es uns notwendig, die Beeinflussung der stromalen Wundheilung durch diese Pharmaka anhand eines aussagekräftigen und quantifizierbaren Tiermodells zu untersuchen [1].

Wichtig erscheint uns, daß die Prüfung an ausgedehnten Hornhautwunden stattfindet (50 mm$^2$). Nur dann ist es möglich, auch geringe Unterschiede festzustellen. Bei kleineren Wunden (button) erfolgt die Heilung der Hornhautwunde so schnell, daß feinere Differenzierungen nicht mehr möglich sind.

## Methodik

Kaninchen (gelb/silber). Trepanation mit 8 mm Trepan (50 mm$^2$), der zentrale Hornhautbezirk wird unter dem Operationsmikroskop bis zu einer Tiefe von ca. 0,15 mm lamellär keratektomiert [2]. Dokumentation und Auswertung des Regenerationsverlaufs durch Planimetrierung von Photogrammen nach Anfärbung mit 1% Fluoresceinlösung.

Die Messungen erfolgen täglich.

Die Kurvenpunkte stellen Mittelwerte aus jeweils mindestens vier Augen dar.

## Substanzen

*Virustatika:* Trifluridin (Trifluorthymidin), 1%ige wäßrige Lösung; Vidarabin, 3%ige Salbe.

*Steroide:* Triamcinolonacetonid, Salbe mit 0,05% und 0,1%; Dexamethasonsulfobenzoat, wäßrige Lösung von 0,05/0,1 und 0,2%; Hydrocortisonacetat, Salbe mit 0,5/1 und 2% (Cortisol).

Die quantitative Bestimmung der stromalen Wundheilung nach lamellärer Keratektomie ist eine brauchbare Methode zur Untersuchung fördernder oder hemmender pharmakologischer Einflüsse auf die Epithelisierung stromaler Wunden.

## Ergebnisse

### Hemmung der Wundheilung durch Steroide (Abb. 1)

Es zeigt sich, daß Dexamethasonsulfobenzoat im Vergleich zu den Kontrollversuchen die Heilung stromaler Wunden nicht hemmt. Triamconolon führt zu einer mäßigen und Hydrocortisonacetat zu einer ausgeprägten Verzögerung der Wundheilung.

### Steroide in Kombination mit Virustatika

Die Kombination von Trifluridin mit jedem der drei geprüften Steroide zeigt eine erhebliche Verzögerung der Wundheilung (Abb. 2, 3), obwohl − wie wir aus unseren früheren Untersuchungen wissen − Trifluridin allein die stromale Wundheilung in dieser Konzentration nicht hemmt.

Vidarabin zeigt allein und in Kombination mit Dexamethason (Abb. 4) oder Triamcinolon keine Verzögerung der Wundheilung.

Die Kombination mit Hydrocortisonacetat führt in der hohen Konzentration von 2% zu einer mäßigen Hemmung, während die Konzentrationen von 0,5% und 1% keine negativen Einflüsse zeigen (Abb. 5).

## Diskussion

Im pharmakologischen Modellversuch haben die geprüften Virustatika/Steroid-Kombinationen unterschiedlichen Einfluß auf die Heilung großer stromaler Wunden. Die aufgezeigten Ergebnisse können insofern eine Anregung zu entsprechenden klinischen Untersuchungen und Beobachtungen bilden.

## Literatur

1. Für ausführliche Literaturzitate siehe Adv Ophthalmol 38 (1979) Karger, Basel

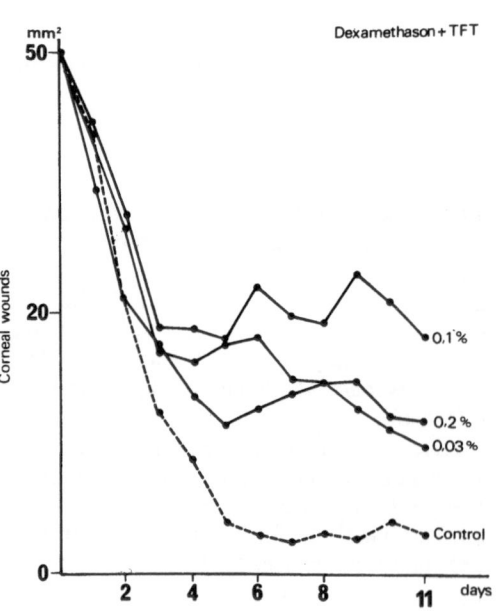

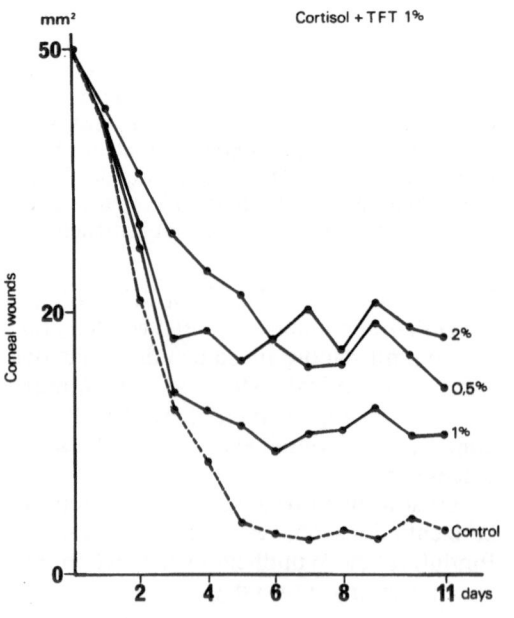

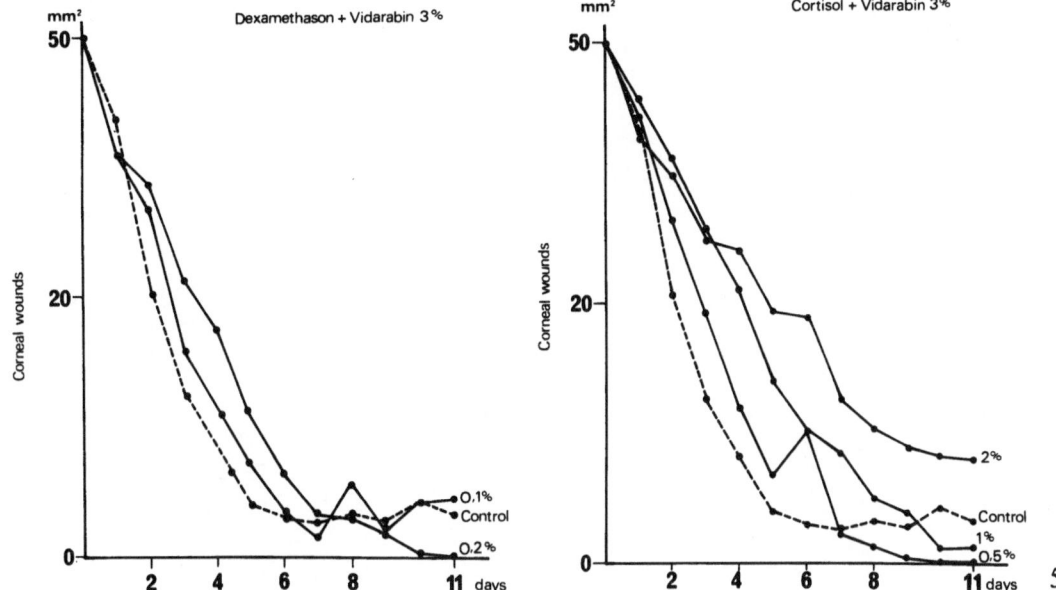

**Abb. 1 bis 5.** Beeinflussung der stromalen Regeneration durch Virustatika und Steroide sowie durch deren Kombinationsbehandlung beim Kaninchen

2. Wollensak I, Kypke W (1965) Albrecht von Graefes Arch Klin Ophthalmol 168:102–115

## Diskussion zum Beitrag S. 287–289

R. Sundmacher (Freiburg)
You said that the combination of Ara-A plus steroids did not inhibit stromal wound healing, whereas TFT plus steroids did. I would like to know what your experimental set-up was and how you measured wound healing.

H. Miestereck (Sauerlach)
We did a half-thickness keratectomie of the cornea and then we measured the closure of this standardized stromal wound.

R. Sundmacher (Freiburg)
I think it is important to stress that you actually measured reepithelization of a stromal wound whereas for stromal wound healing, as I understand it, other models have been applied, e.g. tensile strength.

Sundmacher, R. (Hrsg.):
Herpetische Augenerkrankungen
© J.F. Bergmann Verlag, München 1981

# Trifluorthymidin und bakterielle Hornhautinfektion. Eine tierexperimentelle Studie

W. Behrens-Baumann, U. Weber, R. Ansorg, Göttingen

**Key words.** Trifluorothymidine, bacterial corneal infection

**Schlüsselwörter.** Trifluorthymidin, bakterielle Hornhautinfektion

**Summary.** To investigate the effect of trifluorthymidine on corneal resistance against bacteria, eyes of rabbits were pretreated with TFT and after removal of the corneal epithelium infected with Staphylococcus aureus. An increased affinity for Staphylococcus aureus infection could not be demonstrated after pretreatment with TFT. TFT treatment, however, produced a statistically significant increase of toxic epitheliopathie.

**Zusammenfassung.** An Kaninchenaugen wurde untersucht, ob eine Zunahme von Keratitis durch Staphylococcus aureus nach Gabe von TFT nachweisbar ist. Dabei wurden Gruppen für das Handelspräparat, das Lösungsmittel, TFT in Reinsubstanz sowie für NaCl gebildet.
Eine erhöhte Anfälligkeit der Kaninchenhornhaut für Staphylococcus aureus konnte nicht nachgewiesen werden, wenn mit TFT vorbehandelt wurde. Daneben wurde eine signifikante Zunahme der toxischen Epitheliopathie bei den Gruppen TFT-Reinsubstanz und TFT-Handelspräparat festgestellt.

Der Einfluß der Virostatica auf die Wundheilung der Hornhaut ist inzwischen gut bekannt. Idoxuridin (IDU), Adeninarabinosid. (Ara-A) und Trifluorthymidin (TFT) führen zu biomikroskopisch und histologisch feststellbaren Veränderungen wie Verdünnung des regenerierenden Epithels und Zunahme des intrazellulären Ödems [1].

Dadurch kann es bei Gabe von IDU zu einer verzögerten Wundheilung kommen [10, 11]. TFT scheint diesbezüglich besser vertragen zu werden [4, 12], wenn auch McGill

[8] und Gasset [2] ebenfalls diesen nachteiligen Effekt auf das Epithel feststellten.

Ein Einfluß auf die DNS durch Hemmung der Thymidyl-Synthetase wurde von Heidelberger [3] nachgewiesen. Ein immunsuppressiver Effekt der Virostatica ist daher nicht ausgeschlossen.

Unter dieser Annahme untersuchten Yamaguchi, Okumoto, Stern, Friedlaender und Smolin [14] die Wirkung des IDU auf bakteriell infizierte Kaninchenhornhaut und wiesen eine erhöhte Anfälligkeit gegenüber Staphylococcus aureus nach, wenn die Cornea mit IDU vorbehandelt worden war. Inzwischen ist die therapeutische Überlegenheit des TFT bei Herpes simplex-Infektionen hinreichend bekannt [7, 13], so daß IDU nur noch in seltenen Fällen verordnet wird.

Uns interessierte daher die Frage, ob der für IDU festgestellte negative Effekt bezüglich einer bakteriellen Hornhautinfektion auch für das TFT zutrifft.

## Material und Methode

Verwendet wurden 36 Kaninchen von 3–5 kg Gewicht, deren Hornhäute spaltlampenmikroskopisch regelrecht waren und deren Bindehäute keine bakterielle Infektion aufwiesen.

Es wurden randomisierte Gruppen von je 9 Kaninchen für physiologische Kochsalzlösung, TFT-Reinsubstanz (2 g/200 ml Aqua dest.), Trägersubstanzen (Benzalkoniumchlorid und Oculohydrosol), sowie für das TFT-Handelspräparat (Fa. Dr. Mann, Berlin) gebildet. Zehn Tage lang wurden in beide Augen 5× täglich die entsprechenden Präparationen eingetropft. Am 6. Tag wurde mit einem Hockey-Messer eine Abrasio corneae vorgenommen und unmittelbar anschließend 0,1 ml einer Kultur von Staphylo-

**Tabelle 1.** Versuchsgruppenanordnung

| Gruppe | Substanz |
| --- | --- |
| 1 | 0,9% NaCl |
| 2 | TFT – Reinsubstanz (2 g/200 ml Aqua dest.) |
| 3 | Trägersubstanzen (Benzalkoniumchlorid, Oculohydrosol) |
| 4 | TFT – Handelspräparat (Fa. Dr. Mann, Berlin) |

häute wurden am 11. Tag mit einem Trepan (Durchmesser: 5 mm) entnommen, in 0,25%iger Trypsinlösung (Fa. Serva, Heidelberg) eingebracht und bis zu einer deutlichen Andauung 18–24 Std. geschüttelt (Kreisschüttler, Fa. Köttermann, Henningsen, 60 kpm). Die Suspension wurde anschließend durch Plattieren quantitativ auf Staphylococcus aureus untersucht. Durch Voruntersuchungen wurde abgesichert, daß der Infektionsstamm durch Trypsin in seiner Vitalität nicht alteriert war.

coccus aureus (Stammnummer 7539, Nährboullion mit 1%iger Glucose, Bebrütung 18 Stunden bei 37 °C, ca. $10^8$ bis $10^{10}$ kolonienbildende Einheiten/ml) in den Bindehautsack eingegeben (Tabelle 1).

Die Augen wurden spaltlampenmikroskopisch am 8. und 10. Tag untersucht und der Befund protokolliert. Eine Fotodokumentation erfolgte am 10. Tag. Die Horn-

**Ergebnisse**

Von einer Hornhaut der TFT-Reinsubstanzgruppe konnten 100 kolonienbildende Einheiten des Infektionsstammes gezüchtet werden. In allen übrigen Hornhäuten wurde Staphylococcus aureus nicht nachgewiesen.

Klinisch bestanden unterschiedlich ausgeprägte Epitheltrübungen (Abb. 1–4), die

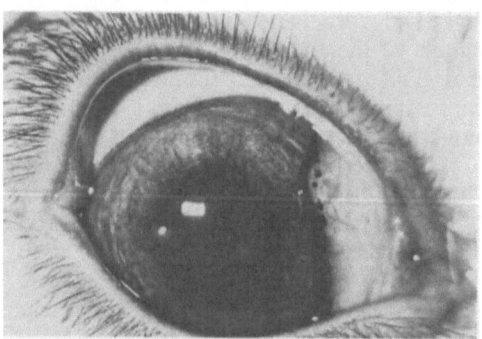

**Abb. 1.** Hornhautbefund bei Kaninchen der Gruppe NaCl

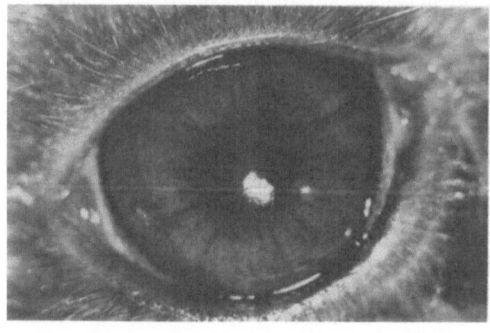

**Abb. 2.** Hornhautbefund bei Kaninchen der Gruppe Trägersubstanz

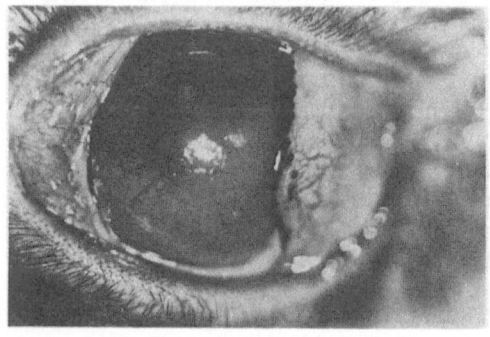

**Abb. 3.** Hornhautbefund bei Kaninchen der Gruppe TFT-Reinsubstanz

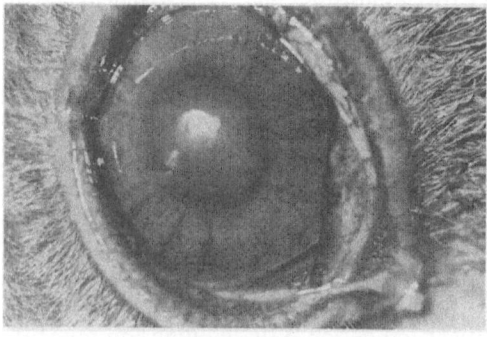

**Abb. 4.** Hornhautbefund bei Kaninchen der Gruppe TFT-Handelspräparat

**Tabelle 2.** Toxische Epitheliopathie der Cornea. Mehrfach-Vergleiche nach Tuckey auf dem 5% Niveau; Stichprobenumfang n = 9

| Gruppenvergleich | Ergebnis | Tuckeysche Spannweitenverteilung |
|---|---|---|
| 1. NaCl/TFT-Handelspräparat | 5,68 > | q 4; ∞ / 95% = 3,63 |
| 2. NaCl/TFT-Reinsubstanz | 4,81 > | q 4; ∞ / 95% = 3,63 |
| 3. Trägerstoff/TFT-Handelspräparat | 4,24 > | q 4; ∞ / 95% = 3,63 |
| 4. TFT-Reinsubstanz/Trägerstoff | 3,38 < | q 4; ∞ / 95% = 3,63 |
| 5. NaCl/Trägerstoff | 1,43 < | q 4; ∞ / 95% = 3,63 |
| 6. TFT-Reinsubstanz/TFT-Fertigpräparat | 0,86 < | q 4; ∞ / 95% = 3,63 |

anhand der Diapositive in eine kontinuierliche Rangliste eingeordnet wurden, wobei dem Untersucher die Gruppenzugehörigkeit nicht bekannt war. Dabei war die Entzündung des stärker affizierten Auges für die Kategorisierung ausschlaggebend.

Die Kruskal-Wallis-Rang-Varianzanalyse[1] (mit Bindungskorrektur) ergab auf dem 5%-Niveau Unterschiede zwischen den Gruppen. Auf dem gleichen Niveau konnten mit der Tuckeyschen Spannweitenverteilung (studentized-range) signifikante Unterschiede zwischen den Gruppen NaCl/TFT-Reinsubstanz, NaCl/TFT-Handelspräparat sowie Trägersubstanz/TFT-Handelspräparat ermittelt werden (Tabelle 2). Dabei war die Intensität der Hornhauttrübung bei der NaCl-Gruppe am wenigsten und bei den TFT-Gruppen am stärksten ausgeprägt. An der Signifikanzgrenze (5%-Niveau) lag der Gruppenvergleich TFT-Reinsubstanz/Trägerlösung, während die Gruppenunterschiede NaCl/Trägerlösung und TFT-Reinsubstanz/TFT-Handelspräparat nicht signifikant waren.

**Diskussion**

Staphylococcus aureus wurde als Testkeim gewählt, da die hierdurch verursachte Keratitis beim Kaninchen spontan in wenigen Tagen abheilt. Eine schädigende Wirkung des TFT müßte durch eine Zunahme der Keratitis und vor allem durch eine erhöhte Keimzahl in der Hornhaut nachweisbar sein.

[1] Für die statistische Auswertung sind wir Herrn Prof. Dr. rer. nat. E. Brunner, Direktor des Institutes für Med. Statistik der Universität Göttingen, zu Dank verpflichtet.

Staphylococcus aureus ist als Testkeim auch deshalb besonders geeignet, da er häufig einen Teil der Bindehautflora beim Menschen darstellt. Wenn TFT die Anfälligkeit der Kaninchenhornhaut für Staphylococcus aureus erhöhen würde, so wäre ein solcher Effekt für die menschliche Cornea ebenfalls möglich.

Während Yamaguchi et al. [14] diese Nebenwirkung des IDU an der Kaninchenhornhaut nachwiesen, konnten wir einen solchen Effekt nach Gabe von TFT nicht bestätigen. Eine erhöhte Keimzahl in der Hornhaut der TFT-Gruppe fanden wir im Vergleich zur Kontrollgruppe nicht.

Daneben stellten wir jedoch einen signifikanten Unterschied bezüglich einer „toxischen" Epitheliopathie zwischen der NaCl-Gruppe und der Gruppe TFT-Handelspräparat und TFT-Reinsubstanz sowie zwischen Trägersubstanz und TFT-Handelspräparat fest, wobei die Intensität der Hornhauttrübung in den TFT-Gruppen am stärksten war.

Da wir den Versuch bereits 5 Tage nach Eingabe von Staphylococcus aureus wegen der mikrobiologischen Untersuchung abbrachen, konnten wir einen späteren, möglichen Rückgang dieser Epitheliopathie in unserem tierexperimentiellen Modell nicht verfolgen.

**Literatur**

1. Foster CS, Pavan-Langston D (1977) Corneal wound healing and antiviral medication. Arch Ophthalmol 95:2062–2067
2. Gasset AR, Katzin D (1975) Antiviral drugs and corneal wound healing. Invest Ophthalmol Visual Sci 14:628–630
3. Heidelberger C, Parsons G, Remy DC (1964)

Syntheses of 5-Trifluoromethyluracil and 5-Trifluoromethyl-2-deoxyuridine. J Med Chem 7:1–5

4. Holtmann HW, Stein HJ (1977) Zur Frage der Epithelregenerationshemmung bei Trifluorothymidin-Behandlung (F₃TDR). Klin Monatsbl Augenheilkd 171:576–579

5. Hyndiuk RA, Charlin RE, Alpren TV, Schultz RO (1978) Trifluridine in resistant human herpetic keratitis. Arch Ophthalmol 96:1839–1841

6. Kaufman HE (1965) In vivo studies with antiviral agents. Ann NY Acad Sci 130:168–180

7. Kaufman HE (1975) Therapy and prophylaxis of herpetic eye disease. Vortrag Univ.-Augenklinik, Freiburg

8. Langston R, Pavan-Langston D, Dohlman CH (1974) Antiviral medication and corneal wound healing. Arch Ophthalmol 92:509–513

9. McGill J, Holt-Wilson AD, McKinnon JR, Williams HP, Jones BR (1974) Some aspects of the clinical use of trifluorothymidine in the treatment of herpetic ulceration of the cornea. Trans Ophthalmol Soc UK 94:342

10. Pollack FM, Rose J (1964) The effect of 5-Iodo-2-Deoxyuridine (IDU) in corneal healing. Laboratory Sciences 71:520–527

11. Puelhorn G, Sosath G, Thiel HJ (1978) The effect of 5-Iodo-2-Deoxyuridine (IDU) and Dexamethasone on corneal wound-healing in the rabbit. Arch Ophthalmol 56:38–52

12. Sundmacher R (1976) Herpestherapie und -prophylaxe, 1. Versuch einer kritischen Wertung. Klin Monatsbl Augenheilkd 169:308–325

13. Sundmacher R (1978) Trifluorothymidinprophylaxe bei der Steroid-Therapie herpetischer Keratouveitiden. Klin Monatsbl Augenheilkd 173:516–519

14. Yamaguchi K, Okumoto M, Stern G, Friedländer M, Smolin G (1979) Idoxuridine and bacterial corneal infection. Am J Ophthalmol 87:202–205

## Diskussion zum Beitrag S. 291–294

O.P. van Bijsterveld (Utrecht)

Why did you choose staphylococci for your study? If you inoculate $10^9$/ml viable, virulent staphylococci in a paracentral wound, you get a central corneal "abscess" on an immunological basis of 30%, but no progressive ulcers.

W. Behrens-Baumann (Göttingen)

Well, I know that Staphylococcus aureus is not very virulent for the rabbit cornea. It is part of the normal flora of the conjunctiva in man. In studying an increased affinity for corneal infection, you should not use a bacteria with high virulence. If you inoculate Pseudomonas aeruginosa, for instance, you will get an infection rate of 60%–100%, which is not a good model for testing an increased affinity for corneal infection after pretreatment with a drug.

O.P. van Bijsterveld (Utrecht)

Yes, but I was not actually referring to pseudomonas; this organism is highly pathogenic for the cornea. You could have taken the pneumococcus, which would have been a suitable micro-organism for this type of study.

W. Behrens-Baumann (Göttingen)

You are right, but Yamaguchi and Smolin did a study with IDU and Staphylococcus aureus. In order to compare this study with ours, we had to use Staphylococcus aureus, too. In general, the level of virulence determines which bacterium is to be used in such a study.

Sundmacher, R. (Hrsg.):
Herpetische Augenerkrankungen
© J.F. Bergmann Verlag, München 1981

# Acyclovir (Zovirax) in the Management of Herpetic Keratitis

B.R. Jones, D.J. Coster, R. Michaud, K.R. Wilhelmus, London

**Key words.** Dendritic keratitis, acyclovir, iodo-deoxyuridine, antiviral drugs – toxicity

**Schlüsselwörter.** Keratitis dendritica, Acyclovir, Joddesoxyuridin, antivirale Medikamente – Toxizität

**Summary.** A double blind randomised trial of topical therapy with 3% Acyclovir (Zovirax) eye ointment, or placebo ointment, each used 5 times daily following treatment of dendritic ulcers by minimum wiping debridement was carried out on 24 men. There were 7 recurrences of microscopic foci of epithelial herpetic disease in the 12 patients treated with placebo but none in the 12 treated with Acyclovir (ACV). A second double blind randomised trial was carried out treating dendritic ulcers with either 3% ACV or 1% IDU ointment. Each ointment was applied 5 times daily until the ulcer was healed, and thereafter for a further 3 days. All ulcers healed within 10 days. There was a trend in favour of ACV but from a logrank analysis of the cumulative frequency distribution curves of healing times. Both medications were equivalent.

These results prove that 3% Acyclovir ointment is an active antiviral in herpetic epithelial ulcers and that it is at least as effective as 1% IDU ointment when used 5 times daily.

Seven of 38 patients using one batch of acyclovir ointment developed minor punctate staining with Bengal rose on the lower third of the bulbar conjunctiva. In two it extended onto the cornea.

**Zusammenfassung.** Vierundzwanzig Männer mit Keratitis dendritica wurden zunächst mit einer minimalen Abrasio („minimal wiping debridement") und anschließend randomisiert und „doppelblind" entweder mit 3% Acyclovir-Salbe (Zovirax) oder Plazebo-Salbe 5× tgl. behandelt. Bei den Plazebo-behandelten Patienten fanden sich 7mal kleine Rezidive, bei den Acyclovir-behandelten überhaupt keine. In einer zweiten Doppelblindstudie verglichen wir die Wirkung von 3% ACV mit der von 1% IDU-Salbe. Die Behandlung erfolgte 5mal tgl., bis die Dendritika abgeheilt war, die Nachbehandlung dann noch drei weitere Tage. Alle Hornhäute waren innerhalb von 10 Tagen abgeheilt. Statistisch ergab sich ein positiver Trend für ACV. Damit ist bewiesen, daß ACV-Salbe ein klinisch wirksames Virustatikum ist, das bei täglich 5maliger Applikation mindestens so gut ist wie IDU-Salbe. Sieben von 38 Patienten, die alle mit einer besonderen Charge ACG behandelt wurden, entwickelten im Laufe der Behandlung eine bengalpositive geringe Konjunctivitis punctata auf dem unteren Drittel der Bulbusbindehaut. In zwei dieser Fälle war auch die untere Hornhaut betroffen.

Acyclovir (ACV), previously known as acycloguanosine or Wellcome 248U, and now produced as Zovirax (Fig. 1) is a purine nucleoside antiviral with an acyclic side chain: it may be regarded as an acyclic analogue of 2'-deoxyguanosine [11]. It has a specific and highly potent antiviral action against type I herpes simplex virus (HSV) in vero cells with a therapeutic ratio of: 3000 [5, 9, 14, 23]. It has a similar activity against type 2 HSV, somewhat less against V-Z virus [2, 15] and other members of the herpes group, but is without action against vaccinia virus, adenovirus and a wide range of RNA viruses.

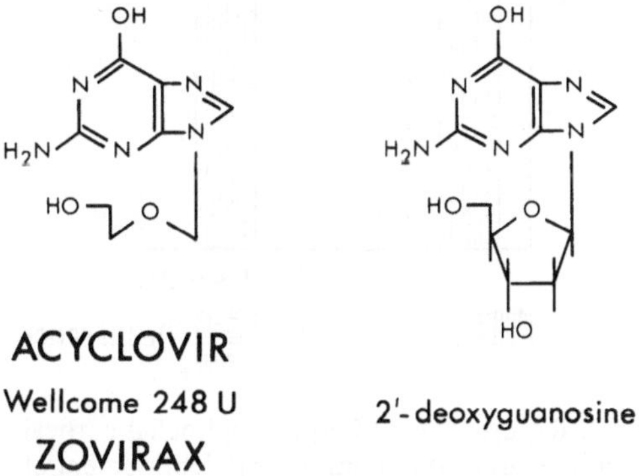

ACYCLOVIR
Wellcome 248 U
ZOVIRAX

2'-deoxyguanosine

**Fig. 1.** Structural formula of Acyclovir showing its resemblance to 2'-deoxyguanosine

295

Highly selective phosphorylation by virus-specified thymidine kinase within HSV infected cells converts it to the active triphosphate form which itself has much greater activity against virus-specified DNA-polymerase than against corresponding host enzymes [11].

Very low toxicity for mamalian cells and several animal species [24] including man, combined with very low ocular toxicity in rabbits [4, 19] and an extremely low level of metabolic degradation after systemic administration [20], make it a promising compound for both topical and systemic herpes virus chemotherapy.

Acyclovir has been shown to be active in several animal models of HSV infection in the cornea [1, 12, 23], the brain [23], skin [10, 13, 18, 21, 23], mucocutaneous areas [21] and dorsal root ganglia [13, 18, 21, 22]. It is also active against B virus (Herpesvirus simiae) in rabbits.

Our clinical experience with acyclovir falls into the following five phases of studies.

1. To prove that ACV has an antiviral effect against clinical HSV infection in man.
2. To compare the efficacy of ACV with that of standard antiviral drugs in topical therapy of dendritic ulcers.
3. To compare the efficacy of ACV with that of standard antiviral drugs in topical therapy of geographic ulcers and deep (stromal) herpetic keratouveitis.
4. To assess intravenous and oral therapy with ACV for deep herpetic keratouveitis and for prevention of recurrences.
5. Cumulative documentation of all cases treated with ACV for possible adverse effects and for recurrence rates.

This paper presents data from 1, 2 and 5.

The first challenge was to prove that the new compound has an antiviral action in a clinical herpesvirus infection in man, whilst exposing the least number of persons to the least quantity of drug. This we did by using the ethically acceptable design of placebo-controlled double-blind randomised trial that we devised first to answer the similar question of human leucocyte interferon [16].

Dendritic ulcers in 24 consecutive men presenting at Moorfields Eye Hospital, and available for follow up, were treated by minimal wiping debridement (MWD) with a sterile cotton-tipped swab. This removes the opaque diseased cells at the ulcer edge or sometimes more widely. It gives rapid relief of discomfort and cures about 50% of cases without chemotherapy [16]. The microscopic foci of epithelial herpetic disease, that recur in 50% of cases, respond very promptly to standard antiviral chemotherapy [16]. Adjunctive treatment with either 3% acyclovir eye ointment or matching placebo was randomly allocated at the time of debridement, on a double-blind basis, for use 5 times daily for 7 days (Fig. 2).

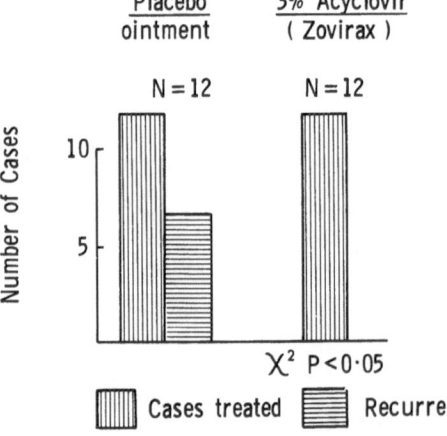

**Fig. 2.** Recurrences of herpetic epithelial corneal ulceration after minimum wiping debridement of dendritic ulcers in patients given adjunctive treatment with either 3% acyclovir or placebo ointment 5 times daily for 7 days

**Table 1.** Incidence of recurrence of epithelial herpetic disease in each treatment group amongst 24 men with dendritic ulcers treated with Minimum Wiping Debridement and randomised adjunctive therapy with either Acyclovir or Placebo

| Adjunctive treatment | Number of patients | Number of recurrences |
|---|---|---|
| 3% Acyclovir | 12 | 0 |
| Placebo | 12 | 7 |
| P = 0.05 (Fisher) | | < 0.005 (Cox) |

**Table 2.** Distribution of 54 patients with small or large dendritic ulcers to ACV or IDU treatment groups

| Ulcer size | Antiviral drug | |
| --- | --- | --- |
| | ACV | IDU |
| small dendritic | 14* | 14* |
| large dendritic | 14 | 12 |
| Total | 28 | 26 |

*one patient in each asterisked group had marked inflammatory reaction at presentation

In the 12 patients who received acyclovir there were no recurrences, whereas there were 7 recurrences within 1 week of debridement in the 12 patients who received placebo ointment [17]. This proved that acyclovir is an active antiviral drug in therapy of human herpetic epithelial keratitis.

Ulcers healed

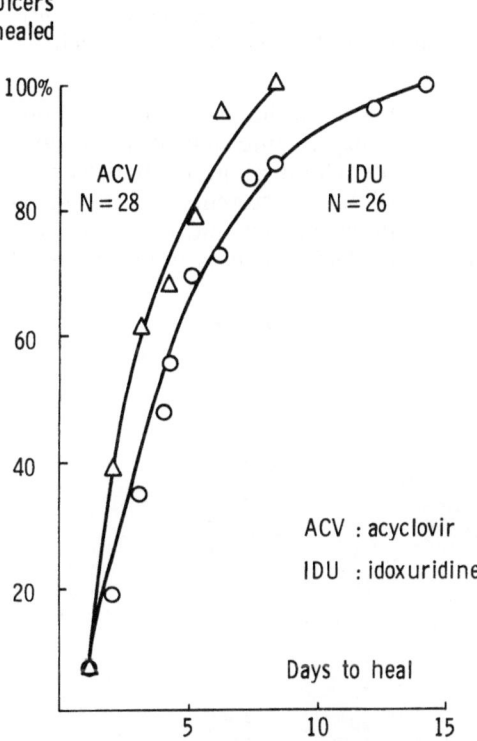

Cumulative frequency distribution of time to cure dendritic corneal ulcers in 54 patients

**Fig. 3.** Cumulative frequency distribution curves for healing times of 54 patients with dendritic ulcers treated with either 3% acyclovir or 1% IDU ointment 5 times daily

The second phase was to compare the efficacy of the new compound with that of standard antiviral as sole antiviral therapy of ulcerative herpetic keratitis. So far, 54 patients with herpetic ulcers have been treated by random double-blind allocation of either 3% acyclovir or 1% IDU eye ointment for use 5 times daily until the ulcer was healed as judged at the slit lamp by absence of epithelial defect demonstrated by staining with fluorescein followed by Bengal rose, and thereafter for a further 3 days.

The cases were closely matched in strata for type of ulcer (geographic or dendritic), size of ulcer, steroid treatment in the previous 3 weeks, and the degree of inflammatory reaction in the cornea and anterior chamber at presentation. Table 2 shows the matching of size of dendritic ulcers between treatment groups in the trial.

The results with these 54 patients with dendritic ulcers were assessed on the basis of the number of days it took for the ulcers to heal, as shown in the cumulative frequency distribution curves (Fig. 2). There were no failures of treatment to heal the ulcers and the patterns of distribution of healing times are very similar with each of the two drugs. A logrank analysis indicates that the difference between the curves was likely to have occurred by chance. Acyclovir 3% ointment is thus at least as effective as 1% IDU ointment: no adverse reaction was observed during the period of therapy with either drug shown in Fig. 3.

The results of treating geographic ulcers will be presented when the series reaches a satisfactory statistical significance. Meanwhile it is interesting to recall that in the previous comparisons between Trifluorothymidine (TFT) and Adenine arabinoside (ARA-A) therapy of herpetic ulcers no difference was demonstrable in treating 100 patients with dendritic ulcers (Fig. 4) whereas a strikingly better response to TFT was demonstrable in only 30 patients with geographic ulcers [8].

It is therefore not surprising that Fig. 3 shows only a trend in favour of ACV for treating dendritic ulcers, which is not statistically significant in this trial treating 54 patients. The results of our current comparative trial treating geographic ulcers will be of especial interest and are awaited with impatience.

One patient whose dendritic ulcer failed to

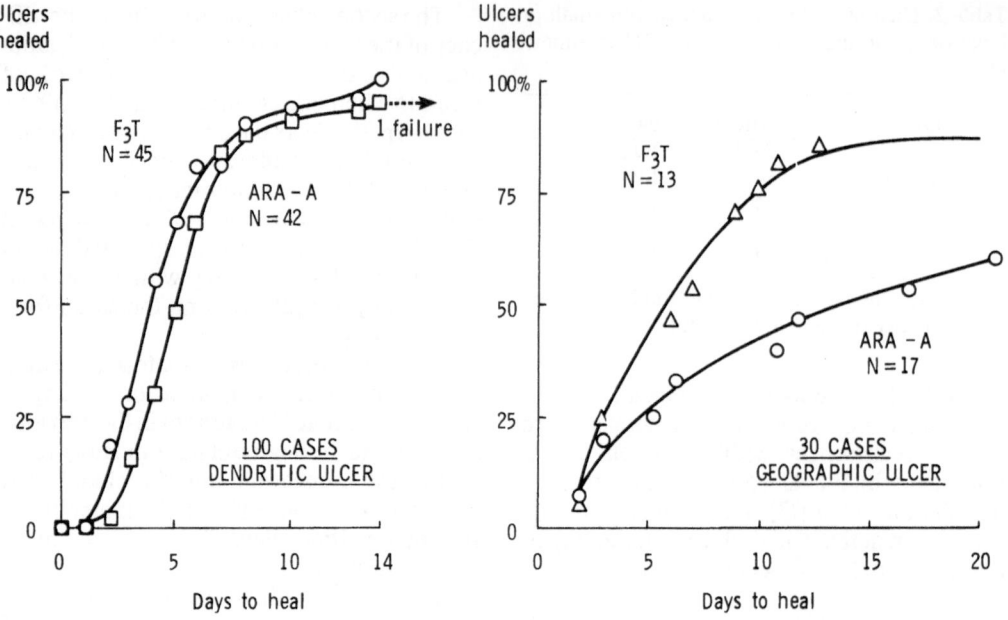

**Fig. 4.** Cumulative frequency distribution curves for healing times of patients with either dendritic or geographic ulcers under treatment with either 3.3% Ara-A ointment or 1% IDU ointment 5 times daily

heal in 14 days on IDU used 5 times daily was treated with ACV ointment: the ulcer healed within 3 days.

The data from in vitro work and animal experimentation suggests that ACV should inhibit herpesvirus replication deep in the corneal stroma, in the uveal tract and optic nerve but may require oral or intravenous administration for this purpose. It may be expected to inhibit recurrences of peripheral lesions during therapy, and may block the release of infective viruses from peripheral

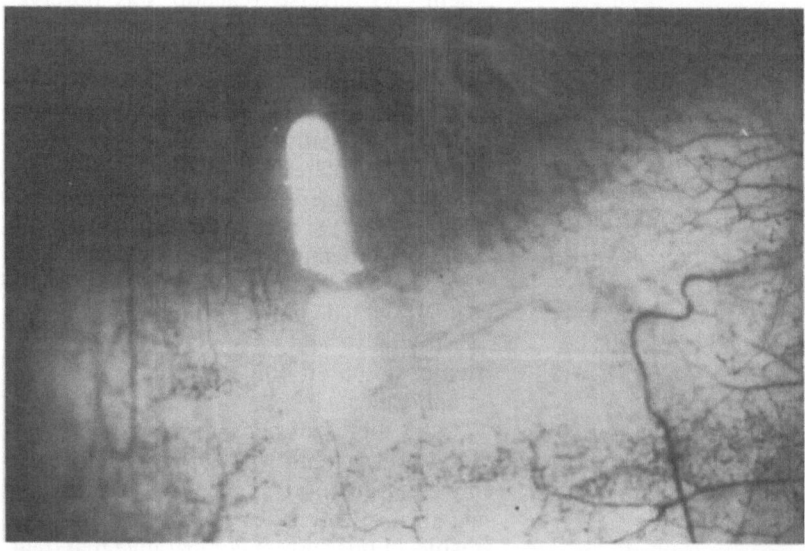

**Fig. 5.** Punctate staining of bulbar conjunctiva with Bengal rose after topical use of 3% acyclovir ointment 5 times daily

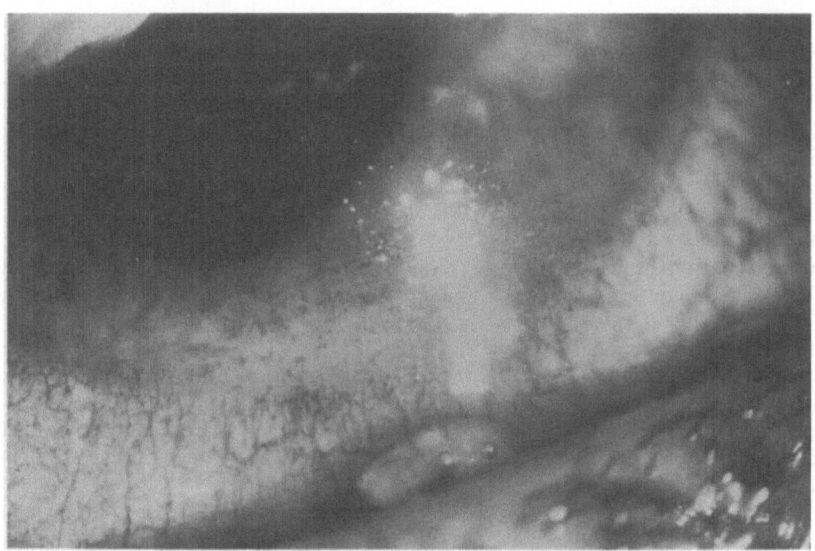

**Fig. 6.** Punctate staining of bulbar conjunctiva with Bengal rose extending over limbus onto cornea. Acyclovir ointment still present as a solid bolus

neurones. Whether it will influence the risk of subsequent recurrence in man, after therapy is terminated remains to be seen.

In our various trials and open observations 89 patients have used ACV ointment 5 times daily, mostly for 7–14 days. No case of contact dermatitis, stenosis of the lacrimal puncta or canaliculi, or of follicular conjunctival reaction has been seen. No epithelial keratopathy or conjunctival abnormality was seen that could be ascribed to the new drug, until the observation of an area of punctate Bengal rose staining of the inferior third of the bulbar conjunctiva in 7 of 38 patients treated with a further batch of ointment (Fig. 5). In two of them it extended across the lower limbus to involve a small area of corneal epithelium (Fig. 6). This represents 18% of the users of this particular batch and 8% of the total number of patients treated with ACV ointment.

This staining with Bengal rose was observed after the following numbers of days of therapy: 3, 3, 10, 12, 14, 15 and 15. The two observations after 3 days occurred in right and left eyes of one patient treated for bilateral herpetic keratitis. In each case the staining disappeared within 3 days of discontinuing ACV treatment. It is tempting to enquire whether it could be due to aggregates of ACV lodging in this area of the lower fornix and causing local overdose; but the true significance of these observations requires further elucidation.

## References

1. Bauer DJ, Collin P, Tucker jr WE, Macklin AW (1979) Treatment of experimental herpes simplex keratitis with acycloguanosine. Br J Ophthalmol 63:429–435
2. Biron KK, Elion GB (1979) Sensitivity of varicella zoster virus in vitro to acyclovir. Antimicrob Agents Chemother Abstr 249
3. Boulter EA, Thornton B, Bauer DJ, Bye A (1980) Successful treatment of experimental B virus (Herpesvirus simiae) infection with acyclovir. Br Med J :681–683
4. Brigden D, Pye A, Collins P, Miranda P de (1978) Preliminary studies with 9-(2-Hydroxyethoxymethyl) guanine (BW 248U administered orally to healthy male human volunteers). Antimicrob Agents Chemother Abstr 74
5. Collins P, Bauer DJ (1979) The activity in vitro against herpes virus of 9-(2-Hydroxyethoxymethyl) guanine (acycloguanosine), a new antiviral agent. Antimicrob Chemother 5:431 436
6. Coster DJ, Falcon MG, Cantell K, Jones BR (1977) Clinical experience of human leucocyte interferon in the management of herpetic keratitis. Trans Ophthalmol Soc UK 97:327–329
7. Coster DJ, Jones BR, Falcon MG (1977) Role

of debridement in the treatment of herpetic keratitis. Trans Ophthalmol Soc UK 97:314–317

8. Coster DJ, Jones BR, McGill JI (1979) Treatment of amoeboid herpetic ulcers with adenine arabinoside of trifluorothymidine. Br Ophthalmol 418–421

9. Crumpacker CS, Schnipper LE, Zaia JA, Levin MJ (1979) Growth inhibition by acycloguanosine of herpesvirus isolated from human infections. Antimicrob Agents Chemother :642–645

10. Descamps J, Clercq E de, Barr PJ, Jones AS, Walker RT, Torrence PF, Shugar D (1979) Relative potencies of different anti-Herpes agents in the topical treatment of cutaneous Herpes Simplex virus infection of athymic nude mice. Antimicrob Agents Chemother Nov:680–682

11. Elion GB, Furman PA, Fyfe JA, Miranda P de, Beauchamp L, Schaeffer HJ (1977) Selectivity of action of an antiherpetic agent, 9-(2-Hydroxyethoxymethyl) guanine. Proc Natl Acad Sci USA 74:5716–5720

12. Falcon MG, Jones BR (1979) Acycloguanosine: antiviral activity in the rabbit cornea. Br J Ophthalmol 63:422–424

13. Field HJ, Bell SE, Elion GB, Nash AA, Wildy P (1979) Effect of acycloguanosine treatment on acute and latent herpes simplex infections in mice. Antimicrob Agents Chemother : 554–561

14. Furman PA, St Clair MH, Fyfe JA, Rideout JL, Keller PM, Elion GB (1979) Inhibition of herpes simplex virus-induced DNA polymerase activity and viral DNA replication by 9-(2-Hydroxyethoxymethyl) guanine and its triphosphate. J Virol :72–77

15. Fyfe JA, Biron KK (1979) Phosphorylation of acyclovir by a thymidine kinase induced by varicella-zoster virus. Antimicrob Agents Chemother Abstr 250

16. Jones BR, Coster DJ, Falcon MG, Cantell K (1976) Topical therapy of ulcerative herpetic keratitis with human interferon. Lancet 2:128

17. Jones BR, Coster DJ, Fison PN, Thompson GM, Cobo LM, Falcon MG (1979) Efficacy of acycloguanosine (Wellcome 248U) against herpes simplex corneal ulcers. Lancet:1:243–244

18. Klein RJ, Friedman-Kien AE, DeStefano E (1979) Latent herpes simplex virus infections in sensory ganglia of hairless mice prevented by acycloguanosine. Antimicrob Agents Chemother :723–729

19. Lass JH, Pavan-Langston D, Park N-H (1979) Aciclovir and corneal wound healing. Am J Ophthalmol 88:102–108

20. Miranda P de, Whitley RJ, Blum MR, Keeney

RE, Barton N, Cocchetto DM, Good S, Hemstreet GP, Kirk LE, Page DA, Elion GB (1979) Acyclovir kinetics after intravenous infusion. Clin Pharmacol Ther 26:718–728

21. Park N-H, Pavan-Langston D, McLean SL (1979) Acyclovir in oral and ganglionic herpes simplex virus infections. Infect Dis 140:802–806

22. Park N-H, Pavan-Langston D, McLean SL, Albert DM (1979) Therapy of experimental herpes simplex encephalitis with aciclovir in mice. Antimicrob Agents Chemother 15:775–779

23. Schaeffer HJ, Beauchamp L, Miranda P de, Elion GB, Bauer DJ, Collins P (1978) 9-(2-Hydroxyethoxymethyl) guanine activity against viruses of the herpes group. Nature 272:583–585

24. Tucker jr WE, Macklin AW, Szot RJ, Clive D (1978) Pre-clinical safety evaluation of Zovirax (BW 248U). Antimicrob Agents Chemother Abstr 64

## Discussion on the Contribution pp. 295–300

L.M.T. Collum (Dublin)
I'd just like to say that we have carried out a double blind control trial, much as Prof. Jones has done and our results are very similar. We had 30 in each group; they were all dendritic ulcers: We didn't include any geographic ulcers in that particular series. They all healed in much the same time scale that Prof. Jones' patients did. I'm just interested to know if any side effects occurred. We had one patient, in fact, who did get punctal tightening or stenosis, and it's interesting that in a paper earlier on, somebody said that a patient using $F_3T$ also got punctal tightening and, of course, IDU is very often associated with that. In a slide later on in my own poster, I have a few comments to make, but I'd just like to say that our results agree entirely with those of Prof. Jones at the moment.

C. Kok van Alphen (Leyden)
I would like to comment that in the old literature I found that the closure of the punctae in herpes was described without the existence of those drugs.

B.R. Jones (London)
There is no doubt that you can get herpetic canaliculitis which results in occlusion of the punctae and the canalicular system; but the appearances that go along with drug-induced changes are very characteristic. You see a broadening of the epithelial zone in the punctum and extending into the canaliculus, the punctum becomes flattened and depressed and filled with thickened epithelium which then meets in the middle to occlude the lumen. If you re-

cognize that early enough, the change is usually reversible. It does seem to be a genuine toxic effect. Unfortunately, we haven't had the courage to biopsy the process.

W.H. Prusoff (New Haven)
Was there any attempt to analyse the two batches of acyclovir. In other words, the presumption would be that the second batch is purer than the first, and then the question would be: Is there a precursor which might be preventing some of the toxicity* which is present in the first batch?

H.E. Kaufman (New Orleans)
That's an optimistic presumption.

B.R. Jones (London)
These studies are going on and it's only a couple of weeks that we have realized this process was occurring, so we don't have data yet.

G. Smolin (San Francisco)
We've seen a great number of reactions to

---

*Punctate staining of conjunctiva and cornea. Ed

preservatives. Were there any preservatives in your acyclovir?

B.R. Jones (London)
Pray tell me what preservatives you use in eye ointments?

G. Smolin (San Francisco)
Benzylkonium chloride. Its required in ointments in the U.S.

B.R. Jones (London)
Has it proven to be effective?

H.E. Kaufman (New Orleans)
No, but it is required.

B.R. Jones (London)
In the eye ointments which are formulated in our hospital, there is no preservative. I do not know at the moment about Acyclovir, perhaps Dr. Ravenscroft could answer this question?

T. Ravenscroft (Beckenham)
The ointment consists of active drug in a bland petrolatum base.

Sundmacher, R. (Hrsg.):
Herpetische Augenerkrankungen
© J.F. Bergmann Verlag, München 1981

# Antiviral Agents in Experimental Herpetic Stromal Disease

E.D. Varnell, H.E. Kaufman, New Orleans

**Key words.** HSV-1 – RE-strain, stromal keratitis, trifluorothymidine, vidarabine

**Schlüsselwörter.** HSV-1 – RE-Stamm, Stroma-herpes, Trifluorthymidin, Vidarabin

**Summary.** A disciform edema or stromal necrosis was produced in New Zealand white rabbits by the mid-stromal injection of the RE strain of herpesvirus. Topical trifluridine and vidarabine monophosphate have been reported to suppress the disease when treatment was initiated before clinical signs of disease were apparent. We investigated the effect of acyclovir on stromal disease using topical ointment and intravenous and subcutaneous injections in comparison with trifluridine and vidarabine treatment.

We found that 1% trifluridine drops were significantly better than subcutaneous acyclovir for preventing the disease when treatment was initiated the day after virus injection and were effective in suppressing disease when treatment was continued. If treatment was discontinued on day 9 after injection, the appearance of stromal disease was merely delayed. Subcutaneous acyclovir was significantly more effective than trifluridine for treatment of symptoms of stromal disease once such symptoms had appeared. Topical treatment with either 3% acyclovir or vidarabine alone had no significant effect on the course of the disease; however, treatment with a combination of both ointments almost completely suppressed the stromal disease.

**Zusammenfassung.** Bei weißen Neuseeland-kaninchen wurde durch die Injektion des Herpes simplex-Virusstammes RE in die Hornhaut-stromamitte entweder ein disciformes Ödem oder eine Stromanekrose erzeugt. Es wurde berichtet, daß lokal gegebenes Trifluorthymidin (TFT) und Vidarabinmonophosphat die Entwicklung solcher Erkrankungen dann verhindern konnten, wenn sie vor dem Auftreten klinischer Symptome gegeben wurden (Arch Ophthalmol 97/727, 1979). Wir untersuchten jetzt die Wirkung von Acyclovir auf diese Stromaerkrankungen und prüften hierbei sowohl die lokale Salbenapplikation als auch intravenöse und subkutane Injektionen im Vergleich mit TFT- und Vidarabinbehandlung. Die einzelnen Testgruppen bestanden aus jeweils zehn Tieren. Alle Bewertungen erfolgten „doppelblind". Die Ergebnisse wurden nach der Kruskal-Wallis-Methode statistisch aufgearbeitet.

Es ergab sich, daß bei Therapiebeginn einen Tag nach der Virusinfektion 1%ige TFT-Tropfen signifikant besser waren als subkutan gegebenes Acyclovir und daß sie den Stromaherpes auch völlig verhindern konnten, wenn die Behandlung lange genug durchgeführt wurde. Wurde die Therapie aber 9 Tage nach der Injektion abgebrochen, so verzögerte man lediglich das Auftreten der Erkrankung. Bestanden zu Therapiebeginn bereits klinische Symptome, so war subkutanes Acyclovir signifikant wirkungsvoller als TFT. Die Lokaltherapie mit 3%igem Acyclovir oder Vidarabin allein beeinflußte den Krankheitsverlauf nicht signifikant. Im Gegensatz hierzu führte aber eine Kombination dieser beiden Salben zu einer fast völligen Unterdrückung der Stromaerkrankung.

## Introduction

At present, there is no specific therapy for herpetic stromal disease. Corticosteroids are used along with antiviral agents for treatment of the inflammation and prevention of recurrences of epithelial herpetic keratitis [2, 9].

Herpetic stromal disease is caused by complex processes. Multiplying virus is usually not found in the stroma. Virus titers are maximal 2 to 3 days after injection and drop to barely detectable levels once disease is apparent, although keratocytes stain with fluorescein-labeled antibody. However, lymphocytes are found near degenerating keratocytes [4]. It has been postulated that the disease is similar to a graft rejection, with the cells that contain viral antigens being re-

303

cognized as foreign. The study of McNeill and Kaufman [3], which showed that early treatment with antivirals suppressed the appearance of stromal disease, indicated that active multiplication of virus is necessary for the initiation of disease.

Animal models for herpetic stromal disease can be made to show disease in immunized animals [10] or in non-immunized rabbits [4, 8], and can produce a transient disciform disease or a necrotizing stromal keratitis. We have chosen to use the model described by Metcalf, McNeill and Kaufman [4], which uses non-immune rabbits in which disciform keratitis appears in 95% of the injected eyes and progresses to a necrotizing keratitis in 10% of these eyes.

We studied the effect of acyclovir [1, 7], an antiviral agent with topical and systemic activity, both alone and in combination with other antiviral agents, on the prevention and treatment of herpetic stromal disease.

## Materials and Methods

New Zealand white rabbits weighing 2 to 3 kg were given intramuscular injections of chlorpromazine (Thorazine, 25 mg/kg) one hour prior to inoculation of the cornea. Corneas were anesthetized by the topical application of proparacaine hydrochloride (Ophthaine,

0.5%) and injected with approximately 0.02 ml of the RE strain of herpesvirus suspension. Both eyes of all animals were injected with virus.

The animals were divided into random treatment groups of 10 rabbits per group. For topical treatment, both eyes of the animal received the same treatment. Eyes were examined by slit lamp biomicroscopy in a blind manner. The stromal disease and iritis were graded on a scale of 0 to 4, as described by McNeill and Kaufman [3].

For topical treatment, 3% ophthalmic ointment of acyclovir (Burroughs Wellcome Research Laboratories), 3% vidarabine (Vira-A®, Parke Davis), or 1% trifluridine in saline was used. For the intravenous and subcutaneous treatments, the sodium salt of acyclovir diluted in Ringer's solution or a suspension of vidarabine in saline was used. Treatment was started the day after virus injection (day 1) when no disease was apparent, day 5 when only epithelial disease was present, or day 7 when stromal disease was beginning to appear.

### Statistical Analysis

For statistical analysis of the scores of severity, Breslow's test was used to compare the treatment groups. If Breslow's test was significant at $p < 0.05$, data were subjected to

**Table 1.** Effect of antivirals in preventing the appearance of experimental herpetic stromal disease

| Treatment | Severity of disease on day after virus injection | | | | |
| | 2 | 5 | 8 | 15 | 19 |
|---|---|---|---|---|---|
| Acyclovir, intravenous 60 mg/kg bid day 1–7 | 0.07 | 0.22 | 0.80 | 1.25 | 1.16 |
| Acyclovir subcutaneous 30 mg/kg bid day 1–7 | 0.02 | 0.32 | 0.65 | 0.65[a, c] | 0.47[a, c] |
| Trifluridine 1% drops, topical 6 times/day day 1–8 | 0.05[a, b] | 0.02[a, b] | 0.02[a, b] | 1.46 | 0.96 |
| Control | 0.05 | 0.80 | 1.47 | 1.81 | 1.18 |

[a] significantly better than control ($p < 0.05$)
[b] significantly better than acyclovir, subcutaneous ($p < 0.05$)
[c] significantly better than trifluridine ($p < 0.05$)
Severity of disease graded from 0–4; values represent average of graded eyes

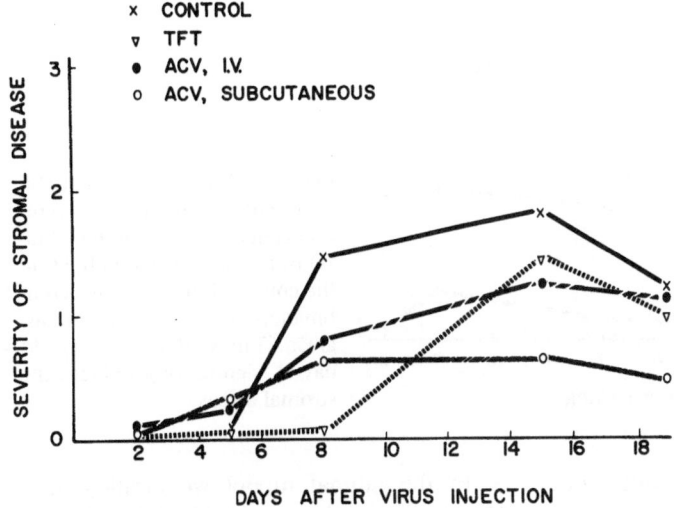

x CONTROL
▽ TFT
● ACV, I.V.
○ ACV, SUBCUTANEOUS

DAYS AFTER VIRUS INJECTION

**Fig. 1.** Seven days after the midstromal injection of the RE strain of herpesvirus into rabbit corneas, untreated control eyes show evidence of disciform keratitis. This stromal disease continues through the 15th day and then subsides in most animals, although some eyes progress to a necrotic keratitis. Trifluridine 1% (TFT) drops given 6 times a day from day 1 to day 8 prevent the appearance of stromal disease; however, when treatment is discontinued, the disease reaches a severity similar to the untreated control eyes. Intravenous treatment with acyclovir from day 1 to day 7 is not effective in changing the course of the disease, but the subcutaneous treatment significantly alters the disease

Gehan's test. Analyses were performed by Jonathan J. Shuster, Ph.D., Department of Statistics, University of Florida, Gainesville, Florida.

## Results

Trifluridine (TFT) was effective in suppressing the stromal disease as long as treatment was continued (Table 1, Fig. 1). In animals administered TFT drops from day 1 through day 8, stromal disease was significantly less than in animals treated with subcutaneous acyclovir at a dose of 30 mg/kg twice a day ($p < 0.05$). However, after TFT treatment was discontinued, the severity of disease rose to a level similar to that in the untreated control group, while the eyes of the animals treated with subcutaneous acyclovir were significantly better than either the TFT-treated or control eyes ($p < 0.05$).

Topical treatment with 3% acyclovir ointment also had an effect on the stromal disease (Table 2, Fig. 2), but the most striking effect was found when a combination of acyclovir and vidarabine (Vira-A) was used ($p = 0.015$). The stromal disease was almost completely suppressed. Combinations of acyclovir and vidarabine, or acyclovir and TFT, started 7 days after injection of the herpesvirus, were not effective in treating stromal disease once

**Table 2.** Topical treatment for the prevention of experimental herpetic stromal disease

| Treatment[b] | Severity of disease on day after virus injection | | | | |
| | 1 | 2 | 7 | 10 | 11 |
|---|---|---|---|---|---|
| Acyclovir 3% and Vidarabine 3% | 0[a] | 0[a] | 0.20[a] | 0.44[a] | 0.12[a] |
| Acyclovir 3% | 0.1 | 0.40 | 1.25 | 1.40 | 1.35 |
| Vidarabine 3% | 0 | 0.05 | 3.05 | 2.27 | 1.75 |
| Control | 0 | 0.08 | 3.00 | 2.88 | 2.88 |

[a] significantly better than acyclovir alone ($p = 0.15$)
[b] all ointments were given 6 times/day from day 1 to day 11
Severity of disease graded from 0–4; values represent average of graded eyes

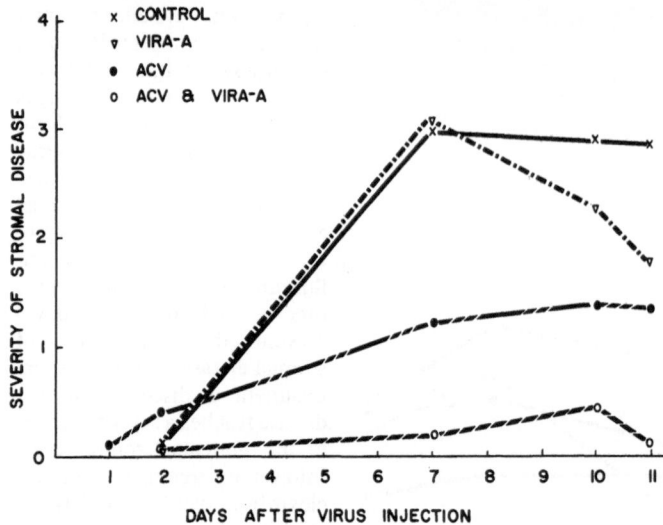

Fig. 2. Topical treatment of rabbit eyes with 3% ophthalmic ointments of either vidarabine (Vira-A) or acyclovir has no effect on the course of disease, but a combination of these ointments, given 6 times a day, from day 1 to day 11, significantly reduces the stromal disease

it was established (Table 3). Trifluridine alone had a transient effect.

## Discussion

Although the relative roles of viral multiplication and viral replication and host reactivity to viruses and antigen in necrotizing stromal keratitis of man are unknown, it is likely from the work of Meyers [5] and others that some viral replication is required but that host reactivity is also a prominent part of the disease. The relative roles may never be clear until effective drugs are found to eliminate the stromal disease.

In the animal model we employed, it appears that viral replication is required in the early phases of infection, and virus titer rises before disease becomes prominent. The titer then begins to fall and is extremely low by the time disease becomes apparent.

In this kind of model, we have shown that trifluridine is effective early in preventing viral replication. Topical acyclovir has some effect, although it appears to be less than that of trifluridine in this rabbit model. Systemic acyclovir is also effective. In humans, acyclovir can be shown to penetrate into the anterior chamber [6], but it must be remembered that these drugs do not work in the aqueous, and the relationship between

**Table 3.** Effect of antivirals in treating established herpetic stromal disease

| Treatment[a] | Severity of disease on day after virus injection | | | | | | |
| | 7 | 9 | 11 | 15 | 16 | 18 | 21 |
|---|---|---|---|---|---|---|---|
| Control | 1.65 | 3.11 | 2.88 | 2.25 | 1.81 | 1.62 | 1.58 |
| Trifluridine 1% and Acyclovir 3% | 0.95 | 2.00 | 2.05 | 2.30 | 1.38 | 1.38 | 1.33 |
| Vidarabine 3% and Acyclovir 3% | 1.35 | 2.55 | 2.45 | 1.85 | 1.60 | 1.55 | 1.44 |
| Acyclovir 3% | 1.05 | 2.40 | 2.35 | 1.90 | 1.50 | 1.38 | 1.44 |
| Trifluridine 1% | 1.40 | 2.05 | 1.80 | 1.68 | 1.50 | 1.18 | 1.00 |
| Vidarabine 3% | 1.15 | 2.30 | 2.30 | 1.94 | 1.61 | 1.38 | 1.16 |

[a] all treatments given 6 times/day from day 7 to day 21
Severity of disease graded from 0–4; values represent average of graded eyes

anterior chamber concentration and efficacy in treating stromal disease is unclear.

One of the most exciting findings of this study is the possibility that combinations of drugs may have an additive or synergistic effect. In this study the use of acyclovir and vidarabine topically gave a significantly greater effect than either drug alone, and although the value of such therapy in the treatment of human disease will not be clear until studies are done, this work does suggest that this combination would be an effective one to try, especially in the early phases of disease. Similarly, the possibility that such combinations might prevent the evolution of stromal disease from initial epithelial infections seems worth evaluating.

**Acknowledgment.** Supported in part by USPHS grants EY02672 and EY02377 from the National Eye Institute, National Institutes of Health, Bethesda, Maryland.

## References

1. Elion GB, Furman PA, Fyfe JA, Miranda P de, Beauchamp L, Schaeffer HJ (1977) Selectivity of action of an antiherpetic agent 9-(2-hydroxyethoxymethyl)guanine. Proc Natl Acad Sci USA 74:5716–5720
2. Kaufman HE, Martola EL, Dohlman CH (1963) Herpes simplex treatment with IDU and corticosteroids. Arch Ophthalmol 69:468–472
3. McNeill JI, Kaufman HE (1979) Local antivirals in a herpes simplex stromal keratitis model. Arch Ophthalmol 97:727–729
4. Metcalf JF, McNeill JI, Kaufman HE (1976) Experimental disciform edema and necrotizing keratitis in the rabbit. Invest Ophthalmol 15:979–985
5. Meyers-Elliott RH, Elliott JH, Maxwell WA, Pettit TH, O'Day DM, Terasaki PI, Bernoco D (1980) HLA antigens in herpes stromal keratitis. Am J Ophthalmol 89:54
6. Poirier RH (1979) Aqueous penetration characteristics of three antiviral compound, trifluridine, Ara-AMP, and acycloguanosine. Ocular Microbiology Group Annual Meeting, San Francisco, Nov. 3
7. Schaeffer HJ, Beauchamp L, Miranda P de, Elion GB, Bauer DJ, Collins P (1978) 9-(2-hydroxyethoxymethyl)guanine activity against viruses of the herpes group. Nature 272:583–585
8. Sery TW, Nagy RM, Nazario R (1972/73) Experimental disciform keratitis. II. Local corneal hypersensitivity to a highly virulent strain of herpes simplex. Ophthalmic Res 4:99
9. Sundmacher R (1978) Trifluorthymidinprophylaxe bei der Steroidtherapie herpetischer Keratouveitiden. Klin Monatsbl Augenheilkd 173:516–519
10. Williams LE, Nesburn AB, Kaufman HE (1965) Experimental induction of disciform keratitis. Arch Ophthalmol 73:112–114

## Discussion on the Contribution pp. 303–307

H.J. Field (Cambridge)
Does this combination of drugs have any synergistic or additive effect in vitro?

E.D. Varnell (New Orleans)
Yes, it does. Dr. Centifanto-Fitzgerald, from our group, has found out that it has at least an additive effect. She hasn't done enough work to find out whether it has a synergistic effect. I believe that Nahmias also presented similar work at the Emory meeting showing that it has an additive effect in tissue culture.

Y.C. Cheng (Chapel Hill)
I just want to comment that we should be careful in using terms concerning antagonistic, additive or synergistic interactions of drugs. Depending on how you evaluate the action of drugs and which system you use, different conclusions can be drawn.

H.E. Kaufman (New Orleans)
It is possible to show that they are synergistic in tissue culture. Here, however, with non-parametric numbers, one can say only that there is a combined, beneficial effect and perhaps be a little vague about what that means.

B.R. Jones (London)
What was the duration of administration of the combination Ara-A/ACV in the experiment where you demonstrated a rather striking effect? Did the treatment continue right through, or was it just for a limited, early period?

E.D. Varnell (New Orleans)
From day one though day 11.

T. Ravenscroft (Beckenham)
What was the dosing frequency in your i.v. study of acyclovir? You gave 16 mg/kg daily?

E.D. Varnell (New Orleans)
We gave 60 mg/kg bid from day one through day 7.

W.H. Prusoff (New Haven)
I was just going to say that in using two drugs and

hoping that they have different sites or different mechanisms of action, we have to be quite careful, because many of these compounds have multiple sites of inhibition. For example, ara-A at the triphosphate level not only inhibits DNA polymerase, but also gets incorporated into DNA; ara-A without being phosphorylated also inhibits S-adenosylhomocysteine hydrolase. This results in a piling up of S-adenosylhomocysteine which now inhibits the methylation reaction so that you don't get methylation or capping of virus messenger RNA. And there are several other enzymes upon which ara-A has an equal effect too. Furthermore, having multiple sites of inhibition is not only characteristic of ara-A; it's characteristic of many compounds.

Sundmacher, R. (Hrsg.):
Herpetische Augenerkrankungen
© J.F. Bergmann Verlag, München 1981

# Treatment of Acute and Chronic Ocular Herpes Infection With Acyclovir

A.B. Nesburn, M.D. Trousdale, Los Angeles

**Key words.** Herpetic keratitis, acyclovir

**Schlüsselwörter.** Herpeskeratitis, Acyclovir

**Summary.** Acyclovir (ACV), an acyclic purine analog 9-(2-hydroxyethoxymethyl) guanine, is a potent antiviral agent with specific inhibitory activity against several members of the herpesvirus group. Antiviral activity of ACV results from a series of phosphorylation reactions, the first of which is catalyzed by an HSV-specific thymidine kinase. The triphosphorylated form of ACV serves as both a substrate and inhibitor of the herpes DNA polymerase.

The effects of ACV on acute and chronic ocular infections induced by Herpes simplex virus type 1, IDU resistant and Ara-A resistant HSV were studied. Acute phase of the disease was reduced dramatically by topical ACV treatment. One HSV strain displayed a difference in drug sensitivity by the in vitro plaque inhibition method and the in vivo rabbit ocular model method of testing. Chronic HSV infected rabbits were given ACV via intravenous and subcutaneous routes for 14–28 days. HSV was isolated from the trigeminal ganglion, midbrain and cerebellum of the chronically infected rabbits when tested 30 days following completion of chemotherapy. Neural involvement varied with the strain of HSV studied.

**Zusammenfassung.** Acyclovir (ACV), das acyclische Purin-Analog 9-(2-Hydroxyethoxymethyl) Guanin, ist ein wirkungsvolles Virustatikum mit spezifischer Hemmwirkung gegenüber mehreren Herpesviren. Die spezifische Wirkung des ACV beruht auf einer Kette von Phosphorylierungsreaktionen, deren erster Schritt durch die HSV-spezifische Thymidinkinase katalysiert wird. Die triphosphorylierte Form des ACV dient dann sowohl als Substrat als auch als Inhibitor der Herpes-DNA-Polymerase.

Die Wirkung des ACV bei akuten und chronischen okulären Herpes simplex-Virus-Typ 1-Infektionen mit IDU-resistenten und ARA-A-resistenten Stämmen wurde untersucht. Die akute Erkrankungsphase wurde durch eine lokale ACV-Therapie eindrucksvoll abgekürzt. Bei einem HSV-Stamm zeigt sich ein deutlicher Unterschied zwischen der Virustatikaempfindlichkeit in vitro (Plaques-Hemmungs-Methode) und den Ergebnissen der in vivo-Testung beim Kaninchenmodell.

Mit HSV chronisch infizierte Kaninchen erhielten ACV intravenös und subkutan für 14–28 Tage. 30 Tage nach Abschluß der Chemotherapie konnte HSV aus dem Trigeminalganglion, dem Mittelhirn und dem Kleinhirn solch chronisch infizierter Kaninchen isoliert werden. Das Ausmaß des neuronalen Befalles war abhängig vom verwendeten HSV-Stamm.

## Introduction

Treatment of acute and recurrent ocular herpetic keratitis is not always successful in part because some strains of herpes simplex virus type 1 (HSV 1) resist the antiviral activity of available drugs. The most commonly used antiviral drugs are Idoxuridine and Vidarabine. Idoxuridine is the generic name of 5-IODO-2-Deoxyuridine. It is frequently referred to as IDU or IUDR. Vidarabine is the generic name of 1-B-Arabinofuranosyladenine. It is frequently referred to as Vira-A or ARA-A. Both of these drugs (IDU and ARA-A) have similar problems involving solubility, toxicity, efficacy and resistance. Another antiherpetic drug soon to be available commercially is triflurothymidine. Triflurothymidine is the generic name of 5-trifluoromethyl-2-deoxyuridine, It is frequently referred to as TFT or $F_3TDR$. Triflurothymidine is a highly soluble and potent drug. Thus far, HSV resistance to TFT does not appear to be a problem. The mechanism of action for IDU, ARA-A and TFT involves the pathway of the DNA synthesis.

Acyclovir, a new antiviral agent being actively investigated, has demonstrated its efficacy in suppressing herpetic keratitis. Acyclovir is the generic name of 9-(2-hydroxyethoxymethyl)guanine. It is frequently referred to as ACV or ACG. This acyclic purine analog has more potent and specific inhibitory activity than other antiviral agents against certain members of the herpesvirus group. The antiviral activity of ACV results from a series of phosphorylation reactions, the first of which is catalyzed by an HSV-specified thymidine kinase. The triphosphorylated form of ACV serves as both a substrate and inhibitor of the herpes DNA polymerase. The favorable properties of ACV which makes it unique is its efficacy, selectivity and specificity for herpes infected cells, low toxicity, good solubility, chemical stability and ability to cross blood-brain barrier. ACV appears to be effective when given topically, orally or parenterally.

It has been known for sometime that many strains of HSV are relatively insensitive to one or more antiviral drugs e.g. Idoxuridine and vidarabine. Here we report the effect of ACV on acute herpetic keratitis induced by drug resistant strains of HSV in the rabbit ocular model.

## Ocular Examination

Eyes were examined daily by the same observer using the slit lamp biomicroscope. The examiner was unaware of the treatment being administered. Grading of epithelial (dendritic and geographic) keratitis was based on the estimates of overall area of lesion involvement. A 0 to 4+ grading system was used, divided into quarter-step intervals below 1+ and half-step intervals above 1+. One plus was equivalent to 25 per cent of the corneal area involved; 2+, 50 per cent; 3+, 75 per cent; and 4+, 100 per cent involvement. Conjunctivitis, corneal clouding and iritis were graded based on clinical severity from 0 to 4+. For each of the three experiments, results of the four treatment groups were studied by one way analysis of variance. Duncan's multiple range test was used to determine which group was significantly different ($p < 0.05$).

## Materials and Methods

### Virus

McKrae strain of HSV was selected because it induces a predictable keratitis, a high incidence of latent CNS infection and a high ocular recurrence rate. McKrae strain is also sensitive to the available antiviral drugs (IDU, ARA-A, TFT and acyclovir). IDU resistant HSV and ARA-A resistant HSV employed in these studies were produced in our laboratory from the parent McKrae strain. McKrae HSV was grown in RK cells in the presence of either 100 Mcgm/ml IDU (Smith kline and french laboratories) or 100 Mcgm/ml ARA-A (Parke-Davis and Co.). Drug resistant strains of HSV-1 were plaque purified 3 times. Drug resistance of these strains was verified by us and Chandler, Seattle, Washington.

### Rabbits

Both eyes of young New Zealand white male rabbits weighing 3–4 kg, were infected with the appropriate strain of HSV and 3 to 4 days following inoculation the eyes were examined. Rabbits then were divided into four groups consisting of 12–26 eyes equally matched on the basis of herpetic corneal epithelial involvement.

### Chemotherapy

Separate experiments using the three virus strains described, were carried out using identical chemotherapy. Treatment began on day 3 or 4 postinoculation and consisted of bilateral topical application (4–6 mm ribbon) of appropriate drug or placebo every 6 hours for about 15 days. Group a was treated with vidarabine (ARA-A, 3% Vira-A ophthalmic ointment). Group b was treated with idoxuridine (IDU 0.5% stoxil ophthalmic ointment). Group c was treated with acyclovir (ACV, 3% zovirax ophthalmic ointment). Group d was treated with a placebo (same carrier used in zovirax ointment). Treatments were coded and were performed in a masked fashion.

### Isolation of HSV from Tear Film and Tissues

Thirty days after the completion of chemotherapy, animals were surgically stimulated to induce viral recurrence and to improve viral isolation rate as previously described in inf. immun. 15:772–775. Tear film samples were taken with cotton swabs at 2 hour intervals for 24 hours following surgical stimulation and inoculated on monolayers of RK cells at 37 °C.

Animals were sacrificed 24 h after stimulation. Corneal epithelial, trigeminal ganglia, midbrain and cerebellar tissues were removed aseptically. The samples were enzymatically dispersed to further enhance detection of latent HSV as described in Proc Sci Exp Biol Med (1980) 163: (in press). Dispersed cells were incubated on secondary RK cell monolayer and examined every other day for cytopathic effects. Negative cultures were passed in RK cells and incubated for at least 2 weeks before being recorded as negative. Identity of all isolates was confirmed by standard microneutralization test using known anti-HSV serum.

## Results

*Experiment 1: Acute Ocular Herpetic Disease Induced by McKrae Strain*

Figure 1 presents the corneal epithelial involvement resulting from McKrae strain HSV infection during antiviral chemotherapy. ACV therapy gave the most favorable results in that corneal involvement was greatly reduced within 24 hours following initiation of treatment. IDU chemotherapy limited corneal involvement slightly more than did ARA-A but less than ACV. As expected, the corneal lesions were most severe in those rabbit eyes receiving the placebo ointment.

In Fig. 1, corneal epithelial involvement is shown for the four treatment groups against the parent McKrae strain of HSV. From the initiation of treatment at day 3, the ACV treated eyes showed a steady decline in corneal involvement. Response to topical therapy with IDU and ARA-A was significantly improved in comparison to the placebo treated eyes from day 6 through 10. There was no significant difference between the IDU and the ARA-A treated eyes during this period. The most striking finding is the steady decline in corneal epithelium involvement with ACV while there was an increase in corneal involvement on days 5 and 6 in the IDU and ARA-A treated eyes although not to the extent of the placebo treated eyes. In this experiment, as well as in the other two experiments which employed ARA-A resistant and IDU resistant HSV, conjunctivitis, iritis and corneal clouding parallel the corneal epithelial involvement (data not shown).

*Experiment 2: Acute Ocular Herpetic Disease Induced by IDU Resistant HSV*

Corneal epithelial involvement resulting from an experimental infection with IDU resistant HSV is presented in Fig. 2. Within 24 hours of ACV treatment corneal involve-

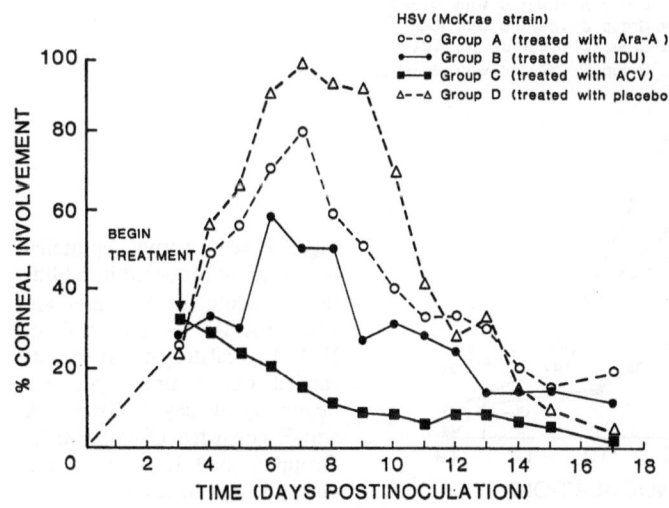

HSV (McKrae strain)
o– –o Group A (treated with Ara-A )
•——• Group B (treated with IDU)
■—■ Group C (treated with ACV)
△– –△ Group D (treated with placebo)

**Fig. 1.** Percent corneal epithelial involvement observed in rabbits during acute ocular infection with McKrae strain of HSV. Each eye was inoculated with $10^5$ pfu without scarification on day 0. Topical drug treatment was carried out 4 times per day beginning on day 3. Each treatment group consisted of 10 animals (20 treated eyes)

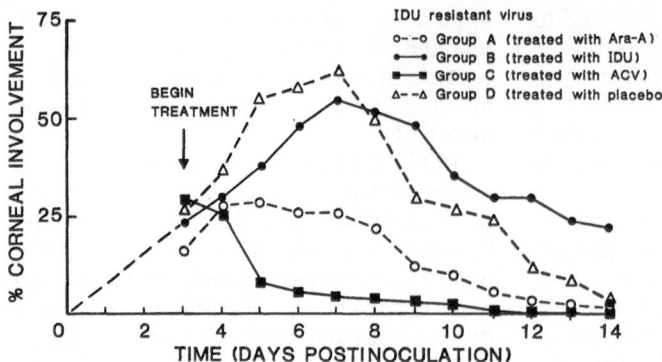

**Fig. 2.** Percent corneal epithelial involvement observed in rabbits during acute ocular infection with IDU resistant strain of HSV. Topical drug treatment was carried out 4 times per day beginning on day 3. Each treatment group consisted of 12 animals (24 treated eyes)

ment started a steady decline. This improvement was significantly better (p < 0.05) than the other treatment groups. Response to ARA-A therapy resulted in significant reduction of corneal involvement by day 5. IDU treatment did not appear to suppress corneal lesions to any significant extent. Corneal lesions in the placebo treated eyes disappeared by day 14, whereas IDU treated eyes remained involved.

Conjunctivitis, iritis and corneal clouding were not significant in animals treated with ACV. However, in the other treatment groups they were significant and paralleled the epithelial lesions.

It appears that IDU resistant strain of HSV employed in this in vivo study was more sensitive than the HSV McKrae strain to the antiviral activity of ACV.

*Experiment 3: Acute Ocular Herpetic Disease Induced by ARA-A Resistant HSV*

Corneal epithelial involvement resulting from ARA-A resistant HSV is presented in Fig. 3. The infection was considerably more advanced before beginning therapy in this study compared to the other two experiments. Treatment was initiated on day 4 instead of day 3. This delay minimized the magnitude of the chemotherapeutic effect of the drugs tested. Corneal lesions in ACV, ARA-A and IDU treated eyes showed favorable responses within 24 hours of initiating therapy. During the first 9 days, regression of corneal lesions treated with antivirals was faster than the eyes treated with the placebo ointment. ACV treatment was the most efficacious (p < 0.05). As in the previous ex-

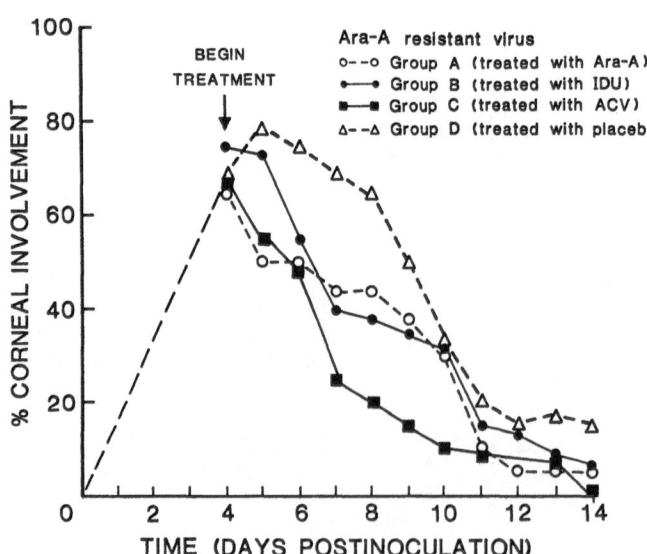

**Fig. 3.** Percent corneal epithelial involvement observed in rabbits during acute ocular infection with an Ara-A resistant strain of HSV. Topical drug treatment was carried out 4 times per day beginning on day 4. Groups A and B consisted of 14 animals. Group C had 12 animals and Group D had 16 animals

**Table 1.** Summary of HSV isolation from rabbits following topical antiviral therapy for acute occular infection

| Experiment # (virus) | # of Rabbits | % of specimens positive for HVS isolation | | | |
| --- | --- | --- | --- | --- | --- |
| | | corneal epithelium | trigeminal ganglia | midbrain | cerebellum |
| expt. 1 (McKrae Strain HSV) | 19 | 26(10/ 38) | 53(20/ 38) | 24( 9/ 38) | 5( 1/19) |
| expt. 2 (IUD resistant HSV) | 26 | 0( 0/ 52) | 71(37/ 52) | 40(21/ 52) | 35( 9/26) |
| expt. 3 (Ara-resistant HSV) | 24 | 19( 9/ 48) | 52(25/ 48) | 50(24/ 48) | 63(15/24) |
| Total | 69 | 14(19/138) | 59(82/138) | 39(54/138) | 36(25/69) |

periments conjunctivitis, iritis and corneal clouding paralleled epithelial involvement.

*Virus Isolation From Experiments 1 to 3*

Table 1 presents a summary of all isolation data from corneal epithelial cells, trigeminal ganglia, midbrains and cerebellar samples. Virus isolation studies were carried out 30 days after the completion of topical ocular chemotherapy, and 24 hours after trigeminal ganglia stimulation.

There were no obvious differences in the rate of HSV isolation between the treatment groups for each test virus. Therefore, data in table 1 was not presented on the basis of treatment. However, there was some variation in the distribution of virus in neural tissue depending on the virus strain employed. For example, when ocular infection was induced with the IDU-resistant strain, virus was detected most frequently in 71% of TG samples. The ARA-A resistant HSV produced the highest rate of virus isolation from cerebellar samples ever encountered in our laboratory (63%).

**Discussion**

Many chemical agents are capable of inhibiting intracellular viral replication. Of these chemical agents with antiviral activity, several including vidarabine and idoxuridine have been proven to be useful in treating herpetic keratitis. Some clinical HSV isolates are known to be resistant to antiviral activity of each of these drugs. In fact, virus resistance to chemotherapy has been recognized for every available drug. Double drug resistance has been observed (Nesburn and Trousdale, unpublished data).

At present, drug resistance is not a major problem because a virus resistant to one drug is usually sensitive to other drugs. However as antiviral drugs are more widely used clinically, more resistant strains are expected to emerge. Because of the potential clinical use of ACV, we wanted to determine the effect of ACV on HSV known to be insensitive to commonly used antiviral drugs.

For the three virus strains employed, ACV was the fastest and most effective drug in suppressing corneal epithelial involvement and conjunctivitis. ACV treated eyes also exhibited less iritis and corneal clouding. Since these parameters parallel the severity of epithelial disease in all treatment groups, it is not clear whether ACV had any direct effect on iritis and stromal disease. As expected, parent McKrae HSV was sensitive to all three drugs. The IDU resistant HSV was also resistant to IDU in the rabbit ocular model. The ARA-A resistant HSV appeared insensitive to both ARA-A and IDU therapy as demonstrated by corneal involvement present on day 10.

In the past, the rabbit ocular model has been a reliable indicator of drug efficacy in treatment of human epithelial keratitis. We would therefore prognosticate that ACV would be an appropriate and valuable drug in therapy of resistant HSV epithelial keratitis in man.

## Conclusion

Topical acyclovir therapy given 4 times a day was significantly more effective than idoxuridine and vidarabine at suppressing acute herpetic ocular disease induced by either sensitive or drug resistant strains of HSV 1. Virus isolation from neural tissues indicated that none of the therapy prevented viral infection of the nervous system.

**Acknowledgment.** Research supported by research grants EY00858, EY02957 and Discovery Fund.

## Discussion on the Contribution pp. 309–314

J. Oh (San Francisco)
In the treatment of the infection, I am wondering if you initiate Acyclovir treatment on postinfection day 1 or earlier, does it block the infection of the ganglia?

M.D. Trousdale (Los Angeles)
I don't know. We have never started chemotherapy as early as 1 day postinfection because viral infection is not evident that early. Our reason for starting antiviral therapy on day 3 postinfection is that it is when the ocular infection is recognizable.

J. Oh (San Francisco)
In our experiments with newborn rabbits, the ganglia are infected with virus as early as 1 day after the skin infection. So, any treatment after that day may not be effective.

H.E. Kaufman (New Orleans)
We did a study in which we began treatment with acycloguanosine about 24 hours after inoculation, and we found that we could prevent ganglionic infection. If treatment was started later than 24 hours, however, we couldn't get rid of the virus either, which is what Dr. Trousdale has reported.

Y.C. Cheng (Chapel Hill)
Is the IDU resistant strain you used in this study a TK⁻ strain?

M.D. Trousdale (Los Angeles)
You would assume that IDU resistant HSV is TK⁻, but we have not yet tested the strains for TK activity.

Y.C. Cheng (Chapel Hill)
It is important to know whether this IDU resistant strain could also induce TK. I am curious whether this IDU resistant strain could induce latency and be reactivated.

M.D. Trousdale (Los Angeles)
Yes, it depends upon your definition of latency. We're able to isolate HSV from trigeminal ganglia by co-cultivation methods at least 30 days postinoculation. We are also able to induce recurrence of HSV into the tear film by surgical stimulation of the trigeminal ganglia.

H.E. Kaufman (New Orleans)
The IDU-resistant strains we found were not TK⁻. The cellular thymidine kinase allows the IDU to work. If the virus drops out thymidine kinase, it doesn't become IDU resistant.

Y.C. Cheng (Chapel Hill)
That I can see, but here you have used the laboratory IDU resistant strain; you are probably using the TK⁻ strain.

Sundmacher, R. (Hrsg.):
Herpetische Augenerkrankungen
© J.F. Bergmann Verlag, München 1981

# Studies of Acyclovir and Ara-AMP Against Herpetic Keratitis in Rabbits

H. Shiota, T. Ogawa, S. Yamane, Tokushima

**Key words.** Herpetic keratitis, corneal epithelial lesion therapeutic assay (CELTA), SEM acyclovir, ara-AMP

**Schlüsselwörter.** Herpeskeratitis, CELTA, Raster-elektronenmikroskop, Acyclovir, ara-AMP

**Summary.** The therapeutic effects of 3% adenine arabinoside 5'-monophosphate (ara-AMP), 3% acyclovir (ACV) and 0.5% 5-iodo-2'-deoxyuridine (IDU) ointment on herpetic keratitis and their toxic effects on normal cornea in rabbits were compared. Ara-AMP showed the strongest antiviral activity, but it produced corneal erosion after 4 days application. Acyclovir showed an equal therapeutic effect to that of IDU and was found to be non-toxic. Acyclovir was, therefore, concluded to be the most effective for treatment of herpetic keratitis.

**Zusammenfassung.** Im Kaninchenmodell untersuchten wir vergleichend den therapeutischen und den toxischen Effekt von 3% Adeninarabinosid Monophosphat (Ara-AMP), 3% Acyclovir (ACV) und 0,5% IDU bei der Herpeskeratitis und bei Normalaugen. Ara-AMP erwies sich als stärkstes Virustatikum, führte aber nach 4tägiger lokaler Anwendung zu Hornhauterosionen. Acyclovir war annähernd so wirksam wie IDU, aber viel weniger toxisch als letzteres. Deshalb schließen wir, daß Acyclovir von den getesteten Virustatika das beste zur Therapie einer Herpeskeratitis ist.

## Introduction

Drugs for treatment of herpetic keratitis should have potent antiviral activity with low toxicity to the host. The effects of two newly synthesised anti-herpetic compounds, acyclovir and ara-AMP, were studied in rabbits with respect to these two points. IDU was used as a control.

## Methods and Materials

### Antiviral Study

Pigmented rabbits weighing about 3.0 kg were used. The technique of multiple micro-trephination [2] and the Corneal Epithelial Lesion Therapeutic Assay or CELTA [4] were used to inoculate herpes simplex virus (HSV) and to assess the therapeutic effects of antiviral compounds, respectively. Rabbits were anesthetised by intravenous injection of pentobarbital sodium (30 mg/kg) and then procaine was given to both eyes by retrobulbar injection. The PH strain of HSV type 1 with a titer of $1.15 \times 10^6$ plaque forming units/ml was inoculated from a fine glass capillary tube of 1.0 mm internal diameter at 25 sites in the cornea of each eye. Ointments of 3% ara-AMP, 3% acyclovir, 0.5% IDU and the vehicle were prepared and applied to one eye of each rabbit in groups of four animals. The other eye was treated with another compound. The treatment was started 48 hours after inoculation and continued every 2 hours during the daytime, 5 times a day for 4 days. The eyes were examined 48 hours after inoculation and then every 24 hours with a photo-slit lamp after applying 1% Bengal rose. Each inoculation site was scored 0 to 4 according to the total circumference infected, and 1 or 2 was added if half or the whole of the cornea enclosed by the circle was ulcerated. The total daily score for each eye was calculated and expressed as a percentage of the score (percentage score) immediately before treatment.

### Toxicity Study

Ointments of 3% ara-AMP, 0.5% IDU and 3% acyclovir were applied to the right eye of 5, 6, and 6 normal rabbits, respectively. Their left eye was treated with vehicle as a control. Ap-

**Table 1.** Percentage scores of severity of herpetic ulcers in rabbit cornea

| Days of treatment | 3% ara-AMP (n = 4) | 3% ACV (n = 4) | 0.5% IDU (n = 4) | Control (n = 4) |
|---|---|---|---|---|
| 0 | 100 | 100 | 100 | 100 |
| 1 | 38.5±10.2 | 67.1±11.2 | 65.5±4.4 | 112.4±18.1 |
| 2 | 34.0± 0.1 | 43.1± 4.4 | 42.3±3.3 | 112.7± 9.4 |
| 3 | 35.3±21.5 | 31.3± 4.5 | 33.2±5.5 | 109.2±20.1 |
| 4 | 73.7±29.3 | 19.7± 5.0 | 19.8±3.1 | 147.8±36.6 |

N.B. Treatment was started 48 hours after HSV inoculation

plications were made every 2 hours during the daytime, 5 times a day. In the ara-AMP treated group, four rabbits were treated for 4 days and one for 7 days. In the IDU- and acyclovir-treated groups, treatments were continued for 21 days. Eyes were examined with a photo-slit lamp every day. At the end of the treatment period, the eyes were enucleated under general anesthesia and sections were examined by light microscopy and by scanning electron microscopy following the method of Takashima [5].

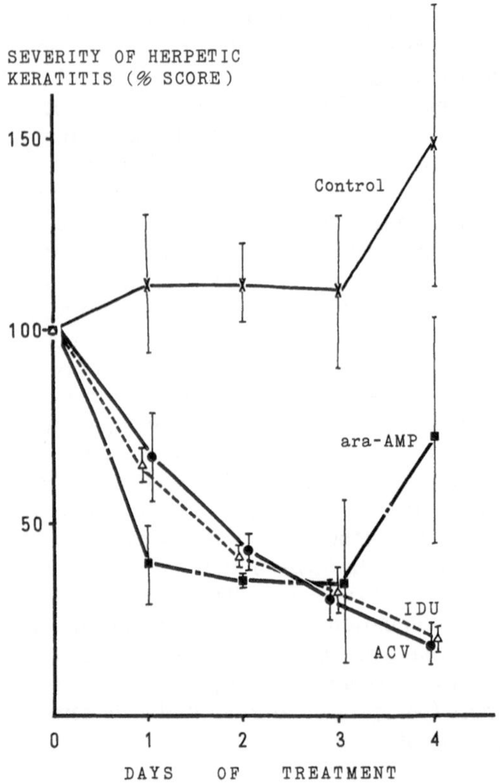

## Results

### Antiviral Study

On examination 48 hours after HSV inoculation, typical dendritic ulcers were seen along the circumference of each infected site. In control eyes, dendritic ulcers developed into large geographic ones by 6 days after inoculation. In eyes treated with 3% ara-AMP ointment, the ulcers became much smaller after 24 hours treatment. But after 4 days treatment, large corneal erosion and diffuse punctate keratitis were seen in all eyes, resulting in a percentage score of 73.7. In eyes treated with 3% acyclovir ointment, dendritic ulcers gradually became smaller and after 4 days treatment the eyes were nearly or completely cured. Eyes treated with 0.5% IDU ointment showed the same clinical improvement as those treated with acyclovir. These results are summarised in Table 1 and Fig. 1.

### Toxicity Study

(a) Ara-AMP treated eyes: After 3 days application of 3% ara-AMP ointment, diffuse punctate keratitis was seen in all eyes and after 4 days application, a large corneal erosion had formed in all eyes. Four of five eyes were enucleated at this stage. Corneal erosion was confirmed histologically and the appearance of the corneal surface by scanning electron microscopy, shown in Fig. 2, indicates degeneration of the corneal

**Fig. 1.** Therapeutic effect of 3% ara-AMP, 3% ACV and 0.5% IDU ointment against herpetic ulcers in rabbit cornea: Treatment was commenced 48 hours after HSV inoculation. Four eyes were subjected to each treatment

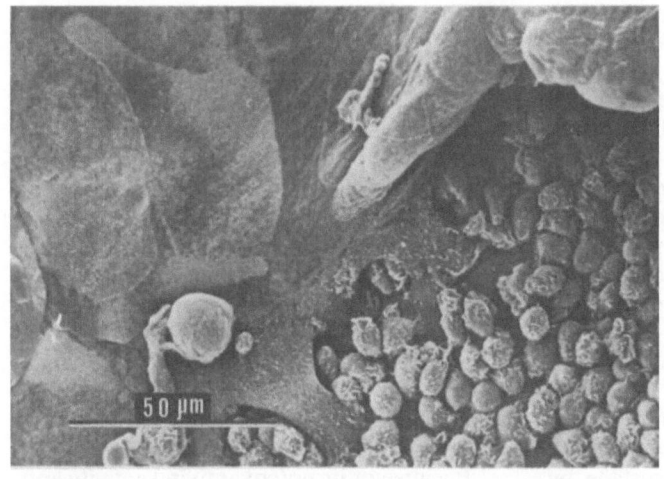

**Fig. 2.** Response of the surface of rabbit cornea after 4 days application of 3% ara-AMP ointment. The epithelium is degenerated and erosion is seen, exposing monolayer cells

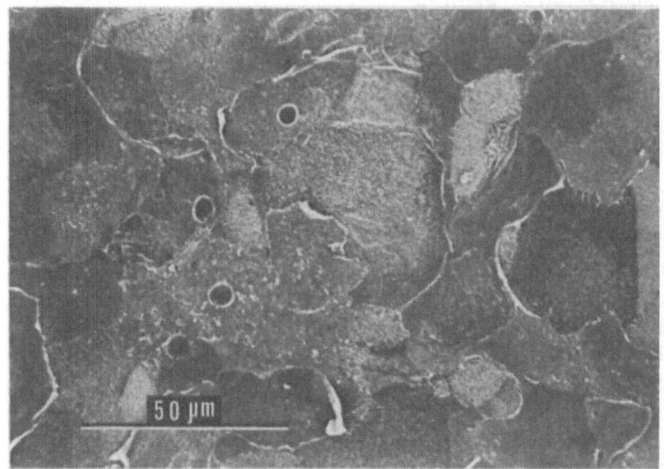

**Fig. 3.** Response of the surface of rabbit cornea after 21 days application of 0.5% IDU ointment. Superficial epithelium is strongly degenerated

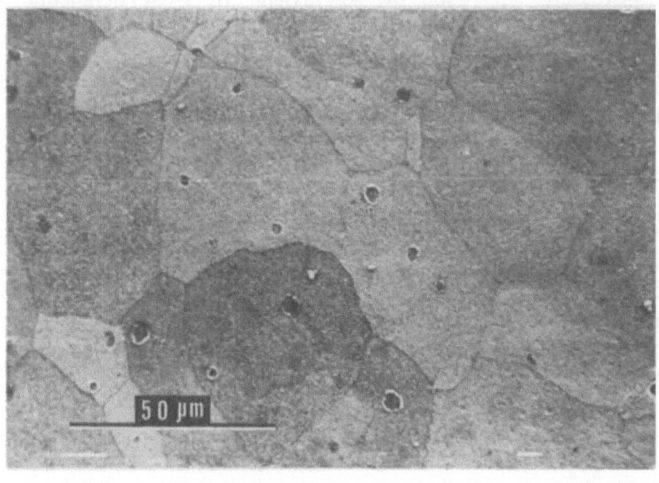

**Fig. 4.** Response of the surface of rabbit cornea after 21 days application of 3% ACV ointment. No particular changes are seen

317

epithelium and erosion. The eye treated with ara-AMP ointment for 7 days showed the same abnormalities.

(b) IDU treated eyes: Diffuse punctate keratitis was sometimes seen in IDU treated eyes and occasionally in control eyes, too. Histological examination revealed that in IDU treated cornea the epithelium was thin and minute erosions were sometimes present. The appearance of the corneal surface by scanning electron microscopy is shown in Fig. 3. Degeneration and peeling off of the superficial epithelium were noted.

(c) Acyclovir treated eyes: No abnormal changes were observed by slit, histological or scanning electron microscopic examination. The appearance of the corneal surface by scanning electron microscopy is shown in Fig. 4.

Control eyes treated with vehicle did not show any significant macroscopic or microscopic changes.

## Discussion

The present comparative studies on the therapeutic effects of 3% ara-AMP, 3% acyclovir and 0.5% IDU ointment on herpetic ulcers in rabbit cornea showed that 3% ara-AMP ointment had the strongest anti-HSV activity. But after 4 days treatment with ara-AMP, large erosions formed probably due to the cytotoxic effect of ara-AMP. To verify this possibility we examined the toxicity of ara-AMP on normal cornea. Again corneal erosion was produced after 4 days treatment, confirming the cytotoxic effect of ara-AMP. However since this side effect was not seen after 2 days treatment and ara-AMP has a very strong anti-HSV activity, application of ara-AMP for 1 or 2 days and then application of a non-toxic compound is one way to use this compound in treatment of clinical herpetic keratitis. Further studies on the relationship between the concentration of ara-AMP and its antiviral effect are necessary.

Another new antiherpetic compound called acyclovir is a guanine derivative [3]. This compound seems to be almost non-toxic to human beings because its action is due to its phosphorylation by a virus-specified thymidine kinase to acyclovir triphosphate, which inhibits viral DNA polymerase [1]. Acyclovir is not phosphorylated appreciably by cellular kinase, and thus is almost non-toxic to host cells. To verify this point, we examined the toxicity of acyclovir in rabbit cornea. No significant abnormalities were observed on application of this compound for 3 weeks. Moreover the therapeutic effect of 3% acyclovir ointment on herpetic ulcers in rabbit cornea appeared to be equal to that of 0.5% IDU ointment. This result on the PH strain of HSV is consistent with our previous findings on the RE strain of HSV [4]. Thus acyclovir has potent antiviral activity against different strains of HSV.

Because of its potent antiviral activity and extremely low toxicity, acyclovir seems to be the best drug for use in treatment of herpetic keratitis.

**Acknowledgments.** We thank Prof. B.R. Jones, University of London, and the Wellcome Research Laboratories, U.K., for providing 3% acyclovir ointment, Parke, Davis & Company for providing ara-AMP and Dr. S. Yamada of this University for help in histological studies.

This study was supported in part by a research grant, No. 457438, from the Japanese Ministry of Education, Science and Culture.

## References

1. Elion GB, Furman PA, Fyfe JA, Miranda P de, Beauchamp L, Schaeffer HJ (1977) Selectivity of action of an antiherpetic agent, 9-(2-hydroxyethoxymethyl)guanine. Proc Natl Acad Sci USA 74:5716–5720

2. Jones BR, Al-Hussaini MK (1963) Therapeutic considerations in ocular vaccinia. Trans Ophthalmol Soc UK 83:613–631

3. Schaeffer HJ, Beauchamp L, Miranda P de, Elion GB, Bauer DJ, Collins P (1978) 9-(2-Hydroxyethoxymethyl)guanine activity against viruses of the herpes group. Nature 272:583–585

4. Shiota H, Inoue S, Yamane S (1979) Efficacy of acycloguanosine against herpetic ulcers in rabbit cornea. Br J Ophthalmol 63:425–428

5. Takashima R (1975) Corticosteroid effects on the corneal surface of rabbits studied by scanning electron microscopy. Jpn J Ophthalmol 19:393–400

Sundmacher, R. (Hrsg.):
Herpetische Augenerkrankungen
© J.F. Bergmann Verlag, München 1981

# The Clinical Use of Acyclovir in the Treatment of Herpes Simplex Corneal Ulceration

J. McGill, P. Tormey, C. Walker, Southampton

**Key words.** Dendritic keratitis, acyclovir, ara-A, resistant ulcers, IDU

**Schlüsselwörter.** Keratitis dendritica, Acyclovir, ara-A, IDU, therapieresistenter Oberflächen-herpes

**Summary.** Thirtyeight patients with herpes corneal ulceration were treated on a randomized double-blind basis with Acyclovir or Vidarabine ointment respectively. The results of this study indicate that Acyclovir is at least as good as Ara-A, and is effective in the treatment of IDU and Ara-A resistant ulcers.

**Zusammenfassung.** Achtunddreißig Patienten mit virologisch bestätigtem epithelialen Herpes corneae wurden in einer randomisierten Doppelblindstudie entweder mit Acyclovir- oder Vidarabin-Salbe behandelt. Die vorliegenden Ergebnisse zeigen, daß Acyclovir mindestens so gut wie Vidarabin ist und darüber hinaus auch bei IDU- und Vidarabin-resistenten Keratitiden wirkt.

Recent advances in the development of herpes simplex virus antiviral drugs have shown that Acyclovir has impressive in vitro and in vivo activity against the herpes simplex virus. In vitro it has been found to have promising antiviral activity [5], with little effect on normal cells, but being preferentially converted to the triphosphate by virally specific thymidine kinase [8], and virally specific DNA polymerase [19]. The drug appears to arrest the development of herpes simplex virus before the stage of passage through the nuclear membrane [3] with reduced viral DNA synthesis causing immature viral particles to be formed [9]. Viral mutants which fail to utilize thymidine kinase have been found to be resistant to Acyclovir [7], so that the possibility of clinical resistance to the drug has arisen.

Acyclovir has been shown to be effective experimentally in the treatment of herpes simplex keratitis in animals [1, 2, 6, 16, 18] and equally as effective as both Idoxuridine and Trifluorothymidine [11]. Also it has been found to be effective in the treatment of experimental skin herpes simplex infection [12].

In man it has been found to be effective in the treatment of herpes simplex corneal ulceration, preventing recurrent herpes infection after minimal debridement of the corneal ulcers [10] and to be as effective as Adenine Arabinoside [20]. It arrests herpes simplex infection when given preferentially to patients with malignant disease [14, 17].

The currently available antiviral drugs, Idoxuridine, Adenine Arabinoside and Trifluorothymidine, are not always successful in the treatment of herpetic corneal ulceration, with side effects of clinical resistance [13] thought in some cases to be due to viral drug resistance (in press), contact dermatitis, and topical toxicity. Thus there is a need for a new highly selective antiviral drug, affecting preferentially virally infected cells with few side effects.

This paper describes the clinical effect of Acyclovir in the treatment, not only of patients with ulcers which were clinically resistant to either Idoxuridine or Adenine Arabinoside (Vira-A) topical treatment, but also compares it to Adenine Arabinoside by means of a double blind coded clinical trial.

Adenine Arabinoside (Vira-A) itself is an effective anti-herpes antiviral [15], with a high cure rate, equally as effective as Trifluorothymidine [4] and effective in cases of either Idoxuridine or Trifluorothymidine resistance. Side effects such as topical toxicity or clinical resistance can occur, so it is of interest to see how Acyclovir compares with it.

## Selection of Patients

Patients with a clinical diagnosis of herpes corneal ulceration, subsequently confirmed by virus isolation, who were attending the Southampton Eye Hospital.

## Treatment

Treatment in the coded controlled trial was randomly assigned to one of the following groups:
a) Acyclovir 3.3%, 5 times day
b) Oc. Adenine Arabinoside 3.3% 5 times day
Stratification of treatment was carried out for age, duration of symptoms and absence or presence of atopy. Records were taken of the size of the ulcer, the presence of any underlying stromal infiltrate or uveitis, or previous corneal ulceration, of any previous antiviral treatment or of any prior steroid treatment.

Patients were seen daily or on alternate days until the ulcer had healed, and then treatment was reduced to 3 times a day for 5 days.

## Investigations

At the initial visit isolates were taken for herpes simplex virus, and at each visit symptoms of pain, grittiness, photophobia, lacrimation were scored on a 0–3+ basis. The size and shape of the ulcer was measured and recorded, and any stromal involvement or associated uveitis was recorded as mild or severe. Associated lid, conjunctival or corneal changes were noted, and any possible adverse drug reaction was looked for.

## Results

### Acyclovir – Adenine Arabinoside Trial

We have treated 38 patients so far in the randomized double blind trial. Adenine Arabinoside was given to 21 patients and 17 received Acyclovir. The presence or absence of atopy had no effect on the final outcome of the healing of the ulcer, all patients had their symptoms for under 2 weeks, and there was an even distribution of patients under and over age 50. The interim results have shown that all patients treated with either antiviral healed, in an average of 6 days for Adenine Arabinoside and 3.6 days for Acyclovir. On follow-up, 4 of the 21 patients treated with Adenine Arabinoside had a recurrent ulcer within 1 month, one of which subsequently became resistant to Adenine Arabinoside, but quickly healed on Trifluorothymidine. Two subsequently developed stromal activity which healed on Adenine Arabinoside and topical steroids. No ulcers recurred after Acyclovir treatment, but two patients subsequently developed stromal activity requiring topical steroid therapy as well (Table 1, 2).

### Idoxuridine Resistant Ulcers

Three patients had ulcers failing to heal with Idoxuridine after at least 2 months' treatment. All ulcers healed when switched to Acyclovir in an average of 4.3 days (Table 3).

### Adenine Arabinoside Resistant Ulcers

Three patients had ulcers which were resistant clinically to Adenine Arabinoside, and which responded favourably to Acyclovir within 7 days (Table 4).

**Table 1.** Distribution of patients in comparative trial of Acyclovir and Adenine Arabinoside

|  | No. patients |
| --- | --- |
| Acyclovir | 17 |
| Adenine Arabinoside | 21 |

**Table 2.** Interim results of treatment of herpes simplex ulcers with either Acyclovir or Adenine Arabinoside

|  | No. patients | No. healed | Av. days to heal |
| --- | --- | --- | --- |
| Acyclovir | 17 | 17 | 3.6 |
| Adenine Arabinoside | 21 | 21 | 6.0 |

**Table 3.** Individual details of patients with Idoxuridine resistant ulcers treated with Acyclovir

| Patient | 1st or Recurrent ulcer | Length of IDU treatment | Days to heal with Acyclovir |
|---|---|---|---|
| 1 | R | 9 months | 4 |
| 2 | R | 2 months | 4 |
| 3 | R | 3 months | 5 |

**Table 4.** Response to Acyclovir of ulcers resistant to Adenine Arabinoside

| Patient | 1st or Recurrent ulcer | Length of Adenine Arabinoside treatment | Days to heal with Acyclovir |
|---|---|---|---|
| 1 | R | | 3 |
| 2 | R | 19 days | 7 |
| 3 | R | | 10 |

## Side Effects to Acyclovir

In all 38 patients have received topical Acyclovir, with a maximum of 4 months' treatment (range 7 days to 4 months).

### Allergy

One patient developed the signs of topical contact dermatitis after 2 weeks' treatment with the ointment, but this quickly settled on cessation of the drug, though investigations are continuing as to whether this allergy was due to the drug itself or the base in which the drug was made up.

### Topical Toxicity

Approximately 20% of the 38 patients have shown very mild punctate epithelial keratopathy, particularly in the interpalpebral fissure on the conjunctiva medially. These signs have not progressed, despite continued treatment, and quickly resolve once treatment has been stopped.

No other side effects to the drug have so far been found, whether it is used either topically or intravenously.

## Conclusions

Acyclovir has been found to be a highly effective antiviral drug in the treatment of herpes simplex corneal infection. It appears to be at least as good as Adenine Arabinoside, and is effective in the treatment of Idoxuridine and Adenine Arabinoside resistant ulcers. Its low toxicity, high effectivity and good ocular penetration may make it an exciting new antiviral drug in the treatment of herpes simplex corneal ulceration.

## References

1. Bauer DJ, Collins P (1978) Activity of 9-(2-Hydroxyethoxymethyl)guanine against herpes virus infections in animal models. Antimicrob Agents Chemother Abstr 73
2. Bauer DJ, Collins P, Tucker WE, Macklin AW (1979) Treatment of experimental herpes simplex keratitis with acycloguanosine. Br J Ophthalmol 63:429–435
3. Collins P, Tisdale SM, Furman PA (1979) Electron microscopic study of the effect of Acyclovir on the In Vitro replication of herpes simplex virus. International Congress of Chemotherapy, Boston, Abstr 253
4. Coster DJ, McKinnon JR, McGill JI, Jones BR, Fraunfelder FT (1976) Clinical evaluation of adenine arabinoside and trifluorothymidine in the treatment of corneal ulcers caused by herpes simplex virus. J Infect Dis Suppl 133: A173–A177
5. Elion GB, Furman PA, Fyfe JA, Miranda P de, Beauchamp L, Schaeffer HJ (1977) Selectivity

of action of an antiherpetic agent 9-(2-hydro-xyethoxymethyl)guanine. Proc Natl Acad Sci USA 74:5716–5720

6. Falcon MG, Jones BR (1979) Acycloguano-sine: antiviral activity in the rabbit cornea. Br J Ophthalmol 63:422–424

7. Field HJ, Darby GK, Wildy P (1979) Patho-genicity for mice of acycloguanosine-resistant mutants of herpes simplex virus. Interscience Congress of Chemotherapy, Boston, Abstr 257

8. Furman PA, Collins P, McGuirt P (1979) The effect of Acyclovir on viral polypeptide syn-thesis in herpes simplex virus type I infected cells. International Congress of Chemothe-rapy, Boston, Abstr 252

9. Furman PA, St Clair MH, Fyfe JA, Rideout JL, Keller PM, Elion GB (1979) Inhibition of herpes simplex virus-induced DNA poly-merase activity and viral DNA replication by 9-(2-hydroxyethoxymethyl)guanine and its tri-phosphate. J Virol 32:72–77

10. Jones BR, Fison PR, Cobo LM, Coster DJ, Thompson CM, Falcon MC (1979) Efficacy of acycloguanosine (Wellcome 248U) against herpes corneal ulcers. Lancet 1:241–242

11. Kaufman HE, Varnell ED, Centifanto YM, Rheinstrom SD (1978) Effect of 9-(2-hydroxy-ethoxymethyl)guanine on herpesvirus-induced keratitis and iritis in rabbits. Antimi-crob Agents Chemother 14:842–845

12. Klein RJ, Friedman-Kien AE, Destefano E (1979) Latent herpes simplex virus infections in sensory ganglia of hairless mice prevented by Acycloguanosine. Antimicrob Agents Che-mother 15:723–729

13. McGill J, Fraunfelder FT, Jones BR (1976) Current and proposed management of ocular herpes simplex. Surv Ophthalmol :358–365

14. O'Meara A, Deasy PF, Hillary IB, Brigden WD (1979) Acyclovir for treatment of muco-cutaneous herpes infection in a child with leu-kaemia. Lancet 2:1196

15. Pavan-Langston D, Dohlman CH (1972) A double blind clinical study of adenine arabino-side therapy of viral keratoconjunctivitis. Am J Ophthalmol 74:81–88

16. Schaeffer HJ, Beauchamp L, Miranda P de, Elion GB, Bauer DJ, Collins P (1978) 9-(2-hy-droxyethoxymethyl)guanine activity against viruses of the herpes group. Nature 272:583–585

17. Selby RJ, Jameson B, Watson JG, Morgen-stern G, Powles RL, Kay HEM, Thornton R, Clink HM, McElwain TJ, Prentice HG, Ross MG, Corringham R, Hoffbrand AV, Brigden D (1979) Parenteral acyclovir therapy for her-pesvirus infections in man. Lancet 2:1267–1269

18. Shiota H, Inoue S, Yamane S (1979) Efficacy of acycloguanosine against herpetic ulcers in rabbit cornea. Br J Ophthalmol 63:425–428

19. Schnipper LE, Crumpacker CS (1979) Mecha-nism of action of the anti-herpes viral agent, acycloguanosine; requirement of viral thymi-dine kinase and DNA polymerase activities. Clin Res 27:356A

Sundmacher, R. (Hrsg.):
Herpetische Augenerkrankungen
© J.F. Bergmann Verlag, München 1981

# Acyclovir (Zovirax) in Herpes Simplex Keratitis

L.M.T. Collum, A. Benedict-Smith, Dublin

**Key words.** Dendritic keratitis, geographic keratitis, disciform keratitis, acyclovir, antiviral drugs – toxicity

**Schlüsselwörter.** Keratitis dendritica, Keratitis geographica, Keratitis disciformis, Acyclovir, antivirale Medikamente – Toxizität

**Summary.** Thirtysix patients with herpetic corneal disease were treated with Acyclovir (Zovirax). The patients were divided into four different clinical groups. The therapeutic effect and the side effects of the drug in each group are discussed. It is suggested that Acyclovir is an effective therapeutic agent in Herpes Simplex Keratitis.

**Zusammenfassung.** Sechsunddreißig Patienten mit Herpes corneae wurden mit Acyclovir (Zovirax) behandelt. Die Beurteilung und Therapie der Patienten erfolgte in vier verschiedenen klinischen Gruppen. Die Therapieergebnisse und Nebenwirkungen werden diskutiert. Wir sind der Ansicht, daß Acyclovir ein wirksames Therapeutikum bei Herpes simplex-Keratitis ist.

## Introduction

Acyclovir (9-(2-hydroxyethoxymethyl) guanine), a purine nucleoside, is recently being used in the treatment of herpes simplex infections in man. It is a guanine derivative with an acyclic side chain and preliminary studies suggest that it holds some promise for the future in the management of herpes virus infections.

The drug treatment of herpes simplex keratitis in man is now well established and agents such as Idoxuridine, Adenine Arabinoside, and Trifluorothymidine are in common usage (Fig. 1). Idoxuridine, introduced in 1962, by Kaufman et al. [10], is still used by many as the standard treatment. It is not, however, universally effective having a failure rate of 16% or more [16] and it does not prevent recurrences [3]. Its side effects, such as S.P.E., punctal occlusion and conjunctival irritation are well documented [16]. In addition it is probably no more effective than mechanical debridement in the management of dendritic ulcers [16, 26].

Trifluorothymidine ($F_3T$), a pyrimidine nucleoside like IDU, has also been extensively used. It was claimed to be more effective than IDU [26] in dendritic ulceration and Coster et al. [5], reported that it was effective in amoeboid ulcers. Because it was more soluble it was also suggested that it might be useful in the treatment of stromal disease. Toxic effects, however, have been recorded [14].

An insoluble purine nucleoside, Adenine Arabinoside, was used by Pavan-Langston and Dohlman [17]. It was shown to be as effective as IDU but McGill et al. [13] pointed out that it has significant side effects.

Comparisons between ARA-A and $F_3T$ suggest that there is no significant difference in their effectiveness [13, 25]. The healing time for these drugs recorded in various trials may, however, vary, depending on the parameters of healing used.

It is apparent, therefore, that a more effective anti-viral drug would be desirable. Acyclovir (Fig. 1) is a soluble agent and preliminary investigations suggest that, as it may be safe to administer it systemically, it may play a significant role in the future, both in the prevention and treatment of herpes simplex keratitis. It is taken up by virus infected cells preferentially and phosphorylated initially to the monophosphate and then to the di and tri phosphates, which are the active agents, by a virus specified thymidine kinase [6]. The triphosphate inhibits DNA polymerase activity by competitively inhibiting the incorporation of deoxyguanosine triphosphate into viral DNA and so interfering with normal viral DNA synthesis. Its in-

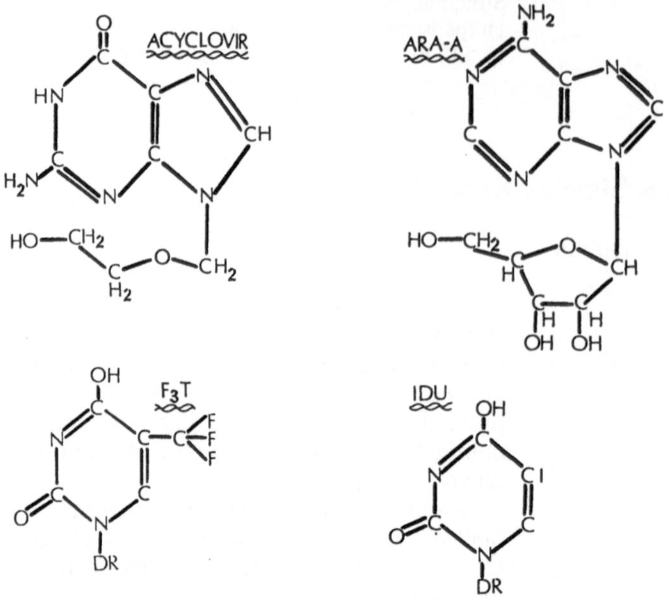

**Fig. 1.** Agents in common usage for the treatment of herpes simplex keratitis in man

hibitory effect on viral DNA synthesis is much greater than its effect on normal cellular DNA synthesis giving, therefore, a preferential effect on virus infected cells, with a relative sparing of normal uninfected cells. In vitro studies, using vero cells infected with herpes simplex type 1 virus, carried out by Schaeffer et al. [19] showed that Acyclovir was ten times as potent as IDU and almost twenty times more potent than $F_3T$. Animal studies showed that it was effective in herpetic corneal ulceration with a minimum of toxic effect [1, 7, 11, 12, 18, 19, 21, 24]. It was used orally in man [2] with no untoward reaction. Systemic herpetic infections in man have been treated by giving Acyclovir intravenously and promising results have been reported [8, 15, 20, 33, 23]. Jones et al. [9] had success in the treatment of dendritic corneal ulceration using Acyclovir ointment and "minimal wiping debridement" and a double blind study of 50 patients showed Acyclovir to be, not alone effective in corneal dendritic ulceration but to be more effective than IDU [4].

**Patients and Methods**

We have used Acyclovir as the treatment of choice in 36 patients with herpes simplex keratitis, as a result of our experiences in our controlled trial. These fell into four groups.

1. Fresh epithelial lesions
2. Epithelial lesions that had failed to respond to other anti-viral agents
3. Epithelial lesions occurring in patients having a combination of steroids and another anti-viral agent for disciform keratitis
4. Patients with fresh complicated keratitis (e.g. combined stromal and epithelial disease)

Patients were seen at least twice weekly in the active stages of the disease, by the same two observers. A full ocular examination was carried out on each occasion. The treatment prescribed for all patients initially was 3% Acyclovir ointment to be used 5 times daily. Most of the patients were also treated with 1% Homatropine.

**Results and Discussion**

Sixteen patients with fresh epithelial lesions were treated with Acyclovir ointment 5 times daily. Three had geographical ulcers while the remainder were dendritics (Table 1). Healing occurred in all but one patient in periods ranging from 2 to 7 days with an average healing time of 3.93 days. The previous use of local cortico steroids did not appear to prolong the healing time. The patient that failed to heal developed a small indolent lesion that was static after the end of 8 days treatment in spite of rapid early improvement. It healed quickly,

324

**Table 1.** Epithelial disease (Fresh)

| Patient | | Lesion | Healing time | Toxicity | Duration of R | Recurrence |
|---|---|---|---|---|---|---|
| | M 30 | D.U. | 5 days | --- | 6 days | --- |
| | F 49 | D.U.(mult) | 4 days | --- | 9 days | --- |
| a | F 56 | Geog.U. | 3 days | --- | 5 days | --- |
| | F 49 | D.U. | 3 days | --- | 14 days | --- |
| | M 77 | D.U. | 4 days | --- | 12 days | --- |
| a | M 27 | D.U. | 3 days | --- | 11 days | --- |
| | F 36 | D.U. | 2 days | stinging | 6 days | --- |
| a | F 72 | D.U. | 4 days | --- | 10 days | --- |
| | M 60 | D.U. | 3 days | S.P.E. | 7 days | --- |
| | M 27 | Geog.U. | 3 days | --- | 13 days | 6/52 |
| | M 30 | D.U.(mult) | 4 days | --- | 7 days | --- |
| | F 48 | D.U. | 3 days | --- | 7 days | --- |
| | M 40 | D.U. | 6 days | --- | 9 days | --- |
| | F 48 | Geog.U. | 7 days | --- | 11 days | --- |
| b | F 24 | D.U. | failed | --- | 8 days | --- |
| | F 62 | D.U. | 5 days | --- | 8 days | --- |

[a] Had local steroids    [b] Ulcer Iodized

however, after iodization. The ointment was generally well tolerated and the only side effects noted were S.P.E. (one patient) and stinging on application of the Acyclovir (one patient). One patient got a recurrence of his dendritic ulcer 6 weeks after finishing his treatment with Acyclovir but this healed again after a further 10 days treatment.

Thirteen patients who had failed to respond to other anti-viral agents, within 4 days, were similarly treated (Table 2). Three had geographical ulcers while the remainder had dendritic lesions. In this group the healing time ranged from 3 to 10 days, with an average of 4.85 days. All patients responded to treatment. Diffuse punctate keratitis was recorded in one patient while two complained of stinging on applying the ointment. One patient complained of excessive watering of the eye which did not cease on discontinuing the treatment. Dilatation of the lacrimal puncta, however, cleared the symptoms. One patient got a recurrence of his ulcer 3 weeks after finishing the treatment and this in turn healed again after 6 days treatment with Acyclovir.

Three patients (Table 2), having a com-

**Table 2.** Epithelial disease (failed alternative treatment)

| Patient | Lesion | Healing time | Toxicity | Duration of R | Recurrence |
|---|---|---|---|---|---|
| a F 22 | D.U.(mult) | 3 days | watering | 6 days | – |
| F 51 | D.U. | 3 days | – | 9 days | – |
| M 40 | Geog.U. | 5 days | – | 8 days | – |
| F 51 | D.U. | 3 days | stinging | 10 days | – |
| M 32 | D.U. | 3 days | – | 12 days | – |
| M 36 | Geog.U. | 7 days | – | 13 days | – |
| M 60 | Geog.U. | 5 days | S.P.E. | 10 days | – |
| F 30 | D.U. | 6 days | stinging | 23 days | – |
| M 61 | D.U. | 10 days | – | 14 days | 3/52 |
| b F 10 | D.U. | 4 days | – | 42 days | – |
| b M 64 | D.U. | 6 days | – | 24 days | – |
| b M 57 | Geog.U. | 5 days | – | 45 days | – |
| F 56 | D.U. | 3 days | – | 8 days | – |

[a] Had local steroids    [b] Ulcers occured while having steroid and other anti-viral agents for Disciform Keratitis

**Table 3.** Complicated keratitis

| Patient | Lesion | Control time | Toxicity | Duration of R | Recurrence |
|---|---|---|---|---|---|
| F 10 | Disciform Keratitis | 22 days | – | 40 days | – |
| M 64 | Disciform Keratitis Iritis | 18 days | stinging | 24 days | – |
| F 24 | Disciform Keratitis Iritis | 34 days | – | 61 days | – |
| [a] M 32 | Disciform Keratitis Iritis Peripheral Furrow. | worsened | – | 4 days | |
| M 42 | Disciform Keratitis | 15 days | – | 46 days | – |
| F 31 | Disciform Keratitis | 18 days | – | 38 days | – |
| M 30 | Disciform Keratitis | 14 days | – | 30 days | – |
| M 57 ... | Disciform Keratitis | 15 days | – | 34 days | – |

[a] Conjunctivectomy, performed

bination of IDU and dilute Betamethazone for disciform keratitis, presented with dendritic ulceration. On discontinuing the steroid the epithelial lesions healed in 4, 5 and 6 days on Acyclovir and they then continued on a combination of dilute steroid and Acyclovir for the stromal disease.

Eight patients with complicated keratitis were treated with Acyclovir (Table 3). Our experiences suggest that Acyclovir is a good alternative to other anti-viral agents such as IDU or ARA-A in disciform keratitis, used in combination with cortico-steroid drops. It has been possible to control seven of the group without having a breakdown of the corneal epithelium. One patient, however, who had a history of severe herpetic keratitis in the past went on to develope a severe Moorenoid lesion which necessitated limbal conjunctivectomy. Initially the Acyclovir ointment was used 5 times daily but we found that once the disease appeared to be controlled it was necessary to use it only twice daily.

## Conclusions

From our experience with these 36 patients with herpes simplex keratitis we suggest that

1. Acyclovir (Zovirax) is effective in fresh epithelial disease.

2. Acyclovir is a useful alternative when other antiviral agents fail to heal epithelial disease.

3. Acyclovir, in conjunction with steroid, can be used in combined keratitis.

4. Acyclovir is relatively non-toxic, the only side effects noted being stinging (four patients), punctate keratopathy (two patients), and epiphora (one patient).

## References

1. Bauer DJ, Collins P (1978) Antimicrob Agents Chemother Abstr 73
2. Brigden D, Bye A, Collins P, Miranda P de (1978) Antimicrob Agents Chemother Abstr 74
3. Carroll JM, Martola EL, Laibson PR, Dohlman CH (1967) Am J Ophthalmol 63:103–107
4. Collum LMT, Benedict-Smith A (1980) Brit J Ophthalmol 64:766–769
5. Coster DJ, MacKinnon JR, McGill JI, Jones BR, Frauenfelder FT (1976) Infect Dis 133: 173–177
6. Elion GB, Furman PA, Fyfe JA, Miranda P de, Beauchamp L, Schaeffer HJ (1977) Proc Natl Acad Sci USA 77:5716–20

7. Falcon MG, Jones BR (1979) Br J Ophthalmol 63:422–424
8. Goldman JM, Chipping PM, Agnarsdottir G, Brigden D (1979) Lancet :820
9. Jones BR, Fison PN, Cobo LM, Coster DJ, Thompson GM, Falcon MG (1979) Lancet : 243–244
10. Kaufman HE, Nesburn AB, Maloney ED (1962) Am J Ophthalmol 67:583–591
11. Kaufman HE, Varnell ED, Centifanto YM, Rheinstrom SD (1978) Antimicrob Agents Chemother 14:842–45
12. Lass JH, Pavan-Langston JH, Park N (1979) Am J Ophthalmol 88:102–108
13. McGill JI, Coster D, Frauenfelder T, Holt-Wilson AD, Williams H, Jones BR (1975) Trans Ophthalmol Soc UK 95:246–249
14. McGill J, Frauenfelder FT, Jones BR (1976) Surv Ophthalmol 20:358–365
15. O'Meara A, Deasy PG, Hillary IB, Brigden WD (1979) Lancet :1196
16. Patterson A, Jones BR (1967) Trans Ophthalmol Soc UK 87:59–84
17. Pavan-Langston D, Dohlman CH (1972) Am J Ophthalmol 74:81–88
18. Pavan-Langston D, Park N, Lass JH (1979) Arch Ophthalmol 97:1508–10
19. Schaeffer HJ, Beauchamp L, Miranda P de, Elion GB (1978) Nature 272:583–585
20. Selby PJ, Jameson B, Watson JG, Morgenstern G, Powles RL, Kay HEM, Thornton R, Clink HM, MacElwain TJ, Prentice HG, Ross MG, Corringham R, Hoffbrand AV, Brigden D (1979) Lancet :1267
21. Shiota H, Inoue S, Yamane S (1979) Br J Ophthalmol 63:425–428
22. Spector SA, Hintz M, Quinn RP, Keeney RE, Connor JD (1979) International Congress of Chemotherapy, Boston, Abstr 256
23. Teare EL, Clements MR (1980) Lancet 1:42
24. Tucker jr WE, Macklin AW, Szot RJ, Clive D (1978) Antimicrob Agents Chemother Abstr 64
25. Bijsterveld OP van, Post H (1980) Br J Ophthalmol 64:33–36
26. Wellings PC, Awdry PM, Bars FH, Jones BR, Brown DC, Kaufman HE (1972) Am J Ophthalmol 73:932–942

## Discussion on the Contribution pp. 323–327

H.E. Kaufman (New Orleans)
Do you think that the punctal stenosis was probably caused by the acyclovir?

L.M.T. Collum (Dublin)
I don't. I think it was more likely due to the virus, as suggested previously.

H.E. Kaufman (New Orleans)
Do you think that the superficial punctate keratitis is caused by the ointment, or are we trying to be optimistic?

L.M.T. Collum (Dublin)
I think it's too early to say. I think we're being perhaps a little optimistic, I want to be as critical as possible of the drug. One has to err in that direction, but it was not a real problem.

H.E. Kaufman (New Orleans)
Do you think the acyclovir had a primary effect on the disciform edema?

L.M.T. Collum (Dublin)
I do, but I think I would like more evidence. We intend to carry on this work and we intend, when we look into the ethics and the other aspect is to use acyclovir perhaps on its own in a controlled study. Now, a lot of people will disagree. As there's such a big immunological factor using it alone, perhaps will not be effective, but there's only one way to find out.

J. McGill (Southampton)
We have used acyclovir in just a few patients, in only those who had disciform keratitis. Using it alone has had no effect at all. We have had to add steroids later on.

L.M.T. Collum (Dublin)
That isn't altogether that surprising.

J. Oh (San Francisco)
This question has nothing to do with this paper. I am a little bit confused as to the pronounciation of this compound. I was told by Dr. Elion at the Wellcome Laboratories that this antiviral is pronounced as (a-sí-klo-vé-ah). Now several speakers in this meeting pronounced it as (a-sí-klo-ver). I am wondering which is the correct pronounciation. I wonder if a person from the Wellcome Laboratories in the audience can help us on this?

T. Ravenscroft (Beckenham)
Acyclovir is the correct pronounciation. The drug will be marketed under the name Zovirax.

Sundmacher, R. (Hrsg.):
Herpetische Augenerkrankungen
© J.F. Bergmann Verlag, München 1981

# On the Mechanism of Anti-Herpes Action of $\underline{E}$-5-(2-Bromovinyl)-2′-Deoxyuridine

E. De Clercq, J. Descamps, Leuven

**Key words.** BVDU, thymidine kinase, DNA polymerase

**Schlüsselwörter.** BVDU, Thymidinkinase, DNA-Polymerase

**Summary.** BVDU [($\underline{E}$)-5-(2-bromovinyl)-2′-deoxyuridine) is an extremely potent and selective inhibitor of HSV 1 (herpes simplex virus type 1) and VZV (varicella zoster virus) replication: in primary rabbit kidney and/or human diploid fibroblast cultures these viruses are inhibited at a drug concentration of about 0.01 µg/ml (0.03 µM). The selective antiherpes activity of BVDU resides in a specific inhibition of viral DNA synthesis, which, in turn, depends on at least two factors: (i), phosphorylation of BVDU by the virus-encoded dThd (deoxythymidine) kinase and, (ii), inhibition of the virus-induced DNA polymerase by the resulting BVDUTP (BVDU 5′-triphosphate). Both viral enzymes appear to contribute to the selective antiherpes action of BVDU. While BVDUTP is a specific inhibitor of HSV 1 DNA polymerase, it remains to be established whether it can also serve as substrate for this enzyme. Unlike 5-halogenated deoxyuridines [i.e. IDU (5-iodo-2′-deoxyuridine)], BVDU does not induce the production of oncogenic RNA viruses in mouse (i.e. BALB/3T3) cell lines.

**Zusammenfassung.** In Zellkulturen (PRK, primäre Kaninchen-Nierenzellen) zeigt BVDU ($\underline{E}$-5-(2-Bromovinyl)-2′-Deoxyuridin) eine hohe Selektivität und antivirale Potenz gegenüber Herpes simplex-Virus Typ 1 (HSV 1). Die Virusreplikation wird bei Konzentrationen gehemmt, die $10^4$mal niedriger als die Konzentrationen liegen, die den normalen Zellstoffwechsel oder das Zellwachstum beeinträchtigen. Die spezifische antiherpetische Wirkung des BVDU scheint mit zwei virusinduzierten Enzymen korreliert zu sein, mit der Deoxythymidinkinase und der DNA-Polymerase. Hierfür spricht, daß BVDU praktisch unwirk-

sam gegenüber TK⁻(dThd-Kinasemangel)-Mutanten des HSV ist, daß es eine starke Bindung an die HSV 1-kodierte dThd-Kinase aufweist ($K_1$ = 0,15 µM (Y.-C. Cheng, persönliche Mitteilung, 1979) und daß es in seiner 5-Triphosphatform (BVDUTP) die HSV 1-DNA-Polymerase schon in einer Konzentration hemmt (2 µM), die wenig oder gar keinen Effekt auf die Aktivität der normalen Zell-DNA-Polymerasen α und β hat (H.S. Allaudeen: persönliche Mitteilung, 1979). In HSV 1-infizierten PRK-Zellen konnte die virale DNA-Synthese mit BVDU-Konzentrationen von 0,3 µM total gehemmt werden, während die normale DNA-Synthese (exponentiell wachsender PRK-Zellen) durch 0,3 mM BVDU nur partiell beeinträchtigt wurde.

Die Vorstellungen über den Wirkungsmechanismus des BVDU sind also sehr ähnlich denjenigen, die man sich vom Acycloguanosin macht: Die Substanz wird in der virusinfizierten Zelle von der viruskodierten dThd-Kinase phosphoryliert, die dann das BVDU allmählich auch von der 5-Mono- zur 5-Diphosphatform überführt. Sobald die 5-Diphosphatform zur 5-Triphosphatform weiter phosphoryliert worden ist (durch zelluläre Kinase(n)), wird das BVDUTP die viruskodierte DNA-Polymerase spezifisch hemmen – wahrscheinlich durch unmittelbare Verdrängung des entsprechenden dTTP.

Es ist nicht gänzlich ausgeschlossen, daß BVDU in DNA eingebaut wird. Der Umstand hingegen, daß BVDU im Gegensatz zu anderen 2′-Deoxyuridin-Derivaten wie IDU (5-Iodo-2′-Deoxyuridin) die Freilassung von endogenen Oncornaviruspartikeln aus latent infizierten Zellen nicht provoziert (z.B. in BALB/c-Mäusezellen (E. de Clercq, H. Heremans, J. Descamps, M. de Ley und A. Billiau, unveröffentlicht, 1979)), deutet darauf hin, daß BVDU entweder überhaupt nicht in zelluläre DNA eingebaut wird oder – falls dies doch geschieht – daß hierdurch keine Aktivierung der entsprechenden Oncornavirusgene provoziert wird.

In recent years several new antiherpes compounds have been developed which have proven to be more potent and/or more selective in their antiherpes activity than the previously established drugs [IDU (idoxuridine, 5-iodo-2'-deoxyuridine), TFT (trifluorothymidine, 5-trifluoromethyl-2'-deoxyuridine), Ara-A (vidarabine, adenine arabinoside, 9-β-D-arabinofuranosyladenine)], and which may therefore be considered as potential candidates for the treatment of herpesvirus diseases. This new generation of antiherpes compounds includes such agents as ara-T (thymine arabinoside, 1-β-D-arabinofuranosylthymine) [3], AIDDU (5'-amino-5-iodo-2', 5'-dideoxyuridine) [41], EDU (5-ethyl-2'-deoxyuridine) and PDU (5-propyl-2'-deoxyuridine) [9, 14, 17, 25], PAA (phosphonoacetic acid) and PFA (phosphonoformic acid) [29, 37, 42, 44], ACG [acyclovir, acycloguanosine, 9-(2-hydroxyethoxymethyl)guanine] [19, 43], BVDU [(E)-5-(2-bromovinyl)-2'-deoxyuridine] [12, 13, 34] and FIAC [2'-fluoro-5-iodoaracytosine, 1-(2-fluoro-2-deoxy-β-D-arabinofuranosyl)-5-iodocytosine] [31, 49]. Of this series, three compounds, namely ACG, BVDU and FIAC, appear to be particularly promising, as they inhibit (herpes simplex virus) replication at concentrations which are lower by several orders of magnitude than those required to inhibit normal cell metabolism [15]. We will now examine the mechanism(s) by which BVDU exerts its selective inhibitory action on HSV replication.

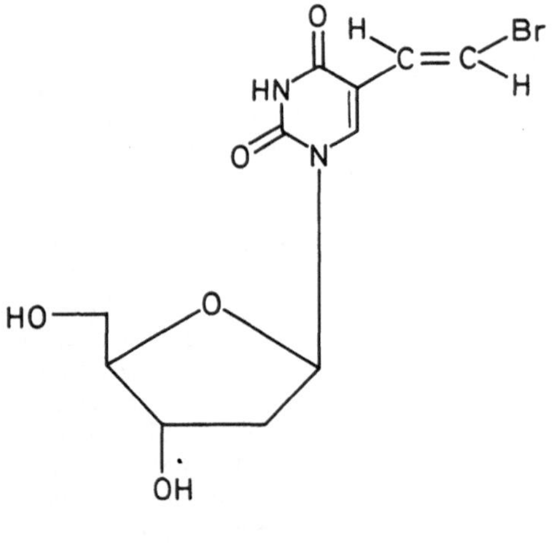

(E)-5-(2-bromovinyl)-2'-deoxyuridine

**Fig. 1.** Structural formula of BVDU

The structural formula of BVDU is depicted in Fig. 1. BVDU can be considered as a close analogue of IDU, the fundamental difference between these molecules being the presence or absence of an ethene bridge that connects the halogen with C-5 of the uracil ring.

In PRK (primary rabbit kidney) or HSF (human skin fibroblast) cell cultures, BVDU inhibited the replication of HSV 1 (herpes simplex virus type 1) and VZV (varicella zoster virus) at extremely low doses: $ID_{50}$ (inhibitory dose-50), 0.008 µg/ml for HSV 1 and < 0.004–0.04 µg/ml for VZV (Table 1). For HSV 2 (herpes simplex virus type 2) replication, the $ID_{50}$ was about 1 µg/ml; and for TK$^-$ HSV 1, a deoxythymidine (dThd) kinase deficient mutant of HSV 1, it was 100 µg/ml (Table 1). In its potency as an anti-HSV 1 or anti-VZV agent, BVDU compared favorably to the other antiviral drugs, i.e. FIAC, ACG, EDU, ara-T, TFT and IDU. However, the latter drugs surpassed BVDU in activity against HSV 2. BVDU was virtually inactive against TK$^-$ HSV 1, which indicates that the compound must be phosphorylated by the virus-induced dThd kinase to exert its antiviral effect. ACG and FIAC were still inhibitory for TK$^-$ HSV 1, although much less so than for TK$^+$ HSV 1, suggesting that these compounds may owe part of their antiherpes activity to mechanisms other than phosphorylation by the viral dThd kinase. PFA, PAA, ara-A and TFT were equally inhibitory to TK$^-$ HSV 1 and TK$^+$ HSV (or VZV) strains (Table 1). Apparently, these compounds do not require phosphorylation by the virus-induced dThd kinase.

The concentration at which BVDU inhibited HSV 1 replication was about 10.000 fold lower than the concentration at which BVDU was found to affect normal cell growth (proliferation) or metabolism (as monitored by the incorporation of radiolabelled 2'-deoxyuridine or 2'-deoxythymidine into DNA) [12, 15]. How then could the selective antiherpes activity of BVDU be rationalized? In attempts to investigate its mechanism of action, we measured the effects of BVDU on DNA synthesis in uninfected (proliferating) PRK cells and (resting) PRK cells which had been infected with either HSV 1 (strain KOS) or HSV 2 (strain G). DNA synthesis was monitored by the incorporation of ($^3$H-methyl)dThd and characterized by CsCl

**Table 1.** Inhibitory effects of BVDU and other anti-herpes compounds on the replication of herpes simplex virus and varicella zoster virus in cell culture

| Compound | $ID_{50}^{a}$ ($\mu g/ml$) | | | |
| | HSV 1 (PRK) | HSV 2 (PRK) | TK$^{-}$ HSV 1 (PRK) | VZV (HSF) |
| --- | --- | --- | --- | --- |
| IDU | 0.13 | 0.3 | > 200 | 0.4 |
| TFT | 0.7 | 0.7 | 0.5 | 1 |
| Ara–A | 7 | 5 | 10 | 2.5 |
| Ara–T | 0.25 | 0.5 | > 200 | 0.04 |
| AIDDU | 26 | 114 | > 200 | 40 |
| EDU | 0.5 | 0.3 | > 200 | 7 |
| PDU | 0.6 | 3 | > 200 | 1 |
| PAA | 13 | 11 | 20 | 20 |
| PFA | 13 | 8 | 20 | … |
| ACG | 0.04 | 0.04 | 7 | 0.4 |
| BVDU | 0.008 | 1 | 100 | < 0.004–0.04 |
| FIAC | 0.017 | 0.05 | 8.5 | … |

[a] Inhibitory dose–50 or dose required to inhibit virus-induced cytopathogenicity by 50%, as compared to untreated virus-infected cell cultures. Virus input: 100 CCID$_{50}$ (cell culture infective dose–50). PRK: primary rabbit kidney; HSF: human skin fibroblast; HSV 1: herpes simplex virus type 1; HSV 2: herpes simplex virus type 2; TK$^{-}$ HSV 1: thymidine kinase-deficient mutant of HSV 1; VZV: varicella zoster virus. Abbreviations for compounds as explained in the text

equilibrium density ultracentrifugation (Fig. 2). BVDU had no effect on normal cellular DNA synthesis (of uninfected, exponentially growing cells), when employed at concentrations of 0.1, 1 and 10 µg/ml; at 100 µg/ml BVDU brought about a 30% reduction of DNA synthesis (after it had been in contact with the proliferating cells for 72 hours) (Fig. 2c). In PRK cells which had been infected with HSV 1 (KOS), BVDU completely shut off DNA synthesis when assayed at a concentration of 1, 10 or 100 µg/ml, and even

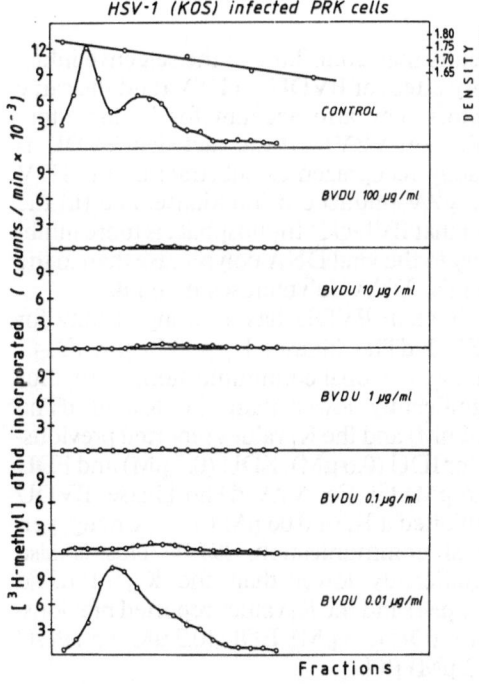

*HSV-1 (KOS) infected PRK cells*

CONTROL

BVDU 100 µg/ml

BVDU 10 µg/ml

BVDU 1 µg/ml

BVDU 0.1 µg/ml

BVDU 0.01 µg/ml

Fractions

**Fig. 2a.** Inhibitory effect of BVDU on DNA synthesis in PRK (primary rabbit kidney) cells infected with HSV 1 (strain KOS). Confluent PRK cell monolayers in 50 mm Falcon plastic petri dishes were infected with HSV 1 (KOS) at a MOI (multiplicity of infection) of 1 CCID$_{50}$ (cell culture infective dose-50) per cell. After 1 h incubation at 37 °C, residual virus was removed and the cells were incubated for 10 h in the presence of ($^{3}$H-methyl)thymidine (10 µCi/0.34 nM/petri dish) and varying concentrations of BVDU (as indicated). The cell cultures were then washed with cold PBS (phosphate buffered saline), frozen, thawed and lysed by addition of 2% SDS, 0.1 M EDTA (pH 8.2) and 0.15 M NaCl, and the lysates were mixed with a CsCl solution of 1.72 g/ml and centrifuged for 72 h at 30,000 rev/min in the swinging bucket rotor (6 × 14 ml) of a MSE superspeed 65 centrifuge. Five-drop fractions were collected from the bottom of the tubes; 2 ml of 5% TCA were added to each fraction, the precipitates were collected on Gelman glass fiber filters (A/E) and assayed for radioactivity in a Packard Tri-Carb liquid scintillation spectrometer. Refractive index was determined for every fifth fraction

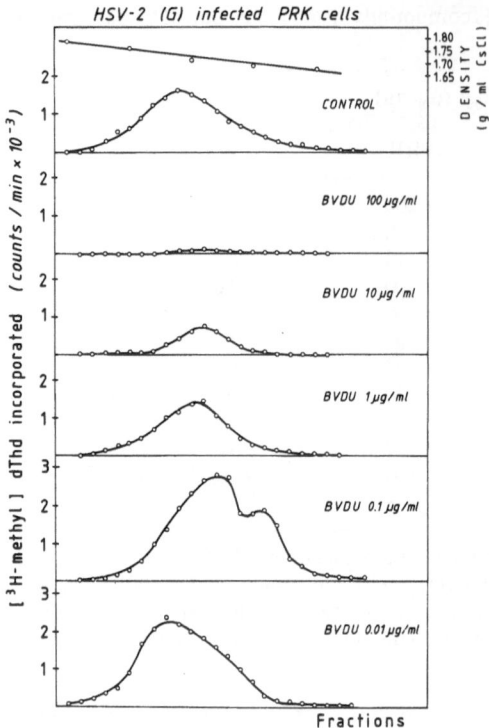

**Fig. 2b.** Inhibitory effect of BVDU on DNA synthesis in PRK cells infected with HSV 2 (strain G). MOI was 0.03 CCID$_{50}$ per cell. Otherwise, the procedure was identical to that applied for measuring HSV 1 (KOS)-induced DNA synthesis (see legend to Fig. 2a)

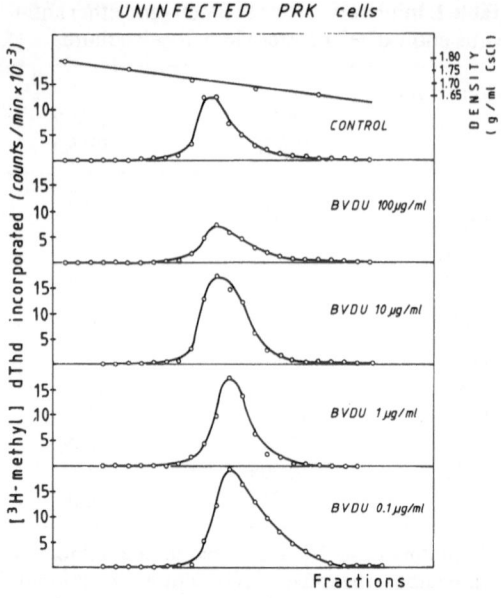

**Fig. 2c.** Inhibitory effect of BVDU on DNA synthesis of uninfected PRK cells. PRK cells were seeded in 50 mm Falcon plastic petri dishes at $10^6$ cells per petri dish and grown up for 72 h in the presence of ($^3$H-methyl)thymidine (10 µCi/0.34 nM/petri dish) and varying concentrations of BVDU (as indicated). At 72 h, when the cell cultures reached about 90% confluency, the cells were washed with cold PBS, frozen, thawed and further processed as explained in the legend to Fig. 2a

at 0.1 µg/ml it achieved a 90% inhibition (Fig. 2a). In these experiments DNA synthesis was measured at 10 hours after virus infection, when synthesis of viral DNA [density: 1.74–1.75 g/ml CsCl (Fig. 2a control)] is assumed to be at its maximum. As could be expected from the difference in ID$_{50}$ of BVDU for HSV 1 and HSV 2 replication (Table 1), BVDU proved significantly less inhibitory for HSV 2 DNA synthesis than for HSV 1 DNA synthesis: in PRK cells which had been infected with HSV 2 (G) there was no reduction in DNA synthesis if BVDU was applied at 0.1 µg/ml; at 1 µg/ml there was only a slight reduction; at 10 µg/ml, DNA synthesis was reduced by 50%; and at 100 µg/ml, BVDU suppressed DNA synthesis almost completely (Fig. 2b).

It would appear, therefore, that the inhibitory effects of BVDU on HSV 1 and HSV 2 replication are mediated by a selective inhibition of viral DNA synthesis. At least two

factors may contribute to the selective inhibitory effect of BVDU on HSV (and the same factors may also account for its inhibitory effect on VZV): (i) the fact that BVDU is readily recognized as substrate by the HSV (or VZV)-induced dThd kinase, and (ii) the fact that BVDU 5′-triphosphate is more inhibitory to the viral DNA polymerase than to the cellular DNA polymerases α and β.

Indeed, BVDU has a strong affinity for HSV 1 dThd kinase: $K_i = 0.15$ µM (Y.-C. Cheng, personal communication, 1979), thus significantly lower than the $K_m$ of dThd (0.6 µM) and the $K_i$ values reported previously for IDU (0.6 µM), EDU (0.7 µM) and PDU (0.6 µM) [8]. For VZV dThd kinase, BVDU exhibited a $K_i$ of 0.06 µM (Y.-C. Cheng, personal communication, 1979). This is also significantly lower than the $K_m$ of dThd (0.4 µM) and the $K_i$ values reported previously for IDU (0.3 µM), EDU (0.3 µM) and PDU (1.2 µM) [10].

Allaudeen et al. [2] found that BVDU 5′-triphosphate was considerably more inhibitory to the activity of HSV 1 DNA polymerase than to the cellular DNA polymerases. For instance, as little as 1 µM of the triphosphate inhibited 50% of the viral DNA polymerase activity while the same amount inhibited only 9% and 3% of the DNA polymerase α and DNA polymerase β activities, respectively. BVDU 5′-triphosphate inhibited DNA synthesis by competing with the natural substrate, dTTP. The $K_m$ of dTTP and the $K_i$ of BVDU 5′-triphosphate for the HSV 1 DNA polymerase were 0.8 µM and 0.22 µM, respectively [2]. ACGTP (the triphosphate of ACG) has also been examined for its inhibitory effect on HSV 1 DNA polymerase [23]: for ACGTP the apparent $K_i$ varied from 0.08 to 1.42 µM, depending on the HSV 1 strain; the corresponding $K_m$ of dGTP (the natural substrate ACGTP is competing with) varied from 0.38 to 1.15 µM.

The picture now emerging for the mode of action of BVDU is, to some extent, reminiscent of that proposed for ACG [19, 23, 24]: BVDU is readily phosphorylated in the HSV- and VZV-infected cell, but not in the uninfected cell. Responsible for this selective phosphorylation is the HSV (or VZV)-encoded dThd kinase, which is endowed with a broader substrate specificity than the corresponding cellular dThd kinase(s) [8]. Since the viral dThd kinase is also endowed with thymidylate kinase activity [5, 6], it may first convert BVDU to its 5′-monophosphate (BVDUMP) and then to its 5′-diphosphate (BVDUDP). BVDUDP would subsequently be converted by a cellular kinase to BVDUTP (BVDU 5′-triphosphate), and, in this capacity, it would attack the viral DNA polymerase, thereby inhibiting the viral DNA polymerase to a significantly greater extent than the cellular DNA polymerases. Thus, according to the model that we propose for the mode of action of BVDU (Fig. 3), two virus-specified enzymes may contribute to the drug's selectivity as an anti-herpes agent, namely dThd kinase and DNA polymerase. While the latter would act as the specific target enzyme for the antiviral action of BVDU, the former would rather serve as the activating enzyme, confining the final action of the compound to the virus-infected cell.

In its mode of action, BVDU differs from the other established antiherpes drugs, IDU, TFT, ara-A, ara-T, AIDDU, EDU, PAA and PFA (Table 2), in that:
- (i) IDU is assumed to exert its primary action subsequently to its incorporation into DNA [38, 39];
- (ii) TFT can also be incorporated into DNA, although its major biological activity, viz. toxicity for rapidly proliferating cells, may be mediated by an inhibition of thymidylate synthetase [11, 28];
- (iii) Ara-A does not require a virus-induced kinase for phosphorylation; it is phosphorylated equally well in the infected as in the uninfected cell, but, once it has been converted to its 5′-triphosphate form, ara-A confers a relatively greater inhibition of viral DNA synthesis than of cellular DNA synthesis [18, 36]; moreover, ara-A is incorporated into (cellular and viral) DNA [36];
- (iv) Ara-T does require phosphorylation by the HSV (or VZV)-encoded dThd kinase to be fully active against these viruses [3, 15] (although Müller et al. contend that it can also be phosphorylated in non-infected cells [35]); as for BVDU, the final target enzyme for ara-T would be the DNA polymerase, although it remains to be seen whether ara-TTP (ara-T 5′-triphosphate), akin to BVDUTP, inhibits the viral DNA polymerase to a greater degree than the cellular DNA polymerases [33, 35]; according to Müller et al. [35], ara-T is incorporated into cellular DNA but not into HSV DNA;
- (v) AIDDU can, like IDU, be incorporated into (cellular and viral) DNA, but, as

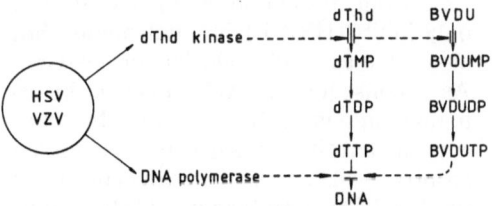

**Fig. 3.** Schematic outline of mechanism of action of BVDU on HSV and VZV replication. The virus-induced thymidine (dThd) kinase serves as the activating enzyme, converting BVDU to its 5′-monophosphate (and, possibly, to its 5′-diphosphate), whereas the virus-induced DNA polymerase acts as the target enzyme for BVDU 5′-triphosphate (formed from the 5′-diphosphate through the aid of an host cell kinase)

**Table 2.** Mechanism of action of anti-herpes compounds

| Compound | Metabolism | Target |
|---|---|---|
| IDU | IDU → IDUMP → IDUDP → IDUTP | IDUTP is incorporated into DNA (as IDUMP) |
| TFT | TFT → TFTMP → TFTDP → TFTTP | TFTMP inhibits dTMP synthetase<br>TFTTP is incorporated into DNA (as TFTMP) |
| Ara-A | Ara-A → Ara-AMP → Ara-ADP → Ara-ATP | Ara-ATP inhibits DNA polymerase (preferentially HSV DNA polymerase) by competition with dATP |
| Ara-T | Ara-T → Ara-TMP → Ara-TDP → Ara-TTP (preferentially in HSV- and VZV-infected cells) | Ara-TTP inhibits DNA polymerase by competition with dTTP |
| AIDDU | AIDDU → AIDDUMP → AIDDUDP → AIDDUTP [only in HSV- (or VZV)-infected cells] | AIDDUTP is incorporated into DNA (as AIDDUMP) (only in HSV-infected cells) |
| EDU (PDU) | EDU → EDUMP → EDUDP → EDUTP | EDUTP is incorporated into DNA (as EDUMP) |
| PAA, PFA | – | PAA and PFA selectively inhibit HSV DNA polymerase by competition with pyrophosphate |
| ACG | ACG → ACGMP → ACGDP → ACGTP [preferentially in HSV- (or VZV)-infected cells] | ACGTP selectively inhibits HSV DNA polymerase by competition with dGTP<br>ACGTP is incorporated into DNA (as ACGMP) and will thereby prevent further elongation of the DNA chain |
| BVDU | BVDU → BVDUMP → BVDUDP → BVDUTP [almost exclusively in HSV- (or VZV)-infected cells] | BVDUTP selectively inhibits HSV DNA polymerase by competition with dTTP |
| FIAC | FIAC → FIACMP → FIACDP → FIACTP [preferentially in HSV- (or VZV)-infected cells] | FIACTP selectively inhibits HSV DNA polymerase by competition with dCTP |

AIDDU is phosphorylated only by the HSV-encoded dThd kinase, this incorporation is restricted to the infected cell [7, 40];
- (vi) EDU is also incorporated into DNA [45], although it has not been demonstrated that EDU (and PDU) need to be incorporated to achieve their antiviral activity;
- (vii) PAA and PFA do not require any processing; they inhibit the DNA polymerase reaction by competition with pyrophosphate [30, 32], and, while HSV 1 DNA polymerase would seem more susceptible to inhibition by PAA and PFA than many other DNA polymerases [29], evidence has been presented that DNA polymerase α is just as sensitive to PAA as HSV DNA polymerase [1];
- (viii) ACG would owe its selectivity as an antiherpes agent to the same factors (virus-induced dThd kinase and DNA polymerase) as postulated above for BVDU [19, 23, 24], but, in addition, ACGTP would not only inhibit HSV 1 DNA polymerase but also serve as a substrate for this enzyme. As a consequence, ACG may be incorporated into viral DNA and thereby act as a chain terminator (since no 3'-hydroxyl group is available for chain elongation) [19];
- (ix) For FIAC insufficient published information is available to fully assess its mechanism of action [31, 49]. It may well conform to the principles outlined for the mode of action of BVDU.

For the majority of the compounds listed in Tables 1 and 2, viz. IDU, TFT, ara-A, ara-T, AIDDU, EDU and ACG, it has been demonstrated that they can be incorporated into (cellular and/or viral) DNA. The incorporation of

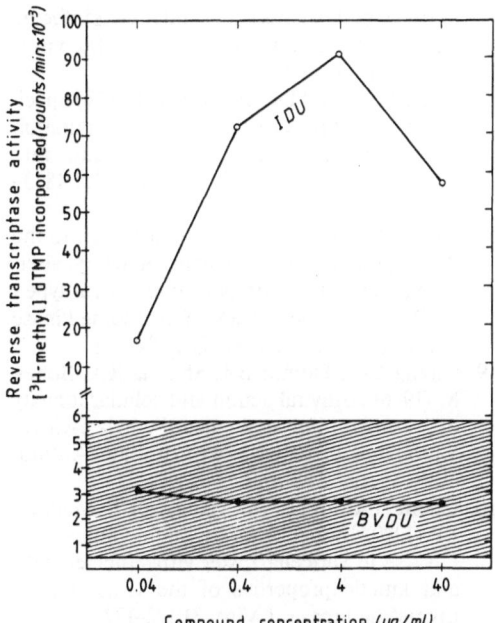

**Fig. 4.** Stimulatory effects of BVDU and IDU on the induction of oncornavirus particles in BALB/3T3 mouse cells. The cells were induced according to the procedure described by Wu et al. [50]. BALB/3T3 cells were seeded in 50 mm Falcon plastic petri dishes at $10^5$ cells per petri dish, grown up for 24 h and then incubated with BVDU and IDU (at the indicated concentrations) for another 24 h, at which time the cell culture fluid (5 ml) was collected (harvest 1). The cells were then incubated in the presence of 1 µM dexamethasone [50] for another 24 h, at which time the cell culture fluid was collected again (harvest 2); the cells were then further incubated in the absence of dexamethasone and the cell culture fluids were withdrawn at the end of the third 24 h incubation period (harvest 3) and fourth 24 h incubation period (harvest 4). All four harvests (20 ml) were pooled and clarified by centrifugation for 10 min at 10,000 g; the virus was then pelleted by centrifugation at 100,000 g for 60 min, resuspended in 20 ml of NT buffer (0.1 M Nacl, 10 mM Tris-HCl, pH 7.4), sedimented again and resuspended in 0.2 ml of NT buffer. Reverse transcriptase determinations were carried out with 75-µl portions of the resuspended virus according to the procedure described by Billiau et al. [4]. $(A)_n \cdot oligo(dT)_{12-18}$ served as template-primer and ($^3$H-methyl)dTTP as substrate [4]. All data represent the average values (per petri dish) for three (BVDU) or six (IDU, mock) separate observations. Mock cell cultures were treated with 1 µM dexamethasone on the second day, as were the BVDU- or IDU-treated cell cultures. The individual values obtained for the mock-treated cell cultures ranged from 316 to 5941 counts/min (▨)

these nucleoside analogues into normal cell DNA may upset the normal functioning of the DNA and elicit a series of undesirable side effects, including the induction of oncogenic viruses (as has been amply demonstrated with IDU [27]). Although circumstantial evidence suggests that incorporation into DNA is a necessary requirement for nucleoside analogues to stimulate oncornavirus release [46], incorporation into DNA is not necessarily complicated by induction of oncornaviruses (as exemplified by EDU [26]). Is BVDU incorporated into DNA, and if it is, does it induce the release of oncogenic RNA viruses? Due to the unavailability of radioactive BVDU it has so far not proven possible to answer the first question. To resolve the second question, BVDU was examined for its potential to activate the release of RNA tumor virus particles from nonproducing BALB/3T3 mouse cells. Under conditions where 0.04 µg/ml of IDU sufficed to induce an appreciable amount of oncornavirus particles [as assessed by virus-associated reverse transcriptase with $(A)_n \cdot oligo(dT)$ as template-primer], BVDU failed to activate such virus particle release, even when assayed at concentrations up to 40 µg/ml (Fig. 4). Even in BALB/3T3 cells which had been infected with HSV 1 (KOS), to ensure proper phosphorylation of the drug (by the virus-induced dThd kinase), BVDU failed to stimulate the production of oncornavirus particles [16]. One may conclude, therefore, that BVDU is either not incorporated into DNA, or, like EDU [26], incorporated to such extent that it does not lead to the expression of oncornavirus genes.

Since the selectivity of BVDU as an antiherpes agent depends on at least two virus-specified enzymes, dThd kinase and DNA polymerase, virus resistance to the drug may arise by mutations at either of these two enzymes. Hence, TK$^-$ mutants of HSV are innately resistant to BVDU (Table 1). TK$^-$ HSV mutants are in fact resistant to all nucleoside analogues that operate according to the "alternative substrate" theory of Cheng [8], which predicts that only those nucleoside analogues that are specifically phosphorylated by the viral dThd kinase may be expected to selectively inhibit HSV replication. One may wonder about the clinical usefulness of nucleoside analogues which are ineffective against TK$^-$ HSV. It would appear, however, that TK$^-$ strains are much less virulent than TK$^+$ strains [21]; they are unable to establish a latent infection in sensory ganglia [47, 48], and, while they can be readily obtained in vitro by passaging the virus in the presence of the drug (i.e. ACG [20]), they rarely arise during treatment in vivo [21]. Thus, the possible occurrence of TK$^-$ HSV strains in clinical situations may have little, if any, impact on the efficacy of HSV TK-dependent drugs such as BVDU or ACG. There are, however, changes at levels other than TK by which the virus could acquire resistance to the drug. Indeed, Field et al. [21, 22] have recently described ACG-resistant HSV mutants, the resistance of which may reside at the DNA polymerase level. One of these ACG-resistant mutants was also resistant to PAA [22]. Whether they are resistant to BVDU is now under study.

# References

1. Allaudeen HS, Bertino JR (1978) Inhibition of activities of DNA polymerase α, β, γ, and reverse transcriptase of L1210 cells by phosphonoacetic acid. Biochim Biophys Acta 520: 490–497
2. Allaudeen HS, Kozarich JW, Bertino JR, De Clercq E (1980) On the mechanism of selective inhibition of herpesvirus replication by (E)-5-(2-bromovinyl)-2′-deoxyuridine (Abstract). Proceedings of the International Conference on Human Herpesviruses, held at Emory University, Atlanta (Georgia), March 17–21
3. Aswell JF, Allen GP, Jamieson AT, Campbell DE, Gentry GA (1977) Antiviral activity of arabinosylthymine in herpesviral replication: mechanism of action in vivo and in vitro. Antimicrob Agents Chemother 12:243–254
4. Billiau A, Heremans H, Allen PT, De Somer P (1976) Influence of interferon on the synthesis of virus particles in oncornavirus carrier cell lines. IV. Relevance to the potential application of interferon in natural infectious diseases. J Infect Dis (suppl) 133:A51–A55
5. Chen MS, Prusoff WH (1978) Association of thymidylate kinase activity with pyrimidine deoxyribonucleoside kinase induced by herpes simplex virus. J Biol Chem 253:1325–1327
6. Chen MS, Summers WP, Walker J, Summers WC, Prusoff WH (1979) Characterization of pyrimidine deoxyribonuclease kinase (thymidine kinase) and thymidylate kinase as a multifunctional enzyme in cells transformed by herpes simplex virus type 1 and in cells infected with mutant strains of herpes simplex virus. J Virol 30:942–945
7. Chen MS, Ward DC, Prusoff WH (1976) Specific herpes simplex virus-induced incorporation of 5-iodo-5′-amino-2′, 5′-dideoxyuridine into deoxyribonucleic acid. J Biol Chem 251:4833–4838
8. Cheng Y-C (1977) A rational approach to the development of antiviral chemotherapy: alternative substrates of herpes simplex virus type 1 (HSV 1) and type 2 (HSV 2) thymidine kinase (TK). Ann NY Acad Sci 284:594–598
9. Cheng Y-C, Domin BA, Sharma RA, Bobek M (1976) Antiviral action and cellular toxicity of four thymidine analogues: 5-ethyl-, 5-vinyl-, 5-propyl-, and 5-allyl-2′-deoxyuridine. Antimicrob Agents Chemother 10:119–122
10. Cheng Y-C, Tsou TY, Hackstadt T, Mallavia LP (1979) Induction of thymidine kinase and DNAse in varicella-zoster virus-infected cells and kinetic properties of the virus-induced thymidine kinase. J Virol 31:172–177
11. De Clercq E, Balzarini J, Torrence PF, Mertes MP, Schmidt CL, Shugar D, Barr PJ, Jones AS, Verhelst G, Walker RT Thymidylate synthetase as target enzyme for the inhibitory of 5-substituted 2′-deoxyridines on mouse leukemia L 1210 cell growth. Molec Pharmacol. In press
12. De Clercq E, Descamps J, De Somer P, Barr PJ, Jones AS, Walker RT (1979) (E)-5-(2-Bromovinyl)-2′-deoxyuridine: a potent and selective anti-herpes agent. Proc Natl Acad Sci USA 76:2947–2951
13. De Clercq E, Descamps J, De Somer P, Barr PJ, Jones AS, Walker RT (1979) Pharmacokinetics of E-5-(2-bromovinyl)-2′-deoxyuridine in mice. Antimicrob Agents Chemother 16: 234–236
14. De Clercq E, Descamps J, Shugar D (1978) 5-Propyl-2′-deoxyuridine: a specific anti-herpes agent. Antimicrob Agents Chemother 13: 545–547
15. De Clercq E, Descamps J, Verhelst G, Walker RT, Jones AS, Torrence PF, Shugar D (1980) Comparative efficacy of different antiherpes drugs against different strains of herpes simplex virus. J Infect Dis 141:563–574
16. De Clercq E, Heremans H, Descamps J, Verhelst G, De Ley M, Billiau A (1981) Effects of E-5-(2-bromovinyl)-2′-deoxyuridine and other selective anti-herpes compounds on the induction of retrovirus particles in mouse BALB/3T3 cells. Molec Pharmacol. In press
17. De Clercq E, Shugar D (1975) Antiviral activity of 5-ethylpyrimidine deoxynucleosides. Biochem Pharmacol 24:1073–1078
18. Drach JC, Shipman jr C (1977) The selective

inhibition of viral DNA synthesis by chemotherapeutic agents: an indicator of clinical usefulness? Ann NY Acad Sci 284:396–406

19. Elion GB, Furman PA, Fyfe JA, de Miranda P, Beauchamp L, Schaeffer HJ (1977) Selectivity of action of an antiherpetic agent, 9-(2-hydroxyethoxymethyl)guanine. Proc Natl Acad Sci USA 74:5716–5720

20. Field HJ, Bell SE, Elion GB, Nash AA, Wildy P (1979) Effect of acycloguanosine treatment on acute and latent herpes simplex infections in mice. Antimicrob Agents Chemother 15: 554–561

21. Field HJ, Darby G (1980) Pathogenicity in mice of strains of herpes simplex virus which are resistant to acyclovir in vitro and in vivo. Antimicrob Agents Chemother 17:209–216

22. Field HJ, Darby G, Wildy P (1980) Isolation and characterization of acyclovir-resistant mutants of herpes simplex virus. J Gen Virol 49:115–124

23. Furman PA, St Clair MH, Fyfe JA, Rideout JL, Keller PM, Elion GB (1979) Inhibition of herpes simplex virus-induced DNA polymerase activity and viral DNA replication by 9-(2-hydroxyethoxymethyl)guanine and its triphosphate. J Virol 32:72–77

24. Fyfe JA, Keller PM, Furman PA, Miller RL, Elion GB (1978) Thymidine kinase from herpes simplex virus phosphorylates the new antiviral compound, 9-(2-hydroxyethoxymethyl)guanine. J Biol Chem 253:8721–8727

25. Gauri KK, Malorny G (1967) Chemotherapie der Herpes-Infektion mit neuen 5-alkyluracildesoxyribosiden. Naunyn Schmiedeberg Arch Pharmakol Exp Pathol 257:21–22

26. Gauri KK, Shif I, Wolford RG (1976) Failure of 5-ethyl-2'-deoxyuridine to induce oncogenic RNA (oncorna) viruses in Fischer rat embryo cells and in Balb/3T3 mouse cells. Biochem Pharmacol 25:1809–1810

27. Goz B (1978) The effects of incorporation of 5-halogenated deoxyuridines into the DNA of eukaryotic cells. Pharmacol Rev 29:249–272

28. Heidelberger C (1975) Fluorinated pyrimidines and their nucleosides. In: Sartorelli AC, Johns DG (eds) Antineoplastic and immunosuppressive agents, part II. Springer, Berlin Heidelberg New York, pp 193–231

29. Helgstrand E, Eriksson B, Johansson NG, Lannerö B, Larsson A, Misiorny A, Noren JO, Sjöberg B, Stenberg K, Stening G, Stridh S, Öberg B, Alenius S, Philipson L (1978) Trisodium phosphonoformate, a new antiviral compound. Science 201:819–821

30. Leinbach SS, Reno JM, Lee LF, Isbell AF, Boezi JA (1976) Mechanism of phosphonoacetate inhibition of herpesvirus-induced DNA polymerase. Biochemistry 15:426–430

31. Lopez C, Livelli T, Watanabe K, Reichman U, Fox JJ (1979) 2'-Fluoro-5-iodo-aracytosine: a potent anti-herpesvirus nucleoside with minimal toxicity to normal cells. Proc Am Assoc Cancer Res 20:183

32. Mao JC-H, Robishaw EE (1975) Mode of inhibition of herpes simplex virus DNA polymerase by phosphonoacetate. Biochemistry 14: 5475–5479

33. Matsukage A, Ono K, Ohashi A, Takahashi T, Nakayama C, Saneyoshi M (1978) Inhibitory effect of 1-β-D-arabinofuranosylthymine 5'-triphosphate and 1-β-D-arabinofuranosylcytosine 5'-triphosphate on DNA polymerases from murine cells and oncornavirus. Cancer Res 38:3076–3079

34. Maudgal PC, De Clercq E, Descamps J, Missotten L, De Somer P, Busson R, Vanderhaeghe H, Verhelst G, Walker RT, Jones AS (1980) (E)-5-(2-bromovinyl)-2'-deoxyuridine in the treatment of experimental herpes simplex keratitis. Antimicrob Agents Chemother 17: 8–12

35. Müller WEG, Zahn RK, Arendes J, Falke D (1979) Phosphorylation of arabinofuranosylthymine in non-infected and herpesvirus (TK$^+$ and TK$^-$)-infected cells. J Gen Virol 43:261–271

36. Müller WEG, Zahn RK, Bittlingmaier K, Falke D (1977) Inhibition of herpesvirus DNA synthesis by 9-β-D-arabinofuranosyladenine in cellular and cell-free systems. Ann NY Acad Sci 284:34–48

37. Overby LR, Robishaw EE, Schleicher JB, Rueter A, Shipkowitz NL, Mao JC-H (1974) Inhibition of herpes simplex virus replication by phosphonoacetic acid. Antimicrob Agents Chemother 6:360–365

38. Prusoff WH, Goz B (1975) Halogenated pyrimidine deoxyribonucleosides. In: Sartorelli AC, Jones DG (eds) Antineoplastic and Immunosuppressive Agents, part II. Springer, Berlin Heidelberg New York, pp 272–347

39. Prusoff WH, Ward DC (1976) Nucleoside analogs with antiviral activity. Biochem Pharmacol 25:1233–1239

40. Prusoff WH, Ward DC, Lin TS, Chen MS, Shaiu GT, Chai C, Lentz E, Capizzi R, Idriss J, Ruddle NH, Black FL, Kumari HL, Albert D, Bhatt PN, Hsiung GD, Strickland S, Cheng YC (1977) Recent studies on the antiviral and biochemical properties of 5-halo-5'-aminodeoxyribonucleosides. Ann NY Acad Sci 284: 335–341

41. Puliafito CA, Robinson NL, Albert DM, Pavan-Langston D, Lin T-S, Ward DC, Prusoff WH (1977) Therapy of experimental herpes simplex keratitis in rabbits with 5-iodo-5'-amino-2', 5'-dideoxyuridine. Proc Soc Exp

Biol Med 156:92–96

42. Reno JM, Lee LF, Boezi JA (1978) Inhibition of herpesvirus replication and herpesvirus-induced deoxyribonucleic acid polymerase by phosphonoformate. Antimicrob Agents Chemother 13:188–192

43. Schaeffer HJ, Beauchamp L, de Miranda P, Elion GB, Bauer DJ, Collins P (1978) 9-(2-Hydroxyethoxymethyl)guanine activity against viruses of the herpes group. Nature 272:583–585

44. Shipkowitz NL, Bower RR, Appell RN, Nordeen CW, Overby LR, Roderick WR, Schleicher JB, von Esch AM (1973) Suppression of herpes simplex virus infection by phosphonoacetic acid. Applied Microbiol 26:264–267

45. Swierkowska KM, Jasinska JK, Steffen JA (1973) 5-Ethyl-2′-deoxyuridine: evidence for incorporation into DNA and evaluation of biological properties in lymphocyte cultures grown under conditions of amethopterine-imposed thymidine deficiency. Biochem Pharmacol 22:85–93

46. Teich N, Lowry DR, Hartley JP, Rowe WP (1973) Studies on the mechanism of induction of infectious murine leukemia virus from AKR mouse embryo cell lines by 5-iododeoxyuridine and 5-bromodeoxyuridine. Virology 51:163–173

47. Tenser RB, Dunstan ME (1979) Herpes simplex virus thymidine kinase expression in infection of the trigeminal ganglion. Virology 99:417–422

48. Tenser RB, Miller RL, Rapp F (1979) Trigeminal ganglion infection by thymidine kinase-negative mutants of herpes simplex virus. Science 205:915–917

49. Watanabe KA, Reichman U, Hirota K, Lopez C, Fox JJ (1979) Nucleosides. 110. Synthesis and antiherpes virus activity of some 2′-fluoro-2′-deoxyarabinofuranosylpyrimidine nucleosides. J Med Chem 22:21–24

50. Wu AM, Reitz MS, Paran M, Gallo RC (1974) Mechanism of stimulation of murine type-C RNA tumor virus production by glucocorticoids: post-transcriptional effects. J Virol 14:802–812

Sundmacher, R. (Hrsg.):
Herpetische Augenerkrankungen
© J.F. Bergmann Verlag, München 1981

# Efficacy of E-5-(2-Bromovinyl)-2'-Deoxyuridine in the Topical Treatment of Herpetic Keratitis in Rabbits and Man

P. Maudgal, E. De Clercq, J. Descamps, L. Missotten, Leuven

**Key words.** HSV, herpetic keratitis, BVDU

**Schlüsselwörter.** HSV, Herpeskeratitis, BVDU

**Summary.** Topical BVDU [(E)-5-(2-bromovinyl)-2'-deoxyuridine] application (i.e. 0.1% BVDU eye drops) has proven to be highly efficacious in the treatment of both epithelial and stromal herpes simplex keratitis, both in rabbits and humans.

**Zusammenfassung.** Die lokale Therapie sowohl der Keratitis dendritica als auch eines Stromaherpes mit 0,1% BVDU-Augentropfen hat sich bei Kaninchen und auch schon bei Patienten als hoch wirksam erwiesen. Bei den Therapieversuchen an Patienten handelt es sich noch nicht um kontrollierte Vergleichsstudien, sondern um offene Pilot-Studien an ausgewählten Patienten.

## Introduction

Several antiherpes agents have been synthesized for the treatment of herpes simplex keratitis. The compounds presently available for clinical use include IDU (5-iodo-2'-deoxyuridine), ara-A (9-β-D-arabinofuranosyladenine) and TFT (5-trifluoromethyl-2'-deoxyuridine). The toxic effect of IDU on the eye is well documented [1]. Ara-A and TFT also cause ocular toxicity, albeit to a lesser extent than IDU [5-7, 10]. The continuing search for more specific antiviral drugs has led to the development of acycloguanosine [9-(2-hydroxyethoxymethyl)guanine] and BVDU [(E)-5-(2-bromovinyl)-2'-deoxyuridine], two compounds which appear to surpass all previously established anti-herpes agents (i.e. IDU, ara-A and TFT), in both potency and selectivity [2, 4].

In primary rabbit kidney and human skin fibroblast cell cultures, BVDU was about 20 times more active than IDU in inhibiting the replication of herpes simplex type 1 virus (HSV 1), whereas it was 60 times less toxic than IDU, as could be judged from the inhibition of [$^{14}$C-2]-deoxyuridine incorporation into the host cell DNA [3]. In primary rabbit kidney cells BVDU proved also more potent and/or more selective as an anti-HSV 1 agent than various other newly developed anti-herpes agents such as phosphonoacetate, phosphonoformate, thymine arabinoside, 5-ethly-2'-deoxyuridine, 5-propyl-2'-deoxy-uridine, 5-iodo-2'-deoxycytidine, 5'-amino-5-iodo-2', 5'-dideoxyuridine, acycyloguanosine and 2'-fluoro-5-iodoaracytosine [2, 4].

In this paper we report on our experience with BVDU in the treatment of herpes simplex keratitis in rabbits and humans.

## Experimental Studies (in Rabbits)

### 1. Prevention of Keratitis

0.5% BVDU ointment applied to the eyes (just after keratitis began to appear) 5 times a day for 5 days suppressed the development of HSV 1 keratitis in rabbits; and, although 0.5% BVDU ointment was more effective than 0.5% IDU ointment, the difference was not statistically significant [9].

### 2. Healing of Established Keratitis

In an open trial, 0.5% BVDU ointment was significantly better than 0.5% IDU ointment in promoting the healing of established HSV 1 keratitis of rabbits [9]. In further double-blind randomized controlled trials we compared the efficacy of (i) 0.1% and 2.5% BVDU ointments, (ii) 0.1% BVDU, 0.1% IDU and 0.5%

IDU ointments, and (iii) 0.1% BVDU and 0.1% IDU eye drops, in the treatment of established HSV 1 keratitis in rabbits. The results of these experiments showed that both IDU and BVDU, whether applied as ointment or drops, significantly reduced the severity of keratitis and that, in its healing effect, BVDU was superior to IDU [8]. The healing effect was slightly more pronounced with 2.5% BVDU ointment than with 0.1% BVDU ointment, but this difference was not statistically significant. On the other hand, the healing effect of 0.1% BVDU ointment was significantly better than that of 0.5% IDU ointment. Also, 0.1% BVDU ointment was superior to 0.1% IDU ointment, but not to a significant level. However, when both drugs were applied as a 0.1% solution, BVDU was significantly more effective than IDU [8].

## 3. Prevention of Deep Stromal Keratitis

Both BVDU (0.1% or 0.5% eye drops) and TFT (1% eye drops), when applied to the eyes from day 1 to day 6 following intrastromal injection of HSV 1, suppressed the development of deep stromal keratitis, and, in this respect, 0.1% BVDU drops proved significantly better than 1% TFT drops.

## 4. Ocular Toxicity

No signs of ocular toxicity were noted after administration of BVDU, whether it was applied as 0.1%, 0.5% or 2.5% ointments, or 0.1% or 0.5% eye drops. IDU and TFT, however, gave rise to punctate epitheliopathy, the former when it was applied as 0.5% ointment, the latter when applied as 1% eye drops.

## Clinical Studies (in Humans)

Encouraged by the results of our experimental studies in rabbits we have recently embarked on the topical treatment of herpetic keratitis patients with BVDU. BVDU 0.1% eye drops were instilled every hour in the eyes of selected patients. Nineteen patients have been treated up to now. Sixteen of these patients had received topical IDU treatment without apparent beneficial effect. Four of these had also tried 3% ara-A ointment. Twelve patients suffered from dendritic keratitis and six others had geographic corneal ulcers. Moderate to severe stromal keratitis was present in all but three new patients. Others had been suffering from recurrent herpetic keratitis for variable periods of time. Eight patients were treated topically with corticosteroids (in addition to IDU or ara-A) at the time BVDU medication was substituted for IDU (or ara-A). Corticosteroid therapy was continued in these patients, as they showed evidence of stromal disease.

The majority of the patients with dendritic keratitis felt marked relief of discomfort after 24 hours of BVDU treatment. The healing time, as judged by the negative fluorescein staining method and the normal glistening appearance of the corneal surface, varied from 2 days to 21 days (average: 7.2 days). Geographic ulcers of five patients healed within an average time of 8.2 days. One patient who had developed a large geographical ulcer despite corticosteroid and IDU treatment, showed marked improvement after IDU was replaced by BVDU, but then developed an indolent corneal ulcer. Two other patients developed corneal edema and bullous keratopathy after their epithelial disease was healed. One of these patients also suffered from recurrent erosions. Both patients remained under corticosteroid therapy when being treated with BVDU.

BVDU exerted a pronounced beneficial effect on stromal keratitis. The stromal inflammation subsided gradually and, in most of the patients the ocular redness disappeared within 1 week of treatment. Of the eight patients who received corticosteroids, three became corticosteroid-dependent while the others could be taken off corticosteroids after 2 weeks to 2 months.

In none of the patients treated with BVDU did we observe any sign of ocular toxicity.

## Discussion

BVDU has proven to be highly efficacious in the treatment of experimental HSV 1 keratitis in rabbits whether it was administered as 0.1%, 0.5% or 2.5% ointment or 0.1% drops, and, in this respect, it was significantly better than IDU [8, 9]. No new lesions appeared during treatment with BVDU, and the existing lesions gradually regressed. Under IDU therapy, the existing lesions progressed before they began to regress and new lesions appeared during treatment. Application of 0.5% IDU ointment provoked punctate epitheliopathy, while BVDU did not produce such (or any other) toxic side effects.

An open clinical trial with BVDU has revealed that the drug (when applied as 0.1% eye drops) is also effective in the treatment of patients with herpetic keratitis that had become resistant to IDU or ara-A therapy. However, the extent of the response varied from one patient to another. BVDU proved also efficacious in patients with stromal herpetic keratitis. This observation is quite interesting, since stromal herpetic disease is thought to be initiated by viral replication and further maintained by an antigen-antibody reaction [11, 12]. From the beneficial effect of BVDU on stromal keratitis, one may infer that the drug adequately penetrates into the corneal stroma.

In neither rabbits nor humans have we observed any untoward effect of BVDU. Two patients, who had suffered from large geographic ulcers, developed corneal edema and bullous keratopathy following BVDU treatment. These complications may probably be attributed to the lack of epithelium attachment.

In conclusion, BVDU appears to be a very potent and non-toxic antiherpes drug which can be recommended for use in the treatment of epithelial and/or stromal herpes simplex keratitis and, in particular, those cases of herpetic keratitis that have become resistant to IDU or ara-A therapy.

## References

1. Binder PS (1977) Herpes simplex keratitis. Surv Ophthalmol 21:313–331
2. De Clercq E, Descamps J, Barr PJ, Jones AS, Serafinowski P, Walker RT, Huang GF, Torrence PF, Schmidt CL, Mertes MP, Kulikowski T, Shugar D (1979) Comparative study of the potency and selectivity of anti-herpes compounds. In: Skoda J, Langen P (eds) Antimetabolites in biochemistry, biology and medicine. Pergamon, Oxford New York, pp 275–285
3. De Clercq E, Descamps J, De Somer P, Barr PJ, Jones AS, Walker RT (1979) (E)-5-(2-Bromovinyl)-2'-deoxyuridine: a potent and selective anti-herpes agent. Proc Natl Acad Sci USA 76:2947–2951
4. De Clercq E, Descamps J, Verhelst G, Walker RT, Jones AS, Torrence PF, Shugar D (1980) Comparative efficacy of different anti-herpes drugs against different strains of herpes simplex virus. J Infect Dis in press
5. Gasset AR, Katzin D (1975) Antiviral drugs and corneal wound healing. Invest Ophthalmol Visual Sci 14:628–630
6. Jones BR (1975) Rational regimen of administration of antivirals. Trans Am Acad Ophthalmol Otolaryngol 79:104–108
7. Laibson PR, Hyndiuk R, Krachmer JH, Schultz RO (1975) Ara-A and IDU therapy of human superficial herpetic keratitis. Invest Ophthalmol 14:762–763
8. Maudgal PC, De Clercq E, Descamps J, Missotten L (1979) Comparative evaluation of BVDU [(E)-5-(2-bromovinyl)-2'-deoxyuridine] and IDU (5-iodo-2'-deoxyuridine) in the treatment of experimental herpes simplex keratitis in rabbits. Bull Soc Belge d'Ophthalmol 186: 109–118
9. Maudgal PC, De Clercq E, Descamps J, Missotten L, De Somer P, Busson R, Vanderhaeghe H, Verhelst G, Walker RT, Jones AS (1980) (E)-5-(2-Bromovinyl)-2'-deoxyuridine in the treatment of experimental herpes simplex keratitis. Antimicrob Agents Chemother 17:8–12
10. McGill JC, Coster D, Fraunfelder TF, Holt-Wilson AD, Williams H, Jones BR (1975) Adenine arabinoside in the treatment of herpetic keratitis. Trans Ophthalmol Soc UK 95: 246–249
11. McNeill JI, Kaufman HE (1979) Local antivirals in a herpes simplex stromal keratitis model. Arch Ophthalmol 97:727–729
12. Metcalf JF, McNeill JI, Kaufman HE (1976) Experimental disciform edema and necrotizing keratitis in the rabbit. Invest Ophthalmol Visual Sci 15:979–985

## Discussion on the Contributions pp. 329–341

T. Ravenscroft (Beckenham)
In the first paper, when you were comparing the activities of the drugs, did you examine one or a number of strains of HSV types 1 and 2, and herpes zoster? Were they fresh isolates or laboratory strains?

E. De Clercq (Leuven)
For HSV type 1 we used 3 laboratory strains and 8 clinical isolates. For HSV type 2 we used 3 laboratory strains and 4 clinical isolates. A number of these laboratory strains, i.e. HSV 1, F, HSV 1 McIntyre and HSV 2 G were obtained from the American Type Culture Collection (ATCC). For VZV we used a clinical isolate.

W.H. Prusoff (New Haven)

If I may refer a question to the second paper. In your third experiment you were comparing, in addition to BVDU, 0.5% and 0.1% IDU. It was interesting that the results are better for 0.1% IDU than for 0.5%. In the fifth experiment, you had worse results for your 0.5% BVDU than for your 0.1%. Can you account for these results?

P.C. Maudgal (Leuven)

The fifth experiment was on stromal keratitis. IDU was not used here. Regarding the third experiment; I did mention that 0.5% IDU ointment produced some punctate epitheliopathy which raised the mean keratitis scores.

W.H. Prusoff (New Haven)

I'm afraid I didn't explain myself very clearly. In the fifth experiment, you compared the effects of 0.5% BVDU, and 0.1% BVDU and the results for 0.5% were worse than for 0.1%. I was wondering why you didn't get a better effect with the higher concentration.

P.C. Maudgal (Leuven)

There is some difference but it is not significant. Under experimental conditions you may have such variations.

W.H. Prusoff (New Haven)

In some of the other slides, however, you had about the same difference which you concluded was significant when you compared BVDU with one of the other drugs.

P.C. Maudgal (Leuven)

In the experiment where I compared 0.5% and 0.1% IDU against 0.1% BVDU, the difference between 0.1% IDU and 0.1% BVDU was not significant. But we must not forget that keratitis was more severe in the BVDU group than in the IDU group at the beginning of therapy.

H.J. Field (Cambridge)

Eric, you expressed surprise that the TK⁻ virus strain B2006 was very sensitive to acyclovir when tested in rabbit kidney cells. I think it is not surprising. If you look at other cell types for instance VERO cells, or human amnion cells, that same strain becomes very resistant. At the opposite extreme, if you measure the resistance of B2006 in a cell which already contains the virus thymidine kinase, then the mutant becomes completely sensitive. This certainly suggests that in your rabbit cells it is a cellular enzyme which is phosphorylating the drug.

E. De Clerq (Leuven)

Yes.

Y.C. Cheng (Chapel Hill)

Eric, it was a beautiful presentation on an interesting compound. Let me ask you one simple question: In your thymidine incorporation experiment with 100 µg/ml, you start to see inhibition of the incorporation of thymidine into DNA. What was the concentration of thymidine you used in this incorporation study?

E. De Clercq (Leuven)

This was extremely low (0.34 nM/petri dish), thus much less than the concentration of BVDU itself.

Y.C. Cheng (Chapel Hill)

I'd like to comment on your radioactive thymidine incorporation into DNA experiments. Thymidine will require to be phosphorylated first by TK in order to get into DNA. In your experiment, thymidine will compete with BVDU. With such low concentration of thymidine and with such high concentration of BVDU in your experiment, you really don't see the incorporation of radioactive thymidine into DNA being inhibited in infected cells. That's a message to indicate that BVDU has poor affinity for the host TK. In contrast, in the viral infected cells, very little of BVDU can inhibit the thymidine incorporation. This indicates that BVDU may be a better substrate for virus TK.

E. De Clercq (Leuven)

Thus, the differential effect of BVDU on thymidine incorporation in virus-infected and uninfected cells may be related to the greater substrate affinity of BVDU for the virus-induced thymidine kinase. This is quite possible.

G. Streissle (Wuppertal)

Dr. De Clercq, do you have information on the effect of BVDU on cytomegalovirus?

E. De Clercq (Leuven)

Yes, this point was checked by H. Schellekens and L.W. Stitz. They found the compound to be inactive against cytomegalovirus, which is not unexpected, because BVDU acts through the virus-induced thymidine kinase and cytomegalovirus does not induce its own thymidine kinase.

Lopes-Cardozo (Amsterdam)

Dr. Maudgal, you mentioned two cases of bullous keratopathy in the open human study with geographic ulcers. Do you ascribe those results to the drug or to unrelated causes?

P.C. Maudgal (Leuven)

It is very difficult to say in this small study if the bullous keratopathy is the result of herpetic disease process or if it was the toxic reaction to the drug. It could be due to either. But all of us know that such problems are frequently encountered, even if with some luck one manages to heal the longstanding geographic ulcers.

Sundmacher, R. (Hrsg.):
Herpetische Augenerkrankungen
© J.F. Bergmann Verlag, München 1981

# The Efficacy of Some Newer Antiherpetic Compounds in the Rabbit Model

J. Wollensak, Berlin

**Key words.** Herpetic keratitis, antiviral drugs, toxicity

**Schlüsselwörter.** Herpeskeratitis, antivirale Medikamente, Toxizität

**Summary.** Phosphonoacetic acid (PAA), Phosphonoformic acid (PFA), two analogous substances, and Trifluorothymidine ointment (TFT) were studied in a rabbit model of herpetic keratitis for their antiviral as well as toxic effects. The preliminary results indicate that PAA and PFA may have a better therapeutic index than TFT ointment.

**Zusammenfassung.** Phosphonoessigsäure (PAA), Phosphonoameisensäure (PFA), zwei Analogsubstanzen, sowie Trifluorthymidin-Salbe (TFT) wurden im Kaninchenmodell auf ihre antivirale Aktivität gegen Herpes simplex-Virus und auf ihre lokale Toxizität überprüft. Die vorläufigen Ergebnisse scheinen zu zeigen, daß PAA und PFA möglicherweise einen besseren therapeutischen Index als TFT-Salbe haben.

Each of us knows, that all the antiherpetic compounds have too many side effects, as can be shown, for example, in the regeneration of the corneal epithelium. For the clinician, the picture of the overtreated herpetic lesion is well known: After the healing of a recent herpetic lesion the epithelium becomes gray, irregular and thickened. Rarely a picture like that of an erosion appears. The cell toxicity is one of the important complications of antimetabolic herpes therapy and is therefore one of the reasons we are searching for other substances. Other problems with antiviral drugs are their inefficiency, their instability and their inability to penetrate the corneal barriers. We heard this today several times.

For our experiments in the rabbit model we used Phosphonoacetic acid (PAA), Phosphonoformic acid (PFA) and analogues substances. As a reference substance Trifluorothymidine (TFT) was used. The cornea test for studies of epithelial regeneration, as well as for herpes virus infection, was carried out according to our own method published previously in 1964–1965. We used an ocular herpes virus strain and the antiherpetic therapy was started as local treatment only after the epithelial lesion could be seen by fluorescein staining. This was usually the case 24 to 36 hours after experimental infection. In the epithelial regeneration test we started as soon as the lesion was induced. In both cases the local treatment was done from 8 a.m. to 10 p.m. every 2 hours. An ointment was then applied for the rest of the night. Progress of the keratitis was recorded by staining the lesion with 2% solution of fluorescein twice daily. The same staining method was used for the regeneration test (also twice daily). Because we do not yet have all of our histological examinations of the experiments, we will not go into the details of interpretation of our results. We will therefore more or less summarize briefly:

Phosphonoacetate has been known for quite a while but the action against herpes viruses was not described until 1973 by Shipkowitz and coworkers [13]. Phosphonoformic acid was first studied by Helgstrand and coworkers in 1978 [4] in skin and in tissue culture. Both PAA and PFA, have been reported to be specific inhibitors to herpes virus DNA polymerase.

In our experiments we could demonstrate that PAA as well as PFA and the analogues substances have almost no influence on the time of regeneration of the epithelium. However, some differences can be seen between the 36th and 72nd hours. In contrast the reference substance Trifluorothymidine (TFT) has a much more toxic effect on the regeneration than the Phosphono-drugs. All substances except the 2% TFT ointment were saturated with nearly 5% solutions. In addition, PFA was a little less toxic then PAA, but the difference is small compared to TFT.

On the other hand, the corneal infection tests do not show as clear results as the epithelial regeneration test. We started three complete experiments with each of the substances mentioned before. For better analysis of the results (we infected one cornea of each rabbit and after visualisation of the herpetic lesion later on) we made five groups in order to test the five presumed antiviral compounds at the same time. As we knew from former experiments, we needed four eyes for each group for a correct evaluation.

In all of the three experiments, PAA showed the best therapeutic effect. It did not matter if the infection dose was high or low or if the scarification of the cornea was primarily made deeper than purely epithelial. PFA was apparently a little more efficacious in low virus dosage infection than the others. PFA showed as good results as TFT. Both analogues substances were not as effective as PAA or PFA. After our experiments PAA seems to be much less toxic then TFT and at the same time we could see better results in the treatment of experimental infection of the rabbit cornea.

# References

1. Gerstein DD, Dawson CR, Oh JO (1975) Phosphonoacetic acid in the treatment of experimental herpes simplex keratitis. Antimicrob Agents Chemother 7:285–288
2. Helgstrand E, Öberg B, Alenius S (1979) Experimental studies on the antiherpetic agent phosphonoformic acid. Adv Ophthalmol 38: 276–280
3. Helgstrand E, Öberg B (1978) Antiviral screening based on cell-free polymerase models and a new selective inhibitor. 10th. Int. Congr. Chemother. 1977. Curr Chemother 329
4. Helgstrand E, Eriksson B, Johansson NG, Lannerö B, Larsson A, Misiorny A, Norén JO, Sjöberg B, Stenberg K, Stening G, Stridh S, Öberg B, Alenius S, Philipson L (1978) Trisodium phosphonoformate. A new antiviral compound. Science 201:819
5. Helgstrand E, Eriksson B, Johansson NG, Lannerö B, Larsson A, Misiorny A, Noren JO,
Sjöberg B, Stenberg K, Stening G, Stridh S, Öberg B, Alenius S, Philipson L (in press) Trisodium phosphonoformate. A new antiviral compound. Science
6. Honess RW, Watson DH (1977) Herpes simplex virus resistance and sensitivity to phosphonoacetic acid. J Virol 21:584–600
7. Leinbach SS, Reno JM, Lee LF, Isbell AF, Boezi JA (1971) Mechanism of phosphonoacetate inhibition of herpesvirus-induced DNA polymerization. Biochemistry 15:426–430
8. Mao JC-H, Robishaw EE (1975) Mode of inhibition of herpes simplex virus DNA polymerase by phosphonoacetate. Biochemistry 14: 5475–5479
9. Meyer RF, Varnell ED, Kaufman HE (1976) Phosphonoacetic acid in the treatment of experimental ocular herpes simplex infection. Antimicrob Agents Chemother 9:308–311
10. Newton AA (1979) Inhibition of the replication of herpes viruses by phosphonoacetate and related compounds. Adv Ophthalmol 38:267–275
11. Overby LR, Robishaw EE, Scheicher JB, Rueter A, Shipkowitz NL, Mao JC-H (1974) Inhibition of herpes virus replication by phosphonoacetic acid. Antimicrob Agents Chemother 6:360–365
12. Reno JM, Lee LF, Boezi JA (1978) Inhibition of herpes virus replication and herpes virus-induced deoxyribonucleic acid polymerase by phosphonoformate. Antimicrob Agents Chemother 13:188–192
13. Shipkowitz NL, Bower RR, Appell RN, Nordeen CW, Overby LR, Roderick WR, Schleicher JB, Esch AM von (1973) Suppression of herpes simplex infection by phosphonoacetic acid. App Microbiol 26:264–267
14. Wollensak J, Klare U (1964) Untersuchungen zur Therapie der experimentellen Keratitis superficialis herpetica. Vergleich mit klinischen Ergebnissen. Albrecht von Graefes Arch Klin Ophthalmol 167:214–224
15. Wollensak J, Kypke W (1965) Hemmung von Epithelregeneration und cornealer Wundheilung beim Kaninchen durch Antimetaboliten. Albrecht von Graefes Arch Klin Ophthalmol 168:102–115

## Discussion on the Contribution pp. 343–344

W.H. Prusoff (New Haven)
Perhaps Dr. Öberg would like to make some comments on the differences between PFA and PAA?

B. Öberg (Södertälje)
The differences we have seen between PFA and PAA are mainly problems with skin toxicity. PAA,

but not PFA, is quite skin toxic, at least in guinea pigs and monkeys. As far as treatment of keratitis goes, I think our results correspond very well to what has been presented by Dr. Wollensak.

The question whether PFA was as effective as trifluorothymidine cannot be answered now since we have not compared these compounds. We have compared IDU and PFA and they had similar activities.

**H.E. Kaufman (New Orleans)**
We haven't worked with the phosphonoformate enough. In our previous studies with PAA, we found it to be comparable to IDU, but not to trifluorothymidine. Of course the experiments were different and the strains were different, but we certainly found trifluorothymidine to be significantly more potent.

**J. Wollensak (Berlin)**
What concentration did you use?

**H.E. Kaufman (New Orleans)**
We used a 1% solution of trifluorothymidine. I can't remember the concentration of PAA.

**J. Wollensak (Berlin)**
The substance was not toxic. The concentrations were in PAA and PFA as high as 5% – nearly saturated solutions – because the toxicity was so low.

**E. De Clercq (Leuven)**
I'am a little bit puzzled by the fact that PAA is such an irritating agent to the skin, and you say it is not irritating to the eye. What was the concentration at which PAA was applied?

**J. Wollensak (Berlin)**
Nearly 5%.

**E. De Clercq (Leuven)**
And this was not irritating?

**J. Wollensak (Berlin)**
No.

**B. Öberg (Södertälje)**
I have one comment concerning the difference in skin and eye toxicity. I think that PAA – and I know that PFA – stays in the upper layer of the skin if you apply the compounds cutaneously. In that way you will have a high local concentration.

In the eye both these compounds are washed away very quickly by the tear fluid and don't build up a high concentration.

**W.H. Prusoff (New Haven)**
This might be a possibility.

Sundmacher, R. (Hrsg.):
Herpetische Augenerkrankungen
© J.F. Bergmann Verlag, München 1981

# Evaluation of Glucosamine in HSV-Keratitis Therapy

R.A. Delgadillo, D.A. Vanden Berghe, A.J. Neetens, W. Van de Sompel, P. Dockx, Wilrijk

**Key words.** Herpetic keratitis, glucosamine

**Schlüsselwörter.** Herpeskeratitis, Glucosamin

**Summary.** Studies with cell monolayers and the use of an animal model for HSV 1 infection demonstrated clearly that glucosamine decreases the multiplication of infectious virus. There is evidence that during the treatment with glucosamine, new glucosamine-tolerant cells are formed in which the virion assembly is affected. However, the viral protein synthesis still occurs so that the immunological anti-HSV 1 reaction is induced. Use of glucosamine in clinical trials shows that glucosamine is a potential antiviral drug.

**Zusammenfassung.** In vitro-Versuche mit Monolayer-Zellkulturen sowie Tierversuche mit einer HSV 1-Keratitis zeigen eindeutig, daß Glucosamin in der Lage ist, die Herpesvirusvermehrung zu reduzieren. Es scheint so zu sein, daß sich während der Glucosamin-Behandlung neue Glucosamin-tolerante Zellen herausbilden, in denen der Zusammenbau des Virus verhindert wird. Die virale Proteinsynthese geht aber dennoch weiter, und entsprechend wird auch eine antivirale Immunreaktion induziert. Die Anwendung von Glucosamin in ersten klinischen Versuchen zeigt, daß es ein potentes Virustatikum ist.

## Introduction

Glucosamine (GN) and other sugar derivates have shown to exert an antiviral effect in tissue cultures and in animal models [1, 2].

Since GN is a natural component of cells, it was of interest to determine whether GN may be useful as an antiviral drug.

## Effect of Glucosamine on Virus Synthesis in Tissue Culture

The mechanism of antiviral action of GN is organ- and tissue-specific and depends on the chemical composition of the extracellular environment [3, 4].

The main effects of GN on virus-infected tissue and organ cultures can be summarised as follows:

a) GN may decrease the viral protein synthesis without affecting the nucleic acid synthesis [5].
b) GN inhibits the assembly of viral nucleocapsid [5].
c) GN impairs the glycosylation of the envelope-glycoproteins resulting in defective viral particles [1].
d) So far, virus mutants resistent to GN have not been detected [5].

A study with virus-infected and mock-infected Vero cells demonstrated that in 3 mM GN the protein synthesis of mock-infected cells is slightly and reversibly affected. On the other hand, the protein synthesis of virus-infected cells is more affected [5]. In order to maintain the action of GN, it is necessary to renew GN in the medium, because it is metabolized by the cells [5]. Long term cultivation of Vero cells in 3 mM GN resulted in a GN-tolerant Vero cell line (GN-t cells). The growth of virus in GN-t cells is different than in normal Vero cells. In GN-t cells the virus yield is drastically decreased even in medium without GN. Nevertheless the total viral protein synthesis is not affected at all. This means that the viral antigens are still present in the infected cells [5].

## Animal Model

Twenty five New Zealand rabbits, under normal ophthalmological conditions, were used in these double blind experiments.

Topical anaesthesia of the cornea of the right eye was performed with 0.4% oxybuprocaine collyrium. A 2 mm diameter sterile millipore filter was applied to the center of the cornea and removed immediateley after contact. This creates an erosion of only the superficial epithelial cell layers as demonstrated by fluorescein test. The lower conjunctival fornix was instilled with 0.1 ml of a semi-purified suspension of herpes simplex virus type 1 (HSV 1) in physiological tris-buffer, pH 7.2 (PTB) with a viral titer of $10^5$ $TCD_{50}$/ml. Two hours after inoculation, 0.1 ml of PTB, alone or containing either 100 mM GN/ml or 150 µg lycorine/ml, was instilled into the lower conjunctival fornix. This treatment was repeated every 2 hours, 5 times during the working hours of each day. The conjunctival inflammation and the morphology of the lesions were evaluated and their patterns recorded schematically. The animals were observed for 28 days.

The virus titer of the conjunctival fluid was determined daily. A conjunctival swab was taken and placed into 1 ml PTB, which was stored at –70 °C until titration of samples. Titrations were carried out on Vero cells [6] and the viral titer was expressed in $TCD_{50}$.

Electron microscopy examinations were carried out as previously described [7, 9].

**Ophthalmological Examination**

Nine rabbits treated with GN as well as con-

trols (16 rabbits) developed a pronounced conjunctivitis beginning the 1st day after inoculation; from the 2nd day on the fluorescein test revealed multiple erosions situated mostly in the central corneal regions. Control animals showed strikingly more erosions and after the 4th day dendritic patterns also appeared (Fig. 1), although the latter did not develop at any time in animals treated with GN (Fig. 2). In controls, the decrease of fluorescein positivity occurred from the 7th day on and became negative on the 14th day, while in GN-treated rabbits, the decrease of fluorescein positivity occurred from the 5th day on and became negative about the 10th day.

About the 18th day, the corneal lesions reappeared. Control animals showed centrally located epithelial corneal erosions with specific dendritic patterns. The infiltration area extended to Bowman's membrane and to the superficial stroma. GN treated corneas showed epithelial fluorescein positive lesions that were not typical for HSV 1. These lesions showed the tendency toward rapid cicatrization without leaving Bowman or stromal opacities. It has to be noted, that during the

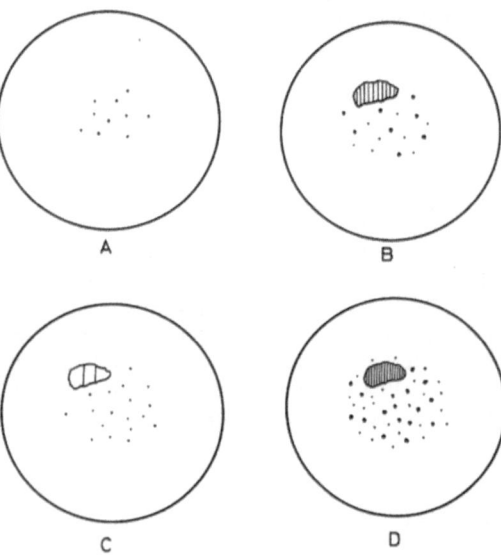

Fig. 2. Schematic drawing of corneal lesions caused by HSV 1 in glucosamine-treated rabbits
A. 2nd day of infection
B. 4th day of infection
C. 5th day of infection
D. 18th day of infection

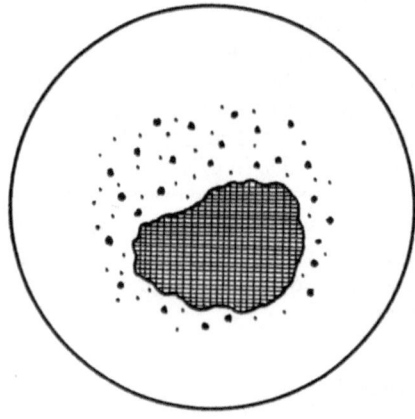

Fig. 1. Schematic drawing of corneal lesions caused by HSV 1 in untreated rabbits on the 5th day of infection

**Table 1.** Influence of glucosamine on herpetic keratitis in rabbits

| Animals | conjunctivitis | fluorescein test | dendritic pattern | Bowman infiltration | stromal inf. |
|---|---|---|---|---|---|
| controls | ++ | ++ | + | ++ | + |
| glucosa-mine treated | ++ | ±→± | − | ±→− | − |

evaluation of the lesions, some Bowman infiltration occurred but faded rapidly and progressively away.

These observations are summarised in Table 1.

**Virus Titration**

In control animals the newly synthesized virus, released into the conjunctival fluid,

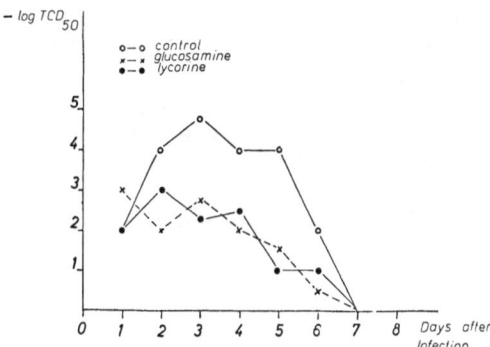

**Fig. 3.** Virustiter in the conjunctival fluid of rabbits with HSV 1 keratitis

increased from the 2nd day on, reaching its maximal titer on day 3; after that, the virus titer decreased progressively, becoming undetectable from the 7th day on until the end of the experiment. In GN-treated animals, except the 1st day, the virus titer of the conjunctival fluid was significantly lower than in controls. Also in this case, no virus was detected from 7th day on (Fig. 3).

During the first 7 days the production of virus GN-treated animals was only 2% of that of the controls.

Electron microscopic examination of the cornea on the 10th day showed HSV nucleocapsids and complete virions in controls stromal cells (Fig. 4). In GN-treated corneas neither nucleocapsids nor virions could be detected (Fig. 5).

Lycorine, an alkaloid isolated from the plant Clivia miniate, also showed antiviral activity. The reduction of virus yield in HSV 1 keratitis (Fig. 3) may be explained, at least in part, by an unspecific cytotoxic effect.

**Clinical Trial [10]**

Patients with superficial epithelial dendritic

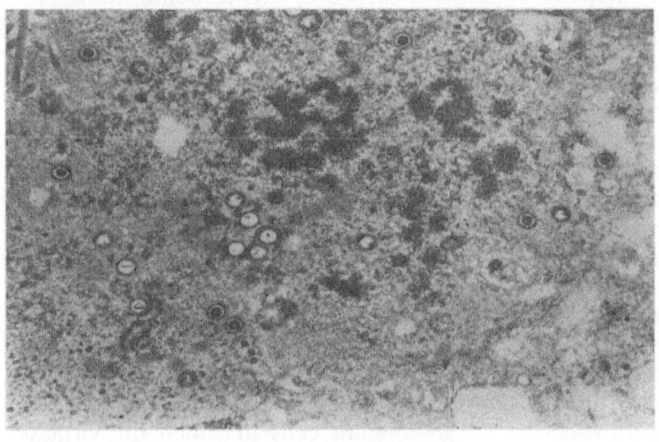

**Fig. 4.** Electron micrograph of stromal cells of untreated HSV 1 keratitis in rabbits. Magnification: 54,000 ×

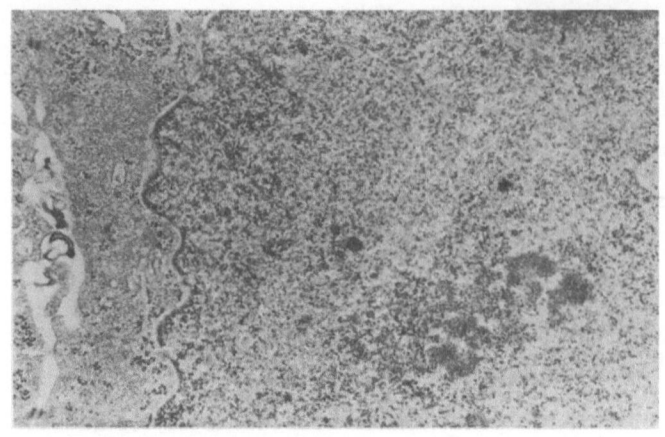

**Fig. 5.** Electron micrograph of stromal cells of glucosamine-treated HSV 1 keratitis in rabbits. Magnification: 40,500 ×

ulcera can be treated in different ways. After heat (physical), ether and iodine (chemical) local treatment, we have used Ara-ac-hx, IDU, PAA, F3T (purine and pyrimidine nucleoside antimetabolites) which are not only inhibitors of HSV 1 but also toxic for the epithelial cells. To heal a HSV lesion with as little loss of transparency of Bowman membrane and stroma as possible and subsequent visual impairment, and in order to obtain a viral epithelial layer, the best method, at least available to us, remains debridement of the total epithelium.

Unfortunately and to our distress, relapses occur, probably because the host cell offers little or no resistance to the virus, and metaherpetic disease of the epithelium develops.

Based on the above in vitro findings and animal experiments, clinical trials were carried out with glucosamine tested in different concentrations for toxicity.

Twenty one patients with primary herpetic keratitis lesions were treated with 100 mM D-glucosamine-containing collyria.

Human spontaneous superficial epithelial dendritic ulcers respond promptly (in 2 or 3 days). Infected epithelial cells swell and merge into larger oedematous vesicles. The epithelium turns greyish with white punctate dots, covering an irregular oval or round area. Presumably only infected cells are influenced by glucosamine, which means that the infected area is larger than may be expected from the dendritic pattern. Nevertheless, the decrease of fluorescein positivity progresses. The epithelium fragments turn into whirled dirty veils, loosely attached to the Bowman

membrane, causing itching and irritation, lacrimation and blepharospasm.

Finally the epithelium may be rejected. At that moment the patient feels better and after a few days a normal epithelial layer regenerates. Little scarring occurs.

These series of events are quite different from that occurring with other topical chemical treatments.

After 3 months a metaherpetic-like relapse occurs and this disease resists more or less treatment with glucosamine but responds quite well to cysteine.

Our follow-up time is only 1 year.

**Discussion**

These studies show that GN improves the clinical course and the degree of lesions of keratitis caused by HSV 1. This may be explained by the drastic decrease of virus multiplication caused by GN as demonstrated by titration of the virus and by electron microscopy. The few corneal lesions observed in GN-treated animals may be the result of a defensive immune response as is discussed below.

The antiviral action of GN in the treatment of herpetic keratitis is based on the following principles:
1) GN inhibits the virus multiplication by affecting mainly the virion assembly.
2) GN still allows the production of viral antigens in infected cells which can explain the immunological reaction in the eye.
3) Prolonged GN-treatment may give rise to GN-tolerant cells in which the virus is

produced at very low titers but showing high content of newly synthesized viral specific proteins.

Since GN drastically inhibits the virus multiplication, it can be expected that little or no virus spreading will occur, e.g. spreading to other corneal epithelial cells, spreading to stromal cells, and eventually spreading to nervous tissues, thus preventing the establishment of latent and recurrent infections.

The presence of infected cells containing viral antigens probably induces an immune response [9] which consists of the local production of anti-HSV 1 IgA and IgG antibodies which may neutralize the spread of the virus extracellularly. This can explain the failure in the detection of HSV 1, which is released in the conjunctival fluid from the 7th day on during the course of the infection. Furthermore, the cellular immune response is represented by the infiltration of lymphocytes, especially T-lymphocytes, plasma cells, polymorphonuclear cells and macrophages. These cells may cause tissue necrosis with subsequent formation of permanent scars. GN-treated corneas contain less infected cells than in controls, and so the areas of immunological shock are also less in number.

# References

1. Scholtissek CM (1975) Inhibition of the multiplication of enveloped virus by glucose derivates. Curr Top Microbiol Immun 70:101–119
2. Floch F, Werner GH (1976) In vivo antiviral activity of D-glucosamine. Arch Virol 52:169–173
3. Delgadillo RA, Vanden Berghe DAR, Van der Groen G, Pattyn SR (1976) Inhibition of the multiplication of enveloped and naked viruses by D-glucosamine. Arch Int Physiol Biochim 84:601–602
4. Delgadillo RA, Vanden Berghe DAR, Van der Groen G, Pattyn SR (1976) Effect of D-glucosamine on the growth pattern of RNA viruses. Arch Int Physiol Biochim 84:1066–1067
5. Delgadillo RA (in press) Antiviral activity of D-glucosamine. Doctoral Thesis. Antwerp University, B-2610 Wilrijk
6. Vanden Berghe DA, Ieven M, Mertens F, Vlietinck AJ (1978) Screening of higher plants for biological activities. II. Antiviral Activity. Lloydia 41:463–471
7. Reynold ES (1963) The use of lead citrate at high pH as an electron opaque stain in electron microscopy. Cell Biol 17:208–212
8. Spurr AR (1969) A low viscosity epoxy resine embedding medium for electron microscopy. J Strastruct Res 26:35–43
9. Metcalf JF, Reichert RW (1979) Histological and electron microscopic studies of experimental herpetic keratitis in the rabbit. Invest Ophthalmol Visual Sci 18:1123–1138
10. Vanden Berghe DA, Neetens JA (1979) D-Glucosamine therapy: A new approach in treatment of human herpetic keratitis. IRCS. J Med Sci 7:84

## Discussion on the Contribution pp. 347–351

R. Wigand (Homburg, Saar)
Does the glucose in the tissue culture medium have an antagonistic effect against your glucosamine effect, or doesn't it matter?

R. Delgadillo (Antwerpen)
Glucose counteracts the antiviral action of glusamine on Vero cells. Uridine monophosphate is also an antagonist of glucosamine. Starting from a Vero cell line, we have been able to select a cell line which shows an increased resistance to glucosamine (GN-t cell line). In GN-t cells, glucose does not counteract the antiviral effect of glucosamine. Another interesting aspect is that in GN-t cells, the poliovirus protein synthesis is not decreased by glucosamine; however, the yield for viral particles is much lower than in Vero cells. In other words, GN-t cells are able to synthesize viral antigens without forming viral particles. We find this effect interesting because, if we treat the patient with glucosamine and the virus production stops, it means that the spread of virus to the trigeminal ganglia, for instance, may be prevented. Virus latency is therefore prevented. In addition, the presence of viral antigens may still induce a normal defensive host-immune response.

W.H. Prusoff (New Haven)
When you measured protein synthesis in the cell, did you look at general protein synthesis or did you look at glycoprotein synthesis specifically?

R. Delgadillo (Antwerpen)
General protein synthesis.

W.H. Prusoff (New Haven)
Well, then you may have had an effect on glycoprotein without seeing it.

R. Delgadillo (Antwerpen)
Yes, it is possible that we may have an effect on glycoproteins, too. However, by measuring the general protein synthesis we arrived at the conclusion that glucosamine affects more specifically

virus-infected cells than noninfected cells. This is an important point.

W.H. Prusoff (New Haven)
The question would be whether the glucosamine is affecting the cellular glycoproteins which in turn affects the penetration of the virus into the cell. Do you know whether the virus is prevented from getting into the cell or where the site of inhibition might be?

R. Delgadillo (Antwerpen)
To my knowledge there are no publications indicating that glucosamine interferes with the penetration of the virus into the cell. In the experiments we performed, the virus was first allowed to come into the cell, and then the glucosamine was added.

W.H. Prusoff (New Haven)
What was your explanation for the effect on the non-eveloppe viruses?

R. Delgadillo (Antwerpen)
It is known that during virus multiplication there is formation of specific viral membranes as in the case of poliovirus-infected cells. The virus biosynthesis is closely associated with these membranes. We think that glucosamine interferes with the synthesis or function of specific viral membranes by inhibiting the glycosylation reactions of the membrane components (glycoproteins or glycolipids). The specific antiviral action of glucosamine is probably due to the fact that in virus-infected cells the up-take of glucosamine is higher than in noninfected cells.

E. De Clercq (Leuven)
There is a more specific glycosylation inhibitor than glucosamine, that is tunicamycin. Have you thought of using this inhibitor in your assays?

R. Delgadillo (Antwerpen)
Sugar derivatives, such a tunicamycin and 2-deoxyglucose could produce abnormal metabolites which may block the cellular metabolism irreversibly. We have chosen glucosamine because it is a normal component of cells. The metabolic effects of glucosamine are quite reversible, because after treatment the remaining glucosamine is easily metabolized.

Sundmacher, R. (Hrsg.):
Herpetische Augenerkrankungen
© J.F. Bergmann Verlag, München 1981

# Trifluorthymidine Sensitivity of Ocular Herpes Simplex Virus Strains

D. Neumann-Haefelin, A. Mattes, R. Sundmacher, Freiburg

**Key words.** Antiviral drugs – resistant virus strains, trifluorothymidine

**Schlüsselwörter.** Antivirale Medikamente – resistente Virusstämme, Trifluorthymidin

**Summary.** Drug resistance in corneal herpes has been frequently reported, and the development of resistance to antimetabolites such as idoxuridine (IDU) and trifluorothymidine (TFT) has been shown with herpes simplex virus (HSV) grown in cell cultures. In this study the TFT sensitivity of corneal HSV 1 isolates was tested in human diploid fibroblast cell cultures. In 28 cases of dendritic keratitis treated topically with TFT, paired isolates revealed no significant change of TFT sensitivity during the course of treatment. Attempts to induce drug resistance by culturing HSV in the presence of TFT failed. Marked cytotoxicity of the drug was observed at concentrations only slightly above that of minimal antiviral activity in the culture system used.

**Zusammenfassung.** Die Resistenzentwicklung gegen antivirale Chemotherapeutika ist ein bekanntes Problem in der Behandlung kornealer Herpeserkrankungen. Experimentell läßt sich Resistenz von Herpes simplex-Viren (HSV) gegen Jod-Desoxyuridin (IDU) in infizierten Zellkulturen erzeugen. Dies wurde kürzlich auch für Trifluorthymidin beschrieben. In den hier dargestellten Untersuchungen wurde die TFT-Empfindlichkeit kornealer HSV 1-Isolate in diploiden menschlichen Fibroblastenkulturen getestet. In 28 Fällen topisch mit TFT behandelter Keratitis dendritica ließ die Untersuchung gepaarter Virusisolate keine signifikante Änderung der TFT-Empfindlichkeit im Verlauf der Therapie erkennen. Auch Versuche der Resistenzerzeugung durch HSV-Kultivierung in Gegenwart von TFT führten nicht zur Entwicklung TFT-resistenter Viren. Für die in den Untersuchungen verwendeten Zellkulturen zeigte TFT eine ausgeprägte Zytotoxizität bei Konzentrationen, die nur knapp über der Schwelle der antiviralen Wirksamkeit lagen.

In our recent clinical studies dendritic keratitis was topically treated with TFT, either alone or in combination with human leukocyte interferon [5]. TFT was selected for different reasons: Its therapeutic efficacy in herpetic keratitis had been shown to be clearly superior to debridement or other chemotherapeutics like IDU [1], and it had revealed low toxicity when topically applied to the cornea [6]. Another advantage of TFT may be the low frequency of drug resistance. Clinical reports of viral resistance towards TFT are rare, and IDU resistance was shown not to be linked with TFT resistance [3].

While efficacy and low topic toxicity of TFT were confirmed by direct clinical observation in our studies, TFT sensitivity of the patients' individual HSV strains was monitored by the investigations reported in this paper.

## Materials and Methods

Paired HSV 1 isolates were obtained from 28 patients who were treated with 1% TFT eye drops five times daily for dendritic keratitis. Some of the patients received additional topical therapy with interferon (two drops containing either $3 \times 10^6$ or $3 \times 10^7$ reference units/ml) once a day. The first isolate was obtained before treatment, the second one as late as possible in the course of TFT therapy.

The virus strains were propagated, titered, and tested for TFT sensitivity in cell cultures of human diploid foreskin fibroblasts [4].

### CPE-Inhibition Test

The cytopathic effect (CPE) of HSV was inhibited by treatment with TFT (0.3, 1, 3, 10, 30, and 100 µg/ml) of cell monolayers in microtiter wells, 60 min after infection with 1, 10, or 100 $TCID_{50}$ of virus.

## Plaque Inhibition Test

HSV plaques were produced in 10 cm² petri dishes (Costar, cluster 6) by adding 2% human serum immune to HSV to the culture medium 60 min after adsorption of 30 to 60 plaque forming units, and after washing the cells. The same medium contained 32, 16, 8, 4, or 2 µg/ml of TFT, or no TFT for the control. Plaques were counted 48 h p.i. after fuchsin staining.

## Virus Yield Reduction Test

Test sets identical to those for plaque inhibition, but without the human immune serum, were frozen (-70 °C) 24 h p.i. and tested for viral infectivity by microtitration [4].

## HSV Cultivation in the Presence of TFT

Virus inocula from those three cultures of one yield reduction set (e.g. containing TFT at 4, 8, and 16 µg/ml) that showed increasing HSV inhibition, were passed three times into subsequent cultures treated with the same TFT dosage. If HSV could be recovered from one of the final cultures, this material was compared with the original isolate by TFT plaque inhibition.

## Results

The CPE-inhibition test proved to be rather insensitive. Antiviral effects and toxic effects could not be reliably separated in the range of 30 µg/ml of TFT. All strains tested appeared to be resistent to 10 µg/ml of TFT at the 10 $TCID_{50}$ level of virus inoculum. Plaque inhibition by TFT was effective at concentrations between 4 and 16 µg/ml, 8 µg/ml being the overall mean concentration resulting in 50% plaque inhibition for all strains. Some differences of the mean inhibiting concentration were observed in subsequent tests and in the results of individual strains tested repeatedly, indicating that the reactivity of cells towards TFT changed. In no instance, however, could any significant difference between paired isolates of one patient be detected, when the viruses were tested in parallel (Table 1).

The virus yield in TFT treated cultures was reduced by 90% or more at those concentrations of the drug required for 50% plaque inhibition. By this method, too, paired isolates were found not to differ from each other (Table 1).

Four virus strains were successfully propagated in the presence of TFT. When the final passage material was compared with the original isolates, however, identical TFT sensitivity patterns were found by plaque inhibition (Table 2).

**Table 1.** Relative TFT sensitivity of paired HSV 1 isolates

| No. of paired isolates | Days of TFT treatment between isolate 1 and 2 | [a]Quotient of TFT concentrations required, with isolate 1 and 2, for | |
|---|---|---|---|
| | | 50% reduction of plaques | 90% reduction of virus yield |
| 2 | 12 | 1 | 1 |
| | | 1.1 | 2 |
| 1 | 11 | 0.9 | 1 |
| 1 | 7 | 0.9 | n.d. |
| | | 1 | 0.7 |
| 3 | 6 | 1 | 2 |
| | | 1 | n.d. |
| 1 | 5 | 0.8 | 0.7 |
| 1 | 4 | 0.9 | n.d. |
| | | 1.1 | 1 |
| 2 | 3 | 1.1 | 1 |
| 4 | 2 | × = 0.9 | n.d. |
| 13 | 1 | × = 1 | n.d. |

[a] Resistance would be indicated by figures significantly smaller than 1

**Table 2.** TFT sensitivity of original HSV 1 isolates and virus passed in the presence of TFT

| Strain | % plaque reduction by TFT | | | |
|---|---|---|---|---|
| | 2 | 4 | 8 | 16 µg/ml |
| 226/6 | 0 | 20 | 90 | 100 |
| "R" | 0 | 10 | 90 | 100 |
| 524/15 | 0 | 40 | 95 | 100 |
| "R" | 0 | 40 | 95 | 100 |
| 919/1 | 0 | 60 | 95 | 100 |
| "R" | 0 | 60 | 95 | 100 |
| 1259/1 | 0 | 50 | 95 | 100 |
| "R" | 0 | 20 | 95 | 100 |

"R" = virus from the third passage in cultures treated with TFT (16 µg/ml) 1 h after infection

## Discussion

Neither in patients nor in vitro, could the occurrence of HSV 1 resistance towards TFT be demonstrated by the present assay system. The low number of patients, whose virus could be isolated over a considerable period of TFT treatment (n = 4 for 1 week or more), may be insufficient to allow general conclusions concerning the genetic stability of TFT sensitivity in HSV 1. However, our data obtained with paired fresh isolates, as well as the results of virus cultivation in the presence of TFT, suggest that resistance does not generally occur as readily as earlier reported [2].

The aim of this study was not to measure absolute TFT sensitivity of HSV 1 isolates. Taking into account the different reactivities of various cell culture systems, one may consider this to be problematic. The small range between antiviral activity and host cell toxicity of the drug, combined with the varying reactivity found in different batches of our cell cultures, taught us that even measurement of relative in vitro correlates for in vivo therapeutic sensitivity may be difficult. However, as we restricted our investigations to parallel comparison of paired viral specimens originating from the same host individual, these problems may not be fully pertinent to the present results.

**Acknowledgment.** This study was supported in part by the Nationales Referenzzentrum für Herpesviren, funded by the Bundesministerium für Jugend, Familie und Gesundheit.

## References

1. Coster DJ, McKinnon JR, McGill JI, Jones BR, Fraunfelder FT (1976) Clinical evaluation of adenine arabinoside and trifluorothymidine in the treatment of corneal ulcers caused by herpes simplex virus. J Infect Dis Suppl. 133: A173–177
2. Gauri KK (1979) Anti-herpesvirus polychemotherapy. Adv Ophthalmol 38:151–163
3. Kaufman HE, Heidelberger C (1964) Therapeutic antiviral action of 5-trifluoromethyl-2' - deoxyuridine in herpes simplex keratitis. Science 145:585
4. Neumann-Haefelin D, Sundmacher R, Wochnik G, Bablok B (1978) Herpes simplex virus types 1 and 2 in ocular disease. Arch Ophthalmol 96:64–69
5. Sundmacher R, Neumann-Haefelin D, Cantell K (1981) Therapy and prophylaxis of dendritic keratitis with topical human interferon. This vol.
6. Wellings PC, Awdry PN, Bors FH, Jones BR, Brown DC, Kaufman HE (1972) Clinical evaluation of trifluorothymidine in the treatment of herpes simplex corneal ulcers. Am J Ophthalmol 73:932–942

## Discussion on the Contribution pp. 353–355

G. Streissle (Wuppertal)
Does this mean that the effect of TFT is not virus-specific but perhaps due to cytotoxic activities?

D. Neumann-Haefelin (Freiburg)
In the culture system used, the cytotoxic effect and the antiviral effect were overlapping, indeed, as we could see in the CPE-inhibition test. Plaque formation and virus yield, however, were clearly restricted by TFT concentrations below the range of cytotoxicity. Resistent mutants would have been discovered, therefore, by these assays.

Y.C. Cheng (Chapel Hill)
I just want to make a comment. I think one of the purposes of this kind of study is to try to find the difference of sensitivity of different virus strains to TFT.

D. Neumann-Haefelin (Freiburg)
Not of absolute sensitivity, but of sensitivity before and after treatment.

Y.C. Cheng (Chapel Hill)
I think for this type of study, it's probably better to use TK⁻ cells as the host. That will give you the answer; and to obtain TK⁻ cells, all you need is to grow cells in the presence of TFT, and I am sure you will eventually get it.

Sundmacher, R. (Hrsg.):
Herpetische Augenerkrankungen
© J.F. Bergmann Verlag, München 1981

# Viral Drug Sensitivity in Cases of Herpes Simplex Ulceration*

J.I. McGill, M. Ogilvie, Southampton

**Key words.** IDU resistance, IDU sensitivity

**Schlüsselwörter.** IDU-Resistenz, IDU-Empfindlichkeit

**Summary.** A survey of patients with Herpes simplex ulcers was carried out. From these ulcers Herpes simplex virus was isolated and the in vitro drug sensitivity of each isolate determined (60 cases) by the plaque inhibition or log dilution techniques. The in vitro sensitivity was then correlated with the patients clinical course and the results showed that:

1. In many cases failure of the ulcer to heal was due to viral drug resistance.
2. Ulcers caused by drug sensitivity viruses healed quickly.
3. Ulcers caused by drug resistance viruses healed slowly, if at all.
4. There was a high incidence of first time ulcers being caused by Idoxurine resistance viruses.

**Zusammenfassung.** Wir untersuchten Patienten mit einem Oberflächen-Herpes. Von den Läsionen wurde Herpes simplex-Virus isoliert und dann die Virusempfindlichkeit jedes Isolates (60 Fälle) gegen verschiedene Virustatika mit der Plaque-Hemmungsmethode oder mit der Log-Verdünnungstechnik geprüft. Die in vitro gefundene Empfindlichkeit wurde dann mit dem klinischen Verlauf bei den Patienten korreliert und dabei zeigte sich:

1. Eine verzögerte Heilung korrelierte oft mit einer Virustatikaresistenz.
2. Dendriticae, die von virustatikaempfindlichen Viren verursacht wurden, heilten schnell.
3. Dendriticae, die von resistenten Viren verursacht wurden, heilten langsam, wenn überhaupt.
4. Es gab einen hohen Prozentsatz von erstmals aufgetretenen Dendriticae, die bereits durch IDU-resistente Viren hervorgerufen wurden.

---

* no paper received

Sundmacher, R. (Hrsg.):
Herpetische Augenerkrankungen
© J.F. Bergmann Verlag, München 1981

# The Clinical Implications of Acyclovir-Resistant Mutants of Herpes Simplex Virus

H.J. Field, Cambridge

**Key words.** Acyclovir, resistant virus strains

**Schlüsselwörter.** Acyclovir, resistente Virusstämme

**Summary.** Herpes simplex viruses readily develop resistance to acyclovir (ACV) in vitro; this would seem to pose a threat to its clinical use. However, the most common mutation leading to resistance results from the virus losing its ability to induce thymidine kinase (TK); the enzyme which activates the drug. Such viruses are attenuated in mice suggesting that the development of resistant viruses in vivo will be comparatively rare, and indeed have not so far been isolated from experimentally infected, ACV-treated animals. However, a highly resistant mutant is described which is TK$^+$ and virulent in mice. But this ACV-resistant virus is very sensitive to a number of other antiherpetic drugs with clinical potential including idoxuridine, trifluorothymidine, Ara A and phosphonoacetic acid.

**Zusammenfassung.** In vitro entwickeln Herpes simplex-Viren sehr schnell eine Resistenz gegenüber Acyclovir (ACV). Hieraus könnte man schließen, daß die klinische Anwendung nicht sehr sinnvoll sei. Das scheint aber in dieser Einfachheit nicht zu stimmen. Die häufigste zur Virustatika-Resistenz führende Mutation ist der Verlust der Fähigkeit des Virus Thymidinkinase zu induzieren, und dieses Enzym – die virusinduzierte Thymidinkinase – ist es ja, die ACV aktiviert. Solche mutierten Viren haben sich in Mäusen bislang als attenuiert (apathogen) erwiesen, was darauf schließen läßt, daß die Entwicklung solcher resistenter Viren in vivo relativ selten sein wird. In der Tat haben wir von ACV-behandelten infizierten Versuchstieren auch bislang nie resistentes Virus isolieren können. Anderseits haben wir aber auch eine hochgradig resistente Mutante erzeugen können, die ihre Fähigkeit zur Thymidinkinasebildung noch hat (TK$^+$) und die für Mäuse weiterhin virulent ist.

Dieses ACV-resistente Virus ist aber sehr empfindlich gegenüber einer Vielzahl anderer klinisch wirksamer Virustatika wie IDU, TFT, Ara-A und Phosphonoazetat.

The selective action of acyclovir (ACV) depends on its phosphorylation by the herpes simplex virus (HSV)-induced enzyme thymidine kinase (TK):

$$\text{HSV TK} \qquad \text{Probably cell enzymes}$$
$$ACV \rightarrow ACVP \rightarrow ACVPP \rightarrow ACVPPP$$
$$\downarrow$$
$$\text{HSV DNA-polymerase}$$

The triphosphate form of the drug then interferes with HSV DNA synthesis.

Mutants which are resistant to the drug arise because the virus loses its ability to induce TK or had changes in the DNA polymerase. Such resistant mutants arise very readily in tissue culture [3] and would seem to pose a threat to the success of this potentially useful compound. However our experiments with an animal model make us optimistic that resistance will not be a widespread problem. Firstly, in experimentally infected mice, treated with ACV no resistant variants have been isolated from the mouse's tissues during or after treatment [1, 2]. The likely explanation for this is that the most common mutation leading the resistance is loss of the virus' ability to induce TK. Such viruses are attenuated in mice [2, 4] and this is particularly marked when the viruses are inoculated into the brain (Table 1). All TK$^-$ viruses tested showed at least 100-fold decrease in virulence by this route.

However, one mutant (Cl(101)P$_2$C$_5$) was found to induce normal levels of TK and this virus retained virulence for mice. This virus was completely resistant in mice undergoing systemic treatment with 50 mg/kg/day ACV (Fig. 1).

**Table 1.** Resistance to ACV, induction of TK, and neurovirulence in mice of four isolates of HSV and several ACV-resistant mutants derived from them by passage in BHK cells in ACV-containing medium

| Virus Strain | $ED_{50}$ ACV ($\blacktriangleleft$ g/ml) by plaque reduction in BHK cells | TK induction (% SC16) | Neurovirulence i.c. inoculation mice (pfu/$LD_{50}$) |
|---|---|---|---|
| HSV 1 SC16 | 0.05 | 100 | 7 |
| SC16$R_1C_1$ | 3 | 1.5 | $3 \times 10^3$ |
| SC16$R_5C_1$ | 7 | 0.2 | $5 \times 10^4$ |
| SC16$R_9C_2$ | <50 | 2.4 | >$10^5$ |
| C1(101) | 0.3 | 38 | 1 |
| C1(101) TK$^-$ | 7 | 0.1 | $2 \times 10^2$ |
| C1(101) TK$^-$p7 | 25 | ND | $2 \times 10^4$ |
| C1(101)$P_2C_5$ | 25 | 78 | 8 |
| C1(101)$P_2C_6$ | 40 | 0.6 | $1 \times 10^2$ |
| H29 | 0.07 | >100 | 1 |
| H29R | 22 | 2.3 | >$10^2$ |
| HSV 2 Bry | 0.15 | 74 | 1 |
| Bry TK$^-$* | 6 | 0.2 | >$10^5$ |
| Bry $P_3C_1$ | 50 | 0.5 | >$10^2$ |
| Bry $P_3C_2$ | 20 | 0.4 | >$10^2$ |

\* BUdR-selected

The sensitivity of this strain ($P_2C_5$) to a variety of antiviral agents was then examined. As can be seen from Table 2., $P_2C_5$ is sensitive to all the agents tested including several drugs with clinical potential.

Since this type of mutant seems more likely to arise in vivo attempts were made to isolate further TK$^+$ resistant viruses. This has been achieved using serum-starved BHK cells which do not favour the growth of TK$^-$ virus. Several further strains have been derived from a different parental virus but which appear to resemble $P_2C_5$. The nature of the resistance of these viruses is still not clear;

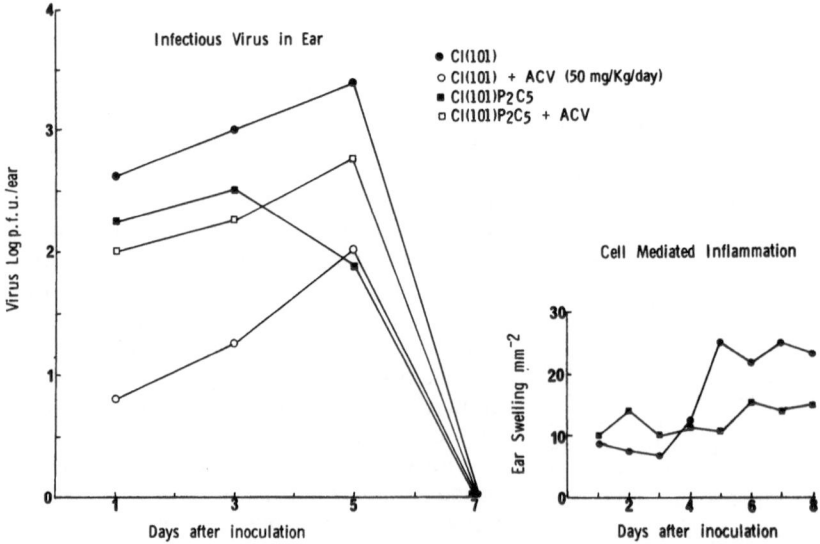

**Fig. 1.** Virus replication and inflammation in the ears of mice following inoculation with $10^4$ p.f.u. wild type or mutant virus and treatment with ACV

360

**Table 2.** Cross sensitivity of ACV-resistant strains of HSV to other anti-herpetic compounds

| | TK-induction % C1(101) | ACV | BVU | IDU | BUDR | Ara T | TFT | Ara A | PAA |
|---|---|---|---|---|---|---|---|---|---|
| C1 (101) | 100 | 1* | 1 | 1 | 1 | 1 | 1 | 1 | 1 |
| C1 (101) TK⁻ | < 0.1 | > 100 | > 100 | > 100 | > 1000 | > 6 | 0.2 | 250 | < 1 |
| C1 (101) P₂C₅ | 100 | > 100 | 1 | 2 | 230 | 0.05 | 0.9 | 9 | 5 |
| C1 (101) P₂C₆ | 1.6 | > 100 | 1 | > 100 | > 1000 | > 6 | 0.7 | 24 | 25 |

* Results are fold increase compared to C1 (101) by a plaque reduction test

ACV   : acyclovir
BVU   : 5 bromovinyl 2′ deoxyuridine
IDU   : 5-iodo-2′-deoxyuridine
BUDR : 5-bromo-2′-deoxyuridine
Ara T  : 1-β-D-arabinofuranosylthymine
TFT   : Trifluorothymine deoxyriboside
Ara A  : 9-β-D-arabinofuranosyl adenine
PAA   : Phosphonoacetic acid

it seems most likely to result from a change in the virus DNA-polymerase although we have little evidence to support this. Alternatively resistance may result from a change in the specificity of the HSV TK.

We believe that resistance to ACV will not be widespread, but with prolonged and repeated treatments surely it will arise. Our results suggest that this problem should be anticipated by investigating sensible routines of polychemotherapy or alternate use of different drugs.

## References

1. Field HJ, Bell SE, Elion GB, Nash A, Wildy P (1979) Effect of acycloguanosine treatment on acute and latent herpes simplex infections in mice. Antimicrob Agents Chemother 15:554–561
2. Field HJ, Darby G (1980) Pathogenicity in mice of strains of herpes simplex virus which are resistant to acyclovir in vitro and in vivo. Antimicrob Agents Chemother 17:
3. Field HJ, Darby GK, Wildy P (1980) Isolation and characterization of acyclovir-resistant mutants of herpes simplex virus. J Gen Virol 49:
4. Field HJ, Wildy P (1978) The pathogenicity of thymidine kinase-deficient mutants of herpes simplex virus in mice. J Hyg 81:267–277

## Discussion on the Contribution pp. 359–361

B.R. Jones (London)
Could you elaborate on your suggestion that the eye might be less discriminating against the mutant viruses.

H.J. Field (Cambridge)
Only the observation that the reports of isolation of resistant viruses from treated patients have come exclusively from the eye and this is also true of animal data using several different antiviral compounds. This may be because these isolates have been pursued more commonly. I am not aware of anyone who has been able to isolate resistant virus from any other site.

G. Streissle (Wuppertal)
What happens if you inject your Acyclovir-resistant TK⁺ mutants into animals? Are they less virulent too?

H.J. Field (Cambridge)
They behave very much like the wild type.

Y.C. Cheng (Chapel Hill)
ACV TP acts as a chain terminator. BVDU is not a chain terminator. Mutation may occur more frequently with a chain terminator; this is, however, just a guess of mine. Did you consider this possibility? Actually, one of the possible side effects of ACV could be that ACV causes more frequent mutations of the virus than a compound like BVDU.

H.J. Field (Cambridge)
I haven't tried to make any mutants resistant to BVDU. Do you know if they arise as readily? I suspect that in vitro spontaneously something like ¹/1000 or ¹/10⁴ viruses are generated which are TK⁻. That is about one TK⁻ virus released for every 10 or so infected cells.

Y.C. Cheng (Chapel Hill)
You mentioned in one statement that it is very easy to get an ACV resistant mutant; one passage in ACV containing medium and you get it.

H.J. Field (Cambridge)
We may be selecting something that's already present. I am not saying that the drug is necessarily mutating the virus. Is that what you are suggesting? There are no grounds to believe that. I really don't know how the rate of development of resistance compares with that to say, IDU. I know it was published in the 60's that some virus strains showed a much higher rate of acquisition of resistance to IDU than other isolates.

H.E. Kaufman (New Orleans)
The IDU-resistant virus we have is not TK⁻.

H.J. Field (Cambridge)
That is consistent with what I would expect.

W.H. Prusoff (New Haven)
There's an increased probability of getting mutants from ACV because you have two good sites where mutations can develop. One is thymidine kinase and the other is DNA polymerase.

H.J. Field (Cambridge)
It seems very much harder to change the DNA polymerase. I had to pass the $TK^-$ mutant B2006 seven times before we got a yield which showed increased resistance – that would be in line with the difficulty of say generating trifluorothymidine resistance.

W.H. Prusoff (New Haven)
But as I recall, and maybe Dr. Öberg could comment on this, the viruses that are resistant to PAA are also resistant to ACV. Is that correct?

B. Öberg (Södertälje)
That is true for some isolates but you can also find mutants resistant to one of the compounds but not to the other. I have a general comment which is a question to the clinicians here. The resistance development is something which we have to consider seriously. I would like to know if anyone has followed a patient by virus isolation before and after treatment and seen a resistance development, and in the next recurrent episode found whether this patient had a resistant or sensitive virus?

J.I. McGill (Southampton)
Yes, we had one patient who's done that. He started off as IDU-resistant and Ara-A resistant and over the year maintained that resistance on various isolates.

H.J. Field (Cambridge)
If I could make a comment to you Dr. McGill. It is about your particular methods for determining resistance. I appreciate that it shows that the virus is resistant, but it gives no information about the degree. Resistance can be a few micrograms/ml or very much greater. In fact, using the very large amount of IDU in your procedure you could be missing more subtle resistance were it arising.

E. De Clercq (Leuven)
Hugh, I was wondering whether $TK^+$ acyclo-guanosine-resistant HSV strains may arise in patients that have been treated with acyclo-guanosine or even occur before treatment is started?

H.J. Field (Cambridge)
We stumbled on our $TK^+$ virus very readily – it was one of half a dozen clones isolated from the second passage of the original isolate in ACV. The two viruses ($P_2C_5$ $TK^+$ and $P_2C_6$ $TK^-$) were "sisters", that is, two clones from the same yield.

E. De Clercq (Leuven)
Might the resistant virus have been present in the HSV stock before you exposed it to acyclo-guanosine?

H.J. Field (Cambridge)
No, I cannot say, but it is possible.

# Different Clinical Experiences

Sundmacher, R. (Hrsg.):
Herpetische Augenerkrankungen
© J.F. Bergmann Verlag, München 1981

# Dendritic Keratitis — a Comparison of Different Therapy Forms With Special Emphasis on Antibody-Therapy

M. Zirm, M. Söser, M. Ogriseg, Innsbruck

**Key words.** Dendritic keratitis, antibody therapy

**Schlüsselwörter.** Keratitis dendritica, Antikörper-Therapie

**Summary.** The therapeutic efficiency of iodine curettage, a therapy using virostatica like IDU, trifluorothymidine or virumerz, has been confirmed already by the statements of other authors. It is apparent, however, that the statistically better effect is obtained using a combined antibody-trifluorothymidine therapy.

**Zusammenfassung.** Die therapeutische Effizienz der Jodabrasio, eine Therapie mit Virustatika wie IDU, Trifluorthymidin oder Viromerz, lassen die bereits von anderen Autoren beschriebenen Aussagen bestätigen. Auffällig ist jedoch der statistisch signifikante bessere therapeutische Effekt einer kombinierten Antikörper-Trifluorthymidin-Therapie.

Until the introduction of idoxuridine (IDU) in 1962 [10], all that the ophthalmologist had at his disposal for the treatment of herpetic keratitis was primarily the application of heat, cold or iodine abrasion. Laibson and Leopold [12] felt that IDU had no better effect therapeutically than "curettage" of the corneal epithelium. It is generally known that after a long period of time IDU has a toxic effect on the corneal epithelium [8]. Wellings et al. [24] published their results regarding treatment of herpes simplex keratitis with the then new medicament trifluorothymidine. At the same time Pavan-Langston and Dohlman [17] reported on another new discovery, adenine-arabinoside (Ara-A). Both trifluorothymidine and Ara-A were described as being more effective than IDU. In spite of numerous optimistic reports in the years following [21], many authors repeatedly made diverging statements about the effectiveness of the various forms of therapy. The cause of this lies for the most part in the assessment of cornea-study findings by different researchers.

The protective effect of gamma-globulins against herpes simplex infections was proven both in tissue cultures and in animal experiments [2]. Experimentally induced herpes simplex infections in animals could also be treated successfully [7]. Herpes simplex viruses were injected into the anterior chamber of rabbits and the period of subsequent iritis was considerably shortened through intraperitoneal doses of gamma-globulins. Experiments using a combination of immunoglobulin therapy and cryotherapy were also successful; the cellular structures were broken open so as to allow the antibody to penetrate into the virus-attacked cell [1]. Therapy attempts with gamma-globulins are recommended for herpetic infections of the cornea by Weg [23], Wittmer [25], Neubauer [15] and Fechner [5].

It is clear to us that complete antibodies are not able to penetrate the cell wall and that since replication of the herpes virus results intracytoplasmatically, it is not possible to influence it. As a result, with knowledge of the humoral and cellular immunoreaction in herpes simplex infections, we have attempted to apply antibody-active immunoglobulin fragments $(F(ab)'_2$-fragments)[a] as a therapy for dendritic keratitis. In a prior report [26] we were able to demonstrate the therapeutic effects on cases of herpes simplex keratitis by means of locally administered eye-drops containing neutralizing antibody fragments. The subjective advantages of this therapy form

---

[a] Gamma-Venin, Behring-Werke, West Germany

(good compatibility and pain-killing) contrasted with a therapy which is not always successful in cases of metaherpetic keratitis. Since therapy with neutralizing antibody fragments regarding dendritic keratitis appeared established, a combined therapy with trifluorothymidine was attempted in order to attain greater effectiveness and hence accelerated recovery.

The present report undertakes to analyze different forms of therapy in cases of dendritic keratitis. Since it deals with a retrospective study, a double blind study is not possible and only objectifiable findings are to be statistically treated.

## Parameters

Therapy form
Duration of therapy until healing of herpetic lesions
Findings prior to application of therapy
Findings after completion of therapy
The healing process
Relapse frequency
Age and sex of the patients

## Forms of Therapy

Group I:    Iodine treatment (monotherapy)
Group II:   Monotherapy using virostatica (IDU, Viru-Merz and trifluorothymidine) 3–5 times daily
Group III:  Combined therapy using curettage and then virostatica (as listed above) 3–5 times daily
Group IV:   Combined therapy using neutralizing antibodies (F(ab)$'_2$ with trifluorothymidine): The local application of this combined therapy took place alternately in intervals of 2 hours

## Patients

We studied 119 patients (79 male/40 female) ranging in age from 1 to 81 years. Care was taken to insure that the factors of age, sex and severity of the infection were distributed equally among each of the therapy groups (I–IV).

## Statistical Analysis

For the computation of how statistically significant the data was, the analysis of variance according to Fisher, and the t-test according to Student and the $Chi^2$-test (as a non-parametric method with qualitative criteria) were used. The resultant degrees of significances are indicated individually.

## Results

### Clinical Manifestations Prior to Applying Therapy

It was impossible to determine all of the cases since data was in part imprecise. We analyzed 101 cases. The range of variation was extremely high (from a few hours to 90 days), and accordingly, the analysis of variance showed no statistically signifant difference between the groups.

### Duration of Therapy

In calculating the necessary duration of therapy some highly significant differences showed up among the groups (Table 1).

Table 1. Survey of therapy duration until symptoms disappeared

| Group | Mean therapy duration | Standard dev. | Range |
|-------|-----------------------|---------------|-------|
| I     | 5.67 d | 3.95 | 2–14 d |
| II    | 9.29 d | 9.77 | 2–36 d |
| III   | 9.43 d | 8.19 | 1–34 d |
| IV    | 5.39 d | 3.72 | 1–18 d |

### Findings Prior to Applying Therapy

Findings in this regard were retrospectively placed in three categories reflecting the severity of infection:
1. Non-severe: superficial herpes lesions with a small degree of spreading.
2. Semi-severe: several herpes lesions or a single herpes lesion spread out over a large area of cornea.
3. Severe: Deep herpes lesions, infiltration, secondary iritis, herpetic ulcer, and as well,

several herpes lesions spread out over the entire cornea.

Analysis according to non-parametric methods showed that the four therapy groups indicated the same development (Chi$^2$: 12.881 with 8 degrees of freedom) and, as such, did not differ from each other regarding the severity of the cases (5% limit: 15.507). As a result, the initial position was the same for all therapy forms.

## Findings After Therapy

Upon completion of therapy the results were categorized as either "satisfactory" or "unsatisfactory". The former refers to complete healing, the latter to cases of infiltration, spreading into deeper layers, short-termed relapses and scar-formation. Significant differences were seen between the individual therapy forms (Table 2).

**Table 2.** Status following therapy

| Groups | Satisfactory | Unsatisfactory | Total |
|--------|--------------|----------------|-------|
| I | 13 (= 56%) | 10 (= 44%) | 23 |
| II | 9 (= 64%) | 5 (= 36%) | 14 |
| III | 28 (= 57%) | 21 (= 43%) | 49 |
| IV | 25 (= 76%) | 8 (= 24%) | 33 |
| Total | 75 (= 67%) | 44 (= 33%) | 119 |

## The Healing Process

In the analysis of the healing process we differentiated between the occurrence or non-occurrence of complications. Complications included premature relapse (up to a month after starting therapy), spreading into deeper corneal layers, and infiltration. Table 3 shows that in 30% of the cases treated with "traditional" therapy forms (group I–III), complications occurred during the healing process. In cases treated with the "new" therapy, only one single case had complications, and these were non-severe.

## Relapse Frequency

The relapses were categorized as either short-term (up to 1 month after starting therapy), mean-term (up to 1 year after starting therapy)

**Table 3.** Complications as %-factor with the different therapy forms

| Groups | No | Yes | Total |
|--------|-----|-----|-------|
| I | 15 (= 65%) | 8 (= 35%) | 23 |
| II | 11 (= 79%) | 3 (= 21%) | 14 |
| III | 33 (= 67%) | 16 (= 33%) | 49 |
| IV | 32 (= 97%) | 1 (= 3%) | 33 |
| Total | 91 | 28 | 119 |

and long-term (after 1 year). In this regard as well, clear differences could be seen between the therapy groups. It must be said, however, that the observation period, especially in the case of therapy group IV, was not quite 1 year in some cases. Table 4 shows a survey of these results.

**Table 4.** Relapse frequency with the different therapy forms

| Groups | No | Yes | Total |
|--------|-----|-----|-------|
| I | 12 (= 52%) | 11 (= 48%) | 23 |
| II | 8 (= 57%) | 6 (= 43%) | 14 |
| III | 39 (= 80%) | 10 (= 20%) | 49 |
| IV | 30 (= 91%) | 3 (= 9%) | 33 |
| Total | 89 | 30 | 119 |

Chi$^2$ with 4 degrees of freedom: 20.129, $p < 0.01$ (highly significant)

In the course of the analysis, it was seen that Group I and II tended to be short- or medium-termed regarding relapses, and that Group III tended to be long-termed. On the basis of the relatively short period of treatment, it was not possible to determine any tendency in the case of the patients treated with neutralizing antibodies.

## Age and Sex

As far as age is concerned, no significant differences could be determined between the individual groups. The somewhat unequal distribution in regard to sex is probably attributable to the relatively small number of cases in Group 2. Table 5 shows a survey of these results.

**Table 5.** Survey of age and sex distribution of the patients

| Group | Number (M/F) | Mean age | Standard dev. | Lowest/highest |
|-------|--------------|----------|---------------|----------------|
| I     | 23 (15/ 8)   | 33.3 a   | 21.24         | 1–75 a         |
| II    | 14 (13/ 1)   | 32.9 a   | 15.55         | 10–59 a        |
| III   | 49 (31/18)   | 33.5 a   | 21.06         | 1–75 a         |
| IV    | 33 (20/13)   | 37.9 a   | 19.83         | 6–81 a         |

## Discussion

In summarizing the above results, we can clearly see that the traditional method of iodine curettage has a short average period of therapy (5.67 d). The formation of corneal lesions can certainly be graded as a disadvantage (mean duration = 3.48 d), and the more frequent relapses (48%) as well. The danger of incomplete healing after iodine treatment is considerably greater than with other therapy forms.

General therapy using *antivirals* indicated a relatively long mean duration of therapy (9.29 d) and a relatively frequent occurrence of relapse (43%). Advantages seen were a relatively low factor of complication (21%) and fewer cases of incomplete healing than with iodine therapy. According to the results of our study, the local application of *neutralizing antibody fragments* with virostatica to the herpes-infected eye offers greater advantages when compared with traditional therapy. These advantages are readily apparent – with a 3% factor of complication, a lower occurrence of relapse (9%) and, especially for the patients, the nonappearance of artificial corneal lesions.

Since the possibility of treatment with trifluorothymidine is generally recognized and attempts at using neutralizing antibodies have often been justifiably rejected, this is the point at which primarily the humoral immunoreaction in herpetic corneal infections should enter into the discussion. Antigenicity decides the outcome of any immunoreaction, for example that of a herpes virus and the capability of the immunosystem to react specifically. In the first case, that of the antigenicity of a herpes virus, we differentiate between the serological characteristics of a type 1, type 2, or an intermediary type. The antigenicity of a virus-capsides has, however,

no connection at all with the pathogenicity of the virus.

In the case of the immunoreactivity of the organism to a specific antigen, there appears to be various dispositions. Chused et al. [3] and Colin et al. [4], for example, reported on an abnormal immunoreactivity in the case of carriers of HLA-B5-antigens in regard to herpes simplex viruses. The original division into cellular and humoral immunoreaction, which appeared to take place independently of each other, can no longer be upheld. Figure 1 shows the interaction between T and B-lymphocytes, macrophages and lymphokines. Metcalf and Reichert [13] were of the opinion that an immunoreaction coordinated with the special conditions in the eye appears to take place in the following manner (Fig. 2): Infection of the cornea with a herpex simplex virus leads to an immigration of lymphocytes from the limbus. These lymphocytes produce lymphokines, which then as a chemotactic factor affect PMN and further lymphocytes. Seven hours after the infection has been artificially induced there are already a few plasma cells to be found at the limbus. Two to 3 days later, the number of PMN is large and, great numbers of plasma cells and lymphocytes are found close to the limbus as well. On the 7th and 8th day PMN and plasma cells predominate. Between the 10th and 20th day, plasma cells and lymphocytes remain at the location of the infection. It is interesting that on the 7th day, numerous immature plasma cells can be seen in close contact with lymphocytes. Lymphocytes are also found in close contact with stromakeratocytes; such conditions increase from the 7th day onwards. It is apparently the case that keratocytes are target cells for T-lymphocytes. The infiltrating PMN lead to enzymatic destruction of collagen, so that through synthesis of a collagen type which is abnormal for the cornea, a permanent scar remains. It should not remain unmentioned that during this time as a result of the virus attack interferon is produced in the cell. Numerous studies were able to show that virus replication is possible also in the presence of interferon. Attempts made to therapeutically apply human leukocyte-interferon [11] did not bring the desired results. Results contrary to the above by Kaufmann are indicated by Jones et al. [9], Neumann-Haefelin et al. [16] and Sundmacher et al. [19]. In a randomized

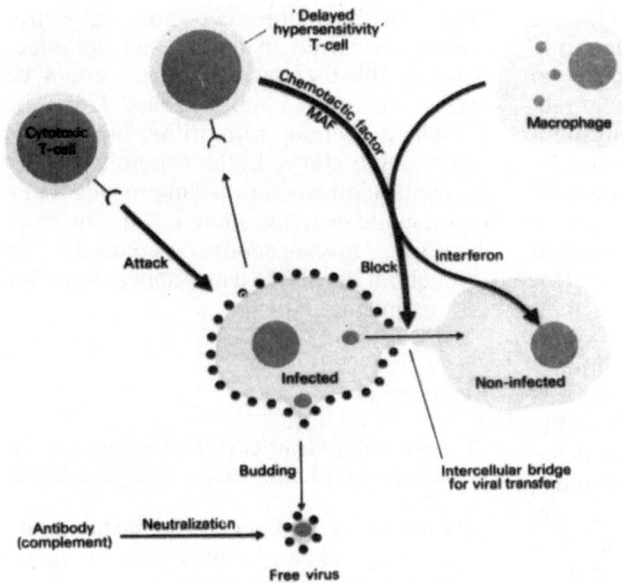

**Fig. 1.** Control of infection by "budding" viruses. Cytotoxic T-cells kill virally infected targets directly after recognition of new surface antigen (. . . . . .) Interaction with a separate subpopulation of T-cells releases lymphokines which attract macrophages to inhibit intercellular virus transfer and prime contiguous uninfected cells with interferon. Free virus released by budding from the cell surface is neutralized by antibody (which, if thymus-dependent, points to yet another contribution by the T-cell to viral immunity). Taken from Roitt I (1977) Essential immunology, 3rd ed. Blackwell

double blind study, Sundmacher et al. [20] applied a combined therapy (iodine abrasion and interferon) and treated dendritic keratitis with human leukocyte-interferon or fibroblast-interferon. Both types of interferon showed the same therapeutic effect. What is not explained, however, is the reason for a combined therapy. Since virus antigens could be demonstrated on the surface of stromakeratocytes [14] and on the surface membranes of rabbit corneal cells in vitro [6], the involvement of a humoral immunoreaction, that is to say the formation of plasma cells, is understandable. However, since virus replication occurs intracellularly, a stimulation of a humoral immunoreaction is pos-

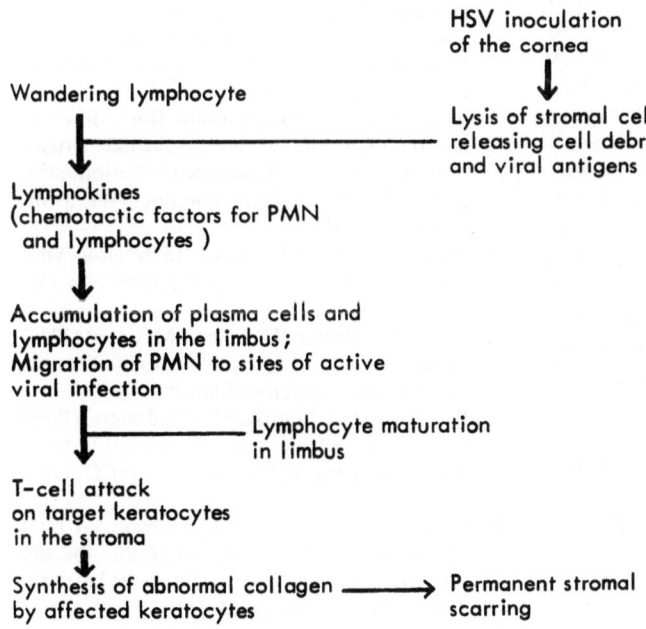

**Fig. 2.** Proposed mechanism for immunopathogenesis of herpetic stromal keratitis in experimental animals. Modified from [13]

sible, but a direct influence on the virus is not. Nevertheless, humoral antibodies do have a definite influence on the course of a dendritic keratitis infection. Sery et al. [18] were able to show that in cases of corneal opacity in rabbits, 81% could be prevented by prior immunization of one eye. Sery attributed this to a local antibody production and a protective effect of herpes antibodies. It appears certain, however, that an immunocomplex is formed which in turn via the complement system (leukotactic factor) leads to increased infiltration of PMN.

The proof that fragments of immunoglobulins are capable of penetrating the cell wall was given by Vollerthun et al. [22] on the basis of animal experiments. Following intravenous injection of gamma-globulins[a], tissue distribution was investigated in the small intestine, kidney, salivary gland and transversely striated muscle of the mouse. The injected preparations were carried out with both peroxidase- and fluoresceinisothiocyanate-marked antibodies. Immunoglobulin fragments were determined in cytoplasm, while native immunoglobulin was located for the most part in vascular and perivascular tissue, but seldomly in cells. Due to the binding of applied tetanus-toxoid to sections of the small intestine in which immunoglobulin fragments were intracytoplasmatically determinable, it can be concluded that the intracellularly determinable immunoglobulin retains its antibody property also in the cell. Tests to determine intracellular F(ab)$'_2$-fragments of an immunoglobulin were carried out 30 minutes, 24 hours, and 4 days after injection. Findings from the small intestine, salivary gland, kidney and transversely striated muscle are similar. Histological preparations showed no indication of shock symptoms and permeability disturbances were not observable either. The investigations confirm that with intravenous injection with the same concentration, the enzyme-treated gamma-globulin, as compared with the native immunoglobulin, leaves the vascular system more quickly and is able to penetrate between, and even into, the cells themselves.

Using these findings as a basis, we undertook for the first time to apply neutralizing immunoglobulin-fragments (F(ab)$'_2$-frag-

ments) to the eye in the form of eye-drops. Since neither objective nor subjective changes occurred in any of the volunteer patients, the therapy experiment could be carried out with a monotherapy [26]. The combined therapy with trifluorothymidine subsequently showed, after 6 months of clinical application, such satisfying results that a report could be made about it [27]. The comparative investigations reported on throughout the above paper appear to justify our optimism.

## References

1. Amoils SP, Maier G (1971) Cryotherapy and autogenous serum therapy. Arch Ophthal 86: 113–114
2. Cheever FS, Daikos G (1950) Studies on the protective effect of gamma globulin against herpes simplex infections in mice. J Immunol 65:135–141
3. Chused TM, Kassan SS, Opelz G et al (1977) Sjogren's syndrome associated with HLA-Dw3. N Engl J Med 296:895
4. Colin J, Chastel C, Saleun JP et al (1979) Herpes oculaire recidivant et antigenes HLA; etude preliminaire. J Fr Ophthalmol 2/4:263–266
5. Fechner PU (1976) Hornhauttherapie. In: Medikamentöse Augentherapie. S 208 ff, Enke, Stuttgart
6. Henson D, Helmsen R, Becker KE et al (1974) Ultrastructural localization of herpes simplex virus antigens on rabbit corneal cells using sheep antihuman IgG antihorse ferritin hybrid antibodies. Invest Ophthalmol 13:819
7. Heyl JT, Allen HF, Cheever FS (1948) Quantitative assay of neutralizing antibody content of pools of gamma globulin from different sections of the United States against the viruses of herpes simplex, lymphocytic choriomeningitis and epidemic keratoconjunctivitis. J Immunol 60:37–45
8. Jones BR (1976) Prospects in treating viral disease of the eye. Trans Ophthal Soc UK 87:537–579
9. Jones BR, Coster DJ, Falcon MG et al (1976) Topical therapy of ulcerative herpetic keratitis with human interferon. Lancet 2:128
10. Kaufmann HE, Martola EL, Dohlman C (1962) Use of 5-iodo-2'-deoxyuridine (IDU) in treatment of herpes simplex keratitis. Arch Ophthal 68:235–239
11. Kaufmann HE, Meyer RF, Laibson PR et al (1976) Human leukocyte interferon for the prevention of recurrences of herpetic keratitis. J Infect Dis 133 (suppl.):A 165

---

[a] Beriglobin and Gamma-Venin, Behring-Werke, West Germany

12. Laibson PR, Leopold HI (1964) An evaluation of double-blind IDU therapy in 100 cases of herpetic keratitis. Trans Amer Acad Ophthal Otolaryng 68:21–34
13. Metcalf JF, Reichert RW (1979) Histological and electron microscopic studies of experimental herpetic keratitis in the rabbit. Invest Ophthalmol Vis Sci 1123–1138
14. Metcalf JF, Helmsen R (1977) Immunoelectronmicroscopic localization of herpes simplex virus antigens in rabbit cornea with antihuman IgG-antiferritin hybrid antibodies. Invest Ophthalmol Vis Sci 16:779
15. Neubauer H (1972) Die medikamentöse Behandlung des Herpes simplex corneae. Bericht über die 71. Zusammenkunft der DOG in Heidelberg 1971. S 273–278
16. Neumann-Haefelin D, Sundmacher R, Skoda R, Cantell K (1977) Comparative evaluation of human leukocyte and fibroblast interferon in the prevention of herpes simplex virus keratitis in a monkey model. Infect Immun 17: 468–470
17. Pavan-Langston D, Dohlman C (1972) A double-blind clinical study of adenine arabinoside therapy of viral keratoconjunctivitis. Am J Ophthal 74:81–88
18. Sery TW, Nagy RM, Nazario R (1972/73) Experimental disciform keratitis. III. Virus infectivity versus hypersensitivity in herpes virus stromal disease. Ophthalmol Res 4:137
19. Sundmacher R, Cantell K, Haug P, Neumann-Haefelin D (1978) Role of debridement and interferon in the treatment of dendritic keratitis. Albr v Graefes Arch Klin Ophthal 207:77–82
20. Sundmacher R, Cantell K, Skoda R, Hallermann CH, Neumann-Haefelin D (1978) Human Leukocyte and Fibroblast Interferon in a Combination Therapy of Dendritic Keratitis. Albr v Graefes Arch Klin Exp Ophthal 208: 229–233
21. Van Bijsterveld OP, Post H (1980) Trifluorothymidine versus adenine arabinoside in the treatment of herpes simplex keratitis. Brit J Ophthal 64:33–36
22. Vollerthun R, Sedlacek HH, Ronneberger H (1977) Gewebeverteilung von nativem und enzymbehandeltem Human-Immunglobulin. Experimentelle Untersuchungen. Dtsch med Wschr 102:684–686
23. Wege K (1963) Behandlung virusbedingter Hornhauterkrankungen mit Gammaglobulin. Klin Mbl Augenheilk 142:970–981
24. Wellings PC, Awdry PN, Bors FH, Jones BR, Brown DC, Kaufman HE (1972) Clinical evaluation of trifluorothymidine in the treatment of herpes simplex corneal ulcers. Am J Ophthal 73:932–942
25. Witmer R (1963) Herpes simplex Keratitis. Ophthalmologica (Basel) 145:312–319
26. Zirm M (1978) Gammaglobulin-Therapie bei Herpes simplex-Augeninfektionen. Die gelben Hefte. Immunbiologische Informationen, XVIII 86–90
27. Zirm M (1979) Immunotherapeutic Tests in Cases of Herpes corneae. Proceeding of the Gamma-Venin-Symposium, Tokyo p 143

## Discussion on the Contribution pp. 365–371

C. Kok van Alphen (Leyden)
I'm afraid I was a bit late because the bus was late. I didn't hear the first part of the paper. Could you explain how the fragments were prepared?

M. Zirm (Innsbruck)
I'm no chemist. The fragments were prepared by the Behring Institute.

C. Kok van Alphen (Leyden)
I'm glad to hear that you still use the old method of debridement, because I think that it is a good method after all.

M. Zirm (Innsbruck)
It is a good method in a very fresh dendritic keratitis.

C. Kok van Alphen (Leyden)
I think the reason why it works is that you take away a lot of diseased tissue although you cannot take away every virus particle, you agree?

M. Zirm (Innsbruck)
Yes. In fact, we made this according to the experience of the director of our clinic who did debridement for 30 years and he wanted me to differentiate between the different forms of therapy. The emphasis of this paper is to show that, among all the possibilities for treating keratitis, debridement is still a possible and certainly an effective treatment. It is also not very expensive.

C. Kok van Alphen (Leyden)
The only bad thing about iodine is that it is rather painful.

M. Zirm (Innsbruck)
It is certainly one of the disadvantages of the therapy that the patients feel pain in the following hours.

P.C. Maudgal (Leuven)
My experience is that if you can get rid of a dendritic ulcer, stromal disease generally doesn't appear. I have treated my patients by making in vivo corneal replicas. Amyl-acetate used in the solution

penetrates up to the superficial stromal layers. Amyl-acetate serves as a fixative, as seen by electron microscopy. So, by making a replica, one fixes the cells as well as the virus. It seems to me that if in this way the superficial lesion, which is the site of virus multiplication, is removed, there is no penetration of virus into the stroma, and the normal healing process of epithelium follows. Making a corneal replica is very effective in treating the dendritic ulcers, but it does not prevent recurrences.

**M. Zirm (Innsbruck)**
We know, of course, that 20% heals by itself, but nobody today would dare not to treat superficial keratitis.

**P.C. Maudgal (Leuven)**
I was talking about recalcitrant disease.

**R. Sundmacher (Freiburg)**
I agree that for the majority of cases you do well when you remove the diseased epithelium. But this solves only part of your problem. The old idea that you only get stromal disease when the virus penetrates from an epithelial lesion into the stroma is not totally wrong, but also not totally right either. Regarding the hypothesis of neuronal HSV latency and the clinical observations of primary stromal disease as well as simultaneous flaring up of HSV disease at multiple sites, it seems more probable to me that the underlying cause for stromal herpes is, in most cases, neuronal HSV shedding to the stroma and not the penetration of virus from a superficial lesion.

**M. Zirm (Innsbruck)**
You can say, of course, that there are other roots of infection.

**D.L. Easty (Bristol)**
With your use of these f (ab) fragments do you have any concern about absorption of immune complexes into the corneal stroma?

**M. Zirm (Innsbruck)**
Our investigations and experiments point to an absorption of immune complexes. We measured the titer of neutralizing antibodies. We were able to see that the local administration of these antibody fragments did not do any harm to the conjunctiva or cornea.

**D.L. Easty (Bristol)**
Did you continue with your antibody treatment over a longer period of time as a prophylaxis?

**M. Zirm (Innsbruck)**
Yes, we believe it is necessary to do it over a period of 7 days.

Sundmacher, R. (Hrsg.):
Herpetische Augenerkrankungen
© J.F. Bergmann Verlag, München 1981

# Zur thermischen Abrasio des Hornhautepithels*

M. Mertz, E. Schierl, U. Papendick, G. Funk, München

**Key words.** Debridement, thermocautery

**Schlüsselwörter.** Abrasio, Thermoabrasio

**Summary.** We reported on our experimental and clinical experiences with a newly developed thermocauter.

The new cauter is constructed according to the thermistor principle: Its tip acts simultaneously as themoapplicator and as thermosensor. In this way, it is possible to measure the actual temperature at the site of application and maintain a predetermined temperature level by electronic feed-back. This guarantees a highly reproducible heat-application.

The healing of corneal erosions after thermodebridement with Wessely's "steam"-cauter and the new thermistor-cauter was investigated using electronical analyzing systems. This led to preliminary results concerning the choice of instrument, temperature and tip size in the rabbit model and in patients. From this we suggested indications for this type of therapy.

**Zusammenfassung.** Bericht über die bei der Entwicklung eines Kauters gewonnenen tierexperimentellen Ergebnisse und klinischen Erfahrungen.

Der neue Kauter arbeitet nach dem Thermistorprinzip: Seine Spitze ist zugleich Wärmeapplikator und Thermofühler, so daß die aktuelle Temperatur unmittelbar am Ort der Koagulation fortlaufend gemessen und durch elektronische Regelung auf einem vorher gewählten Wert konstant gehalten werden kann. Damit ist in hohem Maße eine Reproduzierbarkeit der Wärmeabgabe gewährleistet. Mit Hilfe bildanalytischer Messungen wurden die Abheilungszeiten und -formen der Erosionen nach Koagulation mit dem Dampfkauter nach Wessely bzw. dem neuen Thermistorkauter vergleichend untersucht.

* kein Text eingegangen

Vorgelegt wurden erste Ergebnisse über den Einfluß der Wahl des Instruments, der Temperatur und der Strichdicke, erhoben sowohl am gesunden Hornhautepithel des Kaninchens wie an der herpetisch erkrankten Cornea des Menschen. Die Beobachtungen lassen sich zu einem ersten Indikationskatalog zusammenfassen.

## Diskussion zum Beitrag S. 373

H. Neubauer (Köln)

We know that ophthalmologists are very conservative people, so in Germany, we have had three different ways of doing corneal impregnation and abrasio corneae for the past 20 years: The thermal method, the chemical, and, in later years, the cryo method. The problem is: which of these methods does less harm to Bowman's membrane and the stroma? May I ask for your opinion on the principle of taking off the primary focus of epithelial herpes before treating with antivirals?

W. Böke (Kiel)

Yesterday, when we discussed the principles of antiviral therapy, I was amazed that this way of getting rid of the viruses seems to be almost generally accepted, and that simple debridement seems to have been surpassed. My question is: Is it really preferable to treat a primary superficial lesion by antivirals only, or should one first of all remove the diseased epithelium mechanically? I think – and I would like to have the opinion of antiviral experts on this topic – the best way is to first remove the epithelial lesion, that means removing the virus as far as possible from the cornea. In case we leave the epithelium and we treat with antivirals only, we must be aware of the fact that we still have the virus within the cornea. Certainly, antivirals prevent virus replication, but a recurrence may arise at any time if any condition facilitates the replication. Therefore, I think that the best way is to first remove the epithelium and then treat it with antivirals. I would like to ask those who have a lot of experience with primary antiviral treatment of superficial herpetic keratitis whether they feel that it will be possible, with the newer types of antiviral agents, to completely remove the virus from the epithelium as done by debridement, as long as the virus has invaded only the epithelium.

H. Neubauer (Köln)
This also seems to me to be a very important point concerning the practical treatment. I would be very grateful to some of the experts if they would tell the audience their opinions about a combination of primary epithelial cleaning and local antiviral therapy.

B. Carreras Matas (Granada)
I think there is no doubt that the mechanical removal of the infected epithelial cells is a good start for the therapy with antivirals. But some methods of debridement can easily damage Bowman's membrane and even the stroma, as with iodine, and the endothelium, as may occur with cryotherapy. The results of this may too often be a permanent opacity. I think a method which is strictly limited to the epithelial cells and which permits perfect control of both the intensity and depth of the tissue damage is to be encouraged.

R. Witmer (Zürich)
I think that in the new light of what we know now about the corneal endothelium, every aggressive method of getting rid of the bulk of herpes virus, like cryoapplication or thermocautery, could be potentially dangerous. I can not imagine that a temperatures. What all these methods do is loosen the endothelium, and the same is true for freezing temperatures. All these methods do is loosen the epithelium and facilitate debridement. I think, the simple, old abrasio is the safest method and certainly does the least harm to the endothelium.

M. Mertz (München)
The exposure times must, of course, be so short that they are safe. The aim of therapy is only to coagulate the virus-containing epithelium and leave all non-infected cells in the deeper layers of the cornea unharmed. If you do just mechanical removal without demarcation and coagulation of the diseased cells, you certainly spread virus over the cornea and you are less likely to remove all the virus.

F.M. Polack (Gainsville)
At the University of Florida we prefer to start with antivirals if the epithelial lesion is small. In a large lesion, it's probably better to remove the epithelium before antiviral therapy. Dr. Jones has shown that this will reduce the time of chemical treatment. We have tried thermal cautery and even with a controlled temperature, there is a risk of doing permanent damage to the basement membrane and Bowman's membrane around the ulcer, and also to the deep connective tissue. Cryotherapy is also of some risk to the endothelium if the application is too long, but the use of any devise to remove the epithelium should be localized to the area of disease. Even mechanical scraping can damage the basement membrane and this will bring problems posteriorly.

B.R. Jones (London)
On the principle of the iodine scrub method, it has been my experience that those patients suffer a lot of discomfort in the period after treatment, and in some cases, a chemical keratitis seemed to have been induced. At Moorfields', formerly the custom was to use some wooden "orange stick", which had been sharpened and flattened like a screwdriver so that it was a good instrument for removal of the epithelium, and this stick was dipped into phenol, the phenol blotted off the stick, and then everything that touched the stick coagulated. In spite of these precautions, there was a lot of phenol spread around. The results of this kind of debridement seem to be just as good or just as bad in terms of healing, and certainly the patients had some inflammatory reaction following it. When we had to design a clinical trial system for the evaluation of antivirals, we decided to simply remove the epithelium with a cotton swab applicator, with no chemicals, with the objective of not adding any possible chemical damage to the cornea; and the results were astonishingly good. The ulcers heal almost invariably within 3 days, and there is really no inflammatory reaction following a simple removal. One is, however, left with the phenomenon of microscopic recurrences in about half of the cases within a week of the removal. Maybe they are recrudescences or continuing lesions which were there, but not seen, at the time of removal. It seems to me that the danger of damaging the critical tissues with either heat or cold or chemicals is real and that one first wants to examine the effects of antivirals alone. Antivirals preceded by abrasion is logical. I have been asked many times whether exposing large areas of Bowman's to the application of antiviral drugs risks doing permanent damage to it; but we don't seem to see anything that would suggest that it is a risk if you give antivirals after abrasion.

H. Neubauer (Köln)
I must close this discussion now, but if I may, I would like to add my personal opinion. I see no argument against primary mechanical cleaning of the cornea in epithelial herpes processes. We first use impregnation of the epithelium by ethyliodide (Merck, Germany, Nr. 895 − $C_2H_5J$). Then, it's very easy to take off the impregnated epithelium. We feel that this technique shortens the course of the keratitis and really improves the results of the subsequent antiviral therapy. The Bowman's membrane is less involved and this seems, to me, to be a very important point.

Sundmacher, R. (Hrsg.):
Herpetische Augenerkrankungen
© J.F. Bergmann Verlag, München 1981

# Longitudinal Analysis of Ulcerative Herpetic Keratitis

K.R. Wilhelmus, D.J. Coster, M.G. Falcon, B.R. Jones, London

**Key words.** Dendritic keratitis, stromal keratitis, disciform keratitis, recurrent HSV disease, corticosteroids

**Schlüsselwörter.** Keratitis dendritica, Keratitis disciformis, Stromaherpes, Herpesrezidive, Kortikosteroide

**Summary.** One hundred fifty-two patients with dendritic or amoeboid herpetic ulceration were treated with debridement, vidarabine, or trifluorothymidine. Follow-up extended over a subsequent five-year period. Statistical analysis was used to identify those variables which affected outcome. The recurrence rate for developing a second epithelial ulcer was 40%. The incidence was greater in those patients who had had a previous ulcer and in males. Stromal inflammation occurred in 25% of the patients; no pretreatment factor affected the subsequent occurrence of stromal disease. Over the five-year period two-thirds of the recurrent ulcerations and three-fourths of the cases with stromal inflammation occurred within the first year. A topical corticosteroid was used in 55 patients for a period ranging from 1 month to 5 years with an average duration of use of 1 year. An antiviral medication was used concomitantly with the steroid to prevent recurrent ulceration.

**Zusammenfassung.** 152 Patienten mit Keratitis dendritica oder geographica wurden mit Abrasio, Vidarabin-Salbe oder Trifluorthymidin-Augentropfen behandelt. Die therapeutischen Ergebnisse und die Faktoren, die diese Ergebnisse beeinflußten, wurden statistisch analysiert.
Die durchschnittliche Rezidivrate nach einer ersten Dendritica-Erkrankung betrug 40%. War mehr als ein Erkrankungsschub vorausgegangen oder handelte es sich um Männer, so war die Rezidivgefahr größer. Eine Stromaentzündung – entweder disciform oder interstitiell – beobachteten wir bei 25% der Patienten. Die Stromaerkrankung hing aber von keiner der vorher durchgeführten Behandlungsarten ab. Innerhalb der ausgewerteten Fünfjahresfrist zeigten sich $^2/_3$ der Dendriticarezidive und $^3/_4$ der Stromaerkrankungen innerhalb des ersten Jahres.

Eine lokale Steroidtherapie wurde bei 55 Patienten zwischen einem Monat bis zu 5 Jahren mit einem Durchschnitt von einem Jahr gegeben. Wenn die Steroidapplikation aus 0,01% Prednisolon oder stärkeren Tropfen bestand, so wurde gleichzeitig eine antivirale Therapie dazu verordnet.

The therapy of ulcerative herpetic keratitis consists of mechanical or chemical debridement, a topical antiviral, or a combination of these treatments. However, neither the physical removal nor a pharmacologic interference with the viral replicative cycle will prevent recurrent disease [7]. Because limited information is available on the incidence of recurrences following herpetic keratitis, we have reviewed the course of herpetic eye disease over a five-year period in a group of patients treated for a dendritic or amoeboid corneal ulceration.

## Methods

One hundred fifty-two consenting patients between the ages of 8 and 80 years were treated for a dendritic or geographic corneal ulceration with either mechanical debridement, vidarabine 3.3% ointment, of trifluorothymidine 1% solution during 1974 [2–4]. Following healing of the ulcer, the patients were re-examined in the Virus Clinic of Moorfields Eye Hospital for subsequent complications [8]. All charts were reviewed after a five-year follow-up period to determine the occurrence of recurrent epithelial ulceration, the development of stromal inflammation as manifested by either a disciform or stromal keratitis, and the use of a topical corticosteroid.

The indications for the subsequent use of a topical steroid included the symptomatic presence of active stromal or anterior chamber inflammation. The dosage was graduated

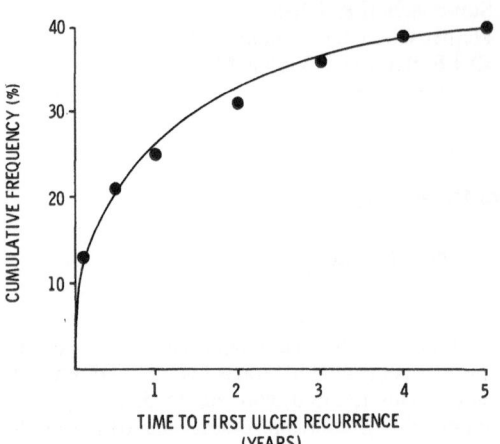

**Fig. 1.** Time to first ulcer recurrence

to the intensity of the inflammation using a half-log dilution series of prednisolone phosphate drops [12].

## Results

### Epithelial Ulcer Recurrence

Figure 1 depicts the cumulative frequency curve of the 61 patients developing their first recurrent dendritic or amoeboid ulceration during the five-year follow-up period. Ten of these 61 patients developed two recurrences during this time, two developed three recurrences, and one patient had four. Twenty

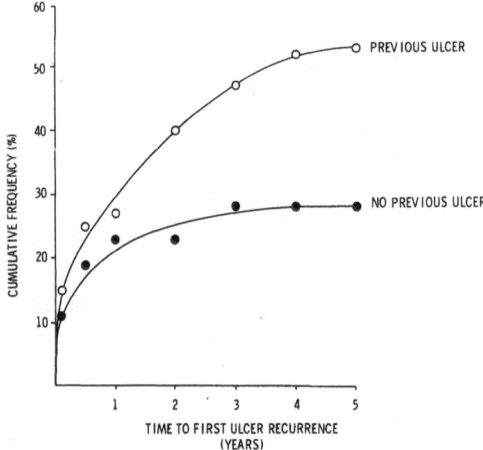

**Fig. 2.** Effect of previous ulcer history on the incidence of ulcer recurrence

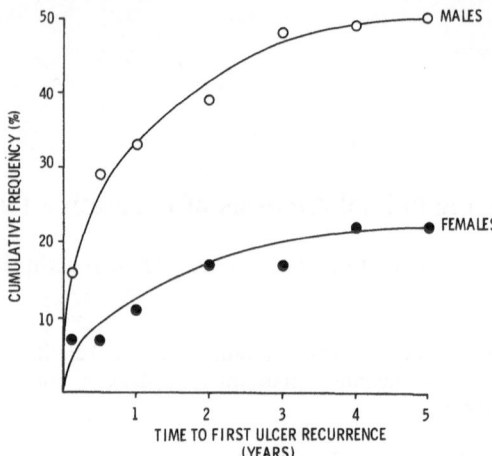

**Fig. 3.** Effect of sex on the incidence of ulcer recurrence

(33%) of these cases occurred during the first month following healing of the initial ulcer; 32 (52%) occurred within the first 6 months. At the end of the 5 years, 40% of the entire population had developed at least one subsequent ulceration.

Those patients with a history of a previous ulcer at their initial presentation were more likely to develop a recurrence (p < 0.005). Figure 2 shows that after 5 years 39 (53%) of all such patients had developed at least one recurrence, whereas only 22 (28%) of those patients who presented with their first ulceration had developed a recurrence.

Similarly, the sex of the patient affected the ulcer recurrence rate (p < 0.005). Forty-nine (50%) of the male patients developed a recurrence within 5 years compared with 12 (22%) of the females. Figure 3 depicts the cumulative frequency curves of recurrences of the male and female patients during the follow-up period.

### Occurrence of Stromal Disease

Stromal inflammation with or without uveitis was subdivided into disciform keratitis and stromal keratitis. The mild subepithelial stromal inflammation associated with the initial ulceration was not included in this classification. Twenty-four (16%) of the patient population developed a subsequent disciform keratitis; 14 (58%) of these occurred within the first month. Fourteen (9%) of the patients developed stromal keratitis during the five-year period. Eleven (79%) of these occurred

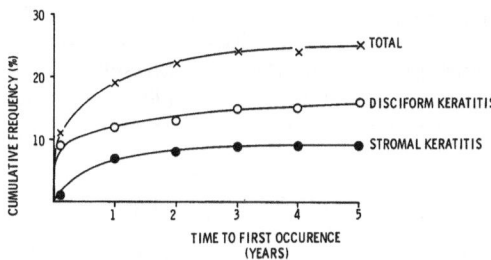

**Fig. 4.** Incidence of subsequent stromal inflammation

within the first 6 months with two cases occurring during the first month, three during the second, and an additional six during the subsequent 4 months. Figure 4 illustrates the time course of the initial development of stromal inflammation. Thirty-eight (25%) of all patients had acquired either a disciform or stromal keratitis within 5 years.

*Use of Topical Steroid*

Thirty-one patients were using a topical corticosteroid when they presented with a herpetic corneal ulceration. The steroid was continued in 25 patients and decreased over the subsequent 2 weeks unless stromal inflammation occurred. Thirty patients were started on a topical steroid following presentation. Sixty-one patients had used a steroid before subsequent stromal inflammation occurred, including those patients who had used a steroid at any time prior to the initial

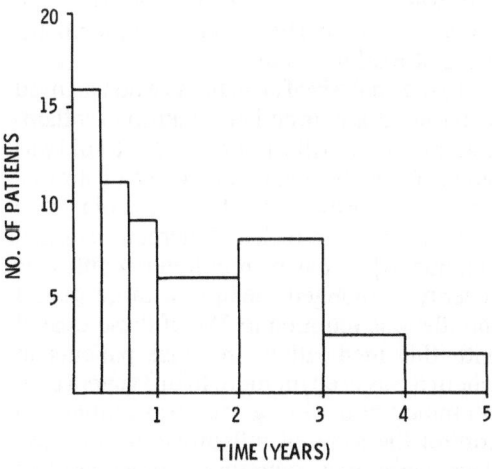

**Fig. 5.** Histogram of total duration of topical steroid use

ulceration. Eighteen (30%) of these patients later developed either disciform or stromal keratitis as compared with 17 (19%) of the 91 patients with subsequent stromal disease who had not previously used any steroid medication (p < 0.0005).

Figure 5 illustrates a histogram of the duration of steroid use in the 55 patients who received this medication following presentation. Sixteen (29%) of these patients used the steroid for less than 3 months, and 36 (65%) received it for less than 1 year. The remaining 19 patients required a steroid for control of stromal inflammation or edema intermittently or continuously for 1 to 5 years total duration of use. The highest concentration of steroid used was 1% prednisolone in eight patients, 0.3% in 13, 0.1% in 18, 0.03% in 11, 0.01% in four and 0.003% in one.

**Discussion**

This study reviewed the course of 152 patients with ulcerative herpetic keratitis over a five-year period with respect to the occurrence of subsequent epithelial ulceration, the development of inflammation, and the utilization of a topical corticosteroid. Cumulative frequency curves were used to represent the time to recurrence, and the effect of various pretreatment factors was assessed by analyzing their chi-square distributions.

The ulcer recurrence rate of the entire population was 40% with over half occurring within the first 6 months (Fig. 1). This incidence compares with previous studies (Table 1) which have reported ulcer recurrence rates from 35% to 71% over two to seven-year follow-up periods. In this series a recrudescence occurred during the first 2 weeks in 46% of those patients treated only with mechanical debridement. If these recrudescent ulcers were excluded, the remaining ulcer recurrences occurred at an average of 351 days following presentation.

Those factors which were associated with ulcer recurrence were the history of a previous herpetic ulcer and the sex of the patients (p < 0.005): patients with a prior ulcer and male patients were more likely to develop a recurrence (Figs. 2, 3). Fifty-three per cent of patients with at least one previous ulcer developed a third recurrent ulcer compared with only 28% of those with no prior history of

377

**Table 1.** Recurrence of herpetic ulceration or stromal inflammation

| Series (no. of patients) | present (152) | Carroll[1] (228) | McGill[7] (35) | Norn[9] (157) | McGill[6] (90) |
|---|---|---|---|---|---|
| Follow-up period (years) | 5 | 2 | 2 | 7 | 7 |
| Recurrent ulcer | 40% | 35% | 71% | 61%[a] | 67% |
| Subsequent stromal disease | 25% | – | 26% | 48%[b] | 26% |

[a] includes observed ulcer recurrences + patients with a history of a previous ulcer
[b] classified as metaherpetic

ocular herpes. Others have also found similar significant differences in the recurrence rates of these two groups. During a two-year follow-up, Carroll et al. [1] reported a recurrence in 43% of those patients with a previous ulcer and 26% of those following their first attack of dendritic keratitis. McGill et al. [6, 7] reported even higher incidences in patients followed for 2 to 7 years.

Similarly, 50% of the male patients developed a recurrence compared with 22% of the females, and those male patients who had had a previous corneal ulcer were more at risk for a recurrence than others. While half of the recurrences of all male patients occurred within the first 6 months following the initial therapy, recurrences in the females occurred at a slower rate: one-third occurred within the first month, but it took up to 1 year for one half of the total to be affected.

No other factor was identified which was directly associated with recurrent ulceration. Because steroid use may predispose to recurrent epithelial disease [10], in this study a concomitant antiviral was prescribed if the steroid concentration was at least 0.01% prednisolone phosphate. Statistical analysis showed that this combination was not associated with an increased ulcer recurrence ($p < 0.1$).

The subsequent occurrence of stromal inflammation occurred in 25% of the population (Fig. 4). Others (Table 1) have also found a similar incidence although one investigator reported an incidence as high as 48% of "metaherpetic" ulcers [9]. Approximately two-thirds of the cases in this study occurred in the form of disciform keratitis, and one-third of the cases of stromal disease occurred as non-disciform stromal infiltrates. The time to first manifestation of stromal inflammation

differed between these two groups. Over one-half of the cases developing disciform keratitis occurred within the first month following resolution of the initial ulcer with the remainder occurring progressively less frequently over the five-year period. On the other hand, only 11% of the cases of stromal keratitis occurred during the first post-treatment month, but 78% had occurred by the end of the first year of follow-up. The different morphologic appearances and the different timings of presentation may imply that these two types of stromal involvement are produced by different immunologic mechanisms [5].

The use of a topical corticosteroid solution was also monitored. Thirty-one patients were taking a steroid at the time of initial presentation which was tapered as rapidly as possible during the treatment period. Twenty-nine per cent of the 55 patients for whom a steroid was prescribed used it for less than 3 months, and 65% used it for less than 1 year (Fig. 5). Of the remaining patients five used it for more than 3 years of total duration.

In the analysis of all patients who had used a steroid at any time before stromal inflammation occurred, the prior use of a steroid was associated with a higher incidence of stromal disease. However, while a steroid may increase the chronicity of herpetic stromal keratitis [11], it may be required to control its severity. Prolonged therapy of more than 3 months was required in 71% of these treated with this medication. In those patients in whom it was used for more than 3 years a concentration of 0.3% or greater was required to control the signs of inflammation. Because these cases may represent a more virulent form of the disease rather than an adverse effect of chronic steroid use and because it

378

was used in all patients in whom persistent disciform or stromal keratitis occurred, the effect of a steroid on the course of the disease in these patients could not be ascertained. The precise indications for steroid use in herpetic keratouveitis as well as further study of the prevention of both recurrent epithelial and stromal disease remain as future prospects in the control of herpetic eye disease.

**Acknowledgments.** Mr. Hugh Donovan, Computer Section, Institute of Ophthalmology, assisted with the statistical analysis, and Mr. Terry Tarrant prepared the graphic tabulations.

## References

1. Carroll JM, Martola E-L, Laibson PR, Dohlman CH (1967) The recurrence of herpetic keratitis following idoxuridine therapy. Am J Ophthalmol 63:103–107
2. Coster DJ, Falcon MG, Cantell K, Jones BR (1977) Clinical experience of human leucocyte interferon in the management of herpetic keratitis. Trans Ophthalmol Soc UK 97:327–329
3. Coster DJ, Jones BR, McGill JI (1979) The treatment of amoeboid herpetic ulcers with adenine arabinoside or trifluorothymidine. Br J Ophthalmol 63:418–421
4. Coster DJ, McKinnon JR, McGill JI, Jones BR, Fraunfelder FT (1976) Clinical evaluation of adenine arabinoside and trifluorothymidine in the treatment of corneal ulcers caused by herpes simplex virus. J Infect Dis (Suppl) 133: A173–A177
5. Jones BR, Falcon MG, Williams HP, Coster DJ (1977) Objectives in therapy of herpetic eye disease. Trans Ophthalmol Soc UK 97: 305–313
6. McGill J, Holt-Wilson AD, McKinnon JR, Williams HP, Jones BR (1974) Some aspects of the clinical use of trifluorothymidine in the treatment of herpetic ulceration of the cornea. Trans Ophthalmol Soc UK 94:342–352
7. McGill J, Williams H, McKinnon J, Holt-Wilson AD, Jones BR (1974) Reassessment of idoxuridine therapy of herpetic keratitis. Trans Ophthalmol Soc UK 94:542–552
8. McKinnon J, McGill J, Jones BR (1975) Summary code for ocular herpes simplex. Br J Ophthalmol 59:539–544
9. Norn MS (1970) Dendritic (herpetic) keratitis. I. Incidence, seasonal variations, recurrence rate, visual impairment, therapy. Acta Ophthalmol (Kobh) 48:91–107
10. Patterson A, Jones BR (1967) The management of ocular herpes. Trans Ophthalmol Soc UK 87:59–84
11. Thygeson P (1967) Chronic herpetic kerato-uveitis. Trans Am Ophthalmol Soc 65:211–226
12. Williams HP, Falcon MG, Jones BR (1977) Corticosteroids in the management of herpetic eye disease. Trans Ophthalmol Soc UK 97: 341–344

## Discussion on the Contribution pp. 375–379

G.O. Waring (Atlanta)
What was the frequency of non-healing epithelial defects or sterile anterior stromal ulceration in this series?

K.R. Wilhelmus (London)
Five patients developed an indolent metaherpetic corneal ulceration. Four of these appeared to be related to toxicity of the antiviral medication.

G. Maass (Münster)
Were the recurrences connected regularly with a reactivation of the herpes virus infection, or did you observe virus shedding during these recurrences? How often did you find an asymptomatic virus shedding in these patients?

K.R. Wilhelmus (London)
We did not perform routine virus culture in these patients.

G.O.H. Naumann (Erlangen)
I think this a a beautiful study, but I have the impression that there is a different usage of the term "dendritic ulcer" on each side of the English Channel. I also noticed in the discussions by Profs. Kaufman and Jones, that they talked about "dendritic ulcers". On our side of the Channel, the term "ulcer" always means destruction of Bowman's membrane and therefore always stromal disease. This difference in terminology might lead to confusion. You mention that you have found, within 5 years, 25% involvement of the stroma. That I interpret as involvement of Bowman's layer and deeper structures. Is that right?

K.R. Wilhelmus (London)
Yes. We defined "ulceration" as any epithelial defect whether or not the underlying stroma was involved. Thus, stromal inflammation may be present without an epithelial ulcer. In this study, stromal involvement was classified into disciform keratitis and irregular non-disciform stromal keratitis.

G.O.H. Naumann (Erlangen)
You also mentioned that you have 6% scars. Could you elaborate on the fact that you find a relatively low percentage of scars in comparison to stromal

involvement; and what do you mean by "stromal involvement"?

K.R. Wilhelmus (London)
By "stromal involvement" I mean active stromal inflammation with the presence of inflammatory cells in the corneal stroma and occasionally in the anterior chamber as well. Stromal scarring may occur after resolution of the active inflammatory process and appears to be due to either altered collagen formation or lipid deposition with or without stromal neovascularization.

W. Böke (Kiel)
Maybe I didn't get it: Did you differentiate recurrences with respect to your treatment?

K.R. Wilhelmus (London)
Yes, a recurrence was defined as an epithelial herpetic ulceration occurring more than 14 days after healing of the initial ulceration.

We analyzed the recurrence rate of a subsequent epithelial herpetic ulceration according to the initial therapy: either vidarabine ointment, TFT solution, or minimal mechanical debridement. With regard to the recurrence rate, no statistical difference was demonstrated among these three treatments.

W. Böke (Kiel)
That is interesting, and it takes us back to the question we had before. Do you think it is of no importance whether one makes a primary debridement or a primary antiviral therapy?

K.R. Wilhelmus (London)
Yes, that is true with regard to the ulcer recurrence rate. However, of those patients who were treated with debridement alone 46% developed a recrudescence of an ulcer or punctate epitheliopathy within the initial 14 days following debridement. Thus, if mechanical debridement is used, an antiviral should also be prescribed to prevent these recrudescent ulcers.

C. Ohrloff (Bonn)
Did you find a relation between steroid therapy and recurrence of keratitis?

K.R. Wilhelmus (London)
The immediate prior use of a topical corticosteroid before the initial ulceration did not statistically predispose to a recurrent ulceration. Similarly, subsequent stromal inflammation was not statistically associated with such steroid use. Interestingly however, if the analysis included all patients who had used a topical steroid at any time before the development of stromal keratitis, an association was demonstrated between steroid use and stromal disease. Additional studies are needed to clarify the indications for the use of a steroid in the treatment of herpetic keratitis.

Sundmacher, R. (Hrsg.):
Herpetische Augenerkrankungen
© J.F. Bergmann Verlag, München 1981

# Trifluorothymidine and Adenine Arabinoside in the Treatment of Dendritic Keratitis

O.P. van Bijsterveld, H.J. Post, Utrecht

**Key words.** Dendritic keratitis, healing criteria, ara-A, trifluorothymidine

**Schlüsselwörter.** Keratitis dendritica, ara-A, Trifluorthymidin Heilungskriterien

**Summary.** In our study no difference between TFT and ara-A in antiviral activity was noted. The average healing time for TFT was 11.14 days and for ara-A 10.54 days. These data differ markedly from those of other studies. This was the result of the use of additional criteria for healing of the lesion. Not only absence of fluorescein staining of the cornea, but also the absence of oedema and cystic changes in the epithelium over the previous ulcer were considered criteria for healing. We found the interval between the first symptoms and commencement of the therapy of greatest importance in the clinical evaluation of antiviral drug efficacy.

**Zusammenfassung.** Wir verglichen Trifluorthymidin und Adeninarabinosid hinsichtlich ihrer antiviralen Wirkung. Beide Medikamente sind bei Keratitis dendritica wirksam. Wir sahen keinen Unterschied hinsichtlich der virustatischen Aktivität. Die durchschnittlichen Heilungszeiten der oberflächlichen kornealen Herpesläsionen waren in dieser Studie anders als in vergleichbaren Studien. Dies lag wahrscheinlich an den anderen Kriterien, die wir für die Heilungszeit anwandten. Sehr wichtig bei der Beurteilung einer antiviralen Aktivität ist die Beachtung des Zeitraums, der zwischen dem Auftreten der ersten Krankheitssymptome und dem Einsetzen der Virustatikatherapie liegt.

In 1972 Wellings et al. [3] investigated the therapeutic effect of trifluorothymidine (TFT) and found this drug to be more effective than idoxuridine (IDU). Pavan-Langston and Dohlman [2] found another antiviral drug, adenine arabinoside (ara-A), also to be more effective than IDU. In addition to being better virustatic agents, less toxic side effects were noted with TFT and ara-A in comparison to IDU [1, 3]. Coster et al. [1] also compared the healing time and rate of healing of dendritic ulcers treated with TFT and ara-A. They could not demonstrate any significant difference in virostatic activity between these drugs.

In this study, the efficacy of TFT and ara-A was reinvestigated in 56 patients with superficial herpetic keratitis. The lesions were considered healed if the epithelium was closed and no edema or cystic changes in the epithelium at the side of the dendrite was noted. The effect of the length of the interval between appearance of the first signs and symptoms of the epithelial lesions and the commencement of treatment and the effect of age on the healing time was also studied. The investigation was carried out in a double blind comparative trial.

## Subjects and Methods

56 patients, 36 males and 20 females participated in the study. The TFT and ara-A treated group consisted each of 28 patients with approximately matching ages and approximately equal male to female ratio. Patients with dendritic keratitis that failed to heal within 23 days, which was our arbitrary limit, were excluded from the study.

Each patient received a coded treatment sequentially. The preparations consisted of either 2% TFT of 3% ara-A ointment in tubes of identical design. The patients were instructed to place 4 to 5 millimeter ointment in the lower cul-de-sac every 4 hours. Usually, also scopolamine 0.2% eyedrops were given once or twice daily. When the dendritic ulcer was healed, treatment was continued for one more week.

Vital staining with fluorescein and rose bengal were used in assessing the corneal epithelial condition. Data were analysed by the analysis of variance technique.

## Results

In Table 1 the average healing times are given, classified according to treatment and sex. The

**Table 1.** Healing time for dendritic ulcers arranged according to treatment and sex

|  | TFT male | female | ara-A male | female |
|---|---|---|---|---|
| Mean | 10.95 | 11.23 | 11.64 | 8.48 |
| number | 17 | 11 | 19 | 9 |

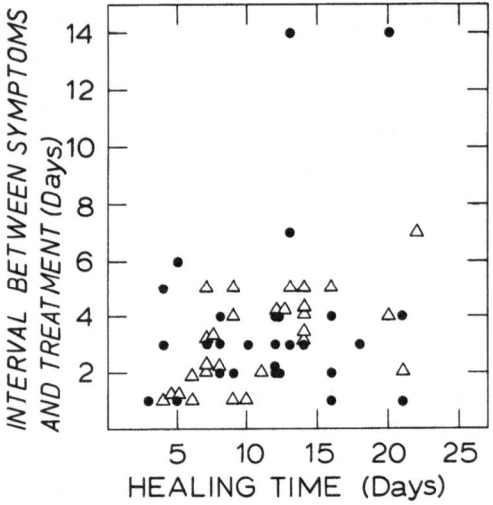

**Fig. 1.** The relationship between the interval between appearance of first symptoms and initiation of the treatment and the healing time: TFT (●) and ara-A (△)

average number of days it took for the dendritic keratitis to heal in the TFT treated group was 11.14 days and for the ara-A treated group this was 10.54 days. The average healing time for males was 11.08 days and for females 10.40 days. Not only were none of the tested mainfactors (treatment, sex and eye) statistically significantly different, but also no difference could be demonstrated in their interactions with the analysis of variance technique.

In Fig. 1 the scatter diagram of the relationship between the number of days that elapsed between the appearance of the first signs and symptoms of the disease and the moment treatment was initiated and the number of days it took for the ulcer to heal is given. The TFT and ara-A treated group did not differ significantly with regard to this interval (Table 2). If the data of the TFT and ara-A treated groups are combined, correlation analysis shows a highly significant positive relationship between these two magnitudes. In Fig. 2, this association is shown for the average values of the data of the interval before treatment was started and the healing time. A second degree curve appears to be a good fit. From the shape of this curve, the importance of early treatment is clearly visible. No significant correlation was found between the age of the patient and healing time. We found both drugs relative safe as judged by rose bengal staining.

## Discussion

We found the average healing time in our study to be considerably longer than that of similar studies. Coster et al. [1] found an average healing time for the ara-A treated group and for the TFT treated group to be respectively 5.13 and 5.75 days. In our study the healing time for the ara-A treated group and

**Table 2.** The relationship of the interval in days between beginning of symptoms and the treatment, and the healing time of the dendritic ulcer

| | Interval prior to treatment (days) | | | | | | | | | |
| | 1 | | 2 | | 3 | | 4 | | ≥ 5 | |
| | TFT | ara-A | TFT | ara-A | TFT | ara-A | TFT | ara-A | TFT | ara-A |
|---|---|---|---|---|---|---|---|---|---|---|
| Mean | 11.25 | 5.00 | 9.5 | 9.4 | 10.75 | 10.5 | 13.8 | 13.5 | 11.0 | 13.5 |
| number | 4 | 5 | 6 | 7 | 8 | 4 | 5 | 6 | 5 | 6 |
| S D | 8.6 | 2.5 | 3.9 | 5.4 | 4.4 | 4.04 | 4.9 | 3.7 | 6.6 | 5.3 |

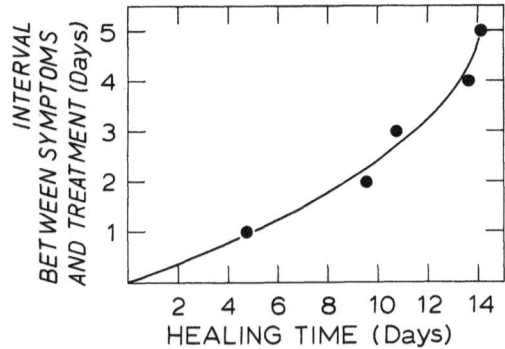

**Fig. 2.** A second degree curve is a good approximation to the type of relationship between the interval before treatment and healing time

TFT treated group was respectively 10.54 and 11.14 days. One of the reasons for this difference could have been the difference in criteria for healing.

The criterium in the study of Coster et al. [1] was absence of fluorescein staining of the epithelium. In our study we also included the absence of cystic or edematous changes in the epithelium in the area of the previous dendritic lesion. Cystic or edematous lesions of the epithelium are often indicative of persistent viral activity and H. simplex virus can be isolated frequently from these lesions, if adequate techniques are used.

As a result of this study, we found the interval between appearance of first signs of herpetic keratitis and the moment treatment was initiated an important parameter in the study of antiviral drugs.

**References**

1. Coster DJ, McKinnon JR, McGill JI, Jones BR, Fraunfelder FT (1976) Clinical evaluation of adenine arabinoside and trifluorothymidine in the treatment of corneal ulcers caused by Herpes simplex virus. J Infect Dis (suppl) 133: A173–A177
2. Pavan-Langston D, Dohlman C (1972) A double-blind clinical study of adenine arabinoside therapy of viral keratoconjunctivitis. Am J Ophthalmol 74:81–88
3. Wellings PC, Awdry PN, Bors FH, Jones BR, Brown DC, Kaufman HE (1972) Clinical evaluation of trifluorothymidine in the treatment of Herpes simplex corneal ulcers. Am J Ophthalmol 73:932–942

**Discussion on the Contribution pp. 381–383**

M. Zirm (Innsbruck)
We experienced great difficulties in finding statistically significant data because many of the first symptoms are misunderstood, not only by patients, but also by the general practitioner. Many cases of dendritic keratitis are therefore incorrectly treated and we have intervals of between one and 90 days in our statistics. We could not use intervals as a statistic parameter and I think this is important in any statistics you do.

O.P. van Bijsterveld (Utrecht)
In the patients treated with a combination of TFT and ara-A there was a good correlation between the interval prior to treatment and the number of days it took the ulcers to heal.

Analyzed separately, there was a poor correlation in the TFT-treated group, but in the ara-A-treated group there was a very strong correlation. This discrepancy could be the result of the difficulty patients and practitioners have in pinning down the moment of infection. One could not expect a 100% correlation, but I think it is worthwhile to at least try to incorporate this parameter in stratified studies.

Sundmacher, R. (Hrsg.):
Herpetische Augenerkrankungen
© J.F. Bergmann Verlag, München 1981

# Unterschiedliche Behandlungsprinzipien bei der herpetischen Keratitis und Keratouveitis und ihre klinischen Ergebnisse

F.J. Rentsch, P. Kihm, H. Liesenhoff, Mannheim

**Key words.** Herpetic keratitis, keratouveitis, trifluorothymidine, corticosteroids, keratoplasty

**Schlüsselwörter.** Herpeskeratitis, Keratouveitis, Trifluorthymidin, Kortikosteroide, Keratoplastik

**Summary.** This retrospective study deals with the efficiency of a combined therapy with Trifluorthymidine and Dexamethasone in cases of herpes keratitis and keratouveitis. Cases which were treated using this therapy are compared with similar cases, which received no steroid or virustatic therapy. Furthermore, some complications following penetrating keratoplasty in herpes cases are demonstrated.

**Zusammenfassung.** In der vorliegenden retrospektiven Studie wird die Effektivität einer Kombinationstherapie von Trifluorthymidin und Dexamethason bei Herpes-Keratitis und Keratouveitis untersucht. Als Vergleichsmaterial dienen die Verläufe von ähnlichen Fällen, die weder Steroide noch Virustatika erhalten hatten. Die Ergebnisse sprechen für die Überlegenheit der Trifluorthymidin-Steroid-Therapie. Darüber hinaus werden einige Komplikationsmöglichkeiten nach durchgreifender Keratoplastik bei Herpes-Patienten aufgezeigt.

Die Behandlung der tiefen Formen der Herpes simplex-Keratitis mit einer Kombinationstherapie von Steroiden und Virustatika scheint sich erst langsam in der Praxis durchzusetzen. Die Gründe hierfür sind vielfältiger Natur. Einmal ist seit langem bekannt, daß Steroide allein eine Verschlechterung der Herpes-Keratitis mit Ausbildung oberflächlicher Ulcerationen, Stromaeinschmelzungen mit Perforation und Sekundärinfektionen herbeiführen können [1–3]. Darüber hinaus war der therapeutische Effekt der IDU-Präparate nicht immer so überzeugend, daß ein zuverlässiger Schutz gegenüber solchen Komplikationen gewährleistet war. Seit der Einführung des Trifluorthymidins, das den IDU-Präparaten hinsichtlich seiner virustatischen Aktivität weit überlegen ist [4], hat sich die therapeutische Ausgangssituation jedoch grundlegend geändert. Klinische Untersuchungen haben gezeigt, daß durch eine Kombination von Trifluorthymidin mit Dexamethason der Krankheitsverlauf der herpetischen Keratitis und Keratouveitis deutlich verkürzt werden kann [5].

In der vorliegenden retrospektiven Studie haben wir die in unserer Klinik behandelten Fälle von schwerer herpetischer Keratitis und Keratouveitis durchgesehen, um die Effektivität der Steroid-Trifluorthymidin-Therapie gegenüber anderen Behandlungswegen zu untersuchen. Darüber hinaus wird über die Ergebnisse nach durchgreifender Keratoplastik bei rezidivierender interstitieller Herpes-Keratitis berichtet.

## Patientengut und Methodik

Aus dem Patientengut wurden insgesamt 30 ähnliche Fälle ausgesucht, die entweder eine Keratitis disciformis, eine interstitielle Keratitis oder eine Keratouveitis mit oder ohne Sekundärglaukom aufwiesen. In der Regel waren bereits ein oder mehrere Schübe einer tiefen Herpes-Keratitis abgelaufen.

Die Patienten wurden in zwei Gruppen aufgeteilt:

*Gruppe A:* 18 Fälle. Die Behandlung bestand ausschließlich oder überwiegend aus medikamentöser Mydriasis, Trifluorthymidin (initial 5× täglich, abfallende Dosierung je nach Befundbesserung) und lokalen Dexamethason-Gaben. Wenn oberflächliche Ulcera vorhanden waren, wurde Dexamethason anfänglich subconjunctival gespritzt. Nach Schluß der Epitheldefekte wurde auf Dexamethason-

385

Tropfen und -Salbe übergegangen. Die Dexamethason-Gaben waren anfänglich hoch (1 Injektion Fortecortin-Kristall s.c. jeden 2.-3. Tag); später wurde die Dosis in Abhängigkeit vom Krankheitsbild allmählich auf 1-2 Tropfen pro Tag reduziert. Bei der Entlassung aus stationärer oder ambulanter Behandlung wurde dem behandelnden Augenarzt die Weiterbehandlung mit niedrigen Trifluorthymidin- und Dexamethason-Gaben empfohlen, bis der klinische Befund einen völligen Entzug dieser Medikamente möglich erscheinen ließ.

*Gruppe B:* 12 Fälle. Hier wurden die Patienten zusammengefaßt, bei denen weder Trifluorthymidin noch ein lokales Steroid angewendet wurden. Die Therapie erfolgte in der Regel durch Mydriasis und unspezifische Salben- bzw. Antibiotika-Gaben. Vereinzelt wurde eine Epithelabrasio mit Jod-Alkohol durchgeführt. Sporadisch waren auch IDU-Präparate eingesetzt worden.

Einige der Fälle der Gruppe B kamen mit einem schweren Keratitis-Rezidiv nach Jahren wieder in die Klinik. Sie wurden dann nach den Prinzipien der Gruppe A behandelt. Sie sind in Gruppe A und B erfaßt.

*Gruppe C:* Umfaßt 8 Patienten, bei denen wegen herpetischen Hornhautnarben (5), perforierten metaherpetischen Ulcera (2) und einer schweren herpetischen Transplantatkeratitis eine durchgreifende Keratoplastik durchgeführt wurde.

Als Kriterien für den therapeutischen Effekt wählten wir in Gruppe A und B den Rückgang der herpetischen Keratitis bzw. der Uveitiszeichen und den Anstieg der Sehschärfe. Auch die Dauer der stationären Behandlung wurde mit berücksichtigt. Ergebnisse:

Der Rückgang des Hornhautödems, der interstitiellen Keratitis, der Uveitiszeichen und die Normalisierung des Augendruckes traten in Gruppe A wesentlich früher ein als in Gruppe B.

Vereinzelt kam es unter der lokalen Steroid-Trifluorthymidin-Therapie zu vorübergehenden Epitheldefekten. In keinem Falle trat jedoch eine schwerwiegende und anhaltende Hornhautulzeration ein.

Die Gruppe C umfaßt die durchgreifenden Keratoplastiken. Der praeoperative Visus lag bei 0,1. Die durchschnittliche Sehschärfe lag nach 10 Monaten bei 0,5. In 5 Fällen kam es zu vorübergehenden immunologischen Transplantatreaktionen, die unter lokaler Steroid-Therapie beruhigt werden konnten.

In einem Falle entwickelte sich eine schwere Keratitis der Wirtshornhaut, die auf den Transplantatrand übergriff. Es kam zur Fadenlockerung, die eine operative Fadennachspannung erforderlich machte. Inzwischen haben wir zwei weitere sehr ähnliche Verläufe nach postherpetischer Keratoplastik beobachtet. Diese Fälle sind in dem oben erwähnten Material nicht enthalten. In allen Fällen war die „marginale Transplantatkeratitis" von flächenhaften Ulzerationen begleitet. Unter einer Kombinationstherapie von Trifluorthymidin und Dexamethason heilten diese Fälle unter Narbenbildung aus.

In zwei Fällen entwickelte sich wenige Tage nach der Fadenentfernung eine schwere Iritis mit Sekundärglaukom. Die Hornhautrückflächenbeschläge, die Iritiszeichen und der Augendruck besserten sich jeweils innerhalb von 1-2 Wochen nach Beginn einer intensiven Dexamethason-Trifluorthymidin-

| | Ausgangsvisus | Visus bei Entlassung aus stationärer Behandlung | Dauer des stationären Aufenthaltes |
|---|---|---|---|
| Gruppe A (n = 18) | 0,26 | 0,65 | 17 Tage |
| Gruppe B (n = 12) | 0,16 | 0,33 | 41 Tage |

Der Anstieg der Sehschärfe war in beiden Gruppen statistisch signifikant. Die Differenz zwischen Ausgangsvisus und Endvisus betrug in Gruppe A knapp 0,4, in Gruppe B 0,17.

Die Dauer der stationären Behandlung war in der mit Trifluorthymidin und Dexamethason behandelten Gruppe A fast 60% kürzer als in Gruppe B.

Therapie. Es traten keine bleibenden Transplantatschäden ein.

**Diskussion**

Unsere Ergebnisse bestätigen, daß die von Kaufman und Mitarbeitern [6] empfohlene

Kombinationstherapie der Herpes-Keratitis mit Steroiden und Virustatika unter enger augenärztlicher Überwachung einen echten Fortschritt darstellt. Dies gilt im besonderen Maße für die Kombinationstherapie von Dexamethason und Trifluorthymidin [5].

Das gute Eindringvermögen von Trifluorthymidin in die Vorderkammer [7] gewährleistet bei gleichzeitiger Steroid-Medikation nicht nur im Hornhautbereich, sondern auch in den tieferen Regionen der vorderen Augenabschnitte einen ausreichenden virustatischen Schutz. Dies ist erforderlich, da zur Behandlung der herpetischen Iritis, Trabeculitis [8] und des Sekundärglaukoms wirksame antiinflammatorische und immunsuppressive Steroidspiegel in der Vorderkammer erreicht werden müssen. Eine rasch einsetzende Steroid-Trifluorthymidin-Therapie war nach unseren Erfahrungen eine der wesentlichen Voraussetzungen, um Augendrucksteigerungen bei Keratouveitis rasch unter Kontrolle zu bringen. Dies steht in Einklang mit den Beobachtungen von Falcon und Williams [9]. Eine zusätzliche Diamox-Therapie kann anfangs erforderlich sein.

Die möglichst früh einsetzende Verminderung der Belastung des Trabekelwerkes mit entzündlichen Exsudaten und Zelltrümmern ist darüber hinaus der beste Weg, um die Entstehung eines lang anhaltenden Sekundärglaukoms zu verhindern.

Unter der Kombinationstherapie von Trifluorthymidin und Dexamethason wurden in unserem Krankengut keine schweren epithelialen Komplikationen beobachtet. Dies steht in Einklang mit den Beobachtungen von Sundmacher [5]. In Fällen, wo eine langfristige Trifluorthymidin-Therapie wegen wiederholter Rezidive erforderlich ist, besteht grundsätzlich die Gefahr toxischer Schäden, die vor allem das Epithel betreffen. Darüber hinaus darf die Möglichkeit einer Resistenzentwicklung der Herpesviren gegen Trifluorthymidin nicht außer acht gelassen werden. Wenn die virustatische Komponente der Trifluorthymidin-Dexamethason-Therapie wegfällt, kann es zu schweren Herpes-Rezidiven kommen [10].

Unter den Komplikationen der Gruppe C erscheinen uns besonders zwei Verlaufsformen bemerkenswert. Es handelt sich einmal um ein Keratitis-Rezidiv, das von der Wirtshornhaut ausgeht und auf die benachbarten Abschnitte des Transplantates übergreift.

Diese Komplikation wird von oberflächlichen Ulzerationen begleitet. Sie zieht meist eine Fadenlockerung nach sich.

Die zweite Komplikation ist eine akut nach der Fadenentfernung auftretende Uveitis. Sie wird als ein Herpes-Uveitis-Rezidiv als Folge der Traumatisierung durch die Fadenentfernung aufgefaßt.

In beiden Fällen führt eine konsequente Steroid-Trifluorthymidin-Therapie zur Befundbesserung. Aufgrund dieser Erfahrungen erscheint es uns ratsam, bei Herpes-Fällen bereits vor der Fadenentfernung Trifluorthymidin und Steroide in niedriger Dosierung zu geben.

## Literatur

1. Kaufman HE, Maloney ED (1961) Experimental herpes simplex keratitis. Am Arch Ophthalmol 66:99–102
2. Thygeson P, Hogan MJ, Kimura S (1953) Cortisone and hydrocortisone in ocular infections. Trans Am Acad Ophthalmol Otolaryngol 57: 64–85
3. Coster DJ, Jones B, McGill JI (1979) Treatment of amoeboid herpetic ulcers with adenine arabinoside or trifluorothymidine. Br J Ophthalmol 63:418–421
4. Pavan-Langston D, Foster S (1977) Trifluorothymidine and idoxuridine therapy of ocular herpes. Am J Ophthalmol 84:818–825
5. Sundmacher R (1978) Trifluorthymidinprophylaxe bei der Steroidtherapie herpetischer Keratouveitiden. Klin Monatsbl Augenheilkd 173:516–519
6. Kaufman HE, Martola EL, Dohlman CH (1963) Herpes simplex treatment with IDU and corticosteroids. Arch Ophthalmol 69:468–472
7. Pavan-Langston D, Nelson DJ (1979) Intraocular penetration of trifluridine. Am J Ophthalmol 87:814–818
8. Hogan MMJ, Kimura SJ, Thygeson P (1964) Pathology of herpes simplex kerato-iritis. Am J Ophthalmol 57:551–564
9. Falcon MG, Williams HP (1978) Herpes simplex kerato-uveitis and glaucoma. Trans Ophthalmol Soc UK 98:101–104
10. Thygeson P, Hogan MJ, Kimura S (1960) The unfavourable effect of topical steroid therapy on herpetic keratitis. Trans Am Soc Ophthalmol 58:245

## Diskussion zum Beitrag S. 385–387

C. Kok van Alphen (Leyden)

I agree that the removal of the suture is a trauma

that can trigger a rejection. It is necessary to increase your cortico-steroid therapy after removal of the suture.

F.J. Rentsch (Mannheim)
With the beginning of the disease, precipitates were not only noted on the transplant but also on the host cornea. Therefore we made a diagnosis of herpes uveitis and not one of graft rejection. Treatment with TFT and dexamethasone was immediately started. In these cases we prefer subconjunctival injections of 4 mg of dexamethasone[a] in com-

---
[a] (Fortecortin solubile, Merck, Darmstadt)

bination with 5 drops of TFT every day. The dose of both medicaments is reduced with improvement.

C. Kok van Alphen (Leyden)
But do you give the same amount just after removal?

F.J. Rentsch (Mannheim)
So far we have given this therapy only in cases where signs of uveitis were present. However, I think we should give TFT and dexamethasone before the removal of the sutures and also for some time thereafter.

# Interferon

Sundmacher, R. (Hrsg.):
Herpetische Augenerkrankungen
© J.F. Bergmann Verlag, München 1981

# Mechanisms of Interferon Action

C. Jungwirth, Würzburg

**Key words.** Interferon – mechanisms of action

**Schlüsselwörter.** Interferon – Wirkprinzipien

**Summary.** Interferons are naturally occurring proteins which can induce an anti-viral state in eukariotic cells, at a very low concentration. They are directed against a variety of animal viruses, including cytocidal and tumor viruses. Interferon produced by cells from animal and human origin has been successfully purified. The molecular mechanism of the antiviral effect of interferon has been studied extensively. Cytocidal viruses are inhibited because viral gene expression is inhibited in interferon-treated cells. Replication of murine RNA tumor viruses, on the other hand, is inhibited by a completely different mechanism. These viruses are inhibited in the late stage of infection either during the assembly or release of progeny virus particles. Besides the drastic antiviral effects of interferon, a variety of anticellular activities have also been detected. At present, the interrelationship between the various effects of interferon is unclear. Of particular interest for potential clinical application are growth inhibitory effects on tumor cells and various effects on the cells of the immune system.

**Zusammenfassung.** Interferone sind natürlich vorkommende Proteine, die in eukaryoten Zellen schon in ganz niedriger Konzentration einen antiviralen Zustand induzieren können. Sie wirken gegen eine Vielzahl von tierischen Viren, sowohl zytozide als auch Tumorviren. Von tierischen oder menschlichen Zellen produzierte Interferone sind erfolgreich gereinigt worden, und man hat die molekularen Wirkungsmechanismen antiviralen Effekte ausführlich studiert. Zytozide Viren werden gehemmt, weil das Interferon die Expression von Virusgenen verhindert. Die Replikation von Maus RNA-Tumorviren wird hingegen durch einen ganz anderen Mechanismus gehemmt. Diese Viren werden in einem späten Infektionsstadium gehemmt – entweder während des Zusammenbaus der Viren oder während ihrer Freisetzung. Neben den ausgeprägten antiviralen Wirkungen hat Interferon auch noch eine ganze Fülle von antizellulären Aktivitäten. Wie diese vielen verschiedenen Interferoneffekte voneinander abhängen, ist zur Zeit noch weitgehend unbekannt. Von besonderem Interesse für eine mögliche klinische Anwendung sind die wachstumshemmenden Interferoneffekte auf Tumorzellen und die verschiedenen Einflüsse auf Zellen des Immunsystems.

Infection of a vertebrate cell with a certain animal virus may inhibit the replication of another virus in the same cell. This well known and often observed virological phenomenon is called viral interference. While studying the mechanism of viral interference among different influenza viruses, Isaacs and Lindemann discovered in 1957 that chorioallantoic membranes from chicken eggs infected with heat-inactivated influenza virus produced a factor which could induce virus resistance in homologous tissue without apparently affecting the viability of this tissue. This factor was called interferon. Naturally, anything which inhibits virus growth without severely damaging the host cell is of interest and the original observation by Isaacs and Lindemann started an active search for interferon-like substances in other virus-cell systems. It is now known that virtually all types of animal viruses and many non-viral compounds can induce interferons in a variety of vertebrate cell cultures and in whole organisms. In prokaryotes interferon-like substances have so far not been detected.

One of the characteristic properties of interferon is its broad spectrum of antiviral activities. In addition, interferons usually have a characteristic defined host range and with some exceptions they are usually more active in homologous rather than in heterologous systems. Virus resistance can develop in a cell only after exposure to interferon for several hours during which time cellular protein synthesis must be possible. The cellular alterations occurring during this time are only partially understood today. However, it has to be assumed that interferon does not act directly but rather via intermediary substances.

Nearly all animal viruses are inhibited by interferon although this can occur to quite different extents. This holds true for cytocidal as well as for tumor viruses. Some viruses are highly sensitive to interferon, for example vesicular stomatitis virus, others are much less so or are nearly resistant to interferon action. It is interesting and also important for the potential clinical application of interferon that virus mutations to interferon-resistance have so far not been detected.

Inhibition of the replication of a cytocidal virus by interferon may result in reduction of the cytopathic effect, protection of host cell metabolism and in some cases, for example the vesicular stomatitis virus infected mouse L cell, it has even been shown by continous passaging in interferon containing medium that the cell may be cured from the virus infection.

Using the antiviral activity as a biological assay, attempts have been made to purify and characterize the interferons induced in different cells and to establish what molecules are responsible for the development of the virus resistant state. Successful purification to chromatographic homogeneity of human and mouse interferon was finally reported in 1979. This has shown that interferons are proteins, in some cases glycoproteins, with an enormous specific activity which explains – in retrospect – the difficulties in purifying them. With respect to the specific activity of the antiviral effect, interferons may be compared to hormones. Except for the extremely high specific activity no unusual properties of the interferon molecules have so far been discovered. In the meantime, amino-acid composition, molecular weight determinations, electrophoretic behaviour and partial sequence work has been carried out. In addition, antibodies which neutralize the biological activity of interferons are now available.

Several virus-cell systems have been analyzed in an attempt to clarify the primary target of the interferon action and the molecular basis of the discrimination between virus and cellular functions. Much valuable information has been accumulated which is of course impossible to report here in detail. Therefore, I shall try to describe the strategy and the results obtained in such studies by analyzing two virus cell systems: First the pox virus infected chick embryo fibroblast cell and then I will describe the action of interferon on the replication of murine RNA tumor viruses.

Interferon has no activity on the extracellular virus particle. Adsorption and penetration of the pox virus particle occurs in interferon treated and untreated chick cells at a comparable rate. So the early steps of vaccinia infection are not the primary target of the anti-viral activity. After the virus particle has penetrated into the cytoplasm and the uncoating process has occurred, the synthesis of virus specific macromolecules which is necessary to build up the viral progeny begins. It is these synthetic reactions of the viral components which are inhibited in the interferon pretreated cell. It has been shown by several techniques that the primary target is the inhibition of virus-specific protein synthesis. The interesting aspect which distinguishes interferon from many other viral inhibitors is the observation that cellular protein synthesis is much less affected and that there is a discrimination between virus specific protein and cellular protein synthesis. This is of course a prerequisite for the protective effect of interferon on the host cell which has been mentioned before.

Under conditions of viral protein synthesis inhibition, pox virus specific mRNA synthesis could still be detected, which suggests an induced translation control system in the interferon treated cell. It is unlikely that a structural alteration of viral RNA is a reason for the inhibition of pox virus specific protein synthesis as no degradation or alteration of the poly A sequences or cap structures of the pox virus messenger RNA has been detected. Attempts have been made to elucidate the molecular mechanism of interferon action by studying the properties of cellfree protein synthesizing systems from interferon treated cells. So far, however, the molecular mechanism of the mRNA specific protein synthesis inhibition in the intact interferon treated cell has not been elucidated by such studies.

Naturally, it has also been attempted to

inhibit the growth of tumor viruses by pretreatment of cells with interferon. It has been established that DNA-tumor viruses, in the lytic cycle are inhibited by the same mechanism as cytocidal viruses i.e. through an inhibition of virus specific protein synthesis. Murine RNA tumor viruses, however, of murine origin are inhibited by a completely different mechanism. In considering which step might be affected in the interferon treated cell, the pecularities of the infectious cycle of RNA tumor viruses have to be considered. When each step – in particular protein synthesis – was studied it was found that the RNA tumor viruses are inhibited by interferon during the assembly process in the final stage of infection which is an intimately cell membrane associated phenomenon. Depending on the RNA tumor virus cell system studied, it is observed that virus particles cannot be released from interferon treated cells or if they can, these particles have a reduced infectivity caused by an altered architecture of the particles. So there are at the moment at least two completely different mechanisms by which viruses may be inhibited in the interferon treated cell. These two mechanisms, however, may finally merge into one, once we understand the interferon system completely.

Originally it was thought that interferon had only antiviral activity; today we know that all types of interferon have in addition to their striking ability to induce virus resistance anticellular or as they are also called nonviral activities. Numerous anticellular activities of interferon have been detected. Detection of such activity in cells involved in the immune response is of particular interest but also of concern in clinical application of interferon. That these activities of interferons were only discovered later than the antiviral activities was due to the fact that the anticellular activities of interferons are usually less drastic and are often only seen at higher concentrations of interferon. In some cases much longer exposure times to interferon are necessary for the development of anticellular activities. Certainly some of these phenomena are interrelated and possibly also related to the antiviral effects of interferon. For example one could imagine that some of the interferon induced alterations of the immune system are related to the proven interferon induced alterations of the cell surface. These alterations of the cytoplasmic

membrane on the other hand may also be the reason for the formation of abnormal RNA tumor virus particles. It will be of interest to study whether all anticellular activities can be detected with pure interferon and particularly at what concentration and after what exposure time the anticellular activities of interferon develop. In this way it may be possible to decide what the true biological importance of interferons are and whether interferons are naturally occurring antiviral compounds with some side effects or are hormones with some regulatory function in cellular physiology whose antiviral activity is only a secondary effect.

## References

1. Vilcek J (1969) Interferon Springer, Berlin Heidelberg New York
2. Finter NB (ed) (1973) Interferons and interferon inducers. North-Holland Publ Co, Amsterdam
3. Baron S, Dianzoni F (eds) (1977) The interferon system. Texas Reports on Biology and Medicine 35
4. Stewart II WE (ed) (1977) Interferons and their actions. CRC, Cleveland
5. Steward II WE (1979) The interferon system. Springer, Berlin Heidelberg New York
6. Gresser I (ed) (1979) Interferon. Academic Press, New York

## Discussion on the Contribution pp. 391–393

Y.C. Cheng (Chapel Hill)
I would first like to make a brief comment. I think that a lot of controversial results which we observed in the past in terms of mechanisms of action of interferon result from the fact that the interferon preparations being used by different laboratories were not pure and had been contaminated. The anti-cell activity and the anti-viral activity of interferon can apparently be dissociated in certain cases as has been reported by several laboratories. Thus, the anticellular and the antiviral substance in "interferon" may not be the same material. I would also like to have your opinion on what the potentiality is of the interferon in potentiating cell transformation by DNA viruses?

C. Jungwirth (Würzburg)
Referring to the first part of your comment: I don't think that the majority of anti-cellular activities of interferons which have been detected are due to

contaminants. We are certain that pure interferon has anti-cellular activity, but not all of the different activities have been tested yet. I know of only a few exceptions where it has turned out that a certain anti-cellular effect was definitely due to an impurity of the interferon preparation. To the second part: The inhibition of transformation of cells in tissue culture by a tumor virus may be due to the well known effect that interferon can inhibit the growth of cells in tissue culture.

Y.C. Cheng (Chapel Hill)

Yes, but what I wanted to ask is − have you considered the possibility that interferon may potentiate the transformation of cells by DNA viruses?

C. Jungwirth (Würzburg)

I was not aware of this effect.

K. Cantell (Helsinki)

There is no evidence that interferon would enhance tumor growth on the basis of clinical studies carried out so far. In addition, there is quite convincing evidence that interferon is a cytostatic agent; pure interferon can inhibit cell division. But interferon differs from all known cytostatic agents in the sense that it can also enhance the activity of the body defense mechanisms such as macrophages and natural killer cells, as Dr. Jungwirth described in his paper.

Sundmacher, R. (Hrsg.):
Herpetische Augenerkrankungen
© J.F. Bergmann Verlag, München 1981

# Human Interferon in Topical Therapy of Herpetic Keratitis

B.R. Jones, London

**Key words.** Interferon, dendritic keratitis, debridement

**Schlüsselwörter.** Interferon, Keratitis dendritica, Abrasio

Dr. Sundmacher has asked me to review our experiences with interferon in topical therapy of herpetic keratitis, and I should like to present this in the light of certain other experiments that explain the evolution of this work, and indeed its slow progress. Finally, I should like to indicate my own guess as to what the future may hold in this field.

Ever since the discovery of interferon by Isaacs and Lindenmann in 1957 [7], it has been attractive to explore the possibility that exogenous interferon may offer wide spectrum antiviral chemotherapy of low toxicity that could be used topically in the eye [2, 6, 25], either in prophylactic or therapeutic mode. Eventually, it has been proved to have some effect on Herpesvirus (HSV) infection in the cornea of man [11, 23]; but the central questions are not why it works so much as why it isn't more effective and how it might be used with greater effect.

The first observation of antiviral effect in man was the demonstration in 1962 that monkey interferon injected into the skin [21] could prevent vaccinia virus lesions at those sites in the skin. From that time I have been under pressure to carry out a placebo-controlled clinical trial on dendritic ulcers, in the hope that the available interferon preparation would work; but without having the assurance from work in a good animal model that the available preparation was sufficiently potent to be expected to work. The recurring dilemma has been whether to rush into clinical trials and risk a series of damaging

negative results, or whether to await data from animal work to guide the clinical trials. We have done both!

Preliminary observations were made with this same preparation of monkey interferon given half hourly when awake to five patients with early ulcerative vaccinial keratitis. In all five patients the ulcers were healing within 24 hours, and in all of the three patients whose eyes were viruspositive on the day treatment was commenced the eye became virus-negative within 24 hours and remained negative on daily culture. On the other hand, one patient not treated with interferon by mistake persisted with ulceration and remained virus-positive for 6 days [8-10, 13]. These observations rather strongly suggested a therapeutic effect but did not prove it.

A randomised double blind placebo controlled trial on dendritic ulcers was begun with this same monkey interferon preparation comparing it with 0.1% Idoxuridine which had just become available for clinical trial.

Either interferon or IDU drops were used hourly by day and 2-hourly by night for three days. Three days was judged to be the earliest time at which ulcers could be expected to show healing if either substance had an antiviral effect, and the longest time for which the supply of monkey interferon would permit treatment! After 3 days treatment the ulcers were healing in two of six patients who received placebo, in four of eight who received monkey interferon and in seven of eight who received IDU [8]. These findings suggested a therapeutic effect from IDU but not from interferon. The trial of IDU versus placebo was extended and provided the first proof of efficacy of this drug in human herpetic keratitis [20]. The trial of monkey interferon was abandoned, the dosage apparently being sufficient to influence the more sensitive vaccinia virus but being insufficient to influence the less sensitive herpesvirus infection in the cornea.

I made a firm resolve to resist pressure for further clinical trials of human interferon until a much more potent preparation was available and there was data from work in animal models to indicate the expectation of a beneficial effect from the dosage schedule to be used with the preparation of interferon available.

The outstanding challenge was therefore to develop a practicable and sensitive quantitative animal model for studying the effects in the cornea of topically applied human interferon.

Using the method of multiple inoculation by microtrephination to calculate the corneal infectivity titre that I had previously used for antiviral studies with vaccinia virus [9] Dr. John Bowbyes, working in Dr. J.D. Bauer's laboratory, adapted the model for use with HSV. With rabbit interferon kindly supplied by Dr. Monto Ho, John Bowbyes demonstrated an apparently linear relation between inhibition of herpetic lesion formation in the rabbit corneal epithelium and the log concentration of rabbit interferon applied topically.

John Bowbyes was followed in this work by James McGill who used human leucocyte interferon (HLI) kindly supplied by Dr. Kari Cantell [1]. To our great delight this also gave a linear relation between inhibition of herpetic lesion formation and log concentration of topically applied human leucocyte interferon (within the range of $6.5 \times 10^4$ to $1.3 \times 10^6$ units/ml available) [7]. Furthermore, this effect in the rabbit corneal epithelium from human interferon was in the same range of magnitude as that from rabbit interferon.

So at last we had a convenient, sensitive and inexpensive model for studying the effect of human interferon on herpesvirus infections in the corneal epithelium, capable of yielding reproducible quantitative data [16, 17]. Further work with this model demonstrated that $\frac{1}{4}$ strength HLI applied four times more often gave less antiviral effect than undiluted HLI in inhibiting lesions when applied at $\frac{1}{4}$ hourly intervals starting 1 hour after HSV inoculation. The antiviral effect was closely related to HLI concentration and not to the total quantity instilled. Furthermore, the effect was not enhanced through increasing the corneal contact time by increasing the viscosity with hydroxyprophylmethyl cellu-

lose. In other experiments the effect was studied of eight applications of drops per day through 2 days starting at 1 hour after inoculation of HSV. Both IDU drops and HLI drops gave marked inhibition of lesion formation when applied eight times a day at hourly intervals. When the eight drops were given each day in a short time at $\frac{1}{4}$ hourly intervals, that is to say within a 2 hour period leaving 22 hours untreated in each 24 hours, IDU had no effect. The HLI effect was however not reduced. A similar antiviral effect was given by one application of two drops of HLI starting 1 hour after inoculation of HSV. The whole effect of HLI appeared to reside in the first drop of HLI applied; furthermore this antiviral prophylactic effect from HLI persists in the rabbit cornea almost undiminished for 24 hours but has gone at 48 hours. These results [16, 17] indicated that optimal prophylactic use would be made of HLI if it were applied only once daily, but were used in the most concentrated form possible, and that a concentration of at least $10^6$ U/ml would probably be required.

With this window into the topical pharmacokinetic and pharmacodynamic behaviour of HLI in the corneal epithelium we were ready to engage in a coded clinical trial [3, 10, 11] using Kari Cantell's preparation of Human Leucocyte Interferon [1]. Because we wished to determine whether an antiviral effect existed or not the trial had to be randomised, coded and placebocontrolled. We had strong data from the animal model of the prophylactic antiviral effect of interferon but no consistent demonstration of effect in therapy of established HSV lesions in animals, so it was necessary that the trial should be designed to detect and measure a prophylactic antiviral effect − if one existed.

These conditions were provided in the type of trial that we have subsequently used to determine whether acyclovir has an anti-HSV effect in man, and in particular on the human cornea [12, 14]. Patients with uncomplicated dendritic ulcers were treated by Minimal Wiping Debridement (MWD) of the diseased epithelial cells at the border of the ulcer, using a sterile cotton tipped swab stick [3, 4, 10, 11]. This gives rapid relief of symptoms, the ulcer heals within a few days and in half the cases so treated this healing is not followed by recurrence or recrudescence during the convalescence. Adjunctive treatment was given with either HLI drops or placebo drops, on a double blind basis, to test efficacy in inhibiting recurrence or recrudescence of corneal epithelial lesions of typical herpetic morphology. Each of the 78 patients in the trial was seen every 24 hours for at least 7 days. After examination at the slit lamp with Bengal rose staining, the coded daily double drop of HLI or matching placebo was instilled each day. All ulcers healed within 48 hours and the majority in 24 hours. In the placebo treated group 49% developed focal recurrences of herpetic epithelial disease, in the low dose interferon group ($33 \times 10^6$ units/ml) 30% development lesions an in the higher dose interferon group ($33 \times 10^6$ units/ml) 20% developed recurrences. The latter recurrence rate is substantially different from the control group and is not likely to have occurred by chance ($x^2$ test: $p < 0.05$).

This demonstration of prophylactic antiviral effect from one daily application of two drops containing HLI, and the way in which the response is related to the concentration of HLI in the drops gives striking confirmation of the validity of extrapolating the predictions from the rabbit model to the clinical situation.

At the same time Sundmacher, Neumann-Haefelin and Cantell [23] published

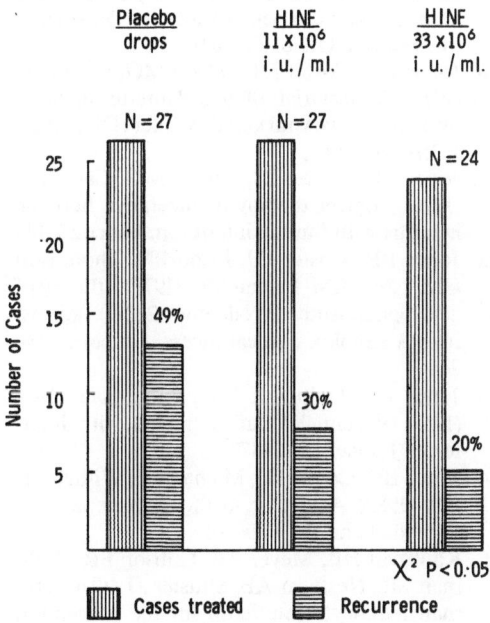

**Fig. 1.** 78 cases dendritic ulcer treated by minimum wiping debridement and adjunctive treatment

their results demonstrating that drops containing HLI $3 \times 10^6$ units/ml, two drops applied twice daily as adjunctive treatment with therapy by thermomechanical debridement beneficially influenced the healing of dendritic herpetic ulcers. These positive results in man and the large scale negative results reported by Kaufman and co-workers [15] using HLI, $6.4 \times 10^4$ units/ml, twice daily as long term prophylaxis to prevent spontaneous recurrence of herpetic keratitis all indicate that a concentration of 1 mega unit per ml. applied to the cornea is on the threshold of prophylactic antiviral effect in man. Results from extensive work in monkeys [18, 22] and rabbits using both human leucocyte interferon and human fibroblast interferon all gives data that is closely concordant with these observations in man. It is not clear whether the 20% recurrences that occurred in our trial with MWD represent recrudescence of herpetic disease in cells already infected and advanced beyond the point that can be influenced by interferon, or whether they represent lesions resulting from more massive infection of cells already inadequately protected by the interferon applied. In the former case higher concentration of interferon would not be expected to inhibit these lesions, whereas in the latter case, the use of more concentrated interferon would be expected to inhibit these lesions. It is clearly desirable to test the efficacy of human interferon further when small quantities of concentrations of 100 megaunits and higher become available.

The possibility that highly concentrated interferon may be useful in therapy of herpetic eye disease remains largely unexplored. Like others [19, 25] we have made some anecdotal observations by treating ulcerative herpetic keratitis with HLI, but apart from establishing its apparent feasability, they do not prove anything. Our own animal work [17] and that of others [22] suggests that currently available concentrations of HLI are unlikely to have a markedly beneficial effect as sole treatment of herpetic ulcers. However, as higher concentrations become available this possibility should be explored first in the rabbit and then in man if indicated by the experimental results.

The other possibility that deserves investigation is that other types of interferon might be preferable for therapy of established herpetic corneal ulcers. Using our Corneal

Epithelial Lesion Inhibition Assay [5] and working in our laboratory with Searle's Human Fibroblast Interferon (HFI) Dr. Geoff Scott has shown that when applied one hour after inoculation of HSV, Searle's HFI and Cantell's HLI are equally potent and, as with HLI, the effect of the HFI resides in the first drop applied and is related to concentration. Surprisingly, however, when the HFI is applied once, at various times before inoculation of HSV, it has no prophylactic antiviral effect. Repeated application of HFI before inoculation tends to overcome this barrier.

These observations suggest that HFI is more rapidly and avidly bound to the superficial epithelial cells of the cornea and does not reach the deeper epithelial cells of the cornea which are the prime target of HSV replication in our models. However, this would be a disadvantage if using HFI for prophylaxis against spontaneous recurrences of herpetic ulcers. On the other hand it might constitute an advantage if treating established lesions. This possibility requires systematic investigation in animal models and, if promising, in coded clinical trials.

From this brief and personal account of one sector of the attempt to develop effective antiviral prophylaxis and perhaps therapy by using human interferon, you will have perceived the dominant role played by the concentration of available preparations of human interferon. Now that sensitive and low cost animal models exist in which to study the action of human interferon in the cornea, the availability of preparations of 10, 100, 1000 or 10,000 mega units per ml. will make possible the experiments that will decide these issues.

The proof that HLI beneficially influences the course of certain tumours in man has created a market with an unjust demand for large scale production of interferon for clinical use. This should catalyze the industrial development of human interferon that is an essential pre-requisite to adequate exploration of its potential use in the eye to control virus infections.

# References

1. Cantell K, Hirvonen S, Mogensen KE, Pyhala L (1974) Human leucocyte interferon: production, purification, stability and animal experiments. In: Waymouth C (ed) The production and use of interferon for the treatment and prevention of human virus infections; proceedings of a Tissue Culture Association workshop, 1973. In vitro: monograph no. 3. Tissue Culture Association, Rockville Md, p 35–38
2. Cantell K, Tommila V (1960) Effect of interferon on experimental vaccinia and herpes simplex virus infections in rabbits' eyes. Lancet 2:682–684
3. Coster DJ, Falcon MG, Cantell K, Jones BR (1977) Clinical experience of human leucocyte interferon in rhw management of herpetic keratitis. Trans Ophthalmol Soc UK 97:327–329
4. Coster DJ, Jones BR, Falcon MG (1977) Role of debridement in the treatment of herpetic keratitis. Trans Ophthalmol Soc UK 97:314–317
5. Falcon MG, Jones BR (1977) Herpes simplex keratitis: animal models to guide the selection and optimal delivery of antiviral chemotherapy. J Antimicrob Chemother (suppl) 3:A83–89
6. Finter NB (1973) Interferons and inducers in vivo. I. Antiviral effects in experimental animals. In: Finter NB (ed) Interferons and interferon inducers. North Holland, Amsterdam, p 295–361
7. Isaacs A, Lindenmann J (1957) Virus interference. I. The interferon. Proc Royal Society (B) 147:258–267
8. Jones BR (1967) Prospects in treating viral disease of the eye. Trans Ophthalmol Soc UK 87:537–579
9. Jones BR, Al-Hussaini MK (1963) Therapeutic considerations in ocular vaccinia. Trans Ophthalmol Soc UK 83:613–631
10. Jones BR, Coster DJ, Falcon MG, Cantell K (1976) Clinical trials of topical interferon therapy of ulcerative viral keratitis. Infect Dis (suppl) 133:A169–A171
11. Jones BR, Coster DJ, Falcon MG, Cantell K (1976) Topical therapy of ulcerative herpetic keratitis with human interferon. Lancet: 2:128
12. Jones BR, Coster DJ, Fison PN, Thompson GM, Cobo LM, Falcon MG (1979) Efficacy of acycloguanosine (Wellcome 248U) against herpes simplex corneal ulcers. Lancet 1:243–244
13. Jones BR, Galbraith JEK, Al-Hussaini MK (1962) Vaccinial keratitis treated with interferon. Lancet 1:875–879
14. Jones BR, Coster DJ, Michaud R, Wilhelmus KR (1980) Acyclovir in the management of herpetic keratitis. This vol.
15. Kaufman HE, Meyer RF, Laibson PR, Waltman SR, Nesburn AB, Shuster JJ (1976) Human leukocyte interferon for the prevention of recurrences of herpetic keratitis. J Infect Dis (suppl) 133:A165–168
16. McGill JI, Cantell K, Collins P, Finter NB,

Laird R, Jones BR (1977) Optimal usage of exogenous human interferon for prevention or therapy of herpetic keratitis. Trans Ophthalmol Soc UK 97:324–326

17. McGill JI, Collins P, Cantell K, Jones BR, Finter NB (1976) Optimal schedules for use of interferon in the corneas of rabbits with herpes simplex keratitis. J Infect Dis (suppl) 133:A13–A17

18. Neumann-Haefelin D, Sundmacher R, Skoda R, Cantell K (1977) Comparative evaluation of human leukocyte and fibroblast interferon in the prevention of herpes simplex virus keratitis in a monkey model. Infect Immun :468–470

19. Pallin O, Lundmark KM, Berge KG (1976) Interferon in severe herpes simplex of cornea. Lancet 1:1187

20. Patterson A, Fox AD, Davies G, Maguire CH, Sellors PJ, Wright P, Rice NSC, Cobb B, Jones BR (1963) Controlled studies of IDU in the treatment of herpetic keratitis. Trans Ophthalmol Soc UK 83:589–591

21. Scientific Committee on Interferon. Effect of interferon on vaccination of volunteers. A report to the Medical Research Council. Lancet 1:873–875

22. Sugar J, Kaufman HE, Varnell ED (1973) Effect of exogenous interferon on herpetic keratitis in rabbits and monkeys. Invest Ophthalmol Visual Sci 12:378–380

23. Sundmacher R, Neumann-Haefelin D, Cantell K (1976) Interferon treatment of dendritic keratitis. Lancet 1:1406–1407

24. Sundmacher R, Neumann-Haefelin D, Cantell K (1976) Successful treatment of dendritic keratitis with human leukocyte interferon. A controlled clinical study. Albrecht von Graefes Arch Klin Ophthalmol 201:39–45

25. Tommila V (1963) Treatment of dendritic keratitis with interferon. Acta Ophthalmol (Kbh) 41:478–482

## Discussion on the Contribution pp. 395–399

H.E. Kaufman (New Orleans)
To review the interferon field very briefly, Barrie Jones' first work on vaccinia was uncontrolled. He used vaccine-immune globulin and other agents in the patients. It would have been premature to conclude at that time that low titer interferon was really effective against vaccinia.

The kind of low titer interferon we used in our human studies was tested in monkeys because there was evidence that homologous interferon had the greatest activity and that similar species were more likely to give similar results. For instance, testing human interferon in the rabbit might give a false low potency. We did find a prophylactic effect in owl monkeys with the low titer interferon,

but I think that Jones' conclusions are correct and that the conclusions from our study were not. Even though we saw a prophylactic effect, it is almost certain now, from later work, that in man, high titer interferon is needed. If it is to be established whether interferon can protect against recurrences of herpes, or perhaps can be therapeutically useful – and I'm a little skeptical of this – there ought to be good clinical trials of really high titer material.

D. Epstein (Stockholm)
You mention that if interferon were used as a sole therapeutic agent, you would have to use high doses; for instance, 10,000 megaunits. Would you comment on the toxicity of that therapy?

K. Cantell (Helsinki)
Perhaps we can come back to this question after Rainer Sundmacher's presentation.

H. Shiota (Tokushima)
I'd like to answer Prof. Jones' question on human fibroblast interferon in rabbits. I started treatment

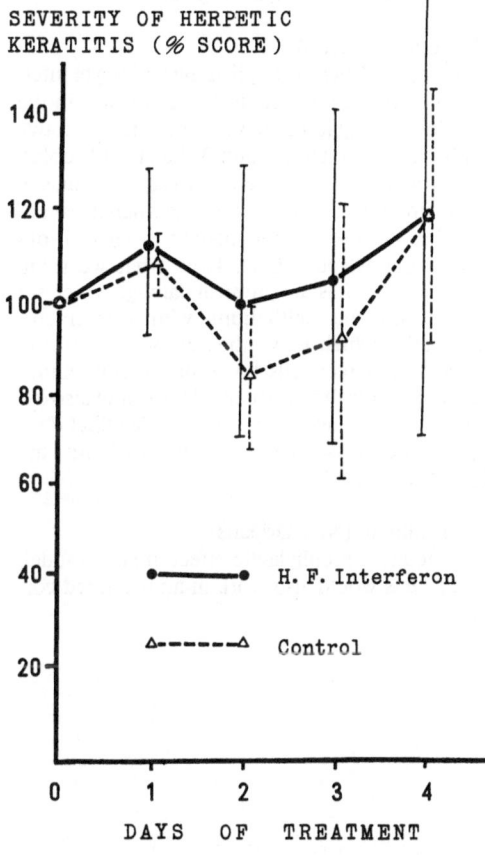

Fig. 2. Treatment was started 48 h after HSV inoculation. No therapeutic effect of human fibroblast interferon was observed against herpetic ulcers in rabbit cornea

upon such eyes with human fibroblast interferon drops with a titer of $10^6$ i.u./ml ten times per day. This is just before treatment. Figure 2 shows on the vertical axis the severity of herpetic keratitis expressed by % score and on the horizontal axis the days of treatment. The bold line shows eyes treated with human fibroblast interferon and the dotted line shows control eyes. You can see that after 4 days of treatment, no therapeutic effect was observed, as is convincing illustrated by the geographic appearance of the lesions after 4 days of treatment with human fibroblast interferon. For established lesions in rabbits, therefore, human fibroblast interferon does not have a therapeutic effect.

R. Sundmacher (Freiburg)
I agree with nearly everything that has been said. Just one question to Prof. Jones: you said fibroblast interferon did not work prophylactically? Maybe I got it wrong, but in our experimental models, which are basically always prophylactic models, we do have a strong prophylactic effect.

B.R. Jones (London)
That is right. When we applied the leukocyte interferon before the virus challenge and it was in the right dose of megaunits, it was completely effective in inhibiting lesion formation. When the fibroblast interferon was applied before virus challenge, it had no prophylactic effect, whereas when it was applied 1 hour after our inoculation of virus, it did have a prophylactic effect. Now what we think happens is that it is the physical damage which we perform on the epithelium with our microtrephination which allows the fibroblast interferon to reach the target cells lower in the epithelium; these are mainly the basal cells. This would also explain why we do not get a prophylactic effect if we apply the fibroblast interferon only once before the physical damage.

H.E. Kaufman (New Orleans)
If you found a prophylactic effect in your model, perhaps this would also work in an ulcerated cornea?

R. Sundmacher (Freiburg)
I think the experimental details are essential. We applied the interferon before infection, then we did the scraping, then we exposed the cells again to interferon and only then was the corneal epithelium infected. Thereafter, again, interferon was applied daily. In this model, which is certainly different from yours, we found the same prophylactic effect for both interferons.

B.R. Jones (London)
Your effect may come from the fibroblast interferon that you put on after the scrape.

R. Sundmacher (Freiburg)
Right. This is possible; but if I understand you correctly, you say that you have found a basic difference in the pharmacocinetic property of human leukocyte and fibroblast interferon to penetrate an intact corneal surface?

K. Cantell (Helsinki)
I think we also have to remember that fibroblast interferon is a more labile molecule than leukocyte interferon. Barrie's explanation may be right, but it is also possible that the fibroblast interferon is destroyed more quickly than leukocyte interferon in vivo.

G. Streissle (Wuppertal)
How do you prevent the spread of virus through tears or by lid movement in your titration experiments?

B.J. Jones (London)
Having made the trephination, we have a little triangle of filter paper and blot the excess inoculum so that it doesn't physically spread. We cannot entirely prevent the spread, and in a given inoculation site about 10% of the infectivity is contamination; and we know that there is that background noise; but when you calculate the 50% infective dosis, and double it, then go to this model where you want to have 100% infection to be on 25 sites, and it works out that you actually get very close to 100%: then, I think, it has validity.

Sundmacher, R. (Hrsg.):
Herpetische Augenerkrankungen
© J.F. Bergmann Verlag, München 1981

# Therapy and Prophylaxis of Dendritic Keratitis With Topical Human Interferon

R. Sundmacher, D. Neumann-Haefelin, K. Cantell, Freiburg, Helsinki

**Key words.** Dendritic keratitis, interferon, debridement, trifluorothymidine, combination therapy

**Schlüsselwörter.** Keratitis dendritica, Interferon, Abrasio, Trifluorthymidin, Kombinationstherapie

**Summary.** Topical human interferon has been used for therapy and prophylaxis of dendritic keratitis in the monkey model and in patients. As yet, an effective long-term prophylaxis of late dendritic recurrences by means of interferon eye drops could not be established. Also, the therapy of dendritic keratitis with interferon *alone* does not seem to offer a clinically relevant therapeutic progress – if it is active at all.

The combination, however, of interferon with either a thermomechanical debridement of the diseased corneal epithelium or with trifluorothymidine eye drops has proven to be more effective than any other monotherapy which we tested.

At the moment, a combination of highly potent human leukocyte interferon ($30 \times 10^6$ units/ml) with trifluorothymidine eye drops has given the best results. Studies are underway to economize the need for interferon in this combination by the factor 10.

**Zusammenfassung.** Die Wirkung lokal applizierten Humaninterferons bei der Therapie und Prophylaxe der Keratitis dendritica wurde sowohl in Affenmodellen als auch bei Patienten untersucht. Eine wirksame Langzeitprophylaxe echter Dendritica-Spätrezidive durch Interferon-Augentropfen hat sich bis heute nicht erreichen lassen. Auch die Therapie der Keratitis dendritica mit Interferon *allein* scheint keine klinischen Vorteile gegenüber anderen eingeführten Verfahren zu bieten, sondern eher schlechter zu sein.

Kombiniert man Interferon aber entweder mit einer Thermo-Abrasio oder mit Trifluorthymidin-Augentropfen, so gelangt man zu Therapieformen, die effektiver sind als alle Monotherapien, die wir untersucht haben.

Augenblicklich haben wir mit einer Kombination eines hochaktiven humanen Leukozyteninterferons ($30 \times 10^6$ E/ml) mit Trifluorthymidin-Augentropfen die besten Ergebnisse. Wir untersuchen ferner, ob man den Interferon-Bedarf in dieser Kombination ohne Wirkungsverlust auf $^1/_{10}$ reduzieren kann.

Most of our experimental and clinical interferon work has been published in German journals which are not everywhere available. We regard it as useful therefore, to present a survey of our work together with some unpublished results.

When we started with a monkey model of dendritic keratitis 6 years ago, we found that even low potent human leukocyte interferon drops at $10^4$ units/ml could prevent exogenous primary herpetic keratitis if given *before* virus inoculation [6, 11]. If, however, interferon was not applied before 6–20 hours after inoculation, it had no effect. This fitted well with the generally accepted idea that interferon acts as a prophylactic antiviral agent which can protect only non-infected cells.

Later, we confirmed the prophylactic action of interferon in the monkey model and also obtained additional data on the dose-response relationship of both leukocyte and fibroblast interferon [7]. The results showed that in our first experiments we had been somewhat lucky in obtaining positive results because interferon drops at $10^4$ units/ml were, in fact, only borderline active. Both interferons, however, inhibited dendritic disease completely at $10^6$ units/ml. Based on these positive results, we were quite optimistic that interferon eye drops could also inhibit dendritic recurrences in humans.

A group with an especially high risk of dendritic *recurrences* are patients treated with steroids for deep herpetic disease which, as we believe, is mostly caused by virus multiplication and then complicated by diverse

401

immune reactions (see Chapter 33). With this high-risk group, we started a randomized controlled clinical study after experiments had shown that even a very intensive topical steroid therapy did not afflict the excellent *prophylactic* action of interferon in the monkey model [15].

We had 40 patients in the study, 20 in each group. All 40 patients received the same standardized steroid regime for a total of 4 months (1st month five drops of dexamethasone 0.1%, 2nd month three drops, 3rd month two drops, 4th months one drop daily). In addition, they were either given coded interferon at $3 \times 10^6$ units/ml one drop daily, or albumine respectively.

Contrary to our expectations, the results of this patient study were completely negative with six virologically proven dendritic recurrences in the interferon group but with only three in the albumine group.

Kaufman and associates had earlier reported on negative experiences with low-titered interferon eye drops for *prophylaxis* of dendritic recurrences in herpes patients not compromised by steroids [3]. Later, another study by Kaufman, this time using an interferon similarly potent to ours, also turned out negative [4].

This leaves us with a striking discrepancy between positive animal studies, which are doubtlessly valid, and negative patient studies which are equally valid. The most likely explanation would be that the animal model did not reflect the pathophysiologic conditions encountered in patients.

In the monkey, we work with an exogenous infection model. The virus is dropped on a scarified corneal epithelium, infecting only those cells which lie overt to the surface and thus have had a chance of being contacted by interferon drops before.

With dendritic keratitis in humans, it seems to be totally different, at least in the majority of cases [1, 5, 9]. Here, we normally deal with endogenous reinfections. The virus travels down the appropriate nerves and is set free among or beneath the basal epithelial cells while the epithelial surface is mostly intact. Under these conditions, topically applied interferon has probably no chance to sufficiently penetrate the epithelial barrier which is sealed by zonulae occludentes and normally keeps off even a lot of low weight molecules, e.g. glucose.

For us, this means that without prior or concomitant damage to the epithelial barrier, the chances of topical interferon *preventing late dendritic recurrences in man* are virtually null, and we have, therefore, given up pursuit of this aim for the moment. This was not difficult as we found, in another controlled clinical study with a comparable patient group, that five drops of trifluorothymidine (TFT) per day completely prevented dendritic complications in steroid-compromised herpes patients [10].

Contrary to these disappointing results with topical interferon prophylaxis, the results of certain forms of interferon *therapy* of dendritic keratitis have turned out to be very promising. Before going into this in more detail, it should be noted, that from all we have learned on interferon action, one would not really expect a tremendous therapeutic effect of interferon, and, in fact, we have not found that interferon *alone* is of advantage in comparison with other established forms of therapy. One such therapy which we have followed up for a few years is simple thermomechanical debridement of the diseased epithelial areas with the aid of an old instrument, the thermocauter of Wessely, the metallic tip of which is heated by internally passing steam. This inexpensive and quite safe form of therapy is highly efficient in at least 80% of patients whose dendrites heal within a week [8]. 20%, however, experience one or more immediate viral recurrences necessitating repeated debridements with an increasing risk of damage to the cornea. Our hope was that it should be possible to prevent these immediate viral recurrences after thermodebridement by adding topical interferon.

The first controlled patient study, however, was again a clear failure [14]. Whether or not interferon was added after debridement made no major difference, and interferon alone looked very much worse than debridement alone. This was not only true for the healing times, but also for the periods of virus-shedding into the cul-de-sac, and we should point out here that all of our clinical studies have been controlled virologically. These negative results were obtained using a low-potent interferon in accordance with our first monkey experiments. We therefore repeated the study with a one hundred times more potent human leukocyte interferon preparation and this time, we achieved a

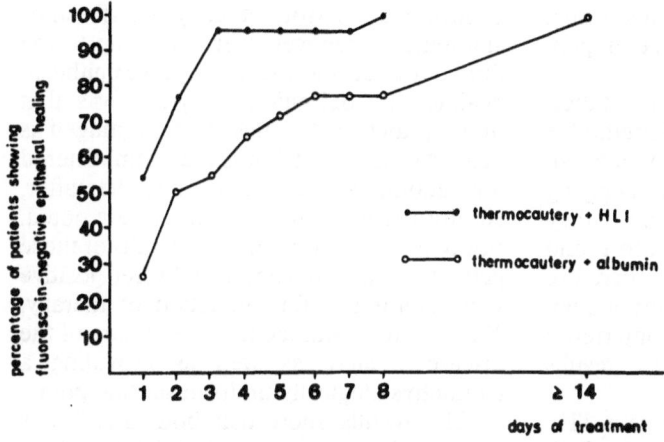

**Fig. 1.** The addition of human leukocyte interferon (HLI) after thermocautery results in significantly quicker healing of dendritic keratitis than after therapy with thermocautery alone (from [13])

clear-cut success, the debridement-interferon group having healed significantly quicker (Fig. 1.) and virus-shedding having stopped significantly earlier (Fig. 2.) than in the debridement-placebo group [12, 13]. Another controlled clinical study established that fibroblast interferon was equally active as leukocyte interferon in this type of combination therapy with thermodebridement [18].

By this time, we had learned that the Moorfields group with Jones had tried a similar therapeutic combination with the difference that they used the totally innocous, though not radical, method of minimal wiping debridement (mwd) together with interferon [2]. They had also achieved a significant amelioration by adding interferon.

They required, however, more potent preparations than we did. We therefore directly compared the role of these two forms of debridement together with interferon [16]. It turned out that in the thermocauter group a second debridement was necessary in only 17% of cases which subsequently healed rapidly, whereas 50% in the mwd group had to be debrided a second time and 33% still a third time. The course in these cases was so prolonged that we performed the third and fourth debridements in the mwd group by thermocautery in order to accelerate healing, and only then the healing curve of the mwd group met that of the thermocautery group. Our conclusion from this study has been that for *therapy* of dendritic keratitis, interferon is

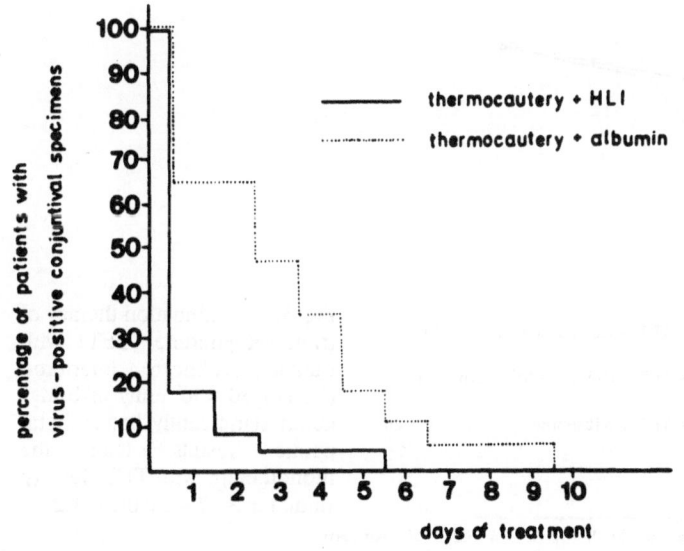

**Fig. 2.** Also, the addition of HLI after thermodebridement reduces the time period of virus shedding into the cul-de-sac significantly (from [13])

403

only meaningful if it can be combined with a therapy which in itself has as much therapeutic potency as possible.

Having come so far, we realized that thermodebridement — though a good method — would not be appreciated by many ophthalmologists, partly because they fear applying surgical methods and partly because they want to avoid additional discomfort and bandaging for their patients. We therefore wondered whether the combination of a potent topical antiviral, together with interferon might bring about equally positive results without discomfort.

The best antiviral as yet available is TFT [20], and we designed a study combining TFT with human leukocyte interferon. Patients with a clinical diagnosis of dendritic keratitis were investigated virologically for the presence of culturable herpes simplex virus in the tear film [13]. All of them received five drops of TFT 1% commercial eye drops[a] daily during waking hours. Further, they were at the beginning of therapy randomly assigned to one of three groups and in addition treated with either albumine, or low-potent interferon ($10^6$ units/ml) or highly-potent one ($30 \times 10^6$ units/ml). They daily received two drops of their coded preparation at 10 minute intervals while resting in a reclined position to ensure that the drops would stay in the cul-de-sac.

Slit lamp examinations as well as virologic

[a] Fa. Dr. Mann, Berlin

controls were performed daily. Interferon or albumine respectively were given up to the third day after fluorescein-negative epithelial healing, the definition of which was that minor punctate stainings were not judged as being "positive". TFT was then administered for 3 additional days and withheld thereafter. No immediate viral recurrences were noted. For final evaluation, only the results of those patients were used who had delivered positive virus cultures before initiation of therapy. This was to guarantee the viral nature of the disease treated, as well as providing a pathophysiologically uniform starting point.

The results show that both interferons enhance the antiviral activity of TFT. But it is only with the most potent interferon ($30 \times 10^6$ units/ml) that a statistically significant improvement is achieved (Fig. 3, 4). Thus, the results of this comparatively large series confirm the results of a smaller study on which we reported earlier [17, 19]. The medium healing times were 3, 4.9, and 6 days respectively. Apart from this it is certainly even more important to stress that in the best group all corneae had healed up to the 4th day.

Further, we would like to draw attention to the point that in this study — as a desirable side effect — we also obtained controlled results for the therapeutic efficiency of TFT alone. These results compare well with those reported in the literature.

We are currently trying to economize the need for interferon in this combination in a randomized controlled clinical study with

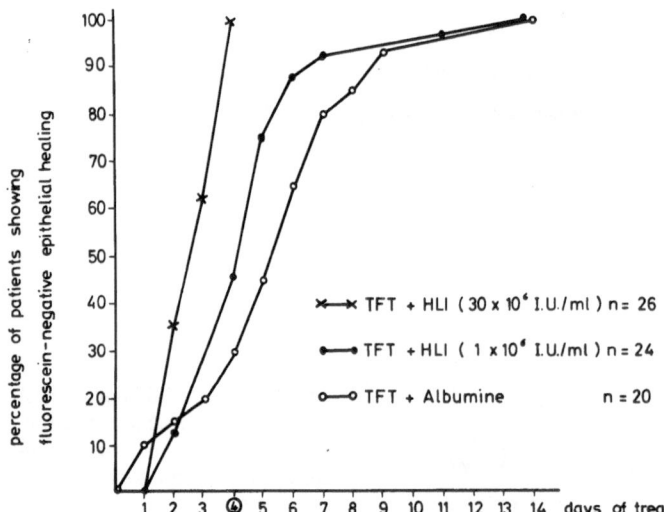

**Fig. 3.** A combination therapy of trifluorothymidine (TFT) with human leukocyte interferon (HLI) at $30 \times 10^6$ units/ml brings about significantly better therapeutic results than the monotherapy with TFT alone (p value for $X^2$ $2 \times 2$ table 0.002)

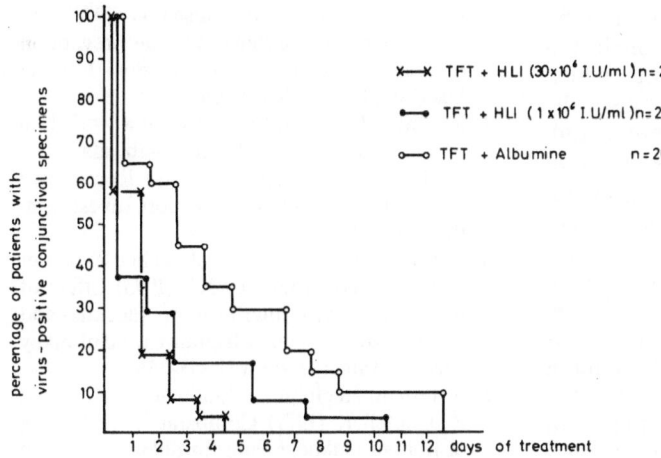

**Fig. 4.** Also, the addition of HLI to TFT reduces the time period of virus shedding into the cul-de-sac significantly (p value of $X^2$ 2 × 2 table 0.01)

two differently potent interferon preparations. As yet, the number of patients is too small to draw valid conclusions whether or not we will succeed in reducing the amount of interferon in this combination by the factor 10, but it looks as if with larger numbers we will still have some difference between the two groups. We have to wait on this because the time factor is directly dependent on how

many practitioners collaborate with us and send not only "preterminal" stages of herpetic corneal disease but also cases of "ordinary" dendritic keratitis. Some of our colleagues are really a great help in this respect and we would like to take the opportunity to thank them.

For a final overview, we present a composite graph in which curves have been combined which we have obtained in controlled

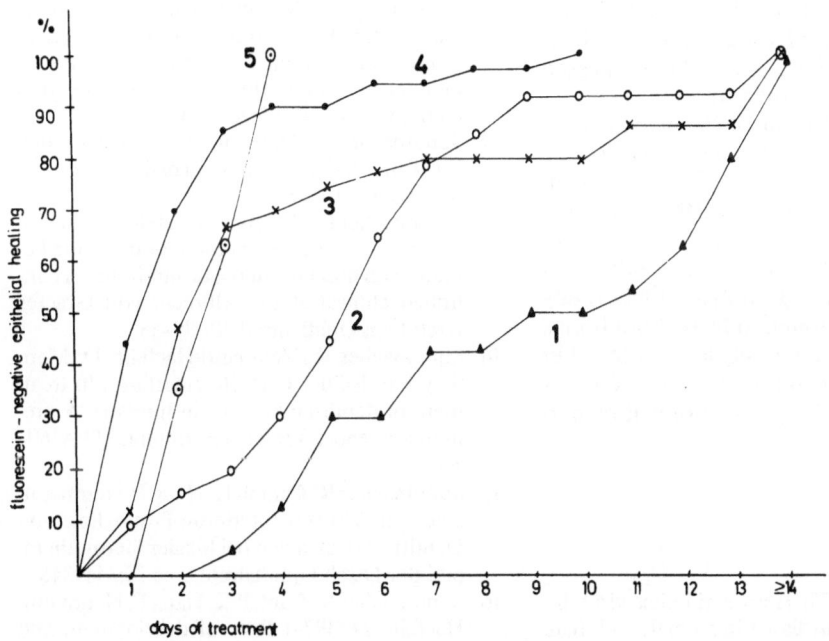

**Fig. 5.** Composite graph of healing curves derived from different randomized, controlled clinical studies of our group. 1: Human leukocyte interferon (HLI, $6 \times 10^4$ IU/ml) n = 16 (ref. 14), 2: Trifluorothymidine (TFT, 1.0%) n = 20, 3: Thermocautery, n = 68 (ref. 8), 4: Thermocautery plus HLI ($3$–$10 \times 10^6$ IU/ml) n = 40 (ref. 13, 16), 5: TFT plus HLI ($30 \times 10^6$ IU/ml) n = 26

patient studies during the last years (Fig. 5). One of us (R.S) has treated and personally followed nearly all of these patients which means that although we cannot statistically compare curves derived from different studies, this graph may nonetheless give us a good clue as to how different forms of therapy compare in respect to epithelial healing. Low potent interferon alone was least effective – if at all (curve "1"). Trifluorothymidine alone takes the next rank (curve "2"). Within the first week after initiation of therapy, it is clearly less effective than thermodebridement alone (curve "3") whereas thereafter, the rest of our patients did better with TFT than with debridement alone. Thermodebridement plus HLI at about $10^6$ units/ml produces a fairly good healing curve (curve "4") which is only surpassed by TFT plus highly potent interferon at $30 \times 10^6$ units/ml (curve "5"). This last curve looks nearly ideal and we are not aware of any other available monotherapy or combination therapy that would have given equally excellent results.

In summary, the *longterm prophylaxis* of late dendritic recurrences by topical interferon gave no positive results and probably will give none. However, the *combination therapy* of dendritic keratitis with either thermodebridement or TFT was so highly effective that it will not be easily met or surpassed by any other form of therapy.

The question we all have, of course, is when will interferon be available to the ophthalmological practitioner? This we cannot answer; but I must confess that I have become more and more reluctant to speak to ophthalmologists about the good effects of interferon because I notice that many colleagues are frustrated to hear about things they cannot reach and easily loose interest in results which they cannot reproduce. We sincerely hope that this symposium will help to change things a little bit.

# References

1. Baringer JR (1975) Herpes simplex virus infection of nervous tissue in animals and man. Progr Med Virol 20:1–26
2. Jones BR, Coster DJ, Falcon MG, Cantell K (1976) Topical therapy of ulcerative herpetic keratitis with human interferon. Lancet 2:128
3. Kaufman HE, Meyer RF, Laibson PR, Waltman SR, Nesburn AB, Shuster JJ (1976) Human leukocyte interferon for the prevention of recurrences of herpetic keratitis. J Infect Dis (Suppl) 133:A165–A168
4. Kaufman HE et al. In: Report of a workshop on herpes infections. NIAID, Bethesda
5. Nesburn AB, Green MT (1976) Recurrence in ocular herpes simplex infection. Invest Ophthalmol 15:515–518
6. Neumann-Haefelin D, Sundmacher R, Sauter B, Karges HE, Manthey KF (1975) Effect of human leukocyte interferon on vaccinia- and herpes virus-infected cell cultures and monkey corneas. Infect Immun 12:148–155
7. Neumann-Haefelin D, Sundmacher R, Skoda R, Cantell K (1977) Comparative evaluation of human leukocyte and fibroblast interferon in the prevention of herpes simplex virus keratitis in a monkey model. Infect Immun 17:468–470
8. Sundmacher R (1976) Herpestherapie und -prophylaxe. I. Versuch einer kritischen Wertung. Klin Monatsbl Augenheilkd 169:308–325
9. Sundmacher R (1977) Die Pathophysiologie der Herpes simplex Rezidive. Klin Monatsbl Augenheilkd 170:613–621
10. Sundmacher R (1978) Trifluorthymidinprophylaxe bei der Steroidtherapie herpetischer Keratouveitiden. Klin Monatsbl Augenheilkd 173:516–519
11. Sundmacher R, Neumann-Haefelin D, Shrestha B (1975) Die Wirkung von Humanleukozyten-Interferon auf experimentelle Viruskeratitiden bei Affen. Albrecht von Graefes Arch Klin Ophthalmol 195:263–270
12. Sundmacher R, Neumann-Haefelin D, Cantell K (1976) Interferon treatment of dendritic keratitis. Lancet 1:1406
13. Sundmacher R, Neumann-Haefelin D, Cantell K (1976) Successful treatment of dendritic keratitis with human leukocyte interferon. A controlled clinical study. Albrecht von Graefes Arch Klin Ophthalmol 201:39–45
14. Sundmacher R, Neumann-Haefelin D, Manthey KF, Müller O (1976) Interferon in treatment of dendritic keratitis in humans. A preliminary report. J Infect Dis (Suppl) 133:A160–A164
15. Sundmacher R, Cantell K, Haug P, Neumann-Haefelin D (1977) Interferon-Prophylaxe von Dendritica-Rezidiven bei lokaler Steroidtherapie. Ber Dtsch Ophthalmol Ges 75:344–346
16. Sundmacher R, Cantell K, Haug P, Neumann-Haefelin D (1978) Role of debridement and interferon in the treatment of dendritic keratitis. Albrecht von Graefes Arch Klin Ophthalmol 207:77–82
17. Sundmacher R, Cantell K, Neumann-Haefelin D (1978) Combination therapy of dendritic

keratitis with trifluorothymidine and interferon. Lancet 2:687

18. Sundmacher R, Cantell K, Skoda R, Hallermann C, Neumann-Haefelin D (1978) Human leukocyte and fibroblast interferon in a combination therapy of dendritic keratitis. Albrecht von Graefes Arch Klin Ophthalmol 208:229–233
19. Sundmacher R, Cantell K, Horn C, Neumann-Haefelin D (1979) Kombinationstherapie der Keratitis dendritica mit Trifluorthymidin and Humanleukozyteninterferon. Ber Dtsch Ophthalmol Ges 76:489–492
20. Wellings PC, Awdry PN, Bors FH, Jones BR, Brown DC, Kaufman HE (1972) Clinical evaluation of trifluorothymidine in the treatment of herpes simplex corneal ulcers. Am J Ophthalmol 73:932–942

## Discussion on the Contribution pp. 401–407

K. Cantell (Helsinki)
Thank you Rainer. I don't think I'm able to predict when interferon will become freely available either, but I can assure you that more interferon will be available this year than last year. The production of interferon is being expanded in many countries.

H.E. Kaufman (New Orleans)
There is additional information that may ameliorate Dr. Sundmacher's pessimism. It is clear that the rabbit has naturally occurring herpes, and after the first infection, develops natural recurrences much like those of humans, and presumably by the same mechanism. It is also clear that interferon inducers can absolutely prevent herpes recurrence in the rabbit for an effective period of 6 to 8 weeks. I've shown this to be true, and Dr. Nesburn, in California, has confirmed it. The mechanism is the same, and if inducers work in rabbits, exogenous interferon ought to work in man. I am more hopeful than is Dr. Sundmacher that it will, in fact, work this way.

For interferon to be active, various processes, such as translational inhibitory protein synthesis, must occur in the cell. It may be that the administration of exogenous steroids interferes with mechanisms in the cell and prevents interferon activity. Then, even though interferon is not active in preventing recurrences of herpes with steroids, it may be active in preventing recurrences in cells that have not had steroids introduced into their metabolic processes. I have no argument with Dr. Sundmacher's data; this is simply another possible interpretation.

R. Sundmacher (Freiburg)
I didn't intend to spread pessimism, otherwise, I wouldn't have started with interferon research. But again, in humans we do have a pharmacokinetic problem with topical prophylaxis, and my bet at the moment would certainly be more against than in favour of a practicable solution. It may also be that steroids in our study did have some negative influence on interferon activity in man, but we have been unable to verify this in the monkey model. Of course, this doesn't prove too much as the steroid influence may be very different in different species.

K. Cantell (Helsinki)
I'm a layman in the field of ophthalmology, but it seems to me that the interferon studies have taught us something. They have taught us how tricky the use of interferon is, how easily negative results are obtained, and that the best results are obtained when interferon is used in combination with an effective therapeutic partner. I recall the study presented yesterday by Dr. Varnell and Dr. Kaufman in which they used a combination of two drugs, ARA-A and acycloguanosine, and got rather striking results. I bet that, in the future, herpetic diseases will be treated more and more with a combination of several drugs and I believe that interferon is one of them.

H.E. Kaufman (New Orleans)
There are, in fact, many experimental studies in the literature, by a variety of workers, which indicate what you just said.

A. Tenner (Wangen)
I would like to ask if somebody has data on the production of interferon in the cornea in infected eyes and whether the production is higher when the tissue temperature is higher? Could the warming of a virus infected eye be of some therapeutic effect?

R. Sundmacher (Freiburg)
This is an interesting idea. However, one should keep in mind that it would certainly be impossible to selectively enhance interferon mechanisms by warming the tissues. You would, at the same time, enhance other, possibly harmful mechanisms. I have been looking around, and I think nobody can as yet answer your question.

Sundmacher, R. (Hrsg.):
Herpetische Augenerkrankungen
© J.F. Bergmann Verlag, München 1981

# Effect of Human Fibroblast Interferon on Dendritic Keratitis

Y. Uchida, M. Kaneko, R. Yamanishi, S. Kobayashi, Tokyo, Kamakura

**Key words.** Human fibroblast interferon, dendritic keratitis, animal models

**Schlüsselwörter.** Human-Fibroblasteninterferon, Keratitis dendritica, Tiermodelle

**Summary.** The therapeutic effect of human fibroblast interferon (FIF) was studied in 21 patients with dendritic keratitis confirmed virologically. FIF or placebo (human albumin) was administered topically four times a day. In a controlled study, five patients treated with $10^6$ u/ml FIF showed improvement, while three of four patients treated with placebo were not cured. In 12 patients, two concentrations of FIF were compared on the basis of double blind method. The effect of $10^6$ u/ml FIF was significantly superior to that of $10^3$ u/ml FIF. Results of animal experiments using the rabbit showed that $2.8 \times 10^6$ u/ml FIF worked in reducing the severity of herpetic keratitis.

**Zusammenfassung.** Wir untersuchten die therapeutische Wirkung von Human-Fibroblasteninterferon (FIF) bei 21 Patienten mit virologisch gesicherter Keratitis dendritica. Die Patienten erhielten viermal täglich einen Tropfen FIF oder Plazebo (Human-Albumin). In einer kontrollierten Pilot-Studie zeigten fünf Patienten, die $10^6$ Einheiten/ml FIF erhalten hatten, eine Besserung, während drei von vier Plazebo-behandelten Patienten nicht geheilt wurden. Bei weiteren zwölf Patienten verglichen wir zwei verschiedene FIF-Konzentrationen in einer Doppelblind-Studie. Die Wirkung von $10^6$ Einheiten/ml war signifikant besser als die von $10^3$ Einheiten/ml. Am Modell der Keratitis dendritica bei Kaninchen zeigte sich, daß man mit $2,8 \times 10^6$ Einheiten/ml FIF den Schweregrad der Keratitis mildern kann.

## Introduction

In the last few years, the progress in production of highly purified human interferon has enabled ophthalmologists to undertake the clinical trials of this agent for viral eye diseases. Effect of human interferon on dendritic keratitis has been studied by several authors [1, 4, 8, 11–13]. Most reports have come to the conclusion that interferon acts prophylactically and has little clinical usefulness in the treatment of established dendritic keratitis, unless other antiviral measures are added.

Leucocyte interferon (LIF) has mostly been studied. In contrast, fibroblast interferon (FIF), an antigenically different one, has appeared in only a few reports [8, 13]. Recently, FIF with the sufficient concentration and purity has become available for clinical trials in Japan. We attempted to study the effect of FIF on dendritic keratitis by topical administration without combining other antiviral procedures. Additionally, we carried out experimental studies to know whether FIF would have therapeutic effect on herpes simplex keratitis in the rabbit.

## Material and Methods

Partially purified FIF was prepared in Toray Basic Research Laboratories as described previously [6].

### 1. Clinical Trials

Twenty-one patients with dendritic keratitis were admitted for investigation. Epithelial scraping materials taken from a small part of the dendritic lesion were examined by the direct method of immunofluorescence for herpes simplex virus antigen. All patients showed positive results. The unscraped area of dendritic figure was subjected to observation.

Patients were treated with solutions of FIF or placebo (human albumin), a drop (0.04 ml) of which was instilled into the conjunctival sac four times a day. In every case a gentamicin eye drop was applied three times a day for preventing bacterial infection. Two trial methods were designed.

a) Nine patients received $10^6$ units ml/FIF or placebo. Samples were coded by two different numbers.

b) Twelve patients received $10^6$ units ml/FIF or $10^3$ units ml/FIF. Samples were coded randomly on the basis of double blind test.

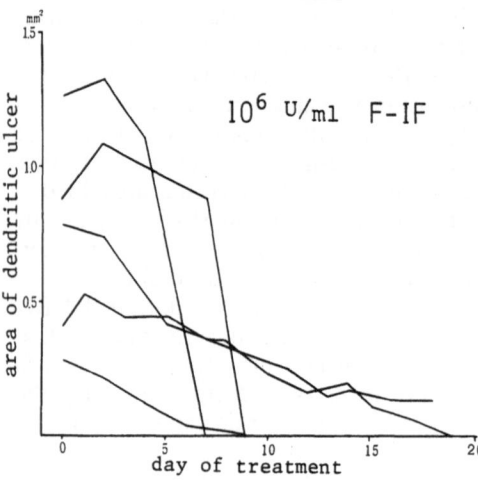

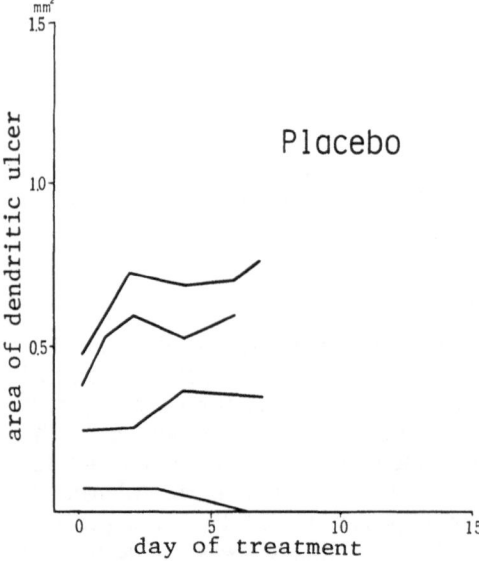

**Fig. 1. a** Results of six cases of dendritic keratitis treated with $10^6$ u/ml FIF assessed by the area of lesion, **b** Four cases treated with placebo

The code was kept by National Institute of Health, Tokyo, and was broken after the results had been evaluated.

Patients were examined every or every other day under a slit lamp microscope after staining the cornea with fluorescein. The dendritic figure was measured by means of a micrometer in Zeiss SM-M slit lamp and an approximate area was calculated in square mm. On the other hand, cure was defined as disappearance of gross staining areas with fluorescein, and evaluation of the effect was expressed in three grades, as good, fair, and poor.

## 2. Animal Experiment

Herpes simplex virus (type 1) isolated from dendritic keratitis and maintained in our laboratory was used. Inoculation to the rabbit cornea was performed by modification of the microtrephination technique of Jones and Al-Hussaini [3] at 17 sites with a viral suspension $1.0 \times 10^7$ PFU/ml. Vials of FIF ($2.8 \times 10^6$ u/ml) and placebo (human albumin) were paired for each rabbit which received FIF in one eye and placebo in the other. One drop (0.01 ml) of the eye lotion was instilled. The investigators were unaware of the identity of the agent being used. All animals were examined once daily for corneal lesions under a slit lamp microscope after staining with 1% rose bengal. Lesions were scored by the criteria of Shiota and associates [10].

## Results

### 1. Clinical Trial

#### a) $10^6$ u/ml FIF vs Placebo

Five patients treated with FIF showed a decrease in the area of lesions and cure was attained in three patients within 10 days and in two patients after 20 days and 36 days of treat-

**Table 1.** Effect of $10^6$ u/ml FIF and placebo on dendritic keratitis

| Effect | good | fair | poor |
|---|---|---|---|
| $10^6$ u/ml FIF | 3 | 1 | 1 |
| placebo | 1 | 0 | 3 |

ment respectively (Fig. 1a). Of four patients who received placebo, one was cured after 7 days, and the other three showed no improvement during 7 to 8 days, and the treatment was changed to IDU (Fig. 1b). Evaluation of the effect was shown in Table 1.

b) $10^6$ u/ml FIF vs $10^3$ u/ml FIF

All six patients in the $10^6$ u/ml FIF group showed a tendency of decrease in the area of lesion. One in the $10^6$ u/ml group and four in the $10^3$ u/ml group showed delayed healing, and they were removed to debridement or

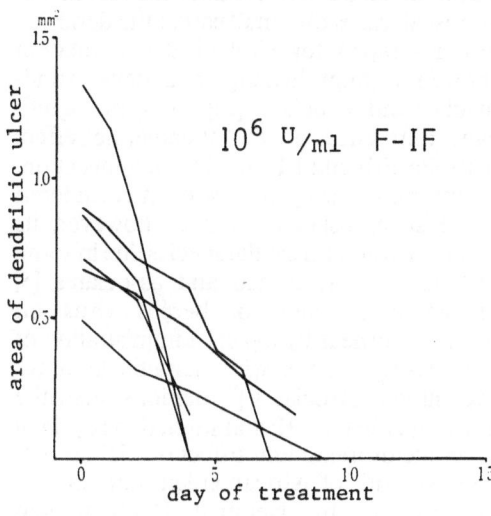

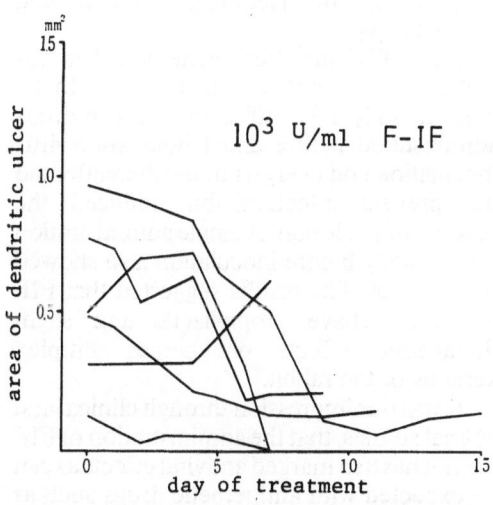

**Fig. 2. a** Results of six cases of dendritic keratitis treated with $10^6$ u/ml FIF assessed by the area of lesion, **b** Six cases treated with $10^3$ u/ml FIF. Double blind study

**Table 2.** Effect of $10^6$ u/ml FIF and $10^3$ u/ml FIF on dendritic keratitis

| Effect | good | fair | poor |
|---|---|---|---|
| $10^6$ u/ml FIF | 5 | 1 | 0 |
| $10^3$ u/ml FIF | 0 | 5 | 1 |

IDU therapy (Fig. 2a, 2b). Evaluation of the effect was shown in Table 2.

## 2. Animal Experiment

Eight rabbits received the eye lotion being tested immediately before and 1 hour after viral inoculation and every 24 hours thereafter. The result of scoring is illustrated in Fig. 3a. All eyes treated with $2.8 \times 10^6$ u/ml FIF exhibited milder clinical manifestations throughout the course as compared with those treated with placebo. Most of the placebo-treated eyes left dense stromal opacities after disappearance of staining areas. In two rabbits treated with only one administration of eye lotion immediately before inoculation, a slight inhibitory effect of FIF upon the lesion was also noted (Fig. 3b).

## Discussion

In our preliminary study, four cases of dendritic keratitis treated with $10^6$ u/ml FIF four times a day showed healing in 8 to 10 days. Therefore, this frequency of application was taken in the present clinical studies. Of four cases received placebo, one showed healing on day 7. This suggests that dendritic keratitis can heal spontaneously in some cases. Except for this case, courses of keratitis were markedly different between the FIF-treated group and the placebo-treated group; in the former, the size of the lesion began to decrease in a few days, and in the latter the lesion continued to progress. The effect was evaluated in three grades, a significant difference was, however, not obtained because of the small number of cases in this trial.

In the second study, six cases which received $10^3$ u/ml FIF showed a tendency of decrease in the area of the lesion, but some took prolonged courses and their treatment was changed to other antiherpetic measures. All six cases treated with $10^6$ u/ml FIF showed a

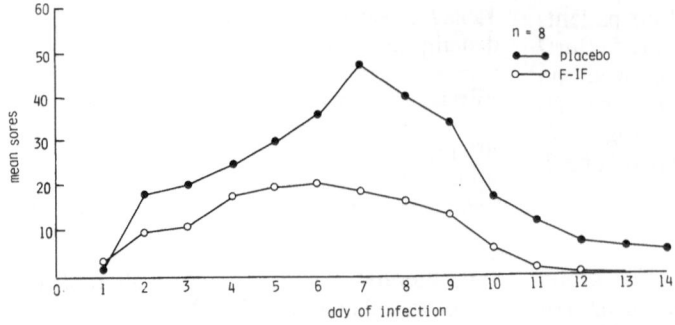

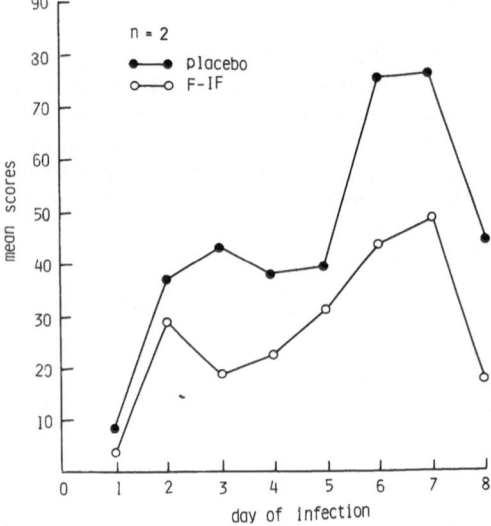

**Fig. 3. a** Results of treatment of herpetic keratitis of the rabbit with $2.8 \times 10^6$ u/ml FIF and placebo determined by mean scores of lesion. Virus inoculation was performed on day 0, and eye drops were administered immediately before and 1 hour after inoculation and every 24 hours thereafter (8 rabbits), **b** A single administration immediately before inoculation (2 rabbits)

favorable response. When evaluation was divided between good and fair, $10^6$ u/ml FIF proved to be more effective than $10^3$ u/ml FIF ($p < 0.05$). It can be concluded that FIF $10^6$ u/ml apparently has a moderate therapeutic effect on dendritic keratitis. FIF $10^3$ u/ml also seemed to inhibit the progress of the dendritic lesion, though slightly.

As for clinical application of interferon in the treatment of dendritic keratitis, Jones and associates [3] reported the necessity of support by minimal wipe debridement, and Sundmacher and associates [10, 11] showed

favorable results following combined thermocautery. The validity of their statement was understood in our trial by the fact that in almost all cases the small part of the dendritic lesion scraped for virological examination showed prompt healing in 2 days. Sundmacher and associates [12] found no significant difference of the therapeutic effect between FIF and LIF in clinical application.

Interferon has generally been considered to be species-specific. Lately, however, its action proved to cross the species line in some instances [2]. Kaufman and associates [5] prevented infection of herpes virus on monkey corneas by topical administration of LIF. Using rabbits with herpetic keratitis, McGill and associates [7] demonstrated the antiviral effect of LIF and studied the optimal schedule of treatment. Effect of LIF on herpetic keratitis of African green monkey was documented by Neumann-Haefelin and associates [9].

As for FIF, the effect on herpetic keratitis of the rabbit has not been documented. In the present study $2.8 \times 10^6$ u/ml FIF eye drops administered before and 1 hour after virus inoculation and every 24 hours thereafter did not prevent infection, but reduced the severity of the lesion. A single administration immediately before inoculation also showed some effect. The results suggested that FIF eye drops have prophylactic and slight therapeutic effects on herpes simplex keratitis of the rabbit.

It was our impression through clinical and animal studies, that the administration of FIF did not have so marked antiviral effects as can be expected with antiherpetic drugs such as idoxuridine and trifluorothymidine. However, there was evidence of accelerated spontaneous recovery of dendritic keratitis following application of FIF.

# References

1. Coster DJ, Falcon MG, Cantell K, Jones BR (1977) Clinical experience of human leucocyte interferon in the management of herpetic keratitis. Trans Ophthalmol Soc UK 97:327–329
2. Desmyter J, Rawls WE, Melnick JL (1968) A human interferon that crosses the species line. Proc Natl Acad Sci USA 59:69–76
3. Jones BR, Al-Hussaini MK (1963) Therapeutic considerations in ocular vaccinia. Trans Ophthalmol Soc UK 83:613–631
4. Jones BR, Coster DJ, Falcon MG, Cantell K (1976) Topical therapy of ulcerative herpetic keratitis with human interferon. Lancet 2:128
5. Kaufman HE, Ellison ED, Centifanto YM (1972) Difference in interferon response and protection from ocular virus infection in rabbits and monkeys. Am J Ophthalmol 74:89–92
6. Kobayashi S (in press) Report of the second international workshop on interferon, New York, April 22, 1979
7. McGill JI, Collins P, Cantell K, Jones BR, Finter NB (1976) Optimal schedules for use of interferon in the corneas of rabbits with herpes simplex keratitis. J Infect Dis (Suppl) 133:A13–A17
8. McGill JI, Cantell K, Collins P, Finter NB, Laird R, Jones BR (1977) Optimal usage of exogenous human interferon for prevention or therapy of herpetic keratitis. Trans Ophthalmol Soc UK 97:324–326
9. Neumann-Haefelin D, Sundmacher R, Sauter B, Karges HE, Manthey KF (1975) Effect of human leucocyte interferon on vaccinia- and herpesvirus infected cell cultures and monkey cornea. Infect Immun 12:148–155
10. Shiota H, Inoue S, Yamane S (1979) Efficacy of acycloguanosine against herpetic ulcers in rabbit cornea. Br J Ophthalmol 63:425–428
11. Sundmacher R, Neumann-Haefelin D, Cantell R (1975) Successful treatment of dendritic keratitis with human leucocyte interferon. Albrecht von Graefes Arch Klin Ophthalmol 201:39–45
12. Sundmacher R, Cantell K, Haug P, Neumann-Haefelin D (1978) Role of debridement and interferon in the treatment of dendritic keratitis. Albrecht von Graefes Arch Klin Ophthalmol 207:77–82
13. Sundmacher R, Cantell K, Skoda R, Hallermann C, Neumann-Haefelin D (1978) Human leucocyte and fibroblast interferon in a combination therapy of dendritic keratitis. Albrecht von Graefes Arch Klin Ophthalmol 208:229–233

## Discussion on the Contribution pp. 409–413

K. Cantell (Helsinki)

Thank you, Dr. Uchida. I think that if you get ten times more potent interferon from the Toray Company your results will be much better.

R. Sundmacher (Freiburg)

I find it quite interesting that you seem to have the same negative therapeutic experiences as Dr. Shiota. Did you use the same interferon?

H. Shiota (Tokushima)

We have been using the same interferon.

Y. Uchida (Tokyo)

We also had the same results as Dr. Shiota's. Forty-eight hours after inoculation, when the lesions had been established, administration of interferon showed no effect. It works mainly for prevention.

R. Sundmacher (Freiburg)

To me it is still not quite absolutely clear whether or not fibroblast interferon has some therapeutic potency of its own – though it can only be a very weak one. We compared fibroblast and leukocyte interferon in a clinical study in a combination therapy with debridement and statistically found no difference between the two interferons. In fact, the fibroblast group looked a bit better. This brings me to the point that we should intensively investigate the proper therapeutic potencies of both interferons, not with the idea of applying interferon as a monotherapy for dendritic keratitis – this would be worse than most of what we have now – but with the idea of better understanding which qualities count most in combination therapies, and which interferon should be preferred.

K. Cantell (Helsinki)

Or maybe different interferons, including immune interferon, will be used together.

H. Shiota (Tokushima)

I just want to make one comment about my work and that of Prof. Uchida. We have been using the same human fibroblast interferon. I started treatment 48 hours after HSV inoculation, which means that the dendrite is clearly established, while Prof. Uchida started treatment 1 to 24 hours after inoculation. He saw either no dendrites or very small ones and the interferon prevented the spreading of HSV to the next cell. However, after 48 hours, when the established lesions were clearly seen, the virus multiplications could not be kept under control by the interferon. Prof. Uchida showed positive results after treating one eye for 1 day, but as he pointed out, the main point is prevention.

Sundmacher, R. (Hrsg.):
Herpetische Augenerkrankungen
© J.F. Bergmann Verlag, München 1981

# Clinical Results of Treatment in Herpes Simplex Ocular Infection (The Effect of Poly I:C on the Inhibition of Ocular Herpes Simplex Virus in Vitro and in Vivo)

A. Romano, R. Stein †, O. Smetana, A. Eylam, M. Weinberg, R. Vulcan, R. Rabinowitz, Tel Aviv

**Key words.** Dendritic keratitis, poly IC

**Schlüsselwörter.** Keratitis dendritica, poly IC

**Summary.** Idoxuridine has long been the standard antiviral chemotherapeutic treatment in cases of epithelial herpes simplex keratitis. During the last few years, additional drugs have been introduced. These are Adenine arabinoside, Trifluorothymidine, and interferon. With IDU, the appearance of resistant virus has been a major problem.

Interferon or inducers of interferon, such as Poly I:C, are considered to be most promising antiviral agents.

Sixty cases with frequent recurrent dendritic keratitis were selected for our research. These patients received Poly I:C treatment and were compared with a control group receiving IDU. The clinical data were compared with laboratory data.

It was found that HSV strains isolated from "primary" infections were more sensitive than those isolated from recurrent infections. No significant changes were found between strains isolated from the same patient during different days of the same recurrence or from different recurrences. There was a high correlation between the minimal inhibitory concentration (MIC) of IDU required for HSV strains in vitro and the response of the patient to IDU treatment. The lysozyme level in tears of patients with HSV eye infection was examined and correlated with the clinical findings and the presence of virus. After termination of treatment with either IDU or Poly I:C, the lysozyme level rose again. Virus was isolated in all 60 patients prior to treatment and a virological follow-up was carried out after initiation of Poly I:C therapy, together with checking of interferon levels and antibody levels in tears and serum. We found that virus isolations failed after a few hours following Poly I:C treatment and there was a definite link between Poly I:C dosage, interferon level in tear fluid, and the so-called refractory state. Fluctuations in tear level of certain immunoglobulins and lysozyme seem to have some determining value as to whether or not one should continue with Poly I:C or interferon therapy.

The increase of IgA and IgG was correlated with dose size and route of administration with Poly I:C. The greatest increase in IgA level occurred when Poly I:C was subconjunctivally administered. Treatment of the infected eye caused a slight enhancement of IgA and IgG antibody levels in the healthy eye. At the end of treatment, 61% of the patients showed a decrease in IgG and 80% of IgA after a 2 week interval.

Our studies will be extended on combinations of Poly I:C and interferon. It may be that these combinations are more advantageous than other kinds of therapy. Interferon, which is difficult to produce in large quantities, should be administered at commencement of treatment in large doses. Poly I:C should then be added as an inducer of interferon whereby the use of initial interferon is reduced and the greatest efficiency is reached.

**Zusammenfassung.** IDU ist lange Zeit das Standard-Virustatikum zur Chemotherapie der Keratitis dendritica gewesen. Insbesondere wegen des Auftretens IDU-resistenter Virusstämme sind in den letzten Jahren einige zusätzliche Virustatika eingeführt worden wie Adeninarabinosid, Trifluorthymidin und Interferon.

Interferon oder Interferon-Induktoren (wie Poly I:C) werden dabei als am erfolgversprechendsten angesehen.

Sechzig Fälle mit häufig rezidivierender Keratitis dendritica erhielten Poly I:C und wurden mit einer IDU-Kontrollgruppe verglichen, wobei klinische Daten mit Laborergebnissen korreliert wurden.

Wir fanden, daß HSV-Stämme, die anläßlich von Ersterkrankungen isoliert wurden, gegenüber IDU empfindlicher waren als Stämme, die anläßlich von Rezidiven isoliert wurden. Stämme, die vom gleichen Patienten während mehrerer Tage im Verlaufe der gleichen Erkrankung isoliert wurden, verhielten sich gleich. Die minimale Hemmkonzentration für HSV-Stämme in vitro korrelierte streng mit dem Ansprechen der jeweiligen Patienten auf die IDU-Therapie. Wir bestimmten auch den Lysozymspiegel in der Tränenflüssigkeit von Herpes-Patienten und korrelierten ihn mit dem klinischen Verlauf und der Anwesenheit isolierbaren Virus. Nach Beendigung der IDU- oder Poly I:C-Behandlung stieg der Lysozym-Spiegel wieder an.

Bei allen 60 Patienten wurde vor Einsetzen der Therapie Virus isoliert, und die virologischen Kontrollen wurden dann unter der Poly I:C-Therapie fortgesetzt. Gleichzeitig bestimmten wir die Interferon- und Antikörperspiegel im Blut und in der Tränenflüssigkeit. Schon wenige Stunden nach Beginn der Poly I:C-Therapie konnten wir kein Virus mehr isolieren; und zwischen der Poly I:C-Dosierung, dem Interferonspiegel in der Tränenflüssigkeit und dem sogenannten Refraktärstadium fanden sich eindeutige Korrelationen. Bewegungen des Lysozym- oder Antikörperspiegels in der Tränenflüssigkeit scheinen einige Bedeutung für die Entscheidung zu haben, wie lange man mit der Poly I:C-Therapie fortfahren sollte.

Ein IgA- und IgG-Anstieg war mit der Poly I:C-Dosis und der Applikationsart korreliert. Den höchsten IgA-Anstieg erzielte man mit subkonjunktivalen Poly I:C-Gaben. Die Behandlung des kranken Auges führte auch im gesunden zu einem geringen Anstieg von IgA und IgG. Innerhalb zweier Wochen nach Behandlungsende zeigte sich dann bei 61% der Patienten ein Abfall des IgG und bei 80% ein Abfall des IgA.

Gegenwärtig studieren wir Kombinationstherapien von Poly I:C mit Interferon. Möglicherweise sind solche Kombinationen erfolgversprechender als alles andere.

Interferon sollte man dabei zu Therapiebeginn in hoher Dosierung geben, danach allmählich Poly I:C hinzufügen und so vielleicht den Bedarf für das schwer erhältliche Interferon reduzieren und dennoch eine optimale therapeutische Wirkung erzielen.

# Keratoplasty

Sundmacher, R. (Hrsg.):
Herpetische Augenerkrankungen
© J.F. Bergmann Verlag, München 1981

# Results of Keratoplasty in Metaherpetic Keratitis

R. Witmer, Zürich

**Key words.** Metaherpetic keratitis, keratoplasty, trifluorothymidine

**Schlüsselwörter.** Keratitis metaherpetica, Keratoplastik, Trifluorthymidin

**Summary.** The comparison of three series of patients treated first by lamellar, second by penetrating keratoplasty without additional treatment, and third with penetrating keratoplasty combined with postoperative treatment with TFT, seems to indicate that much better results may be obtained with the latter combination.

**Zusammenfassung.** Es werden drei Patientengruppen miteinander verglichen. Eine erste Gruppe von 30 Patienten aus den Jahren 1965–1974 wurde wegen einer schweren, z.T. ulzerativen herpetischen Keratitis mit einer lamellären Keratoplastik behandelt. Im Verlaufe der Jahre zeigte sich, daß über 80% der Patienten im Transplantat oder neben dem Transplantat wieder Rückfälle ihrer herpetischen Keratitis durchgemacht haben. Entsprechend waren die funktionellen Resultate in dieser Gruppe sehr schlecht.

Aufgrund dieser schlechten Erfahrungen mit der lamellären Keratoplastik wurden im Verlaufe des gleichen Zeitabschnittes von 1965–1974 60 Patienten mit perforierender Keratoplastik behandelt, wobei sich zeigte, daß auch bei diesen Patienten die Zahl der Rezidive über 50% betrug. Die funktionellen Resultate waren aber doch wesentlich besser als in der Gruppe mit lamellärer Keratoplastik.

Eine dritte Gruppe von nur 22 Patienten wurde während der letzten 3 Jahre mit einer perforierenden Keratoplastik behandelt und erhielt gleichzeitig postoperativ prophylaktisch während 3–12 Monaten Trifluorothymidin 3× täglich 1 Tropfen einer 1%igen Lösung. Unter diesen Patienten ist bis jetzt nur in 2 Fällen ein Rezidiv der Keratitis aufgetreten.

Es scheint also, daß die lamelläre Keratoplastik eine schlechte Behandlungsmethode der tiefen

Keratitis herpetica ist, die perforierende Keratoplastik ergibt bessere Resultate, es ist möglich, daß eine konsequente prophylaktische postoperative Behandlung mit Trifluorothymidin die Resultate noch weiter verbessern wird.

Keratoplasty in metaherpetic keratitis is still indicated despite the use of potent virostatic drugs. It may be done for functional reasons, or for therapeutic reasons in case of descemetocele or spontaneous perforation, and it may even be done in rare cases for cosmetical reasons (Table 1).

There is still some controversy whether lamellar or penetrating keratoplasty should be performed. In our hands lamellar grafts have done so poorly during the last 15 years, that we have almost completely abandoned this technique. But the recurrence rate in perforating keratoplasty was very high too. We therefore started treating all our patients with transplants for herpetic keratitis with Trifluorothymidine (TFT) postoperatively (Bigar).

I would like to compare three series of patients suffering from severe herpetic keratitis and treated with either lamellar or penetrating keratoplasty without additional vivostatic treatment, and a third group with

**Table 1.** Indication for lamellar and penetrating keratoplasties in herpetic keratitis

| indication | lamellar | penetrating | total |
|---|---|---|---|
| functional | 3 | 12 | 15 |
| therapeutical ulcerative keratitis | 20 | 35 | 55 |
| descemetocele spont. perforation | 7 | 13 | 20 |
| total | 30 | 60 | 90 |

**Table 2.** Number of lamellar ☐ and penetrating ▨ keratoplasties in herpetic keratitis

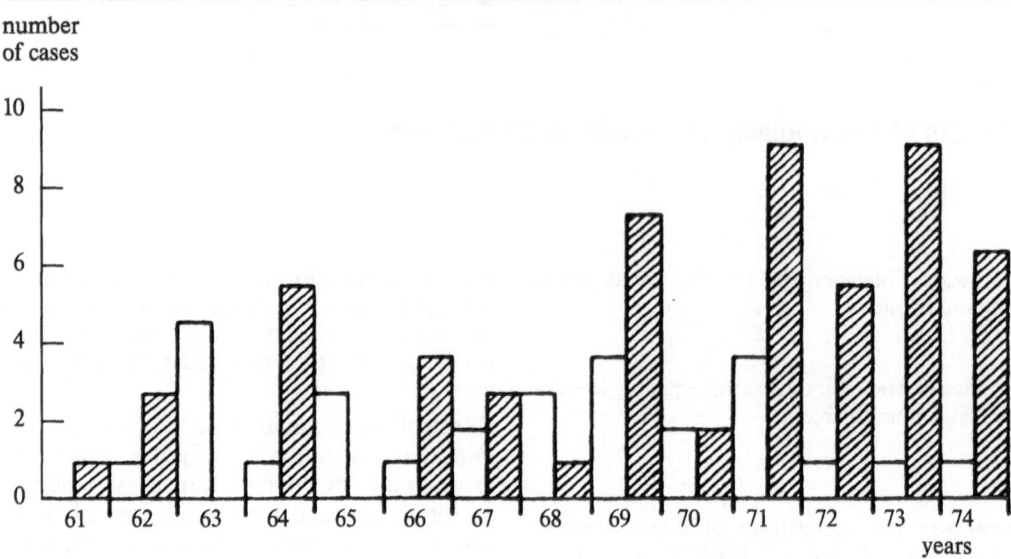

penetrating transplants and postoperative treatment with Trifluorothymidine.

**Lamellar Keratoplasty**

For many years, we treated some of our patients with herpetic keratitis by lamellar keratoplasties, since we thought that this procedure was less dangerous and a penetration of virus into the deeper parts of the eye would not occur during surgery. But in quite a few cases with either large descemetoceles or spontaneous perforation in an active phase of the disease, lamellar grafts were not possible and penetrating transplants therefore had to be performed. During these approximately 15 years we had the definite impression, that our lamellar grafts were doing rather poorly compared with the results of penetrating keratoplasties. It is for this reason that the number of penetrating keratoplasties increased steadily and lamellar grafts were done less frequently (Table 2).

Among the 30 patients with lamellar grafts the final number of recurrences after several years of observation was very high (Table 3). Of 30 eyes 26 (87%) operated upon developed a new dendritic ulcer or deep stromal keratitis. Most of these recurrences occurred within 1 year after the operation [1]. Many of these patients had been treated with IDU immediately after the onset of symptoms. Of these eyes 23 had been operated either for

**Table 3.** Number of recurrences and functional results of lamellar keratoplasties for herpetic keratitis

| indication | recurrences | | | functional results | |
|---|---|---|---|---|---|
| | | − | + | good | poor |
| functional | 3 | 0 | 3 | 0 | 3 |
| therapeutical | | | | | |
| ulcerative keratitis | 20 | 4 | 16 | 5 | 15 |
| descemetocele | 7 | 0 | 7 | 3 | 4 |
| total | 30 | 4 | 26 (87%) | 8 | 22 |

observation time 3–14 years

420

**Table 4.** Number of recurrences and functional results of penetrating keratoplasties for herpetic keratitis

| indication | recurrences | − | + | functional results good | poor |
|---|---|---|---|---|---|
| functional | 12 | 7 | 5 | 8 | 4 |
| therapeutical | | | | | |
|   ulcerative keratitis | 35 | 12 | 23 | 16 | 19 |
|   descemetocele or | | | | | |
|   spont. perforation | 13 | 9 | 4 | 10 | 3 |
| total | 60 | 28 | 32 (53%) | 34 | 26 |

observation time 3–14 years

therapeutical or tectonic (descemetocele) reasons. It was therefore very likely that not all virus infected material had been removed by the surgical procedure. The final functional results were very disappointing: 12 grafts were more or less opaque with poor vision and only eight remained clear with improved visual acuity.

Our clinical impression therefore was confirmed by this analysis of our data.

## Penetrating Keratoplasty

During the same time period 60 eyes were operated for a severe herpetic keratitis by penetrating keratoplasty. Again the indication for surgery was mostly therapeutical or tectonic (descemetoceles and spontaneous perforation, n = 21) and a few for optical reasons (n = 7). The number of recurrences in this group of patients was 32 (53%) despite intensive treatment in most cases with IDU (Table 4). 23 occurred during the first year after the operation.

Apart from these herpetic recurrences the eyes with penetrating keratoplasties suffered a number of other complications, like allograft reactions in 13 cases and secondary glaucoma in ten cases.

The final functional results were a little better than in the previous group: 26 were cloudy, with poor vision and 34 had improved vision. Among the 12 eyes operated upon for optical reasons only eight achieved better vision after the operation. We could not demonstrate a significant difference of the recurrence rate among lamellar and perforating keratoplasties performed during an active ulcerative stage of the disease or during a clinically inactive stage.

## Penetrating Keratoplasty With Additional Postoperative Treatment With TFT

During the last 3 years we have been treating all our patients with penetrating keratoplasty after herpes during the postoperative period with an additional local treatment of TFT 1%

**Table 5.** Results of penetrating keratoplasty in herpetic keratitis with postoperative treatment with Trifluorothymidine

| indication | recurrence keratitis | iritis | functional result good | poor |
|---|---|---|---|---|
| functional | 8 | | 8 | 0 |
| therapeutical | 14 | 2 | 2 | 14 | 0 |
| total | 22 | 2 (10%) | | |

observation time 1–3 years

eye drops three times daily over a period from 3–12 months. The number of patients is still small (22), and the time of observation is short (maximal 2 years), but the results so far are very encouraging. Only two patients have experienced a definite herpetic recurrence. Two patients suffered from a rather severe iritis, which was most probably herpetic in nature, but the grafts remained clear. All recurrences (keratitis and iritis) healed within a short time by increased topical medication with TFT and steroids. Functional results, therefore, are very good so far in this last group (Table 5).

## Discussion

The results of these three groups seem to show, that lamellar keratoplasty is absolutely unsatisfactory, but penetrating transplants too may undergo recurrences in a very high percentage (53%). It seems, however, that penetrating keratoplasty in combination with postoperative prophylactic treatment with TFT yields much better final results. We must admit, that we have no comparable group of patients treated with lamellar grafts and additional TFT. Furthermore, we have seen that in two patients apparently a herpetic iritis occurred without keratitis despite this treatment. The spreading of virus particles into the uvea could not be inhibited or abolished by the drug.

As far as final functional results are concerned, they turn out to be a little better than the rate of recurrences. This would indicate that a recurrence in a lamellar or penetrating transplant does not necessarily lead to complete cloudiness of the graft and loss of vision. In quite a number of cases, topical treatment with either IDU or TFT in combination with steroids may prevent opacification and therefore improve vision.

## Reference

1. Bigar F (1979) Adv Ophthalmol 38:110–115

## Discussion on the Contribution pp. 419–422

D. Epstein (Stockholm)
Prof. Witmer, you mentioned that you use TFT for a long period of time after the operation, but you didn't give us any indication as to what guidelines you have for how long it should be applied and why.

R. Witmer (Zürich)
We give TFT 1% three times daily as a routine for at least 3 months, preferably longer, up to 6 months until it is time to remove the suture. If, however, we find the already described signs of epitheliopathy, we reduce the dosage or stop it.

D. Epstein (Stockholm)
But some you have treated for a year, you said. Is that because the sutures were left in for a year?

R. Witmer (Zürich)
We gave some patients TFT once or twice a day over 1 year. We know that the recurrence rate is higher during the 1st year after keratoplasty.

A. Korra (Alexandria)
What is the best time to intervene surgically and would TFT affect the viability of the graft? Would it affect post-operative wound-healing if you give it immediately after operation?

R. Witmer (Zürich)
We prefer to operate on a quiet eye. We did not have the impression that TFT has any effect on the survival of the graft. The wound healing was normal under topical administration of TFT.

If we have to operate during an active stage of the disease because of a perforating ulcer, we give TFT immediately after the operation.

C. Kok van Alphen (Leyden)
I saw those slides with the precipitates on the endothelium. Are you sure that it was herpes iritis? Couldn't it have been a rejection, or a combination of both?

R. Witmer (Zürich)
The typical allograft reaction always leads to a swelling of the stroma and one can see a line of lymphocytes precipitates on the endothelium. If the cornea remains clear and we see many pigmented precipitates all over the corneal endothelium, then they must stem from the iris. Therefore it is very likely that we are dealing with a herpetic iritis.

B.R. Jones (London)
Our experience with lamellar grafts for herpetic keratitis has been just like yours, and for a long time we had given it up because of the high incidence of recurrent stromal disease. So far as the penetrating grafting was concerned, it seemed to us that the effect of excising the diseased stroma had, in fact, moved the patient from being at a high risk of recurrence to being in a category much the same as a patient coming with just an epithelial ulceration –

rather than with epithelial ulceration on stromal disease. So perforating keratoplasty did seem to improve the prognosis for recurrences. We had been in the habit of using IDU after grafting for as long as we were giving steroids, and over a period of many years, we became aware of the fact that we were inducing a tremendous amount of damaging disease in the epithelium leading to vascularization and other problems in the graft. Therefore, for many years it has been our policy not to use antivirals post-operatively after grafting except when the patient is on a heavy regimen of steroid therapy. In this way, we feel sure that we have reduced the complications that come from toxicity of antivirals, and I feel very concerned about the widespread use of trifluorothymidine over a long period of time after grafting because, I feel sure, if it becomes popular, it is at risk of producing a harvest of toxicity. I would like to ask you what you mean by "prophylaxis"? Do you mean a period of treatment that deals with, say, residual herpes virus in stromal keratitis, because it is not technically possible to do a complete excision? In other words, a shortish course of treatment; or do you mean a continued blanket of antiviral cover over a long period of months or years? I think it is *that* concept which gets people in our part of the world into a lot of trouble.

R. Witmer (Zürich)
We have not done any prophylactic treatment with IDU in former series of penetrating keratoplasties. We therefore have not seen proliferation of blood vessels. The most dangerous period is the time of the removal of the suture, which is normally 6 months after the operation. If we get over that stage without complications we reduce and finally stop topical administration of TFT.

I would like to stress, however, that we treat all our patients with topical steroids as well. Usually three times daily one drop of dexamethasone 1%, after 2 months only twice daily, and after 4 months once daily until the removal of the sutures.

H. E. Kaufman (New Orleans)
Barrie Jones told me some time ago about some of his complications using antivirals, specifically IDU. My experience has been identical to Dr. Witmer's in regard to keratoplasty after herpes. The lamellar keratoplasty patients have done poorly and the penetrating keratoplasty patients have done well. It has proven to be a mistake to use steroids after surgery without an antiviral cover. If abused, trifluorothymidine can produce toxicity, but we've seen no major problems with post-keratoplasty patients.

Sundmacher, R. (Hrsg.):
Herpetische Augenerkrankungen
© J.F. Bergmann Verlag, München 1981

# Penetrating Keratoplasty for Herpes Simplex Keratitis

C. Foster, Boston

**Key words.** Herpetic keratitis, keratoplasty

**Schlüsselwörter.** Herpeskeratitis, Keratoplastik

**Summary.** Eighty-two transplants in 61 eyes of 58 patients with various forms of herpetic corneal disease were analyzed. Corneal transplantation for herpes simplex keratitis in eyes that were not heavily vascularized, nor actively inflamed, nor actively ulcerating was highly successful. This was also true for HSK eyes with chronic or recurrent immune disciform edema. Penetrating keratoplasty for re-establishment of the integrity of the globe after HSK stromal ulceration and corneal perforation was routinely associated ultimately with graft clouding. Management of such perforations or impending perforations with lamellar patch grafts or with cyanoacrylate tissue adhesive, with later penetrating keratoplasty for visual rehabilitation was highly successful. HSK with concomitant sicca syndrome, atopy or ocular rosacea seemed to be associated with an especially poor prognosis, with a particularly high incidence of postoperative persistent epithelial defects and graft clouding due to surface failure. The preoperative status of donor corneal epithelium did not affect this complication incidence.

**Zusammenfassung.** Die perforierende Keratoplastik nach Herpes simplex-Keratitis ist umstritten und wohl auch nur mäßig erfolgreich gewesen. Frühere Nachuntersuchungen von Transplantaten bei Herpespatienten an der Massachusetts Eye and Ear Infirmary zeigten an Hand von 20 Fällen, die zwischen 1960 und 1968 operiert worden waren und mindestens 2 Jahre nachuntersucht werden konnten, nur eine 40%-Erfolgsquote, wenn man diese nach der Klarheit der Transplantate beurteilte. Diese durchschnittliche Erfolgsquote war auch kaum davon beeinflußt, wie aktiv die Erkrankung präoperativ war und welche Vaskularisation bestand. Eine spätere Analyse von 20 Fällen, die zwischen 1970 und 1972 operiert wurden, berichtete dann über eine 80%-Erfolgsquote, wobei dem Vaskularisationsgrad, der entzündlichen Aktivität und dem Umstand, ob es sich um ein erstes oder um ein Re-Transplantat handelte, eindeutige prognostische Bedeutung zukam. Diese verbesserte Erfolgsquote wurde auf eine subtilere Operationstechnik und bessere postoperative Nachsorge zurückgeführt.

Wir analysierten 60 perforierende Keratoplastiken, die von 1970–1978 an der Massachusetts Eye and Ear Infirmary nach Herpeskeratitis operiert und mindestens 2 Jahre nachuntersucht worden waren. Unsere Ergebnisse stimmen prinzipiell mit obigem Bericht überein; wir möchten aber noch einige Aspekte vertiefen und besonders betonen. Zusätzlich zu der Analyse von präoperativen prognostischen Faktoren und zur Evaluierung der Bedeutung prä-, intra- und postoperativer Therapie, waren wir auch an den Langzeitkomplikationen wie Katarakt, Glaukom und zystoidem Makulaödem interessiert, die trotz eines klaren Transplantates zu einem funktionell blinden Auge führen können. Außerdem haben wir nach möglichen Verbindungen mit gewissen HLA-Phänotypen (insbesondere auch DR) und der Wahrscheinlichkeit einer unabweisbaren Immunreaktion geschaut. Wir fanden, daß 100% aller Transplantate, die in klinisch ruhigen Augen und nicht-vaskularisierten Hornhäuten durchgeführt wurden, erfolgreich waren. 50% aller Transplantate, die in stark vaskularisierten Hornhäuten eingenäht wurden, erlitten eine Abstoßungsreaktion mit Transplantateintrübung, dies auch, wenn das Auge zum Operationszeitpunkt „ruhig" war. 75% aller wegen drohender Perforation operierten Augen entwickelten eine Abstoßungsreaktion mit Transplantateintrübung. Wenn man bei drohender Perforation zunächst mit Cyanoacrylatklebern oder lamellären Transplantaten arbeitete und die perforierende Keratoplastik erst nach Beruhigung des Auges durchführte, so war die Prognose erheblich besser. 50% der Re-Keratoplastiken bei Herpespatienten erlitten vielfache Immunreaktionen mit Transplantateintrübungen. 60% aller Augen, die im akuten Entzündungszustand – gewöhnlich wegen tiefer einschmelzender Infiltrate – operiert wurden, hatten nach 2 Jahren noch funktionsfähige klare Transplantate.

Einige Begleiterkrankungen gestalten die Prognose für ein erfolgreiches Transplantat erheblich schlechter. Hierzu gehören Atopien, Sicca-Syndrome und Akne rosacea. 100% solcher Patienten mit erheblichen Begleiterkrankungen erlitten Immunreaktionen mit Transplantateintrübungen spätestens nach 2 Jahren.

Ob die Prognose in solchen Fällen besser ist, wenn man – wie früher einmal vorgeschlagen – frisches Spendermaterial mit lebensfähigem Epithel transplantiert, haben wir in dieser Studie nicht ermittelt. Dies mag theoretisch bei Patienten nützlich sein, die kein normales peripheres Epithel haben, von dem man eine schnelle und normale Wiederbedeckung des Transplantates erwarten kann. In solchen Fällen würden wir eine ABO-Typisierung des Spenders und Empfängers empfehlen, um hiermit die Möglichkeit einer epithelialen Abstoßungsreaktion zu reduzieren. Meistens wird es aber empfehlenswerter sein, die Antigenmenge durch Entfernung des Spenderepithels zu reduzieren.

Bei den Fällen mit schlechterer Prognose scheint ein ganz wesentlicher Faktor für das funktionelle Spätergebnis die Erfahrung des Ophthalmochirurgen mit der postoperativen Therapie zu sein, was insbesondere die Anwendung von Corticosteroiden, Mydriatika und antiinflammatorischen Substanzen, die nicht zu den Steroiden gehören, umfaßt.

Herpes simplex keratitis (HSK) is the leading cause of corneal blindness in developed countries, and in the United States it is the most common cause of unilateral blindness (Dawson, 1976; Valenton, 1977). Many patients with HSK ultimately receive corneal transplants for visual restoration, for re-establishment of the integrity of the globe after ulceration and perforation, or for removal of antigenic/neoantigenic material from the cornea which has served as a stimulus for persistant or repeated immunologic inflammatory episodes of keratitis. While the prognosis for successful outcome after penetrating keratoplasty for herpetic keratitis improved during the period 1960–1972 (Langston, 1975), certain forms of herpetic keratitis appear to be particularly susceptible to graft failure after penetrating keratoplasty. It is the purpose of this paper to report our analysis of penetrating keratoplasties in patients with various forms of herpetic corneal disease.

**Methods and Materials**

Eighty-two transplants in 61 eyes of 58

patients with various forms of herpetic corneal disease performed at the Massachusetts Eye and Ear Infirmary between January 1970, and January 1978 form the basis of this report. The average length of time post keratoplasty at the time of analysis was 4.3 years. All other cases which could not be analyzed completely because of inadequate information or because of a postoperative follow up period of less than 2 years were excluded. The basic technique of penetrating keratoplasty was similar in all eyes with respect to use of surgical microscope, suturing technique, etc. Sutures were either 23 µ monofiliment nylon (interrupted or continuous) or 9–0 silk (interrupted). These variables, along with graft size, status of donor epithelium (intact or absent), intraoperative synechial sweep, intraoperative use of steroids and mydriatics and adjunctive surgery (lens extraction, vitrectomy) were the intraoperative study parameters. Preoperative study parameters included history (ocular, including ocular surface status, intraocular inflammation, previous graft, previous ulceration/perforation, and glaucoma history/and general medical history, including atopy), signs of sicca syndrome or ocular rosacea, corneal status (inflammation, vascularization, ulceration, perforation, disciform edema). Postoperative study parameters included postoperative medical management (topical and systemic steroids, mydriatics, non-steroidal anti-inflammatory agents, antiviral agents, anti-glaucoma medication) and outcome parameters (graft clarity, visual acuity, recurrence of HSK, graft rejection episodes, cataract, glaucoma, retinal detachment, cystoid macular edema).

In the data analysis each transplant was treated as a separate case. To determine whether or not certain outcomes were independent of preoperative status, operative technique, or postoperative management, two-way contingency tables were formed. One of two analyses was then performed. If the minimum expected value in any cell of the contingency table was greater than or equal to 5, the Chi-square test (with Yates' continuity correction for $2 \times 2$ tables) was used. If the expected value in any cell of the contingency table was less than 5, Fisher's exact test of independence was used. If the probability of either test was less than 0.05, the test was judged significant at the 5% level of confidence and the outcome (e.g. graft clarity) was judged *not* independent of the condition examined (e.g. corneal perforation).

## Results

The outcomes of the 82 transplants were sorted into two categories: cloudy graft or clear graft. Table 1 shows the overall percentage of clear grafts in this series, as well as the percentage of clear grafts in various preoperative categories. Successful outcome, in terms of clear transplant, was achieved in a very high percentage of HSK patients with either chronic or recurrent immune (disciform) edema or in HSK patients with quiet, nonvascularized, nonulcerating scarred corneas. Deep, extensive vascularization, active stromal ulceration, and/or active inflammation at the time of surgery were each associated with a significantly worse long range prognosis. The most striking example of poor prognosis associated with preoperative ocular status is seen in the 16 corneas which received penetrating keratoplasties for perforations. None of these grafts were clear 2 to 8 years after transplant. The operations were successful in re-establishing the integrity of the perforated, inflamed, ulcerating corneas. And some of these transplants remained clear for many months (21 months in one case); but at the time of our analysis all were cloudy. Repeat grafts for vision failed in 93% of these cases. Equally striking was the finding for per-

forated eyes that were managed initially with lamellar patch grafting or with cyanoacrylate tissue adhesive with subsequent penetrating keratoplasty 6 to 24 months after the ocular inflammation had subsided. 11 of the 13 penetrating grafts performed in eyes managed in this way were clear at the time of our analysis.

Patients who had sicca syndrome, atopy (especially eczema), and/or ocular rosacea in addition to HSK appeared to do less well than patients without these concomitant diseases. The development of postoperative persistent epithelial defects in these patients was particularly troublesome. The P values for the Chi-squared and for Fisher's exact test performed on the data sorted into the contingency tables for graft clarity are shown in Table 2. The number of patients in the sicca syndrome, atopy and rosacea categories is small, and the P value does not reach significance at the 5% confidence level. The trend, however, is clear. The Chi-squared P values emphasize the difference in prognosis for patients grafted acutely for corneal perforation compared to those who are managed with glue or with patch grafting, with subsequent penetrating keratoplasty in the quiescent state. Similarly, there is a significantly better prognosis for patients with either disciform HSK or with quiet scars as compared to other forms of HSK (with active inflammation, ulceration and deep, extensive vascularization).

Table 3 contains the contingency table for graft clarity versus operative technique. We

**Table 1.** Percentage of clear grafts after penetrating keratoplasty for HSK

| Preoperative ocular status | Percentage of clear grafts |
|---|---|
| All categories, combined | 39% |
| Noninflammed, nonulcerating, nonvascularized | 90% |
| Disciform edema | 80% |
| Deep, extensive vascularization | 35% |
| Active inflammation | 15% |
| Active ulceration | 15% |
| Sicca syndrome | 11% |
| Ocular rosacea | 11% |
| Atopy | 10% |
| Perforation | 0% |
| Perforation/Integrity restored by penetrating graft: | |
|     subsequent penetrating graft for vision | 7% |
| Perforation/Integrity restored by tissue adhesive or patch graft: | |
|     subsequent penetrating graft for vision | 85% |

**Table 2.** Contingency tables for test of independence between preoperative ocular status and graft clarity

| Preoperative ocular status | Graft | | Test | P Value |
|---|---|---|---|---|
| | Cloudy | Clear | | |
| Active stromal ulceration | 23 | 4 | $X^2$ | p < 0.005 |
| No stromal ulceration | 27 | 28 | | |
| Perforation | 16 | 0 | $X^2$ | p < 0.001 |
| No perforation | 34 | 32 | | |
| Perforation/Glue or patch graft | 2 | 11 | Fisher | p < 0.0001 |
| Perforation | 16 | 0 | | |
| Perforation/Glue or patch graft | 2 | 11 | Fisher | p < 0.01 |
| Perforation/PK | 5 | 1 | | |
| Sicca syndrome | 8 | 1 | Fisher | p = 0.08 |
| No sicca syndrome | 42 | 31 | | |
| Atopy | 9 | 1 | Fisher | p = 0.08 |
| No atopy | 41 | 31 | | |
| Ocular rosacea | 8 | 1 | Fisher | p = 0.08 |
| No ocular rosacea | 42 | 31 | | |
| Intraocular inflammation | 42 | 17 | $X^2$ | p < 0.005 |
| No intraocular inflammation | 8 | 15 | | |
| Aphakic | 4 | 3 | Fisher | p = 1.000 (N.S.) |
| Phakia | 46 | 29 | | |
| Previous transplant | 20 | 6 | $X^2$ | p = 0.08 |
| No previous transplant | 30 | 26 | | |
| Previous rejection | 11 | 3 | $X^2$ | p = 0.24 |
| No previous rejection | 39 | 29 | | |

**Table 3.** Test for independence between operative technique and graft clarity

| Operative technique | Graft | | Test | P Value |
|---|---|---|---|---|
| | Cloudy | Clear | | |
| No intra-op steroids | 27 | 19 | $X^2$ | 0.8023 |
| Intra-op steroids | 23 | 13 | | |
| No intra-op dilatation | 31 | 16 | $X^2$ | 0.3993 |
| Intra-op dilatation | 19 | 16 | | |
| No intra-op synechial sweep | 27 | 21 | $X^2$ | 0.4165 |
| Intra-op synechial sweep | 23 | 11 | | |
| Donor epithelium off | 34 | 20 | $X^2$ | 0.7844 |
| Donor epithelium on | 16 | 12 | | |
| No lens extraction | 35 | 28 | $X^2$ | 0.1179 |
| Lens extraction | 15 | 4 | | |
| No vitrectomy | 38 | 31 | $X^2$ | 0.0268 |
| vitrectomy | 12 | 1 | | |

**Table 4.** Test for independence between postoperative management and graft clarity

| Postop management | Graft | | Test | P Value |
|---|---|---|---|---|
| | Cloudy | Clear | | |
| Routine topical steroids | 7 | 8 | $X^2$ | 0.3350 |
| Intense topical steroids | 21 | 24 | | |
| No systemic steroids | 21 | 18 | $X^2$ | 0.3012 |
| Systemic steroids | 29 | 14 | | |
| No mydriatics | 7 | 2 | Fisher | 0.4711 |
| Mydriatics | 43 | 30 | | |

were unable to show any significant effect of the various intraoperative parameters listed, with the exception of vitrectomy. We found no significant correlation between graft size (7–9 mm) or suture type on graft clarity. No postoperative management techniques were shown to have a statistically significant effect (Table 4).

Thirty-eight of the 82 cases (46%) had at least one episode of transplant rejection. Twenty-seven of these 38 cases (71% of all eyes experiencing at least one rejection episode) eventually had cloudy grafts due to rejection. Nine grafts were hazy at the time of our analysis due to surface failure and 13 were cloudy because of endothelial failure that could not definitely be ascribed to rejection. One graft was cloudy due to damage from recurrent HSK (Table 5). All conditions analyzed in the preoperative, operative and postoperative parameters appeared to be independent of the frequency of graft rejection episodes, surface failure or endothelial failure of unknown cause. In particular, our data do not support the notion that use of fresh donor corneas with intact epithelium reduces the incidence of postoperative persistent epithelial defects in patients with HSK.

Although the data do not reach statistical significance, there is nearly a 2 : 1 incidence of rejection in our HSK patients who had previously rejected a transplant, compared to those without previous rejection (Table 2). The incidence of recurrent infectious HSK in corneal transplants in this series was 6.1% (five of the 82 cases).

Table 6 shows the concomitant ocular problems in patients with clear transplant but with visual acuity less than 6/6. Cataract, glaucoma and cystoid macular edema were the causes of decreased vision in these cases.

**Table 5.** Cause of graft clouding in 50 transplants

| Cause | Number of cases |
|---|---|
| Endothelial rejection | 27 |
| Endothelial failure not definitely ascribable to rejection | 13 |
| Surface failure | 9 |
| Recurrent HSK | 1 |

**Table 6.** Concommitant ocular pathology in patients with clear transplants but with visual acuity less than 6/6

| Ocular pathology | Number of cases | |
|---|---|---|
| | Visual acuity | |
| | 6/9–6/24 | 6/30–6/120 |
| Cataract | 8 | 3 |
| Glaucoma | 5 | – |
| Cystoid macular edema | 5 | – |

Twenty-nine of the 32 eyes with clear grafts had visual acuity of 6/24 or better.

## Discussion

The analysis of questions as complex as multifactoral effects on outcome of a surgical procedure, performed on many patients (each with a unique preoperative ocular status) by several different surgeons, is difficult. We are currently attempting to compose a more sophisticated computer program capable of performing multivariate analysis on our data. The data are imperfect, however. For example, the preoperative sensation thresholds of the ocular surface (conjunctiva and peripheral cornea) and tear secretion levels may be important prognostic factors, especially regarding development of persistent epithelial defects postoperatively. But we were rarely able to obtain such data from the medical record.

Results of the analysis of these cases, nonetheless, suggest that certain factors are associated with eventual graft failure after penetrating keratoplasty for HSK, while other factors or constellations of factors appear to be associated with a more favorable outcome. We find that corneal transplantation for HSK in eyes that are not heavily vascularized, nor actively inflamed, nor actively ulcerating is highly successful. In eyes with chronic or recurrent immune, disciform, HSK but without significant intraocular inflammation or vascularization, corneal transplantation was also very successful, in terms of clear grafts, good visual acuity, and cessation of the episodes of disciform edema.

Our results also suggest that penetrating keratoplasty for re-establishment of the integrity of the globe after HSK stromal ulceration and corneal perforation may not be the ideal approach if visual restoration is also a goal. Lamellar patch grafting or cyanoacrylate gluing of perforations, with prolonged convalescent periods to allow cessation of all inflammation, followed by penetrating keratoplasty was a much more successful approach in our series.

Although the data do not reach statistical significance, the trend suggesting poorer prognosis in HSK patients who also have sicca syndrome, atopy, or ocular rosacea is clear. And we wish to emphasize that in our clinical experience these diseases set the stage of potential additional problems after corneal transplantations for HSK, with persistent epithelial defect and eventual graft clouding secondary to surface failure the major complications. Aggressive management of these concomitant diseases (as was done in the 3 successful cases in this series) is important.

Data analysis of the effect of the various intraoperative and postoperative management techniques was the most unsatisfactory part of this study because of the multivariate nature of the relationships. Our clinical impression is that intraoperative systemic and subconjunctival steroid, subconjunctival mydriatic cocktail injection, lysis of synechiae, and aggressive steroid, mydriatic and non-steroidal anti-inflammatory therapy post-operatively are important management techniques in poor prognosis cases with synechiae and vascular instability and extreme intraoperative and postoperative inflammation. The data analysis in this report does not show a dependence of outcome on these factors. We will await with great interest the results of the multivariate analysis of this question.

We are able to state, on the basis of results presented here, that the development of a persistant epithelial defect postoperatively did not depend upon whether donor epithelium was present on the transplant tissue. This might be an important finding if the concept of reducing foreign antigenic stimulus by removal of epithelium from corneal grafts (particularly in patients at higher risk for transplant rejection) were supported by definitive evidence that such a reduction is associated with a decreased incidence of rejection episodes. At the very least, however, the surgeon who believes no normal peripheral recipient corneal epithelium capable of resurfacing a graft in an HSK patients exists, and who, therefore, wishes to transplant healthy donor epithelium with the graft, should probably not transplant across the ABO barrier. ABO antigens are extremely potent transplant antigens, and corneal epithelium is rich in them [2]. Epithelial rejection with development of a persistent epithelial defect in a case like that just described would clearly negate the surgeon's original intention.

**Acknowledgment.** Supported in part by Grant EY03063 (Foster) from the National Institute of Health. Reprint request to Doctor Foster, 20 Staniford Street, Boston, MA, 02114 USA.

# References

1. Dawson CR, Togni B (1976) Herpes simplex eye infections: Clinical manifestations, pathogenesis, and management. Surv Ophthalmol 21:121-135
2. Foster CS, Allansmith MR (1979) Lack of blood group antigen A on human corneal endothelium. Am J Ophthalmol 87:165-170
3. Langston RHS, Pavan-Langston D (1975) Penetrating keratoplasty for herpetic keratitis: Decision-making and management. Int Ophthalmol Clin 154:125-140
4. Valenton MJ, Tan R, Abendanio, Nievera L (1978) Causes of corneal ulceration. Phil J Ophthalmol 10:64-69

Sundmacher, R. (Hrsg.):
Herpetische Augenerkrankungen
© J.F. Bergmann Verlag, München 1981

# Keratoplastik bei Herpes corneae. Vergleich zwischen klinischem und histopathologischem Befund an 100 Augen

H. Knöbel, E.N. Hinzpeter, G.O.H. Naumann, Hamburg

**Key words.** Herpetic keratitis, keratoplasty, histopathology

**Schlüsselwörter.** Herpeskeratitis, Keratoplastik, Histopathologie

**Summary.** One hundred corneal buttons obtained during penetrating keratoplasty for sequelae of herpetic disease were examined histologically and the findings compared with the preoperative clinical interpretation of "activity". In one third of the so-called inactive chronic corneal scars of quiet and clinically non-inflamed eyes, definite signs of a chronic keratitis were found histologically. The histological diagnosis is, therefore, more important for evaluating the prognosis of keratoplasty in herpetic disease.

**Zusammenfassung.** Die klinischen präoperativen Befunde bei 100 Augen mit herpetischer Keratitis wurden mit den histologischen Diagnosen verglichen. Dabei ließ sich feststellen, daß in ⅓ der Augen, die klinisch eine „inaktive" Narbe zeigten, histologisch deutliche Zeichen einer chronischen Keratitis nachzuweisen waren. Der histopathologische Befund ist somit aufschlußreicher für die „Aktivität" des Herpes corneae und sollte eher als der präoperative klinische Befund genommen werden, als prognostisch wichtiger Faktor für die Auswertung der Ergebnisse bei perforierender Keratoplastik bei dieser Erkrankung.

## Einleitung

Humane Herpes simplex-Viren stellen in Mitteleuropa die häufigste Ursache für entzündliche Hornhautnarben mit Visusminderung dar. Eine Keratoplastik aus optischer Indikation wird möglichst im „inaktiven" Intervall durchgeführt. Bei therapieresistentem Verlauf oder Per-forationsgefahr muß dagegen das erkrankte Hornhautareal exzidiert werden und eine kurative Keratoplastik wird erforderlich. Früher wurde die Prognose der Keratoplastik bei Herpes corneae als ungünstig beurteilt, während man heute die Aussichten im ganzen für besser hält [1–3, 5, 9, 10, 12, 14, 17].

Die Angaben über postoperative Komplikationen beim Herpes corneae weichen erheblich voneinander ab. Es fällt auf, daß ein Bezug auf eindeutige, präoperative Kriterien meistens fehlt, die für die Prognose einer Keratoplastik von Bedeutung sein könnten.

Im folgenden berichten wir, wie bemerkenswert klinische und histopathologische Befunde differieren.

## Material und Methoden

Zwischen 1960 und 1975 wurden an der Universitäts-Augenklinik Hamburg insgesamt 878 perforierende und lamelläre Keratoplastiken durchgeführt, davon 100 wegen eines Herpes corneae bzw. metaherpetischen Zustandes. Diese sollen hier ausgewertet werden.

Die insgesamt 100 präoperativen, klinischen Befunde wurden an Hand der Krankengeschichten ausgewertet und in drei Gruppen eingeteilt (Tabelle 1):

Gruppe 1 „Inaktive Narbe": Hornhauttrübung bei reizfreier Bindehaut

**Tabelle 1.** Präoperativer Befund

| Gruppe 1 | „inaktive" Narbe | 66 |
|---|---|---|
| Gruppe 2 | „aktive" chronische Keratitis | 18 |
| Gruppe 3 | ulcerative Keratitis | 16 |
| | insgesamt | 100 |

und Vorderkammer sowie intaktem Hornhautepithel;

Gruppe 2 „Aktive chronische Keratitis":
Zum Zeitpunkt der Keratoplastik bestanden ein „rotes Auge", Epitheldefekt und/oder Parenchymtrübungen sowie ein Vorderkammerreizzustand;

Gruppe 3 „Ulcerative Keratitis": Bei dro-

**Tabelle 2.** Histologischer Befund

| Gruppe A | nicht vaskularisierte Hornhautnarbe | 31 |
|---|---|---|
| Gruppe B | vaskularisierte Hornhautnarbe | 20 |
| Gruppe C | chronisch-diffuse Keratitis | 43 |
| Gruppe D | granulomatöse Reaktion gegen die Descemetsche Membran | 6 |
| | insgesamt | 100 |

**Tabelle 3.** Vergleich zwischen klinischem und histopathologischem Befund

| klinisch | histologisch | |
|---|---|---|
| *inaktive* | | |
| Narbe | nicht vaskularisierte Hornhautnarbe | 30 |
| | vaskularisierte Hornhautnarbe | 20 |
| | chronisch-diffuse Keratitis | 15 |
| | granulomatöse Reaktion gegen die Descemetsche Membran | 1 |
| | | 66 |
| *aktive* chronische | | |
| Keratitis | nicht vaskularisierte Hornhautnarbe | - |
| | vaskularisierte Hornhautnarbe | 1 |
| | chronische-diffuse Keratitis | 16 |
| | granulomatöse Reaktion gegen die Descemetsche Membran | 1 |
| | | 18 |
| ulcerative | | |
| Keratitis | nicht vaskularisierte Hornhautnarbe | - |
| | vaskularisierte Hornhautnarbe | - |
| | chronisch-diffuse Keratitis | 12 |
| | granulomatöse Reaktion gegen die Descemetsche Membran | 4 |
| | | 16 |
| | insgesamt | 100 |

hender oder bereits erfolgter Perforation lagen tiefe Parenchymdefekte vor.

Die Diagnose eines Herpes corneae bei den sogenannten „inaktiven" Fällen stellten wir aus der Anamnese von rezidivierenden Dendriticafiguren. Viruskulturen wurden nicht durchgeführt.

Die bei der Keratoplastik gewonnenen 100 Hornhautscheibchen wurden nach makroskopischer Begutachtung in Bioloid eingebettet und 8 μ-Schnitte mit Haematoxylin-Eosin und PAS gefärbt. Es erfolgte eine Nachuntersuchung dieser histologischen Schnitte nach bestimmten Gesichtspunkten und folgender Gruppeneinteilung (Tabelle 2, 3):

Gruppe A Nicht vaskularisierte Hornhautnarbe *ohne* entzündliches Infiltrat;

Gruppe B Vascularisierte Hornhautnarbe *ohne* entzündliches Infiltrat;

Gruppe C Chronisch-diffuse Keratitis;

Gruppe D Granulomatöse Reaktion gegen die Descemet'sche Membran.

**Ergebnisse**

Von 100 Augen boten präoperativ 66 klinisch eine reizfreie „inaktive" Narbe. 18 Augen wiesen noch eindeutige Zeichen einer floriden Kerato-Uveitis auf. 16 Augen hatten eine tiefe, ulcerative Keratitis, die eine tektonische Keratoplastik à chaud erforderte, 6 von ihnen waren bereits perforiert (Tabelle 1).

*Die histologische Untersuchung* erbrachte in 51 Fällen der 100 gewonnenen Hornhautscheibchen eine nicht vaskularisierte oder vaskularisierte Hornhautnarbe mit Epithelunregelmäßigkeiten, Defekten der Bowmanschen Membran und Zusammensinterung der Stromalamellen, aber *ohne* entzündliche Infiltrationen und mit normaler Descemet'scher Membran und regelrechtem Endothel. 43mal fiel histologisch eine chronische Keratitis mit lymphozytärer Infiltration aller Stromaschichten auf, 6mal wurde eine granulomatöse Reaktion gegen die Descemet'sche Membran beobachtet (Tabelle 2).

*Der Vergleich zwischen klinischem und histopathologischem Befund* ließ an den 100 Augen erkennen, daß in 66 Fällen, bei denen klinisch eine reizfreie Narbe beschrieben worden war, 30mal histologisch eine nicht vaskularisierte und 20mal eine vaskularisierte Hornhautnarbe bestand. 15mal zeigte sich je-

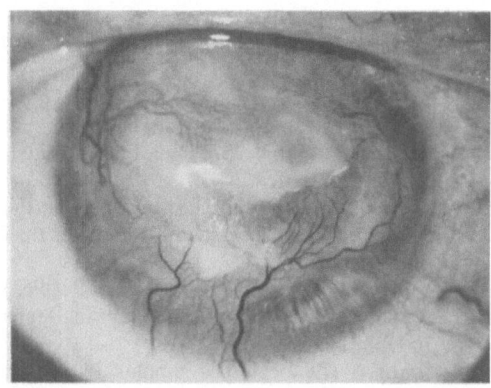

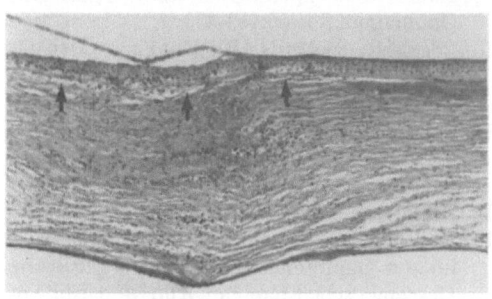

**Abb. 1a, b.** Scheinbar „inaktive" vaskularisierte Hornhautnarbe bei Herpes corneae
OD, 58jähriger Mann (E.S) **a** Klinik: man beachte das reizfreie Auge **b** Histologisch: „floride Keratitis"
Defekte der Bowmanschen Membran (Pfeile)
Auflockerung des Stromas mit Gefäßen, diffuse lymphozytäre Infiltration. PAS × 83 UKE Nr. 370/68

doch eine chronisch-diffuse Keratitis (Abb. 1a und b), 1mal sogar mit granulomatöser Reaktion gegen die Descemet'sche Membran.

Die klinisch als „aktive" chronische Keratitis eingeteilten 18 Hornhäute wiesen 16mal eine chronisch-diffuse Keratitis, 1mal eine granulomatöse Reaktion gegen die Descemet'sche Membran und 1mal sogar eine vaskularisierte Hornhautnarbe auf.

Bei den 16 Augen mit einer klinisch tiefen Ulceration war histologisch 4mal eine granulomatöse Reaktion gegen die Descemet'sche Membran vorhanden und 12mal eine chronisch-diffuse Keratitis zusätzlich zu den Stromadefekten (Tabelle 4).

## Diskussion

Die Prognose der Keratoplastik bei Herpes corneae hängt ab vom präoperativen Befund, der operativen Technik und der postoperativen Behandlung. Um auszuwerten, inwiefern der präoperative Status von Bedeutung ist, erschien es uns wichtig, zunächst einmal festzustellen, ob eine Beziehung zwischen dem klinischen und histologischen Befund besteht, um dann in einer zweiten Untersuchung die Korrelation zwischen präoperativem Befund und Erfolg der Keratoplastik sicherer bewerten zu können. Es ist bekannt, daß in den Fällen, die zum Zeitpunkt der Operation eine „aktive" herpetische Erkrankung aufweisen, die Neigung zum Herpesrezidiv auf dem Transplantat, zur endothelialen Dekompensation durch Uveitis und zu Wundheilungsproblemen erhöht vorhanden sind [10]. Dagegen soll nach Polack und Kaufman [11] der Erfolg in den sogenannten klinisch „inaktiven" Fällen dem der Keratoplastik bei Keratokonus entsprechen.

Wir konnten feststellen, daß der klinische Befund nur dann dem histologischen entsprach, wenn eine aktive Entzündung vorhanden war. Bei allen präoperativ gereizten Augen waren dementsprechend mit einer Ausnahme histologisch Entzündungszellen im Stroma nachweisbar. Die Fälle, die klinisch eine tiefe ulcerative Keratitis aufwiesen, zeigten in besonders hohem Ausmaß eine *granulomatöse Reaktion gegen die Descemetsche Membran*. Diese Reaktion ist als erworbene Autosensibilisierung gegen die durch Herpesviren angegriffene Descemetsche Membran und gegen die Endothelzellen anzusehen, analog der phakoanaphylaktischen Uveitis und sympathischen Ophthalmie. Das Aufsplittern der Descemetlamellen führt dann zur Descemetocele und schließlich zur Perforation [4, 8, 15, 16, 18].

Dieser bei der tiefen ulcerativen herpetischen Keratitis sehr häufige Befund sowie der experimentelle Nachweis von Viren in den Stromakeratozyten und im Endothel sind der Grund, warum wir eine perforierende gegenüber einer lamellären Keratoplastik bei einer chronischen herpetischen Keratitis bevorzugen.

Auffallend war der *Unterschied zwischen klinischem und histologischem Befund* bei den Fällen der Gruppe I, die klinisch als „inaktive" Hornhautnarben bei reizfreiem Auge imponierten. Hier zeigten von 66 Hornhäuten 16 eine unerwartete diffuse, vorwiegend lymphozytäre Infiltration, eine davon sogar mit einer granulomatösen Reaktion gegen die Descemetsche Membran. Diese Diskrepanz entspricht etwa den Untersuchungen von Hogan [7], wo $\frac{1}{3}$ der klinisch inaktiven Hornhäute Entzündungszellen enthielten.

Zusammenfassend ist anzunehmen, daß in etwa $\frac{1}{3}$ der klinisch *„inaktiven"* Hornhautnarben nach Keratitis metaherpetica wahrscheinlich noch Herpesviren innerhalb der Keratozyten, im Epithel und auch gelegentlich im Endothel mit histologischen Zeichen einer chronischen Keratitis zu finden sind. Diese Diskrepanz zwischen den klinischen und histologischen Diagnosen erscheint uns hinsichtlich der Prognose der Keratoplastik von Wichtigkeit. In einer weiteren Untersuchung wollen wir über die Langzeitergebnisse der 100 Keratoplastiken berichten.

**Danksagung.** Wir danken Frl. E. Portwich für die Herstellung der histologischen Schnitte und Frl. I. Hadlock für die Anfertigung der klinischen Fotografien.

# Literatur

1. Castroviejo R (1968) Keratoplastik. Thieme, Stuttgart
2. Dawson C, Togni B (1968) Structural changes in chron. herp. ker. Arch Ophthalmol 79:740–747
3. Ffooks O, Pickering A (1971) Role of penetrating grafts in herpetic keratitis. Br J Ophthalmol 55:321–330
4. Green WR, Zimmerman LE (1967) Gran. Reaction to Descemets membrane. Am J Ophthalmol 64:555–558
5. Hallermann W (1965) Ergebnisse der Keratoplastik bei Herpes. Klin Monatsbl Augenheilkd 146:161–171
6. Hinzpeter EN, Naumann GOH (1977) Transplantation of the cornea. Handbuch der Allgemeinen Pathologie. Springer, Berlin Heidelberg New York, S 403–438
7. Hogan MJ (1957) Corneal transplantation in the treatment of herp. disease of the cornea. Am J Ophthalmol 43:147–157
8. Hogan MJ, Kimura SJ, Thygeson P (1963) Pathology of herpes simplex keratoiritis. Trans Am Ophthalmol Soc 61:75–99
9. Kimura S (1962) Herpes simplex uveitis: A clinical and experimental study. Trans Am Ophthalmol Soc 60:440–470
10. Pfister R, Richards HE, Dohlman C (1972) Recurrence of herpetic keratitis in corneal grafts. Am J Ophthalmol 73:192–196
11. Polack F, Kaufman HE (1972) Penetrating keratoplasty in herpetic keratitis. Am J Ophthalmol 73:908–913
12. Rintelen F (1964) Ophthalmologica 147:255
13. Roll P, Hanselmayer H (1976) Die Ultrastruktur der granulomatösen Reaktion gegen die Descemet'sche Membran. Klin Monatsbl Augenheilkd 168:819–824
14. Schenck H, Kunze R (1960) Klin Monatsbl Augenheilkd 136:663
15. Stock W (1939) Pathologische Anatomie des Auges, Enke, Stuttgart
16. Vogel MH, Naumann G (1970) Die granulomatöse Reaktion gegen die Descemet. Ber Dtsch Ophthalmol Ges 71:35–41
17. Witmer R, Iwamoto R (1968) Electron microscopic observations of herpes-like particles in the iris. Arch Ophthalmol 79:331–337
18. Wolter JR, Johnson FD (1971) Acquired autosensitivity to degenerating Descemet's membrane in a case with anterior uveitis in the other eye. Am J Ophthalmol 72:782–786

Sundmacher, R. (Hrsg.):
Herpetische Augenerkrankungen
© J.F. Bergmann Verlag, München 1981

# Prognosis and Management of Corneal Transplantation for Herpetic Keratitis*

## L. Cobo, D.J. Coster, N.S.C. Rice, B.R. Jones, London

**Key words.** Herpetic keratitis, keratoplasty

**Schlüsselwörter.** Herpeskeratitis, Keratoplastik

**Summary.** A retrospective review was undertaken of 132 penetrating keratoplasties performed at Moorfields Eye Hospital between 1967 and 1978 for the purpose of determining significant prognostic factors, as well as an appraisal of postoperative morbidity and management. This was a period of generally uniform surgical and postoperative care, with postoperative care delivered at the same institution. In general, the surgical technique consisted of continuous monofilament suturing of the donor tissue without the removal of donor epithelium. Eighty-six percent of donor buttons were between 6.5 and 8.0 mm. Postoperative management consisted of cycloplegics and high dose topical corticosteroids without antiviral cover, tapered over a period of 12 months. Episodes of allograft rejection were treated with subconjunctival injection of dexamethasone or betnesol and intensive topical dexamethasone therapy, again without antiviral cover. Herpetic recurrences in the postoperative period were managed with topical antivirals. Ninety-nine of the 132 keratoplasties were performed in clinically uninflamed eyes with corneal scarring due to prior herpetic disease or prior failed keratoplasty. Thirty-three penetrating keratoplasties were performed in inflamed eyes, 15 with either a perforation of descemetocele, and 18 with chronic inflammation which was non-responsive to medical therapy. For the entire group of 132 keratoplasties, life table analysis revealed a survival rate of a clear graft of 64% at two years and 62% at 5 years. The cause of graft clouding was determined in the 47 keratoplasties which ultimately failed. Allograft rejection was the most frequent cause of

* The following is presented as a summary of the complete paper which shall appear in the Archives of Ophthalmology (Chicago)

graft opacification, responsible for 64% of cloudy grafts. The course of eyes undergoing allograft rejection was frequently complicated. Seventy-nine percent of eyes undergoing allograft rejection did not recover clarity despite steroid intensive therapy, with herpetic recurrence and bacterial superinfection frequently developing after the onset of rejection. Early graft failure accounted for 13% of clouded grafts. Epithelial herpetic recurrences were the third most frequent cause of a clouded graft (11%). Less frequent causes of a clouded graft were stromal herpetic disease (4%), elevated intraocular pressure (4%), spontaneous perforation (one case), and fungal keratitis (one case).

The major prognostic factors were preoperative corneal vascularization and the presence or absence of inflammation. The rate of allograft rejection at 5 years was found to be 16% in avascular recipient corneas, 30% in partially vascularized corneas, and 54% in cases where the recipient cornea was fully vascularized. This trend towards increasing rates of rejection with increasing degrees of corneal vascularization was found to be significant. Likewise, the prognosis for penetrating keratoplasties performed in uninflamed eyes was significantly better than that for an eye which was actively inflamed at the time of surgery. The survival rate by life table analysis indicated that 69% of keratoplasties in uninflamed eyes were clear 2 years, as opposed to 44% in eyes which were actively inflamed at the time of surgery. The only significant difference noted was an increased rate of early graft failure in eyes which were actively inflamed at the time of surgery. This was defined as a failure of the graft to clear postoperatively. No significant difference was found relative to allograft rejection or herpetic recurrence.

An increased rate of recurrent epithelial herpetic disease was noted in eyes undergoing steroid intensive therapy for allograft rejection. Thirty-two percent of eyes undergoing allograft rejection developed epithelial herpetic recurrences within 4 months, as opposed to a recurrence rate of 6% at 4 months in eyes which were uncomplicated by allograft rejection. Neither group received antiviral cover while on steroid intensive therapy. The epithelial herpetic recurrence rate was shown to increase with time, with rates noted of 15% at 1 year, 18% at 2 years, and 22% at 4 years. Because of the inordinately high recurrence rate in eyes undergoing rejection, antiviral cover is recommended for steroid intensive therapy in this situation. In the uncomplicated postoperative keratoplasty on topical corticosteroids, herpetic recurrence would not appear to relate to topical steroid use, and should be avoided because of potential toxicity for donor epithelium.

Finally, an additional group of 14 eyes undergoing lamellar keratoplasty between 1959 and 1970 was reviewed. Thirteen of these lamellar keratoplasties subsequently opacified (average 38 months; range 1–144 months). Only one has remained clear, with a visual acuity of 6/36. The most frequent cause of failure of these keratoplasties was recurrent stromal herpetic disease and interface vascularization. Virtually all of these eyes became fully vascularized, and the prognosis for subsequent keratoplasty was diminished, with only 45% retaining a clear graft at 2 years.

**Zusammenfassung.** Wir untersuchten retrospektiv den Verlauf nach 132 Keratoplastiken, die zwischen 1967 und 1978 am Moorfields Eye Hospital durchgeführt worden waren, um sowohl prognostisch wichtige prä-operative Merkmale zu bestimmen als auch einen Überblick über die post-operativen Komplikationen und ihre Behandlung zu gewinnen. Während dieses Zeitraumes wurden Operation und Nachbehandlung annähernd gleichartig gehandhabt, und die Nachbehandlung lag in den Händen des Krankenhauses selbst. Meistens wurden die Transplantate mit einer fortlaufenden Monofilament-Naht eingenäht und das Spenderepithel mit transplantiert. Sechsundachtzig Prozent der Transplantate maßen zwischen 6,5 und 8,0 mm. Postoperativ wurden Cycloplegica zusammen mit hoch-dosierten Steroiden lokal gegeben, die über 12 Monate abgebaut wurden. Zusätzliche Virustatika gab es nicht. Intermittierende Immunreaktionen wurden mit subkonjunktivalen Dexamethason- oder Betnesol-Injektionen zusammen mit einer intensiven Dexamethason-Tropfen-Therapie behandelt. Auch hierbei gab es keine zusätzlichen Virustatika. Herpesrezidive wurden mit lokalen Virustatika therapiert. Neunundneunzig der 132 Keratoplastiken wurden an klinisch „ruhigen" Augen durchgeführt, die Herpesnarben aufwiesen oder bei denen bereits eine Keratoplastik fehlgeschlagen war. Dreiunddreißig Keratoplastiken fanden an entzündeten Augen statt; 15 hatten eine Descemetozele oder eine Perforation, und 18 wiesen eine chronische, therapie-refraktäre Entzündung auf. Für alle 132 Transplantate zusammen ließ sich die Häufigkeit eines klaren Transplantates mit 64% nach zwei Jahren und 62% nach fünf Jahren bestimmen. Bei den 47 endgültig eingetrübten Transplantaten wurde nach den Ursachen geforscht. Eine Immunreaktion stellte mit 64% der eingetrübten Scheibchen den Hauptgrund für das Transplantatversagen dar. Der post-operative Verlauf solcher Augen war oft kompliziert. Neunundsiebzig Prozent von ihnen gewannen auch nach Einsetzen einer intensiven Steroidtherapie ihre Klarheit nicht zurück, wobei auffiel, das Herpesrezidive und bakterielle Superinfektionen sich häufig der Immunreaktion aufpropften. Eine mangelhafte Entquellung des Transplantates unmittelbar postoperativ war in 13% für das negative Ergebnis verantwortlich. Am dritt-häufigsten waren epitheliale Herpesrezidive (11%). Weniger häufig waren ein Stromaherpes-Rezidiv (4%), ein erhöhter intraokularer Druck (4%), eine spontane Perforation (einmal) oder eine Pilzinfektion (einmal) für den ungünstigen Ausgang verantwortlich.

Die wichtigsten prognostischen prä-operativen Kriterien waren das Ausmaß einer Vaskularisation und einer klinisch diagnostizierbaren Entzündung. Die Häufigkeit von Immunreaktionen war bei gefäßfreien Hornhäuten innerhalb von 5 Jahren nur 16%, bei mäßig vaskularisierten Hornhäuten 30% und in total vaskularisierten 54%. Diese Korrelation zwischen Vaskularisationsgrad und Gefahr einer Immunreaktion war statistisch signifikant. Die Langzeitprognose war auch dann besser, wenn das Auge prä-operativ klinisch nicht entzündet war. Die statistische Hochrechnung ergab, daß prä-operativ reizfreie Augen nach 2 Jahren noch in 69% der Fälle ein klares Transplantat haben, prä-operativ entzündete aber nur in 44%. Der einzige signifikante Unterschied zwischen beiden Gruppen war allerdings nur ein frühes Transplantatversagen, d.h. die Transplantate entquollen unmittelbar postoperativ nicht recht. Bezüglich Immunreaktionen oder Herpesrezidiven gab es keinen Unterschied.

Augen, die wegen einer Immunreaktion intensiv mit lokalen Steroiden behandelt wurden, erlitten häufiger Herpesrezidive. Dies war bei 32% solcher Augen innerhalb von 4 Monaten der Fall, während Rezidive im unkomplizierten Verlauf innerhalb von 4 Monaten nur in 6% auftraten. Beide Gruppen hatten keinen antiviralen Schutz erhalten. Die Rezidivrate nimmt mit den Jahren langsam zu. Sie beträgt 15% nach 1 Jahr, 18% nach 2 Jahren und 22% nach 4 Jahren. Wegen der ungewöhnlich viel größeren Gefahr eines Rezidivs in Augen, die wegen einer Immunreaktion besonders intensiv mit Steroiden behandelt werden, empfehlen wir in dieser Situation einen zusätzlichen antiviralen Schutz. Hingegen bei sonst komplikationslosem Verlauf empfehlen wir das nicht, weil in diesen Fällen keine Korrelation zwischen Steroid-Dosierung und Herpesrezidiven erkennbar war und weil die zusätzlichen Virustatika eine erhebliche potentielle Gefahr für das Spenderepithel darstellen.

Wir untersuchten auch die Verläufe nach 14

Augen, die mit einer lamellären Keratoplastik versorgt worden waren (1959–1970). Dreizehn dieser Transplantate trübten nach durchschnittlich 38 Monaten (1–144) ein. Ein einziges blieb mit einem Visus von 6/36 klar. Die häufigste Ursache für das Trübwerden waren rezidivierender Stromaherpes und Vaskularisationen an der Wirt-Spender-Grenze. Praktisch alle diese Augen vaskularisierten vollständig, was die Prognose für eine spätere perforierende Keratoplastik ungünstig beeinflußte (nur 45% der nochmals Operierten hatten nach 2 Jahren ein klares perforierendes Transplantat).

Sundmacher, R. (Hrsg.):
Herpetische Augenerkrankungen
© J.F. Bergmann Verlag, München 1981

# Differential Diagnosis of Post-Keratoplasty Complications in Herpes Patients

R. Sundmacher, Freiburg

**Key words.** Herpetic keratitis, keratoplasty – differential diagnosis of complications

**Schlüsselwörter.** Herpeskeratitis, Keratoplastik – Differentialdiagnose der Komplikationen

**Summary.** Herpes recurrences in the graft are widely considered to be the main threat to perforating corneal transplants in herpes patients. Although such recurrences do occur, the incidence is probably relatively low. More frequent are herpetic recurrences outside the graft, and even much more decisive for graft damage are immune reactions. Many other factors may further contribute to graft failure.

**Zusammenfassung.** Im allgemeinen wird angenommen, daß Herpesrezidive im Transplantat die Hauptgefahr bei perforierenden Hornhauttransplantaten wegen Herpes darstellen. Obwohl es solche Rezidive natürlich gibt, sind sie nach unseren Beobachtungen relativ selten. Viel häufiger findet man Herpesrezidive in der Wirtshornhaut außerhalb des Transplantates, hier allerdings meist als stromale Entzündung oder Endotheliitis.

Sehr viel entscheidender für das Klarbleiben oder Eintrüben des Transplantates sind Immunreaktionen vor allem gegen Transplantatendothel. Daneben muß man bei der post-operativen Überwachung solcher Patienten besonders auf Schäden durch eine Keratokonjunctivitis sicca, durch Glaukom und durch Fadenlockerungen achten.

It has been commonly believed that herpetic recurrences in the graft represent the main threat for corneal transplants in herpes patients. Our experience, taken from a 4 year prospective survey, does not support this assumption.

A lot of controversy stems from the uncertainty as to whether or not one can make a sound clinical differential diagnosis between graft rejection and herpetic recurrence. We believe that in a majority of cases differential diagnosis is in fact no major problem, and we would, therefore, like to present our diagnostic criteria and have them discussed.

Figure 1 has been designed as a simplified "memo-scheme" of postkeratoplasty complications with emphasis on the relative importance of each single event. We have purposely

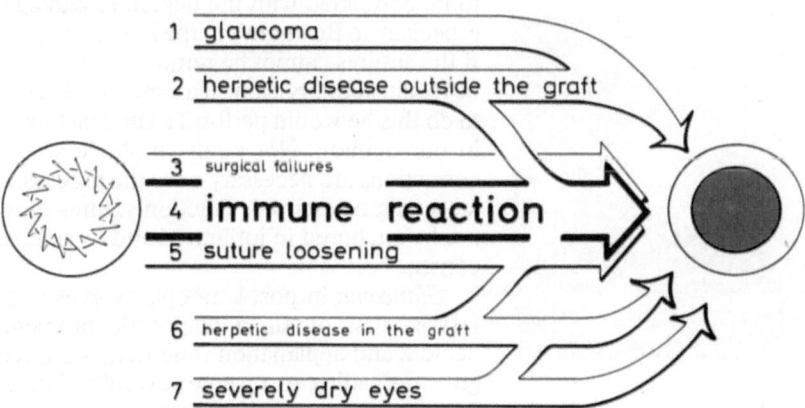

**Fig. 1.** Major pathways to graft failure after keratoplasty for herpes

not inferred figures and statistics in this presentation because before doing this one should have followed a fairly large number of patients prospectively for many years, and this study is still underway. On the other hand, giving simple percentages of complications would not suit the purpose of this paper either, as some complications are relatively frequent, but not so dangerous as others which may be rare. The graph, therefore, represents our current accumulated experience as to the overall danger of single complications which, of course, is a function of different factors like incidence, localization, aggressiveness, diagnostic problems, availability of therapy, responsiveness to therapy, and others.

Our current conclusion is that like in other types of disease which require perforating keratoplasty, immune reactions, especially against the endothelium of the transplant, represent the major threat towards graft clarity [1, 6, 7]. Herpetic diseases in the graft, however, cause only a small percentage of definite graft failures. We feel that the relative sparing of the graft itself from herpetic recurrences is well explained by the neuronal hypothesis of herpes simplex virus latency and recurrence, which makes it appear logical that the virus has great difficulties in reaching structures of the transplant other than just its borders, once the sensory nerves of the cornea have been cut during operation. Regrowth of nerves is considerably slow in these patients. On the other hand, herpetic diseases *outside* the graft should be as frequent as before operation.

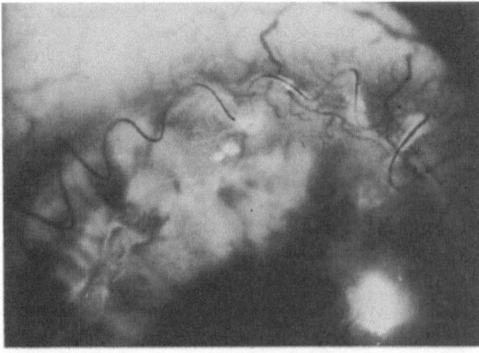

**Fig. 2.** Suture loosening in an area where the host cornea is heavily vascularized and has lost its normal structure

Going into some more detail, we would like to comment on the single topics of Fig. 1 with special emphasis on the differential diagnosis of herpetic recurrences and immune reactions.

*Surgical failures* (Fig. 1/3) may cause a variety of undesirable side effects, e.g. faulty adjustment of the graft, glaucoma, surgical endothelium damage, or most often, primarily low quality of the graft which either does not deturge after surgery or becomes only borderline compensated because of too few and/or malfunctioning endothelial cells. These cells are often barely visible due to a fluctuating corneal edema. The preoperative quality control of the graft's endothelium with the aid of the specular microscope is unfortunately not as feasible as necessary at every clinic and in every country. In Freiburg, for example, we rarely get transplants earlier than 12 hours post mortem for legal reasons, which limits the use of the specular microscope considerably. We therefore have most often to rely on our "clinical experience" when accepting or refusing a transplant for keratoplasty. The long-term results, though, are good, but could certainly be even better if we would not now and then pick up a transplant with low endothelial quality. At the moment it does not appear that the legal situation will become any better. The contrary may be true and may lead in the future to an increasing number of failing grafts due to "legal insufficiency".

*Suture loosening* (Fig. 1/5 and 2) with subsequent irritation, infiltration and vascularization may lead to stromal necrosis and trigger an immune reaction. Its incidence seems to be correlated with the degree of damage, especially to Bowman's in the host cornea [3]. If the sutures cannot be removed, they must be readjusted surgically. If a surgeon hesitates to do this he would perform a surgical failure in our opinion. Not rarely, multiple suture corrections are necessary once the process of loosening has started. Traction sutures must not be anchored in infiltrated and weak host cornea.

*Glaucoma* in post-keratoplasty eyes (Fig. 1/1) is, first of all, a diagnostic problem. Schiötz and applanation tonometry do often give misleading or divergent results. Therefore, digital estimation of the intraocular pressure is still an inevitable, additional diagnostic criterion in this special situation and should never be missed at the regular controls of transplant patients. Provided that eyes with uncontrolled glaucoma have been primarily excluded from surgery, one will mostly have to deal with eyes that start to develop a chronic secondary glaucoma after herpes or that start to escape medical control of an established glaucoma. In both cases, the intraocular pressure will be borderline in the beginning which makes diagnosis even more difficult. If there is any doubt as to the development of a glaucoma, efforts should be made to lower the intraocular pressure by medical means. Apart from chronic glaucoma, acute secondary glaucoma may accompany recurrences of herpetic endotheliitis or iritis (see Chapter 33 and below).

The most frequent complication in keratoplasty eyes after herpes is a *keratokonjunctivitis sicca* (Fig. 1/7). *Severely dry eyes,* ultimately leading to graft failure, are relatively rare with herpes. Moderately dry eyes with severe – though transitory – epithelial problems, however, are quite common. The clinical picture may vary from slight to moderate to severe superficial punctate staining and erosions. Not rarely, *pseudodendrites,* commonly misdiagnosed as viral dendrites, arise (Fig. 3). We believe that misinterpretation of these pseudodendrites, which present a microstructure totally different from that of true viral dendrites, has been the major source of the belief that dendritic recurrences in the graft are common after keratoplasty for herpes. We have virologically controlled all pseudodendrites

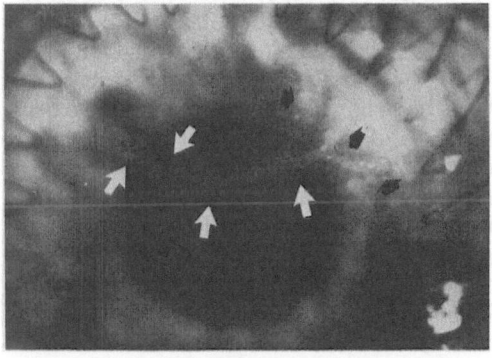

**Fig. 3.** Pseudodendrites may arise because of complex surface problems and keratokonjunctivitis sicca after herpes. They have nothing to do with a true viral dendrite

and true viral dendrites during the last years and have found that pseudodendrites are far more frequent than viral lesions. If these pseudodendrites are treated with antivirals, as is often the case, then the condition will worsen. If this occurs, frequently a diagnosis of "refractory dendritic keratitis" is made and the antiviral therapy augmented, which finally may result in gradual "dissolving" of the epithelium with clouding of the stroma and functional loss of the transplant. Thus, dry eye problems should always be suspected after keratoplasty for herpes; therefore we routinely combine artificial tears and appropriate ointments together with the otherwise necessary therapy postoperatively as a prophylactic measure against epithelial loosening.

*Herpetic diseases in the graft* (Fig. 1/6), *herpetic diseases outside the graft* (Fig. 1/2) *and immune reactions* (Fig. 1/4) will be considered together, because, with the exception of dendritic recurrence, their pathophysiology is very similar and leads to similar clinical pictures.

Theoretically, *dendritic recurrences* could be expected to occur either in the epithelium of the host cornea where the nerve endings are still intact or at the margin of the graft epithelium where the nerves terminate – at least during several months post-operatively. Interestingly, we have not as yet found a verified viral dendrite in the host epithelium, but all true dendrites have manifested themselves in the epithelium of the graft along the suture line (Fig. 4). One may speculate that the cut and slowly regenerating nerve endings in this area shed virus more easily than terminal nerves in the host cornea, and also that the epithelium along the suture line is often especially irritated and may thus provide a site of minor resistance for a viral attack. Therefore, at least in the first months after operation, the localization of a "dendrite" may, in addition to its microstructure, help in the differential diagnosis between a viral dendrite and a pseudodendrite. Pseudodendrites are preferentially localized horizontally, viral dendrites along the suture line. This does not preclude that many months or years after operation, true viral dendrites may be found in every part of the transplant depending on how complete re-innervation of the transplant has taken place. Viral dendrites in the graft are treated like any other dendritic

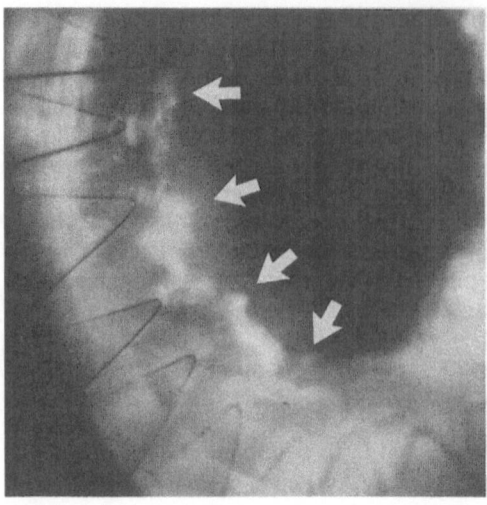

**Fig. 4.** Virologically verified recurrence of dendritic keratitis in the epithelium of the graft along the suture line; the underlying stroma is already slightly infiltrated

keratitis and have the same prognosis unless they are primarily combined with stromal disease.

*Stromal infiltrates* can theoretically be either recurrences of interstitial herpetic keratitis or stromal immune reactions. The

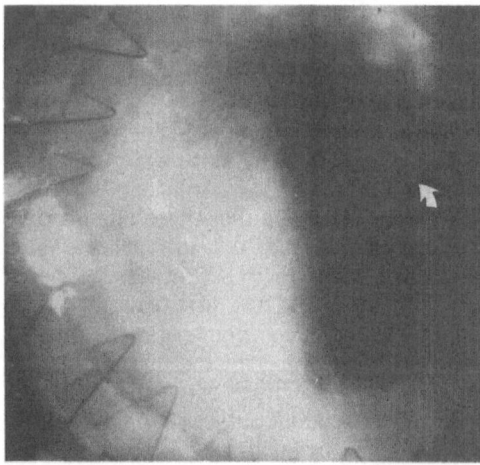

**Fig. 5.** (Same eye as in Fig. 4) The interstitial herpetic keratitis which, in this case, has been associated with a recurrence of dendritic keratitis from the beginning, has extended to nearly half of the transplant, the rest of it still being relatively unaffected. (Arrow: photographic artefacts)

biomicroscopy of the infiltrate can't reveal structural etiologic pecularities, because in both cases immunocompetent cells together with polymorphonuclear cells attack keratocytes which express foreign antigens on their surface – either herpetic ones or transplantation antigens. We nonetheless believe, that in most cases a differential diagnosis is possible. First, it is noteworthy that up to now we have never seen an unequivocal stromal immune reaction *without* an endothelial immune reaction in *nonherpes* patients. This allows the conclusion that an isolated stromal infiltrate (without concomitant endothelial disturbance) represents an interstitial herpetic keratitis. The second criterion would be the localization of the infiltrate. If it is exclusively found in the host cornea, it cannot be of the graft rejection type and, therefore, is most probably herpetic. We would assume the same etiology for infiltrates extending from the host into the donor stroma. With infiltrates confined exclusively to the graft stroma, the diagnostic likelihood speaks more for a herpetic event if stromal involvement is far more pronounced than endothelial disease as outlined above. This is illustrated in Fig. 5 (same eye as Fig. 4): An interstitial herpetic keratitis has added to the virologically proven dendritic keratitis. The endothelium of the graft is only secondarily involved, which is indicated by the clear parts of the graft to which the destructive stromal process has not yet extended. In summary, stromal infiltrates are probably herpetic in most cases. Whether or not in the course of this event a stromal immune reaction is additionally triggered is not very important from the point of therapy which should consist of a combination of antivirals together with steroids.

The pathophysiological similarity between herpetic and homograft reactions also exists at the *endothelial level:* Immunocompetent cells attack endothelial cells which either express viral antigens or transplantation antigens. In the first place, we deal with an *herpetic endotheliitis* (see Chapter 33), in the second with an *immune reaction against donor endothelium.* Consequently, no basic difference between both reactions can be found with the specular microscope because a difference exists only on the macromolecular level. But here again, two diagnostic criteria may help in the differential diagnosis. First, an endotheliitis, which is confined ex-

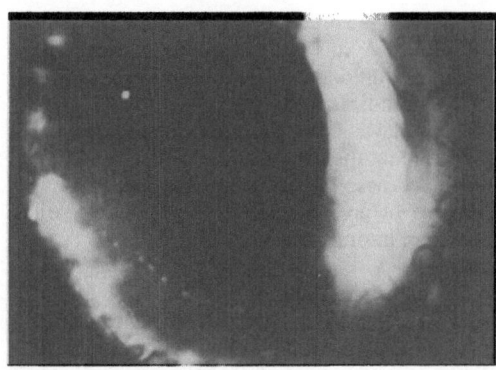

**Fig. 6.** Endothelial rejection line

clusively to the host endothelium, cannot be a homograft rejection and is most probably a herpetic recurrence. We would assume the same etiology for processes which extend from the host onto the donor endothelium. Vice versa, an endotheliitis confined exclusively to the donor endothelium most probably represents a homograft reaction. Theoretically, although a central herpetic endotheliitis (= disciform keratitis) would look identical, we consider the possibility of such an event to be very small, because the attacking virus in this cases must have come via the acqeous (the nerves as normal pathways for the virus being cut), and this would only appear to be possible if some additional acute herpetic process shed large amounts of virus into the acqeous (e.g. concomitant focal herpetic iritis). We have not come across such a case in our series. The

general conclusion, therefore, would still be that an endotheliitis confined exclusively to the donor endothelium is nearly always a homograft reaction. This may in some cases be further substantiated by the second diagnostic criterion which is the rejection line named after *Khodadoust* [2] (Fig. 6). This line we find exclusively in graft rejections, and I would like at this point, to give credit to the work of *Polack* [4, 5] who, to my knowledge, was the first to describe these rejection lines consisting of immune cells. It should be noted, however, that the *rejection type with diffusely scattered pocks of immune cells* is probably more common than the type with a clear-cut line [6] and often, the localized precipitates, which are diagnostic, are hidden behind a severe edema and can only eventually be seen if therapy is effectively initiated and the edema subsides [7] (Fig. 7). If diagnosed early enough, it should nearly always be possible to efficiently treat immune reactions and thus save or regain the graft's clarity.

Many ophthalmologists will find it useless to occupy themselves with the problems of differential diagnosis between immune reactions and herpetic recurrences in corneal grafts because they always combine antivirals with steroids. We have hesitated doing this and tried to treat immune reactions only with steroids in order to reduce the stress on the epithelium, which is often feeble anyway because of sicca problems. During all these years, we have had only one patient who developed dendritic complications in the course of steroid treatment of homograft rejection. In this particular case, treatment was excessively high-dosed and long, so that it would appear reasonable to reserve an antiviral cover – e.g. with five drops of trifluorothymidine per day – for those patients who are at an especially high risk of dendritic recurrences in the course of high-dosed topical steroid therapy.

Finally, it may be useful to mention that an *iritis* does not generally bring about diagnostic difficulties. The precipitates are passively scattered on the endothelium of either origin. They do not consist of cells which attack the endothelium, and thus the endothelium remains functioning with the overlying cornea transparent. Normally no major damage to the endothelium is visible with the specular microscope. If it is a focal herpetic iritis, which is relatively rare (see Chapter 33),

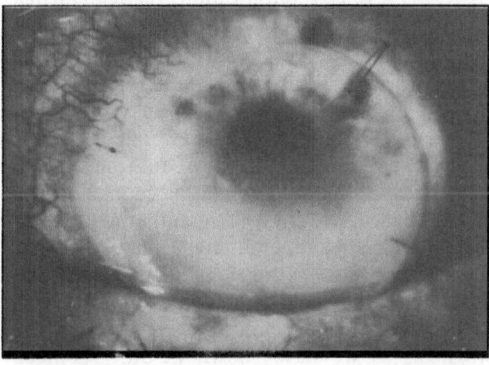

**Fig. 7.** Acute endothelial rejection by diffusely scattered pocks of immune cells which, due to gross corneal swelling, cannot be visualized in this stage of the disease

therapy should consist of antivirals plus steroids. If it is an "ordinary" iritis without any special features, only steroids should be given, as in these cases we have as yet never found live herpes simplex virus in the acqeous.

## References

1. Ciba Foundation Symposium 15 (new series) (1973) Corneal Graft Failure (B.R. Jones, President), Elsevier, Excerpta Medica, North Holland, Amsterdam London New York
2. Khodadoust AA, Silverstein AM (1969) Transplantation and rejection of individual cell layers of the cornea. Invest Ophthalmol Visual Sci 8:180–195
3. Mackensen G, Haug HP, Horn Ch, Sundmacher R, Witschel H (1978) Nahtlockerung nach Keratoplastik und Korrekturmöglichkeiten. Klin Monatsbl Augenheilkd 173:700–707
4. Polack FM (1965) Inhibition of immune corneal graft rejection by Azathioprine (Imuran). Arch Ophthalmol 74:683–689
5. Polack FM (1966) Modification of the immune graft response by Azathioprine. Surv Ophthalmol 11:545–553
6. Sundmacher R (1977) Immunreaktionen nach Keratoplastik. Klin Monatsbl Augenheilkd 171:705–722
7. Sundmacher R, Müller O (1980) Spaltlampenmikroskopie des Hornhautendothels im Spiegelbezirk. Ber Dtsch Ophthalmol Ges 77: 943–950

## Discussion on the Contributions pp. 425–444

R. Sundmacher (Freiburg)
As we are running late in time, I would ask you not to begin with a detailed discussion on the various diagnostic parameters outlined, as these would certainly require intensive discussions. The main purpose, for which I designed this poster, was to stress that immune reactions constitute the major cause for graft failure, also in herpes patients, and that everybody can diagnose the majority of immune reactions very easily. You only have to apply the broad knowledge accumulated on this topic by various authors; a good start to study the problem would be to read the proceedings of the excellent Symposium on Corneal Graft Failure presided by Prof. Jones some years ago in London.

F. Hoffmann (Berlin)
You say, Dr. Sundmacher, that the localization of precipitates is important for the differential diagnosis. If the precipitates are located only on the donor cornea, this indicates an immunoreaction, but if, in addition, they are found on the recipient cornea, it indicates an iritis.

Nowadays, there is some evidence that transplanted endothelial cells move towards the recipient cornea. Is it not possible to explain the presence of precipitates on the recipient cornea also as an immunoreaction?

R. Sundmacher (Freiburg)
Now, what you touch on is an important aspect and may be a real possibility. But I doubt whether this sliding over of donor endothelium goes so far that it interferes with the diagnostic criteria outlined here; and for didactic purposes, I would prefer to stick to the definitions which I have outlined unless you present clinical data which prove the contrary. Finally, it is of course, not only the distribution of the precipitates which gives you the diagnostic clue but also the functional behaviour of the cells of which the precipitates are comprised. If they attack donor endothelium, which you can see from the resultant gross corneal edema or the endothelial swelling observable by specular microscopy [7] you can be pretty sure that – with the unlikely exception of a focal herpetic endotheliitis – you are dealing with an immune reaction.

G.O.H. Naumann (Erlangen)
I think we are all in general agreement that the prognosis of penetrating keratoplasty is better, the quieter the eye is at the time of surgery. Therefore the histological studies are relevant for an evaluation of therapy, because they show lymphocytic infiltrates as signs of active keratitis in clinically apparently inactive corneal scars after herpetic keratitis. Whether this is due to virus or some immune reaction is an open question, but it may support the indication for local steroid therapy.

As to Dr. Foster. We are quite in agreement that we would not do surgery on a particularly bad red eye. No sane surgeon would try keratoplasty in the cornea with the diffuse infiltrate in all diameters. However, the figures you showed on the bad prognosis of keratoplasty in perforated herpetic ulcers is an argument in favor of doing active surgery just *before* such a perforation occurs. I believe the peculiar clinical entity of a granulomatous reaction to Descemet's membrane – that we can recognize clinically – is the precursor of corneal perforation. If this is a circumscribed process, it facilitates, at least technically, surgery and the prognosis as we have shown in our Tübingen series. With 16 eyes, with a follow-up of 2 years, we had no difficulties under steroids and antiviral cover of 1–2 TFT.

The final point. I was surprised by the large size of the grafts shown in the Boston series. Certainly it would be desirable to excise as much diseased tissue as possible, but I believe, although I do not have the figures at the moment, that the incidence of graft reaction may be less if you use a smaller graft and stay away from the limbus. Perhaps, with a size of 7 mm or less, if at all possible, even if the optical results are less satisfactory, I think the incidence of homologous graft reaction is less and you will have less problems with suture fixation in an area of the cornea with damaged Bowman's membrane. I would like to know if any of the surgeons have figures showing that smaller grafts are less prone to corneal immune reaction.

### G. Smolin (San Francisco)
We've been told that the absence of corneal sensation is a poor prognostic sign. In your data does the presence or absence of corneal sensation have any prognostic value?

### C.S. Foster (Boston)
I agree with you, Gill. It was simply impossible for us to discover all of the things that we would have liked to have known about the patients from the medical record. One of those things was the preoperative corneal sensation status. Another was the preoperative Schirmer value.

### F.M. Polack (Gainesville)
In 1972, Kaufman and I published the results of 50 cases of keratoplasty in herpetic keratitis and we made the point that the results of lamellar keratoplasty were usually poor. Since then we have done only penetrating keratoplasty in herpetic-infected corneas. I think that even though graft rejection is a leading cause of graft failure, we prefer to keep antiviral coverage, especially in patients using steroids, because if viral reactivation develops at the same time as graft rejection, there is a better chance for graft survival. It is very likely that the two processes may occur at the same time – the immune graft reaction and the herpetic reactivation. Perhaps the latter triggers the graft reaction. I think the information presented by Dr. Naumann is very interesting and this is another reason why we should cover grafts with antivirals, even though these patients seem to have inactive herpes. They do have latent herpetic infection, and viral particles have been shown by electron microscopy by Dr. Dawson. This is a finding against lamellar grafts since infected tissue may persist below the graft.

### M. Cobo (Miami)
I would like to respond to the comments with respect to the routine use of antivirals postoperatively. As I mentioned in the presentation of our data, I believe that a zone of ambiguity exists where one cannot be certain if one is dealing with herpetic recurrences or graft rejection. In either case, antiviral cover would certainly be warranted on a prophylactic basis while treating the patient with corticosteroids. However, in our series the observed recurrence rate of epithelial herpetic disease of 15% in the first year would seem to argue that it would not be reasonable to treat the other 85% of the patients with antivirals which are potentially toxic. You will note that no mention was made of persistent epithelial defects in our series because none occurred. This is opposed to the series that Dr. Foster presented as well as to the earlier series of his co-worker, Dr. Pavan-Langston, where epithelial defects persisted in some 25%–40% of the patients. I think one should be careful with the potential toxic effects of prophylactic antivirals.

### C.S. Foster (Boston)
One comment regarding persistent epithelial defects. Dr. Langston, on the basis of her previous study from Mass Eye and Ear, began to use only fresh donor material with intact, healthy epithelium for grafting herpetics, and many of us began to do likewise. In the analysis of our data which didn't come out during this presentation, we were unable to demonstrate any particular, beneficial effect by retaining donor epithelium – from the standpoint of graft clarity or persistent epithelial defect development post-operatively. I think retention of donor epithelium is a double-edged sword. If one imagines that reducing total antigenic load to a young, healthy person with an "energetic" immune system might be of some benefit, then one might want to think twice about including epithelium in these grafts. I think it is very much an open question.

### H.E. Kaufman (New Orleans)
All of these papers have shown the difficulties in operating on acutely inflamed eyes. However, sometimes there is no choice, and, in that case, I would recommend the procedure suggested originally by Drs. Aaronson and Moore, as difficult as it may seem.

If one must operate on an acutely inflamed, herpetic eye, or a perforated eye, it appears that giving systemic steroids for 3 or 4 days quiets things down before surgery and makes surgery safer. I think that small, quiet perforations can be glued, and big holes cannot be glued. It is difficult to compare that sort of series.

In general, the common causes of epithelial defects, as Dr. Polack pointed out, are lagophthalmos or lack of tear flow, and these problems are very common after herpes infection. We use antiviral agents routinely after grafts for herpes, and we never send a patient home with an epithelial defect.

C.S. Foster (Boston)

One last emphasis on Doctor Kaufman's comments is that two of the most crucial factors in relating to ultimate favorable outcome in corneal transplantation in patients with herpes simplex keratitis appears to involve keeping the surface happy with fluid postoperatively and with the aggressive use of systemic and topical antiinflammatory agents, steroidal and nonsteroidal. The meticulous attention to all contributing details which might conspire against a favorable outcome, and the appropriate aggressive management of such problems is essential.

# Zoster Ophthalmicus

Sundmacher, R. (Hrsg.):
Herpetische Augenerkrankungen
© J.F. Bergmann Verlag, München 1981

# A Controlled Trial of Intravenous Therapy With Adenine Arabinoside (Ara-A) in Ophthalmic Zoster

R.J. Marsh, R. Laird, A. Atkinson, A. McD. Steele, B.J. Jones, London

**Key words.** Ophthalmic zoster, ara-A

**Schlüsselwörter.** Zoster ophthalmicus, ara-A

**Summary.** A blind trial was carried out on the effect of intravenous Adenine Arabinoside 10 mg per kg for 7 days on ophthalmic zoster. Twenty-four patients were admitted to the study. Its effects were studied on healing of the rash, postherpetic neuralgia and the development of ocular complications. Patients were randomly allocated on three criteria (1) severity of the rash, (2) length of time they had suffered from the rash before treatment and (3) whether ocular complications were apparent at presentation.

More rapid resolution of mucus in the tear film was the only statistically significant finding in favour of Ara A. Clinically there appeared to be faster healing in the rash, quicker resolution of conjunctival hyperaemia, less likelihood of episcleritis and postponement of corneal sensitivity loss in those treated with Ara A. The treatment was well tolerated and no serious adverse effects were recorded.

**Zusammenfassung.** In einer „Blind-Studie" untersuchten wir die Wirkung von Adeninarabinosid (10 mg/kg Körpergewicht i.v., Therapiedauer 10 Tage) bei 24 Patienten mit Zoster ophthalmicus. Beurteilungskriterien waren die Abheilung der Hauteffloreszenzen, das Verhalten einer post-zosterischen Neuralgie sowie die Entwicklung oculärer Komplikationen. Die Randomisierung erfolgte unter Berücksichtigung 1) der Ausbildung der Effloreszenzen, 2) der bereits verstrichenen Krankheitsdauer und 3) ob schon oculäre Beteiligung nachgewiesen werden konnte oder nicht.

Die einzige nachweisbare signifikante Wirkung von Ara-A war ein schnelleres Verschwinden des zähen Schleims in der Tränenflüssigkeit. Man hatte auch den Eindruck, daß die Effloreszenzen schneller abheilten, die Konjunctivitis schneller abklang, eine Episcleritis weniger häufig war und die Reduktion der Hornhautsensibilität nicht ganz so stark ausgeprägt war, wenn Ara-A gegeben wurde. Dies war aber nicht signifikant. Die Behandlung wurde gut vertragen und ernsthafte Nebenwirkungen konnten wir nicht feststellen.

## Introduction

Ophthalmic zoster is a viral disease leading to severe neurological and ocular complications, responsible for severe morbidity and persisting debility. About 10% of patients develop, later on in the disease, marked postherpetic neuralgia, corneal scarring or anterior segment necrosis. It would appear that these changes are primed in the acute phase of the disease, and develop fully in the convalescent phase. This being so, it would seem logical that they might be averted by control of the varicella/zoster virus replication at the very onset of the disease. Therefore, a systemic safe effective antiviral agent, easily crossing the blood/ganglion barrier, delivered at this time should be of enormous value in therapy.

Two antiviral agents have been used systemically in the past: Idoxuridine (IDU) and Cytosine arabinoside. The former has proved too toxic for systemic use, and the latter has had mixed reports of success, with the placebo proving more effective in therapy of systemic zoster in the most recent double-blind controlled trial [8]. Recently a new systemic antiviral agent, Adenine arabinoside, has been developed [1, 2] and has been reported to have few side effects [10]. It has proved effective against DNA viruses, including varicella and herpes simplex [3–7] and has favourable reports in the therapy of herpes zoster in the immunosuppressed [9].

In view of the large number of cases of herpes zoster passing through our hands, we decided to set up a clinical trial to decide on the effect of the drug in a presumed immunologically competent group.

## Methods

All new patients presenting at Moorfields Eye Hospital, City Road, London, with moderate to severe ophthalmic zoster were invited to participate in the trial. We excluded those patients with a rash duration of over 14 days and those who were pregnant.

The objectives of the study were to assess the effect of intravenously administered Adenine arabinoside (Ara-A) at a dose of 10 mg/kg per day over a seven-day period on the following features of ophthalmic zoster:

1. visual acuity
2. duration of cutaneous ulceration and degree of subsequent scarring
3. duration and intensity of post-herpetic neuralgia
4. scleritis/episcleritis
5. corneal sensation
6. keratitis
7. iritis and iris atrophy
8. glaucoma
9. external ocular motor palsy

The trial was designed as controlled and single-blind. Allocation to treatment groups was by stratified randomisation with the object of making the treated and control groups comparable in terms of the following three variables:

1. time of presentation after onset
   a. 1–3 days
   b. 4–7 days
   c. 8–10 days
   d. 11–14 days
2. severity of rash
   a. mild vesicular
   b. severe vesicular
   c. haemorrhagic
3. distribution of rash
   a. ocular involvement
   b. no ocular involvement

Comparability in respect of other variables, such as age, sex and presence or severity of other clinical features, had to depend on random factors.

We felt the experiment could not be made double-blind because it would have been ethically not permissible to have administered large volumes of intravenous fluid each day for a week to patients in the control group.

The result of random allocation of treatment was communicated only to the house surgeons (interns) who were to administer it in the mornings. The authors examined the patients in the afternoon when the infusion had been removed. In so far as this device was successful in keeping the authors ignorant of the treatment group, the trial could be called single blind.

On admission to the trial, a full medical and ophthalmic history and examination were carried out. We documented the phase of the rash as vesicular, pustular or crusty. Its severity was scored as nil (0), mild (1), moderate (2), severe with haemorrhages (3), and the oedema as nil (0), mild (1), ipsilateral (2), or bilateral palpebral fissure narrowing (3). Its distribution was noted as nasociliary, lid margin or neither. The degree of pigmentation and pitting with regard to scarring were recorded in four grades from nought to three. Other features were similarly scored at every examination. These included the degree of oedema, the bulbar and tarsal conjunctival hyperaemia, episcleritis/scleritis, corneal tear film mucus, the severity of corneal epithelial stromal lesion and iritis. Other features to be included were the corneal sensitivity (assessed centrally, and in four quadrants, using the aesthesiometer of Cochet and Bonnet). The degree of iris atrophy was marked as absent, small chinks, sphincter atrophy, and massive atrophy. The pupil reaction was recorded and the applanation. The fundi were examined and the external ocular movements assessed. Neuralgia was scored in five degrees as absent, mild, moderate, severe and very severe. Finally, any adverse reactions were recorded. Observations were to be made and recorded three times during the 1st week, twice in the 2nd and once each in the 3rd and 4th weeks, and again during the 3rd and 6th months.

A number of special investigations were carried out including photographs of full face, side face and close-up of the lids, blood analyses, and chest X-ray. To avoid unnecessary repetition, a copy of the check-list is attached.

All patients were treated with Neocortef ointment three times daily to the affected areas of skin, Terra-Cortril spray to the scalp and Distalgesic tablets to provide analgesia as required. Steroid, mydriatic and antibiotic drops were used as indicated by previous experience with ophthalmic zoster.

The 200 mg/ml drug suspension as supplied was diluted 500-fold in Dextrose saline for intravenous infusion, warmed so as to aid solution and administered once daily intravenously in sufficient volume to provide 10 mg/kg of body weight, i.e. 25 ml/kg. Treatment was continued in the absence of adverse affects for 7 consecutive days.

Each patient was shown a written statement setting out the design and objectives of the trial and invited to participate or not.

## Results

Twenty-five patients were initially accepted for the trial on the basis of clinical criteria and allocated to the treatment group according to scheme for stratified randomisation. One patient, however, declined to sign the consent form and was therefore dropped. Another patient, after he had been allocated to a treat-

ment group, was found to be suffering from hypertension and left ventricular hypertrophy of sufficient severity to contra-indicate large volumes of intravenous fluid. This patient was therefore relegated to the control group.

Figure 1 shows the distribution of the patients to the treatment and control groups by age.

One patient in the control group had suffered zoster in another part of the body previously, one in the treatment group had suffered Crohn's disease 3 years before and another pulmonary tuberculosis 1 year previously.

Table 1 shows the distribution and severity of the variables upon which the stratification was based at the time of presentation.

This shows that the distribution between groups is as equal as it can be with such small numbers, except in the case of three patients who had mild vesicular zoster without ocular involvement 4 to 7 days before admission to the trial. All three were allocated to the Ara-A treatment group. These three patients were scrutinised to see whether the clinical course was such as to influence the outcome of the trial.

*Deviation From the Protocol*

Inevitably, dealing with out-patients for a 6 month period, there were some irregular intervals between assessments. Appointments were missed either due to patients forgetting, not wanting to come, or being physically unable to come. There was particularly poor attendance at the second visit during the 2nd week and precisely at the 6th month. The analysis therefore had to be adjusted such that the former was ignored and all observations during the 4th and 5th months were aggregated with month 6. One of the

ara-A 6 men 7 women
control 4 men 7 women

years of age

**Table 1.** Stratified randomisation of patients to Ara-A and control groups

| | Time of presentation | | | | Severity | | | Ocular involvement | |
|---|---|---|---|---|---|---|---|---|---|
| | 1–3 days | 4–7 days | 8–10 days | 11–14 days | mild vesicular | sev. vesicular | haemor-rhagic | present | absent |
| Ara-A Group | 4 | 9 | 0 | 0 | 8 | 5 | 0 | 10 | 3 |
| Control Group | 2 | 8 | 1 | | 5 | 6 | 0 | 10 | 1 |

patients in the control group died on day 7. Death was caused by myocardial infarction of which the patient had had a previous attack in 1973. The last assessment was carried out on the day of death.

Efficacy was judged on the basis of the following variables: changes in the visual acuity of the affected eye, rash duration, severity and oedema and scarring. Other variables included the incidence severity and duration of conjunctivitis, keratitis, corneal anaesthesia, iritis, glaucoma, optic neuritis, ocular motor palsies and post-herpetic neuralgia. The object of the trial was, of course, to determine the effect of Ara-A and not to record the natural history of the disease. Thus the patients in whom a given feature is absent throughout can provide no useful information, variables that are not influenced by the disease are valueless and similarly variables that are not influenced by the treatment. For these reasons it was unprofitable to pursue the analysis of many of the supposed indices of effect. Consequently, the rash and neuralgia were the key parameters in the sense that they were not only clinically important but likely to be demonstrably influenced by effective therapy.

### Visual Acuity in the Affected Eye

No relevant effect was seen here.

### Rash

Nearly all patients had a vesicular eruption when first examined. Fig. 2 shows the time course of the rash from the vesicular to the crusting phases of the disease.

No patient in the Ara-A treated group had vesicles after the second day of treatment or pustules later than day 4. The earliest time at which no skin lesions were recorded was day 7. In the control group vesicles persisted in one patient until the fifth day of treatment and pustules in another until the seventh. The earliest time at which no skin lesions were recorded was day 14.

These results do seem to suggest that the rash cleared more quickly in the Ara-A treatment group.

No significant effect was found on the degree of severity of the rash. This may be explained by difficulty in estimating the degree of severity.

### Oedema and Scarring

No real difference was found between the two groups.

### Conjunctivitis

Tables 2 and 3 show the effect on tarsal and bulbar conjunctivitis. There was a suggestion of more rapid resolution in the Ara-A group: five members of which achieved a sustained zero rating during the first 7 days compared with only one in the control group.

### Episcleritis/Scleritis

There was no difference between the two groups.

### Cornea

There was less mucus in the tear film in the

**Table 2.** Resolution of Bulbar hyperaemia

| Treatment Group | 1st Week | 2nd Week | 3rd Week | 4th Week | 5th Week | Over 14 |
|---|---|---|---|---|---|---|
| Ara-A | 5 | 1 | 2 | 1 | 0 | 3 |
| Control | 0 | 3 | 1 | 3 | 1 | 3 |

**Table 3.** Resolution of Tarsal hyperaemia

| Treatment Group | 1st Week | 2nd Week | 3rd Week | 4th Week | 5th Week | 6th Week | Over 14 |
|---|---|---|---|---|---|---|---|
| Ara-A | 2 | 3 | 0 | 1 | 0 | 2 | 3 |
| Control | 0 | 0 | 1 | 4 | 0 | 0 | 5 |

**Table 4.** Resolution of precorneal mucus film

| Treatment Group | 1st Week | 2nd Week | 3rd Week | 4th Week | 5th Week | 6–14th | Over 14 |
|---|---|---|---|---|---|---|---|
| Ara-A | 2 | 3 | 0 | 1 | 0 | 2 | 3 |
| Control | 0 | 0 | 1 | 4 | 0 | 0 | 5 |

Ara-A group and Table 4 shows when a sustained zero rating was reached.

*Corneal Sensation*

A suggestion that Ara-A can delay the development of sensory loss even though there is no evidence that it can prevent it.

*Iritis, Intra-ocular Lesions, Optic Disc, Retina and Neuralgia*

There is nothing to suggest an effect of treatment.

*Adverse Experiences*

Five patients of the Ara-A group and four of the control group experienced adverse symptoms. The symptoms occurring in the former can be divided into those occurring during treatment with Ara-A and those occurring subsequently. The former occurred in four patients including one syncope and emesis of moderate severity on day 1, one moderate left-sided hearing loss on day 3, one headache of unspecified severity on day 4 and one case of mild nausea and vomiting on day 1 followed by mild nausea on day 2. The only severe

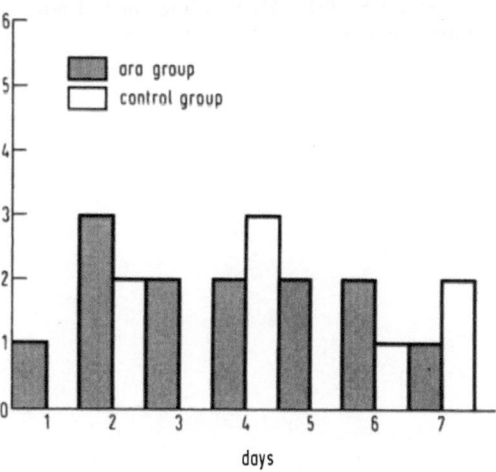

days

"adverse" experience was the nausea and vomiting that affected one patient on days 12 and 13 (5 days after the last administration of Ara-A).

*Clinical Laboratory Determinations*

Unfortunately a significant number of results were unavailable or wrong, due to difficulties in handling blood samples. So far as they go there was no evidence of drug related toxicity.

**Discussion**

It was disappointing that neither the severity nor the duration of neuralgia was demonstrably diminished by the administration of Ara-A. This may well mean that intra-neural virus is inaccessible to the drug and that would be consistent with the observation of some other workers: that localised zoster responds less favourably to treatment with Ara-A than varicella and disseminated zoster. The presence of a number of differences between the treated and control groups that seem to suggest a favourable influence of Ara-A without reaching an acceptable level of statistical significance may suggest either that a larger group of patients should be treated or that a larger dose of the drug should be given.

Of the twenty variables analysed only one has shown a statistically significant difference between treated and control groups, i.e. resolution of precorneal mucus. This could easily occur by chance.

The balance of the evidence is in favour of more rapid healing of the rash, quicker resolution of conjunctival hyperaemia, less likelihood of scleritis and episcleritis developing, postponement of corneal sensitivity loss, quicker healing of corneal epithelial lesions and less likelihood of increased intra-ocular pressure.

The treatment was well tolerated and no serious adverse effects were recorded.

**Table 5.** ARA-A Zoster trial moorfields eye hospital (check sheet)

Name  ....................................................  Hosp. No.  .......................................  Trial No.  ...........................

| Day of Observation | Pre Treat | Day 2 | 4 | 6 | 7 | 9 | 13 | 21 | 28 | 3 months | 6 months |
|---|---|---|---|---|---|---|---|---|---|---|---|
| Date | | | | | | | | | | | |
| History | x | | | | | | | | | | |
| Ophth. Exam | x | x | x | x | x | x | x | x | x | x | x |
| Photos | x | x | x | x | | x | | | | | |
| Urinalysis | x | x | x | x | x | | | | | | |
| Hb. W.B.Cs. ESR film L.F. Ts 'strip | x | | | | x | | | | | | x |
| Enzymes cholestrol Blood sugar | x | | | | x | | | | | | |
| Adverse effects | x | x | x | x | x | x | x | x | x | x | x |

# References

1. Lee WW, Benitez A, Goodman L, Baker BR (1960) Potential anticancer agents XL. Synthesis of the B-anomer of 9-(D-arabinofuranosyl) adenine. J Am Chem Soc 82:2648–2649
2. Reist EJ, Benitez A, Goodman L, Baker BR, Lee WW (1962) Potential anticancer agents LXXVI. Synthesis of purin nucleosides of B-D-arabinofuranose. J Org Chem 27:3274–3279
3. Privat de Garihle M, De Rudder J (1964) Effet de deux nucleosides de l'arabinose sur la multiplication des virus de l'herpes et de la vaccine en ailture allulaire. CR Acad Sci (D) (Paris) 259:2725–2728
4. Freeman G, Kuehn A, Sultanian I (1965) Response of tumorigenic viruses and of cells to biologically active compounds. I. methods for determining response and application of methods. Cancer Res (Suppl 40) 25:1609–1625
5. Freeman G, Kuehn A, Sultanian I (1965) Tumorigenic virus and cell responses to biologically active compounds. II. Pharmacologic specificity in cell-virus relationships. Ann NY Acad Sci 130:330–342
6. Schabel jr FM (1968) The antiviral activity of 9-B-D-arabinofuranosyladenine (ara-A). Chemotherapy 13:321–338
7. Miller FA, Dixon GJ, Ehrlich J, Sloan BJ, McLean jr IW (1968) The antiviral activity of 9-B-D-arabinofuranosyladenine (ara-A). I. Cell culture studies. Antimicrob Agents Chemother :136–147
8. Stevens DA, Jordan GW, Waddell TF, Merigan TC (1973) Adverse effect of cytosine arabinoside on disseminated zoster in a controlled trial. N Engl J Med 289:873–878
9. Luby JP, Johnson MT, Buchanan R, Ch'ien LT, Whitley R, Alford CA (1975) Adenine arabinoside therapy of varicella-zoster virus infections. In: Pavan-Langston D, Buchanan RA, Alford CA (eds) Adenine arabinoside: an antiviral agent. Raven, New York, pp 237–245
10. Keenay RE (1975) Human tolerance of adenine arabinoside. Ref 9, pp 265–273

Sundmacher, R. (Hrsg.):
Herpetische Augenerkrankungen
© J.F. Bergmann Verlag, München 1981

# A Double-Blind Controlled Trial of Therapy With Levamisole in Ophthalmic Zoster

R.J. Marsh, L. Olsen, R. Weatherhead, B.R. Jones, London

**Key words.** Ophthalmic zoster, levamisole

**Schlüsselwörter.** Zoster ophthalmicus, Levamisol

**Summary.** A double-blind controlled study was carried out to determine the effect on ophthalmic zoster of Levamisole at a dose of 150 mg for 3 days a week over a 6 month period. The same criteria were judged as for the Ara-A trial. Fifty-two patients were admitted to the trial of which 15 had to be excluded from the analysis. The only statistically significant finding in favour of Levamisole was more rapid resolution of mucus in the tear film. There was less rapid healing of the rash in the Levamisole patients than those taking the placebo. A significant number of adverse reactions were noted in both groups.

**Zusammenfassung.** In einer „Doppelblind-Studie" untersuchten wir den Einfluß von Levamisol auf den Verlauf eines Zoster ophthalmicus. Die Dosierung war 150 mg an drei Tagen pro Woche über einen Zeitraum von 6 Monaten. Der Beurteilung lagen die gleichen Kriterien zugrunde wie in der Ara-A Studie (S. 449ff). Von 52 initial teilnehmenden Patienten konnten schließlich 37 ausgewertet werden. Die einzige statistisch belegbare Levamisol-Wirkung war das schnellere Verschwinden des zähen Schleims aus der Tränenflüssigkeit. Die Effloreszenzen verschwanden bei den Levamisol-Patienten sogar weniger schnell als bei den Plazebo-Behandelten. In beiden Therapiegruppen wurde eine größere Anzahl von „Nebenwirkungen" festgestellt.

## Introduction

For some time there has been a distinct clinical impression that many patients developing zoster, especially the elderly, have impaired immunity. Certainly patients suffering from zoster with systemic spread of the rash have a high incidence of reticuloses, neoplasms and immunosuppression [3]. Unfortunately proof of impaired immunity is rarely obtained prior to the development of the disease. After the rash resolves many of the ophthalmic zoster patients develop chronic and relapsing ocular complications with features suggestive of defective immunity. However, there seems to be no difference between the neutralising antibody response of these patients and those without ocular complications. The only hint of scientific evidence for defective immunity in uncomplicated zoster is a defect detected in the monocytes during the acute phase of the disease [5]. Assuming a basis of defective delayed immunity it would be worthwhile assessing a drug that would reinforce it. Levamisole presents itself as such a drug [4].

It has been shown to have an immunopotentating effect following the observation that cows receiving Levamisole developed enhanced immunity for suboptimal brucella vaccine. The effect principally occurs when existing host defence mechanisms are impaired. Levamisole particularly restores T cell and macrophage function (especially to antigen previously encountered), but has little effect on the B cell humoral antibody system. There was a large body of clinical evidence which suggested that the immunopotentiating effect of Levamisole may have been of benefit in chronic persistent infections and a report confirmed this in chronic upper respiratory tract infections in children [6].

## Methods

All new patients presenting at Moorfields Eye

Hospital with moderate to severe Ophthalmic Zoster were invited to participate in the trial. We excluded those patients with a rash duration of over 10 days and those who were pregnant.

The objectives of the study were to assess the effect of orally administered Levamisole at a dose of 150 mgm. daily for 3 days a week over a 6 month period on the following features of ophthalmic zoster:

1. Visual acuity
2. Duration of cutaneous ulceration and degree of subsequent scarring
3. Duration and intensity of post herpetic neuralgia
4. Scleritis/episcleritis
5. Corneal sensation
6. Keratitis
7. Iritis and iris atrophy
8. Glaucoma
9. External ocular motor palsy

The trial was designed as controlled and double-blind. Allocation to treatment groups was by stratified randomisation with the object of making the treatment and control groups comparable in terms of the following variables.

1. Time of presentation after onset:
   a. 1– 3 days
   b. 4– 7 days
   c. 8–10 days
2. Severity of rash:
   a. mild vesicular
   b. moderate vesicular
   c. severe vesicular
3. Significant ocular involvement at presentation:
   a. present
   b. absent

Comparability in respect of other variables, such as age, sex and presence or severity of other clinical features had to depend on random factors.

The result of random allocation of treatment was revealed to the pharmacist who accordingly dispensed Levamisole or placebo tablets to the patients.

On admission to the trial the same history, examination and documentation were carried out as for the Ara-A trial. Observations were made at the same intervals. The same special investigations were carried out with the addition of blood examinations at weeks 2, 3 & 4 and months 3 & 6. Adverse reactions were carefully recorded.

All patients were treated with the same conventional therapy as in the Ara-A trial. The Levamisole and placebo tablets were given at a dose of 150 mgm. daily for 3 days a week for 6 months in the absence of adverse affects. Each patient was shown a written statement setting out the design and objectives of the trial and invited to participate or not.

## Results

Fifty-two patients presented to the trial. Fifteen patients were excluded from the analysis, 3 of which failed to take their tablets reliably, 3 failed to keep an adequate number of follow-up appointments and 9 had toxic side effects preventing them from completing the trial. This left 37 patients for the analysis. Figure 1 shows the distribution of patients to the treatment and control groups by age. Three patients in the placebo group had suffered general disease including one case of hypertension, one of diabetes mellitus and one had had a rodent ulcer.

Five patients in the Levamisole group had suffered general disease. One had diabetes mellitus, one tuberculosis twenty years previously, two had bronchitis and congestive heart failure and one had thyroid disease.

Table 1 shows the distribution and severity of the variables upon which the stratification was based at the time of presentation. Only global totals are given for stratified randomisation. Eighteen combinations were possible but statistically there were too few patients in the study to merit detailed stratifi-

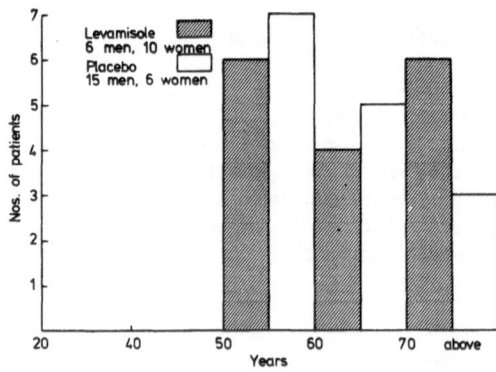

**Fig. 1.** The distribution of patients to treatment and control groups by age

456

**Table 1.** Stratified randomisation

| | Time of presentation (in days) | | | Severity of rash | | | Ocular involvement | |
|---|---|---|---|---|---|---|---|---|
| | 1-3 | 4-7 | 8-10 | Mild | Moderate | Severe | Present | Absent |
| Levamisole | 2 | 11 | 3 | 2 | 12 | 2 | 13 | 3 |
| Placebo | 2 | 16 | 3 | 5 | 11 | 4 | 16 | 2 |

cation and this report concerned itself with global totals and not individual strata levels.

### Deviations From the Protocol

There were some irregular intervals between assessments as occured in the Ara-A trial and for precisely the same reasons. However, no serious deviations from the protocol took place. Patient drop-outs and exclusions will be dealt with later on. Efficacy was judged on the same variables as for Ara-A with the same exclusions of clinically unimportant data.

### Visual Acuity

No relevant effect was seen here.

### Rash

Figure 2 shows the time course of the rash from the vesicular to crusting phases of the disease. This suggests a more rapid resolution

of the rash in the Placebo group than Levamisole. However, the nature of the data does not allow simple hypothesis testing and therefore no statistical significance is attached to speed of resolution.

### Oedema and Scarring

No real difference was found between the two groups.

### Conjunctivitis

Table 2 records the progress of tarsal hyperaemia and here there is a suggestion of more rapid resolution in the Levamisole group, four members of which achieved a sustained zero rating on or before day 7 compared with none in the Placebo group. There was no difference between the two groups as far as bulbar hyperaemia was concerned.

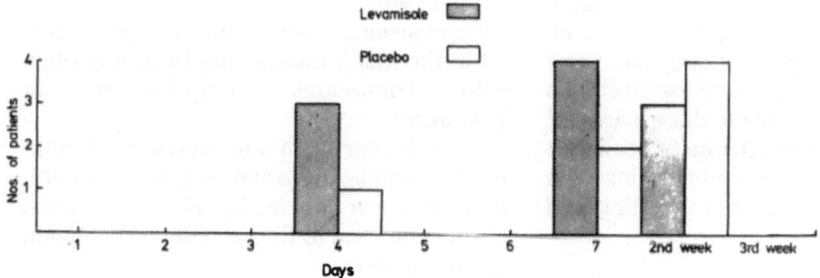

**Fig. 2.** Time course of rash from vesicular to crusting phase

**Table 2.** Resolution of tarsal hyperaemia

| Treatment Group | Week 1 | Week 2 | Week 3 | Week 4 | Week 5 | Week 6 | Over 12 |
|---|---|---|---|---|---|---|---|
| Levamisole | 4 | 1 | 3 | – | 2 | – | 5 |
| Placebo | – | 3 | 3 | – | 3 | 1 | 9 |

**Table 3.** Resolution of pre corneal mucus film

| Treatment Group | Week 1 | Week 2 | Week 3 | Week 4 | Week 5 | Week 6 | Over 12 |
|---|---|---|---|---|---|---|---|
| Levamisole | 2 | 2 | 1 | – | 2 | – | 7 |
| Placebo | – | – | 4 | 2 | – | – | 7 |

*Precorneal Mucus*

Table 3 provides details of the mucus in the tear film. Omitting the patients who scored zero throughout and counting those from each group who achieved a sustained score of zero on or before day 14 a significant difference in favour of Levamisole appears.

*Episcleritis/Scleritis, Keratitis, Corneal Sensation, Iritis and Iris Atrophy, Glaucoma and External Ocular Motor Balsy*

There were no significant differences between the Levamisole and placebo treatment groups.

*Adverse Experiences*

The nine patients removed from the trial due to toxic effects included six on Levamisole and three on Placebo. Thirteen patients completing the trial had adverse reactions, five on Levamisole and eight on Placebo. The complications of those taking Placebo were three cases of nausea, three of neutropenia, one of parasthesia in legs and feet, one flu-like illness, one of vomiting, one of body pains and one a rash (concurrently taking tegretol). The Levamisole group included three cases of drowsiness and depression, one of headache and nausea, four of abdominal pains with diarrhoea, two of nausea and vomiting and one of a rash.

*Clinical Laboratory Determinations*

As mentioned above three patients on the placebo developed neutropenia. These were mild and in two cases sporadic. The third case developed at 1 month and was present at every subsequent month until the tablets were terminated at the 6th. There were no abnormalities in the Levamisole group.

**Discussion**

It was disappointing to see that Levamisole too had no effect on either the severity or duration of post-herpetic neuralgia. Like Ara-A it had a statistically significant action only on the resolution of mucus in the tear film and a clinically significant action on tarsal hyperaemia. Unlike Ara-A there was a more rapid healing of the rash in the placebo group.

Adverse reactions were of a significant number in both groups. It is difficult to explain all those occurring in the placebo group. Many of them were taking analgesics concurrently and many of the symptoms described may occur during the natural course of convalescent Ophthalmic zoster. The three cases of neutropenia were hard to explain although in severe zoster neutropenia and lymphopenia can occur naturally. The absence of this finding in the Levamisole group, however, might suggest some protective action exerted by this drug. Levamisole has well recognised complications including: nausea, gastric intolerance, central nervous stimulation, nervousness, irritability, insomnia, a 'flu-like syndrome, skin rashes and granulocytopenia [7]. A higher incidence of gastro intestinal discomfort, most pronounced in the first 3 months has been described with continuous administration of Levamisole.

This is why we administered it intermittently. Complications appear to be more common in cancer patients [2]. The search must clearly continue to find an effective antiviral agent in Zoster.

However, if viral replication is confined to the onset of the disease and if the later lesions are, as seems likely, due to immunologically mediated reactions not dependent on the presence of live virus, the results will not prove useful unless the drug is administered at the very onset of the disease [1]. Furthermore an effective anti-anergic drug would be complimentary in the successful treatment of Zoster.

**Acknowledgments.** We would like to thank Parke-Davis for their help with the Ara-A trial and Janssen Pharmaceutical Ltd. for the Levamisole trial. It is a pleasure to thank Miss J. O'Regan for secretarial assistance.

# References

1. Marsh RJ (1976) Ophthalmic herpes zoster. Br J Hosp Med :609–618
2. Parkinson DR, Jerry LM, Shibata HR, Lewis MG, Cano PO, Capek A, Mansell PW, Marquis G (1977) Complications of cancer immunotherapy with Levamisole. Lancet 1:1129–1132
3. Stevens DA, Merigan TC (1972) Interferon, antibody & other host factors in herpes zoster. J Clin Invest 51:1170
4. Thienpont D, Vanparijs OFJ, Raeymaekers AHM, Vandenberk J, Demoen PJA, Allewijn FTN, Marsboom RPH, Niemegeers CJE, Schellekens KHL, Janssen PAJ (1966) Tetramisole (R8299) a new, potent broad spectrum anthelmintic. Nature 209:1084
5. Twomey J, Gyorkey F, Norris SM (1974) The monocyte disorder with herpes zoster. J Lab Clin Med 83:768–771
6. Eygen M van, Znamensky PY, Heck E, Raymaekers I (1976) Levamisole in prevention of recurrent upper respiratory tract infections in children. Lancet 1:382–385
7. Willoughby DA, Wood C (1977) Levamisole in rheumatoid arthritis. For Immunother 2: 7–12

Sundmacher, R. (Hrsg.):
Herpetische Augenerkrankungen
© J.F. Bergmann Verlag, München 1981

# The Use of Acyclovir in the Treatment of Herpes Zoster Ocular Infections

J. McGill, C. James, P. Hiscott, T. Worstman, M. Larkin, Southampton

**Key words.** Ophthalmic zoster, acyclovir

**Schlüsselwörter.** Zoster ophthalmicus, Acyclovir

**Summary.** Eighteen patients with ocular herpes zoster involvement were treated with either topical Acycloguanosine (n = 13) or intravenous therapy (n = 5). The preliminary results compare favourably with the results of therapy reported in the literature. Only one patient required topical steroids. Further controlled studies are required.

**Zusammenfassung.** 18 Patienten mit okulärer Beteiligung bei Zoster ophthalmicus wurden mit Acycloguanosin behandelt, 13 mit Lokaltherapie und 5 intravenös. Die Therapieergebnisse erscheinen im Vergleich mit den in der Literatur berichteten Ergebnissen günstig; endgültige Schlußfolgerungen werden aber erst nach kontrollierten Studien möglich sein. Besonders ermutigend ist, daß nur ein Patient mit lokalen Steroiden behandelt werden mußte.

## Introduction

Herpes zoster ophthalmicus is a severe, painful disease, showing much variation in the extent of its clinical involvement. In the acute phase it is often associated with much toxicity, and the dreaded complications of postherpetic neuralgia and ocular involvement are common.

Ocular involvement can lead to severe damage and visual loss. Steroids have an established place in the treatment of ocular involvement, but treatment is often unsatisfactory and, in some cases, fails to prevent ocular damage. Also, this form of treatment has severe drawbacks, not only due to the ocular side-effects of steroids, but due to the need to continue treatment to prevent recurrences. If steroid treatment is stopped too soon, not only can the ocular involvement recur, but corneal opacities can appear with subsequent lipid deposition infrequently taking place, resulting in severe visual loss [7].

So far, no topical antiviral has been shown to have a definite effect in the treatment of herpes zoster ophthalmicus. There is thus the need for a drug which actively suppresses ocular involvement and prevents recurrent ocular disease.

### Acyclovir − Acycloguanosine (9(2-Hydroxy-oxymethylguanine) (Welcome)

Acyclovir is an acyclic nucleoside with a high specificity for virally infected cells and little effect on uninfected cells [4]. Biron and Elion in 1979 [2] examined, by means of the plaque reduction technique, the sensitivity of herpes zoster virus to Acyclovir and found that although it was less sensitive to Acyclovir than herpes virus, there was still irreversible inhibition of plaque formation by non-toxic drug doses of Acyclovir. The formation of the triphosphate form of the drug, specific to viral infected cells, and not normal cells, by means of viral thymidine kinase, leads to inhibition of herpes simplex and zoster DNA viral synthesis [5, 6].

Experimentally Acycloguanosine has an effect on herpes simplex cutaneous, ocular and encephalitic infections, and it has also been stated to have an effect on varicella zoster virus, cytomegalo virus and the herpes B virus [1, 10].

Acyclovir has a high solubility, can be given intravenously, and as it is catabolised only to 5%, practically all the compound is present in the active form [1, 10], with no sign of any systemic toxicity [3]. Preliminary clinical results in herpes zoster infection in immu-

461

nosuppressed patients have been encouraging [9].

In view of these properties, and the promising experimental results, it was decided to test clinically the effect of Acycloguanosine in the treatment of herpes zoster ophthalmic infections by means of an open trial using both the intravenous and the topical form of the drug.

## Patient Selection

Patients were treated with Acyclovir for herpes zoster infection provided they were over 16 years of age and not women of childbearing potential. They were treated with intravenous Acyclovir 5 mg/kg tds for 5 days if they had herpes zoster involvement of the ophthalmic division of the trigeminal nerve, with ocular involvement, and with a skin rash of less than 72 hours duration, and at the vesicular stage or earlier. If they had ocular herpes zoster complications and the skin rash had developed, they were treated with topical ocular ointment (3.3%) Acyclovir five times a day.

Those patients on intravenous therapy were admitted and the remainder were treated on an out-patient basis.

At each visit a note was taken of the stage of the skin rash and the degree of pain present. Satellite lesions were searched for. From the eye point of view, patients were asked for symptoms of pain, grittiness, photophobia, and lacrimation, and these were scored on a 0–3+ basis. The rash was scored on a 0–4 basis (Table 1). The conjunctiva was examined for hyperaemia, the presence of follicles, papillae, thickening, scarring, or

**Table 1.** To show presenting symptoms of patients with skin and ocular involvement treated with I.V. Acyclovir

|  | Rash | Pain |
|---|---|---|
| Patient 1 | 3 | 2 |
| 2 | 3 | 3 |
| 3 | 2 | 2 |
| 4 | 4 | 3 |
| 5 | 2 | 3 |

Key: Rash Score. 1 Scanty/Discrete, 2 Profuse Discrete, 3 Semi-confluent, 4 Confluent. Pain Score. 0 none, 1 mild, 2 moderate, 3 severe

keratinisation. The corneal epithelium was examined for the presence or absence of ulceration, scarring, and the stroma for the presence of infiltration, oedema, or vascularisation. If uveitis was present it was scored as either mild or severe. Note was taken of any iris involvement, whether the pupil was active or not, or whether there was evidence of atrophy of iris tissue. The clarity of the lens and the fundal appearance, and the presence or absence of any extraocular muscle palsy, was noted.

At the initial visit, skin and ocular lesions were cultured for herpes zoster virus, and during the course of intravenous treatment, daily skin cultures were taken.

The patients' antibody response was monitored by means of measuring the IgG, IgM and IgA titres, using the membrane fluorescence reciprocal titre.

## Results

Eighteen patients with ocular herpes zoster involvement were treated in this series, of whom five had intravenous therapy and 13 topical ointment. Eight were male, ten female, and their ages varied from 25 years to 83 years.

*Intravenous Treatment*

Table 1 shows the initial presenting symptoms of the five patients having intravenous therapy. The rash was scored on a 0–4+ basis and pain on a 0–3+ basis. Follow-up has been for a maximum of 47 weeks. Four had ocular involvement within the first 2 days of treatment, but this settled within 5 days, and in all five the skin rash crusted within 5 days, with resolution of the pain.

Two patients developed mild post-herpetic neuralgia which has since gradually subsided. The patient with no initial ocular involvement, patient 3, subsequently developed a herpes zoster disciform keratitis which quickly settled within 2 weeks on topical ointment. None have since had a recurrence of their ocular involvement.

In three patients antibody levels were measured, and in all three there was a rise in IgG titre (Table 2). Herpes zoster virus could be isolated up to the 4th day of treatment in the three patients cultured (Table 3).

**Table 2.** Antibody levels during and after intravenous Acyclovir treatment

| | | Membrane fluorescence reciprocal titre | | |
| | | IgG | IgM | IgA |
|---|---|---|---|---|
| Patient 3 | Day 5 | 16 | 8 | 8 |
| | 66 | 256 | 8 | 8 |
| Patient 4 | Day 0 | 512 | 8 | 8 |
| | 5 | 1024 | – | 8 |
| | 45 | 256 | 8 | 8 |
| Patient 5 | Day 2 | 8 | 8 | 8 |
| | 66 | 8 | 8 | 8 |

**Table 3.** To show herpes zoster viral isolation rates during course ofe intravenous Acyclovir treatment

| Patient 3 | Day 1 + ve |
|---|---|
| | 2 + ve |
| | 3 + ve |
| | 4 + ve |
| | 5 – ve |
| Patient 4 | Day 1 + ve |
| | 2 + ve |
| | 3 + ve |
| | 4 + ve |
| | 5 – ve |
| Patient 5 | Day 1 + ve |
| | 2 + ve |
| | 3 – ve |

*Topical Treatment*

Thirteen patients developed the late complication of ocular involvement after the skin rash had subsided. These were treated with topical ointment 3.3% Acyclovir five times a day (Table 4).

Ten patients had peripheral dendritic corneal ulceration normally associated with herpes zoster infection [11]. These healed in an average of 5.2 days. Ten patients had uveitis which settled within 19 days average, and eight patients developed a herpes zoster stromal reaction, either a disciform reaction or localised infiltrate, which settled in an average of 11 days. Two further patients developed episcleritis which settled in an average of 25 days. Of this group of 13 patients, only two required the additional use of steroids, one patient (number 7) had severe

**Table 4.** To show outcome of 13 patients with herpes zoster ocular involvement treated with topical 3.3% Acyclovir ointment. Average follow-up 20.3 (range 8–47) weeks

| | Number | Days to heal |
|---|---|---|
| Ulcer | 10 | 5.2 |
| Stromal involvement | 8 | 11.7 |
| Episcleritis | 2 | 24.5 |
| Uveitis | 10 | 19.2 |
| 2° Glaucoma | 3 | 28.3 |

No recurrences

herpes zoster kerato-uveitis which developed prior to any skin rash, having developed 15 years ago, herpes zoster ophthalmicus. At the time of presentation she had a severe reaction in the same area which failed to adequately settle on topical Acyclovir; with the addition of steroids and ocular hypotensive treatment the kerato-uveitis and secondary glaucoma settled. Patient 6 had prior steroid treatment before Acyclovir was started, and it was not possible to wean off the steroids and replace them with Acyclovir alone.

The average follow-up was 18 weeks (range 5 to 45 weeks). No patient has had a recurrence of herpes zoster ocular involvement after a course of topical treatment. One of the five treated with intravenous therapy developed an ocular recurrence which settled on topical ointment, and has not recurred after 7 weeks.

The duration of topical treatment varied from 5 weeks to 16 weeks without any signs of toxicity, apart from two patients developing a mild punctate epithelial keratopathy in the interpalpebral fissure, on the conjunctiva only. This quickly settled when the treatment was tailed off.

**Discussion**

Herpes zoster ophthalmicus is a variable disease affecting different patients to different degrees of severity. Therefore it is difficult in an open trial such as this to draw any definite conclusions as to the effectiveness of the Acyclovir in the treatment of herpes zoster.

However, it would appear that for all patients treated with topical Acyclovir, and four of the five treated with intravenous Acyclovir, the ocular involvement subsided, and so far in a comparatively short follow-up period there have been no recurrences. Particularly impressive have been the resolution of stromal involvement, episcleritis, and uveitis.

Previous workers have found that the corneal ulcers take up to 11 days to settle [8], and that the kerato-uveitis can grumble on for many months [7]. The results reported here compare favourably with these figures.

Whilst the intravenous therapy successfully controlled the skin and ocular manifestations of the disease, it had no effect on the antibody levels, which is important, as it means that Acyclovir can arrest the disease without affecting the immune response. Thus treated patients do not have an increased chance of further attacks which they would have had if the drug had affected the disease process before the immune response had developed.

Only one patient required topical steroids, and in no patient, once topical treatment had been stopped, have their been any signs of recurrence of the diseases as so frequently happens in steroid-treated patients, though a longer follow-up period will be necessary to be definitely sure of this.

The absence also of widespread topical toxicity after prolonged treatment is of significance; it bears out the claim that the drug only affects virally infected cells. Further controlled trials with this drug are required, particularly comparing it with topical steroids in the treatment of herpes zoster ocular involvement.

## References

1. Bauer DJ, Collins P, Tucker WE, Macklin AW (1979) Treatment of experimental herpes simplex keratitis with acycloguanosine. Br J Ophthalmol 63:429–435
2. Biron KK, Elion GB (1979) Sensitivity of varicella zoster virus in vitro to acyclovir. Antimicrob Agents Chemother Abstr 249
3. Brigden D, Bye A, Collins P, Miranda P de (1978) Preliminary studies with 9-(2-hydroxyethoxymethyl)guanine (BW248U) administered orally to healthy male human volunteers. Antimicrob Agents Chemother Abstr 74
4. Elion GB, Furman PA, Fyfe JA, Miranda de P, Beauchamp L, Schaeffer HJ (1977) Selectivity of action of an antiherpetic agent, 9-(2-hydroxyethoxymethyl)guanine. Proc Natl Acad Sci USA 74:5716–5720
5. Furman PA, St Clair MH, Fyfe JA, Rideout JL, Keller PM, Elion GB (1979) Inhibition of herpes simplex virus-induced DNA polymerase activity and viral DNA replication by 9-(2-hydroxyethoxymethyl)guanine and its triphosphate. J Virol 32:72–77
6. Fyfe JA, Biron KK (1979) Phosphorylation of acyclovir by a thymidine kinase induced by varicella-zoster virus. Antimicrob Agents Chemother Abstr 250
7. Marsh RJ (1976) Ophthalmic herpes zoster. Br J Host Med June, 609–618
8. Piebenga LW, Laibson PR (1973) Dendritic lesions in herpes zoster ophthalmicus. Arch Ophthalmol 90:268–270
9. Selby PJ, Jameson B, Watson JG, Morgenstern C, Powles RL, Kay HEM, Thornton R, Clink HM, McElwain TJ, Prentice HG, Ross MG, Corringham R, Hoffbrand AV, Brigden D (1979) Parenteral acyclovir therapy for herpesvirus infections in man. Lancet 2:1267–1270
10. Schaeffer HJ, Beauchamp L, Miranda P de, Elion GB, Bauer DJ, Collins P (1978) 9-(2-hydroxyethoxymethyl)guanine activity against viruses of the herpes group. Nature 272:583–585
11. Marsh RJ, Fraunfelder F, McGill JT (1976) Herpetic corneal epithelial disease. Arch Ophthalmol 1899–1902

Sundmacher, R. (Hrsg.):
Herpetische Augenerkrankungen
© J.F. Bergmann Verlag, München 1981

# Trials With Interferon in Ophthalmic Zoster

R. Sundmacher, D. Neumann-Haefelin, K. Cantell, Freiburg

**Key words.** Ophthalmic zoster, interferon

**Schlüsselwörter.** Zoster ophthalmicus, Interferon

**Summary.** 24 patients with ophthalmic zoster were treated either 5 or 10 days with $3 \times 10^6$ units of leukocyte interferon or albumine intramuscularly in addition to a standard therapy consisting of topical steroids plus mydriatics. This controlled pilot study showed some reduction of the iritis severity index by interferon, the longterm overall course, however, was not impressively altered by the interferon regime. We would expect interferon to be more effective in a combination with a systemic antiviral which in itself has been proven to be effective against zoster (acycloguanosine?). Furthermore, a therapeutic regime for zoster should consider that presumably quite early immunologic hyperreactivity may cause more damage than viral cytolysis.

**Zusammenfassung.** 24 Patienten mit Zoster ophthalmicus erhielten zusätzlich zu der bei uns üblichen lokalen Steroid-Mydriatika-Therapie für 5 bzw. 10 Tage intramuskuläre Injektionen von $3 \times 10^6$ Einheiten Leukozyteninterferon oder Albumin. In dieser kontrollierten Pilot-Studie zeigte sich zwar eine günstige Interferon-Wirkung hinsichtlich des Schweregrades der Iritis; auf lange Sicht gesehen war der therapeutische Eindruck vom Interferon aber nicht überzeugend. Wir würden dennoch erwarten, daß Interferon in Kombination mit einem systemischen Virustatikum, was selbst nachgewiesenermaßen bei Zoster wirksam ist (Acycloguanosin?) eine erheblich bessere Wirkungschance hat. Darüber hinaus sollte man bei der Zostertherapie auch nicht vergessen, daß wahrscheinlich immunologische Überreaktionen mehr Schaden anrichten als virale zytolytische Prozesse und daß deshalb auch eine dosierte Immunsuppression Bestandteil einer Kombinationstherapie sein sollte.

It has been our experience that zoster keratouveitis benefits from topical steroid therapy, irrespective of whether or not epithelial foci still exist. This constitutes a marked difference to dendritic keratitis. Since we have treated zoster patients who have ocular involvement starting at the time of the first symptoms with cycloplegia plus dexamethasone eye drops (0.1%; the steroids being tapered out over a long time), we have no longer observed severe sequelae like necrotizing keratitis, severe corneal scarring, persistent or recurrent corneal defects, or severe glaucoma [2]. If, however, the steroid regime is started too late, is under-dosed, or is stopped too early, steroids may indeed not be of major value as indicated in Duke-Elder's System of Ophthalmology [1].

Our hypothesis for the steroids' effect would be that after an initial immunosuppression with consequent endogenous reinfection by zoster virus, immune reactions supervene and lead to immune disease. Immunocytolysis is probably much more dangerous than viral cytolysis, a phenomenon which we also encounter in deep herpetic diseases, e.g. disciform edema (see pp. 203ff.).

On the other hand, it is likely that zoster virus either persists in peripheral tissues for quite some time or is repeatedly shed from sensory neurons.

**Table 1.** Set-up of interferon-trial in zoster-patients

| Duration of treatment | Interferon (HLI) $3 \times 10^6$ units i.m. per day | Albumine i.m. |
|---|---|---|
| 5 days | 3 patients | 3 patients |
| 10 days | 9 patients | 9 patients |
| Comparative evaluation | 9 patients | 12 patients |

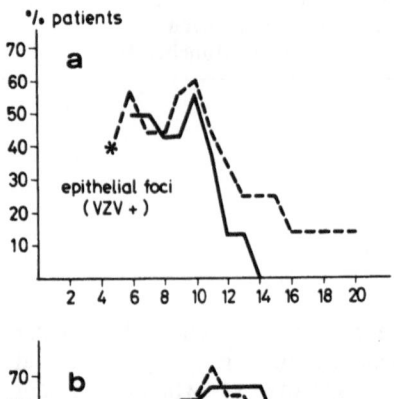

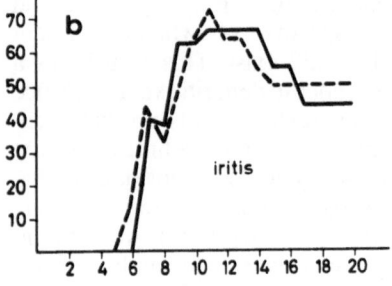

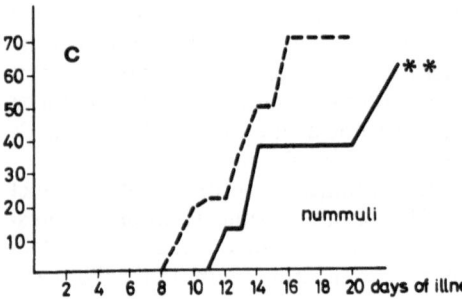

**Fig. 1.** Ocular involvement of 21 patients with ophthalmic zoster; in addition to topical steroid therapy, nine of them received human leukocyte interferon intramuscularly (−), and 12 albumine (----). (*/**: not all patients could be clinically evaluated very early and very late in the course of the disease)

We were, therefore, interested in studying whether or not an *additional systemic interferon therapy* might further improve the therapeutic results.

Twenty-four zoster patients with established or threatening ocular involvement (Hutchinson's sign) were treated identically with topical steroids (five drops of dexamethasone 0.1% per day). Additionally, they received either human leukocyte interferon or albumine intramuscularly on a random, double-blind basis.

A first series of six patients was treated for 5 days. Because no marked difference could be found, another series of 18 patients was treated over a prolonged period of 10 days. After the termination of this additional interferon or placebo therapy, topical therapy with steroids was carried on as indicated above. For comparative evaluation we had nine patients treated with interferon and 12 patients treated with albumine (Table 1).

No major difference was found as to the incidence of epithelial viral disease (Fig. 1a), iritis (Fig. 1b), or nummular keratitis (Fig. 1c). The appearance of nummuli, however, was deferred in the interferon-treated patients (Fig. 1c). Also, when scoring the severity of the individual cases of iritis and calculating a severity index for both groups, the interferon group looked somewhat better (Fig. 2).

### Conclusions

1. An additional medium-dosed, systemic interferon therapy started at day 6 of the illness (range: day 2−day 10), does not markedly improve the course of the disease. In the end, all eyes quieted to the same degree, and the incidence and se-

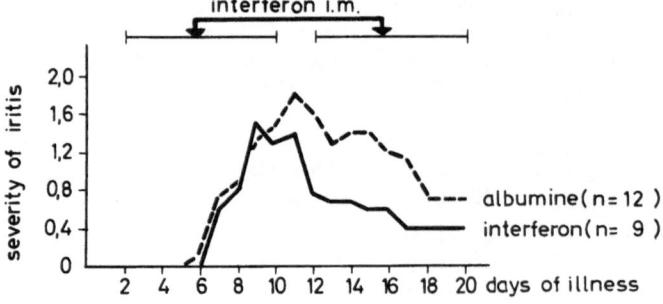

**Fig. 2.** While the *incidence* of iritis was equal in both treatment groups, the *severity* of iritis was somewhat lower in the interferon group

466

verity of nummuli were about equal in both groups. Taking into account the cost of interferon, the tested interferon regime cannot generally be recommended.

2. On the other hand, additional systemic interferon does seem to have exerted some positive effects which are indicated by a quicker subsiding of iritis and slower appearance of nummuli. This points to the possibility that the interferon was in itself active but has been applied inadequately-either the dosage, onset of therapy, or duration of therapy.

3. Analogous to our excellent results from a combined interferon treatment of dendritic keratitis consisting of an antiviral plus interferon (see pp. 401ff), we would suspect that a combination of an efficient systemic antiviral together with systemic interferon might bring about a therapeutic break-through for all kinds of zoster, not only ophthalmic. Acycloguanosine seems a promising substance for clinical testing in such a combination.

## References

1. Duke-Elder S (1965) System of ophthalmology, Vol VIII, 1. Kimpton, London, pp 340–346
2. Sundmacher R (1980) Zoster ophthalmicus, klinische und therapeutische Aspekte. Klin Monatsbl Augenheilkd 176:481–482

## Discussion on the Contributions pp. 449–467

**E.E. Kritzinger (Birmingham)**
I'd like to ask Mr. Marsh about side effects from Ara-A. Was it nerve or middle ear deafness?

**R.J. Marsh (London)**
The case of deafness was probably present before Ara-A was taken and so we cannot claim it to be a clinically significant finding.

**G. Grabner (Wien)**
I am very astonished to hear about your high rate of gastro-intestinal complications. How did you prescribe the levamisole? With our treatment schedule (3 × 50 mg for 3 days, repeated every 14 days for a total of five times; white blood count measured before and during the treatment at monthly intervals) we had no side effects at all in nearly 150 patients (herpes labialis and cornealis), except for one patient who complained of unspe-

cified cardiac sensations that resolved after discontinuing the treatment. We found no depression of the white blood count, either.

**R.J. Marsh (London)**
I think British patients must be neurotic about their bowels because both the placebo and the levamisole group reported about 20% gastro intestinal complications. We had three cases of depressed white cell counts but they were in placebo patients. The reasons for this are discussed in the text. We had been advised to give the dosage of levamisole over Friday, Saturday and Sunday every week for six months because we were told by Janssen that continuous administration in a three month period caused a greater number of gastrointestinal complications.

**P. Wright (London)**
That must also depend on the other drugs one is taking for analgesia and so on.

**G.O.H. Naumann (Erlangen)**
How often can you culture zoster virus in ophthalmic zoster – both in intraocular and corneo-epithelial involvement? In zoster, the case for the virus travelling down the neuron is very convincing for the ophthalmic pathologist because of the almost pathognomonic ciliary neuritis we have seen in the more than 25 eyes studied histologically.

**R. Sundmacher (Freiburg)**
As far as the eye is concerned, we have as yet only cultured zoster virus from epithelial lesions of the cornea. We have been unsuccessful in culturing it from the acqueous in cases of intraocular involvement, although I am sure that it is there. With the coarse punctate or dendritic lesions of the cornea in the acute stage of disease, there is no difficulty in getting virus.

I would like to know Dr. McGill's opinion about *late* recurrences of iritis after zoster: do you feel that they are viral or rather non-viral? Then, perhaps a short question to Dr. Marsh: What is the underlying cause for this very sticky and harmful mucus in zoster patients which you would not find in any other viral disease of the conjunctiva I know of?

**J. McGill (Southampton)**
The origin of the intraocular involvement must have a viral basis. Whether there is an immunological aspect, I don't think people can answer. The fact that it is suppressed by steroids but returns when you stop steroids may be of significance here. We have, as you have, been able to culture virus from the epithelial corneal lesions and skin lesions after 4 days after the onset of the rash, but no further.

R.J. Marsh (London)

If I can comment on the etiology of the iritis. It seems that this is definitely primed by the virus, but whether chronic iritis is dependent on the continuing presence of the virus is hard to say. But there is no doubt that the iritis in zoster is a vasculitis. The reason for the increased amount of mucus in the tear film, I think is dependent on co-existing conjunctivitis. I would like to criticise some papers reporting culturing varicella-zoster virus from corneal lesions. I do not see how you can isolate from the cornea alone unless you are isolating cells and testing with fluorescein antibody. Using a cotton wool applicator to culture inevitably means absorbing tears and where there are vesicles around the lesions they are bound to shed virus into the tear film.

R. Sundmacher (Freiburg)

To successfully isolate zoster virus, you should first of all isolate virus-loaded cells because zoster virus is very labile and looses infectivity shortly after being set free from a cell. So, with normal swabs of the conjunctiva you will not be very successful. We tried to isolate zoster virus from corneo-conjunctival washings. This too, seems to be rarely if ever, effective. Therefore, when you isolate zoster virus from epithelial pieces of the cornea which you have obtained by debridement with a knife − as we do − then you can be pretty sure that the isolated virus stems from the epithelium and does not constitute a pick-up from the tear-film.

B.R. Jones (London)

Many years ago, before the zoster virus was grown, I had taken scrapings of the corneal epithelium and they showed intranuclear inclusions demonstrating the typical zoster site of pathology in the epithelium.

L.M.T. Collum (Dublin)

I was very interested listening to this. Mr. McGill made a comment yesterday when I was talking about the disciform treatment or the treatment of stromal disease in HS, but he didn't think the acyclovir on its own was going to be helpful there. In this sort of disease that we are talking about, with stromal edema, and cells in the anterior chamber, I would suggest that we are talking about two different things and that the herpes simplex form is more immunological and this one may be more viral, when one compares one with the other.

R. Sundmacher (Freiburg)

I could show a series of slides which I prepared for tomorrows endothelial workshop in Zürich. In zoster, as in herpes simplex, you find an endotheliitis. In zoster, however, the course seems to be slower, more variable and perhaps more benign than in simplex. I believe, however, that both are basically viral with secondary immune reactions.

468

Sundmacher, R. (Hrsg.):
Herpetische Augenerkrankungen
© J.F. Bergmann Verlag, München 1981

# Corneal Perforation in Herpes Zoster Ophthalmicus Caused by Eyelid Scarring With Exposure Keratitis

G.O. Waring, M.B. Ekins, California

**Key words.** Ophthalmic zoster, corneal exposure, keratopathy, eyelid, corneal perforation

**Schlüsselwörter.** Zoster ophthalmicus, Keratopathia e lagophthalmo, Lidbeteiligung, Hornhautperforation

**Summary.** We present four cases of corneal perforation in herpes zoster ophthalmicus. In all cases, corneal exposure, hypesthesia, and treatment with topical corticosteroids caused the perforation. Corneal perforation can occur without zoster keratouveitis. Vigorous early prophylaxis such as tarsorrhaphy, lubrication, and soft contact lenses can prevent these disasters.

**Zusammenfassung.** Wir berichten über vier Patienten mit einer Hornhautperforation nach Zoster ophthalmicus. In allen Fällen verursachten ein ungenügender Lidschluß mit Hornhautexposition, Hypaesthesie und lokale Steroidbehandlung diesen schweren Verlauf. Eine Hornhautperforation kann auch ohne Zoster-Keratouveitis eintreten. Nur mit energischen und frühzeitig einsetzenden Maßnahmen wie Tarsorrhaphie, Salbenabdeckung und weichen therapeutischen Kontaktlinsen kann man solch eine schwere Komplikation abwenden.

For more than a century, ophthalmologists have reported corneal perforation as a sequel to herpes zoster ophthalmicus [1-8]. We report four cases of corneal perforation occurring three to 23 months after the onset of herpes zoster ophthalmicus, and emphasize seven factors that predisposed to corneal dissolution and perforation (Tables 1, 2):

1. Cicatricial retraction of upper eyelid causing corneal exposure.
2. Neurotrophic keratopathy.
3. Keratoconjunctivitis sicca with or without systemic connective tissue disease inducing corneal epithelial abnormalities.
4. Systemic immunosuppression predisposing to microbial keratitis.
5. Topical glucocorticoids decreasing collagen synthesis and resistance to infection.
6. Zoster vasculitis causing iridocyclitis and corneal edema.
7. Zoster keratitis.

Each of these factors alone may be insufficient to cause corneal perforation, but in combination they can be destructive. Thus, we emphasize two points: 1) corneal perforation can occur without zoster keratouveitis, and 2) prophylactic measures like early tarsorrhaphy [9–12], conjunctival flap [13], frequent artificial tears, topical antibiotics, and the judicious use of therapeutic high water content soft contact lenses and corticosteroids can prevent corneal perforation [10, 12, 13].

Although herpes zoster ophthalmicus is not a common problem, the herpes zoster virus causes 1–2% of all dermatologic disease and 7% of this is ophthalmic [14].

## Case Reports

### Case 1

This 76 year old woman had rheumatoid arthritis with keratitis sicca, diagnosed by reduced Schirmer strip wetting, since 1957. In January, 1977, at the age of 73, she developed herpes zoster of the ophthalmic and maxillary branches of the right trigeminal nerve. When she was referred to the University of California, Davis, Medical Center three weeks later, she had marked eschar formation and scarring across the right forehead, upper lid, and cheek with mild involvement of the tip of her nose (Fig. 1). The skin was crusted and bleeding, the lid margins were irregular, and the lashes matted and rubbing the cornea. Visual

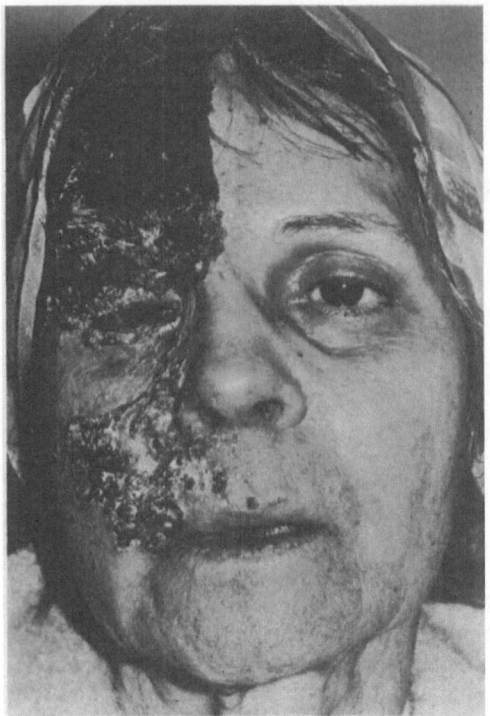

**Fig. 1.** Case 1. Herpes zoster of the ophthalmic and maxillary divisions of the right trigeminal nerve demonstrating eschar formation of the affected skin, including a few crusted vesicles on the tip of the nose, three weeks after onset

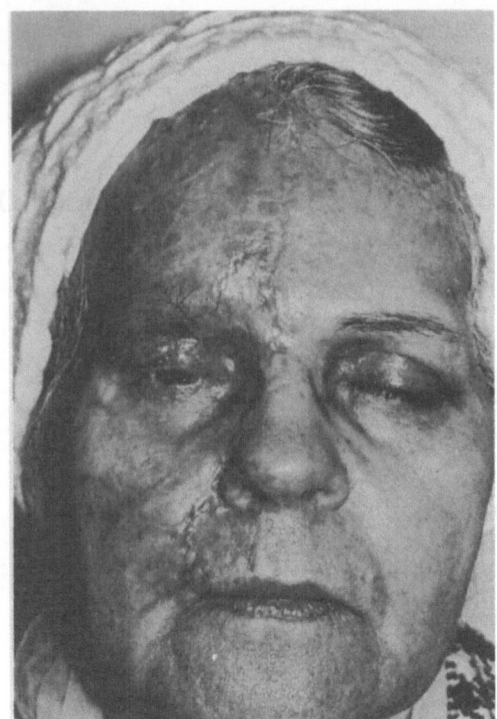

**Fig. 3.** Case 1. The right eyelids do not close centrally despite the medial and lateral tarsorrhaphies. The involved skin is scarring and healing

acuity was count fingers at three feet. There were epithelial erosions of the central one-third of the cornea and mild stromal edema without infiltration. Corneal sensation was markedly reduced and intraocular pressure was 24 mm Hg with the MacKay Marg tonometer. Examination of the left eye was normal.

A plano T soft contact lens was inserted in the right eye and 3% gentamycin and 1% atropine drops were prescribed. Over the next ten days the cornea beneath the central

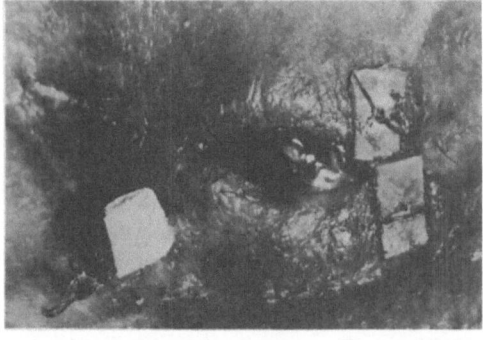

**Fig. 2.** Case 1. Medial and lateral tarsorrhaphies of the scarred right eyelids

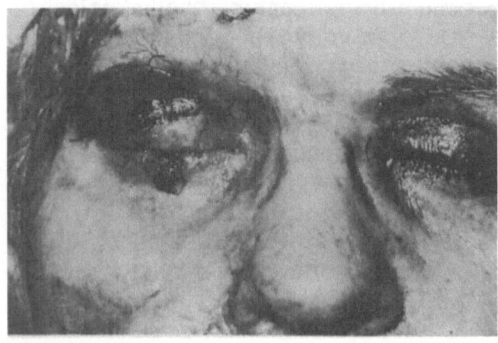

**Fig. 4.** Case 1. A skin graft has been performed to lower the right upper eyelid

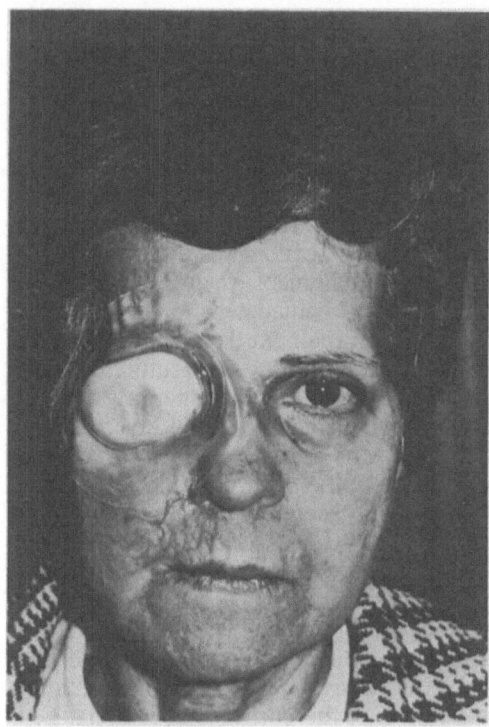

**Fig. 5.** Case 1. An occlusive bubble helps protect the cornea

erosion began to thin; 10% acetylcysteine drops and polyvinyl alcohol artificial tears were added. Another ophthalmologist gave her dexamethasone 0.1% eye drops every two hours, and when we next saw her, she had an hypopyon ulcer with cicatricial retraction of

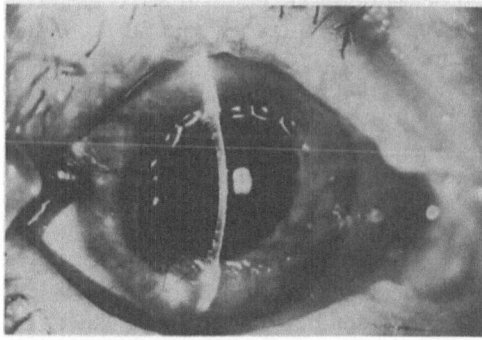

**Fig. 6.** Case 1. The right cornea perforated and a penetrating keratoplasty, sector iridectomy, lensectomy, anterior vitrectomy and lateral tarsorrhaphy have been performed

the right upper eyelid. The contact lens was removed; the ulcer was cultured; and a lateral tarsorrhaphy was performed. The erosion progressed and three days later, a medial tarsorrhaphy was done (Fig. 2). Cultures of the corneal scrapings were negative; cultures of the contact lens grew Candida parasilosis, Torulopsis glabrata, and a penicillium species. Despite the tarsorrhaphies, the eyelid would not close centrally (Fig. 3), so another plano T soft contact lens was inserted and a skin graft performed to lower the right upper eyelid (Fig. 4). Even though blood vessels began to grow toward the corneal erosion, there was continued thinning and scarring of the anterior stroma, and in spite of a central tarsorrhaphy and an occlusive bubble (Fig. 5), the cornea perforated six weeks later. A 7.5 mm penetrating keratoplasty with sector iridectomy, lensectomy, anterior vitrectomy, and a lateral tarsorrhaphy were performed (Fig. 6).

Despite additional skin grafting and tarsorrhaphies, the donor cornea developed an epithelial defect, then a dense central infiltrate that vascularized. Six months after the graft was performed, the central cornea was keratinized, and for the succeeding two years, the tarsorrhaphies remained secure, the eyelid scarring ceased, and there have been no changes in the cornea. Her intraocular pressure is controlled with topical 0.5% timolol. She has also suffered from a post-herpetic neuralgia.

Light microscopy of the host corneal button revealed absent epithelium and basement membrane and full-thickness stromal scarring with acute and chronic inflammatory cell infiltrates. Centrally the stroma was thin, Descemet's membrane absent, and uveal tissue formed the posterior corneal surface. Elsewhere, Descemet's membrane was intact but endothelial cells were not seen.

*Case 2*

A 72 year old white male had a history of congestive heart failure, hypertension and untreated borderline diabetes mellitus. On Thanksgiving Day, 1977, at age 69, he developed right herpes zoster ophthalmicus affecting the tip of his nose. His vision was 6/12 in the right eye and he developed a punctate epithelial keratopathy; oral and topical corticosteroids were started. On December 3, he developed a cellulitis of the right side of his face that improved with nine days of intravenous penicillin. Right upper eyelid scarring prevented complete eyelid closure. He was readmitted to the hospital on December 20 with a Staphylococcus aureus abscess of the right upper lid that required incision and drainage and systemic antibiotics. By mid-January, he had a paretic right pupil, punctate epithelial keratopathy of the inferior one-third of his cornea, and diminished corneal sensation. He developed a corneal erosion and subsequent stromal thinning, treated with artificial tears, topical antibiotics and corticosteroids, and night-time patching.

In mid-March, he was referred to the Corneal and External Disease Clinic of the University of California, Davis, Medical Center with a corneal perforation in the erosion. The right upper lid was scarred, exposing the hypesthetic cornea (Fig. 7). There was neither corneal infiltrate nor sign of active keratouveitis. The left eye was normal. Cyanoacrylate adhesive and a plano T soft contact lens were

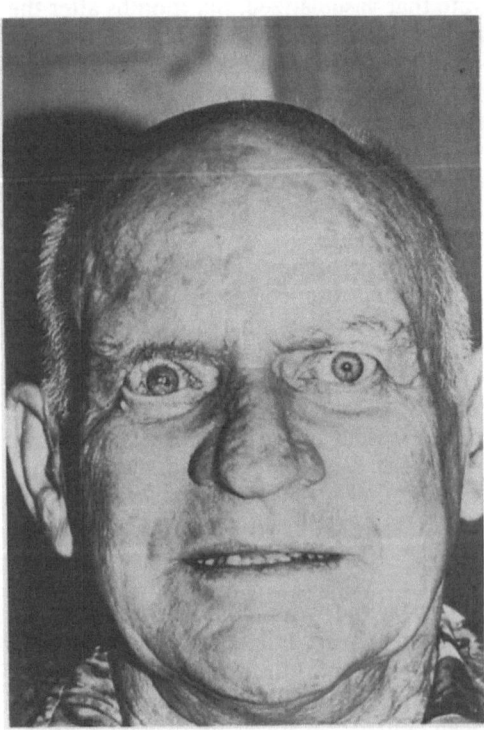

**Fig. 7.** Case 2. Full face view demonstrating right upper eyelid retraction and inferior sterile corneal thinning with perforation

applied, a lateral one-third tarsorrhaphy performed, and topical 1% atropine, neomycin-polysporin-polymyxin combination, and 3% gentamycin eye drops with a night-time occlusive bubble prescribed. A week later, the glue and the contact lens were gone, but the anterior chamber was formed. The inferior cornea was thin and the epithelial defect persisted. His medication was then changed to 0.5% chloramphenicol eye drops and artificial tears. The soft contact lens was replaced but fell out again the next day. He underwent a levator disinsertion and Frost suture. Because the cornea thinned further inferiorly over the next month, medial and lateral tarsorrhaphies were done and another plano T soft contact lens inserted; the ulcer began to vascularize. Prednisolone acetate 0.12% eye drops were added. The corticosteroids were quickly tapered to once daily and he was left with a rapidly maturing cataract, a vascularizing corneal scar, a soft contact lens, and medial and lateral tarsorrhaphies. A year and a half after the onset of his illness, ocular inflammation was minimal, the cornea was epithelialized, and he was maintained on only artificial tears.

### Case 3

A 62 year old white female was bedridden with severe, advanced rheumatoid arthritis complicated by vasculitis, Sjögren's syndrome, instability of the first and second cervical vertebrae, subluxation of both hips and the right knee, and decubitus ulcers. Her disease has been controlled with Chlorambucil 4 mg daily, a therapeutic dose which has kept her white blood count at 2,000 cells/ml and her lymphocyte count at 800 cells/ml.

In early December, 1978, at the age of 61, she developed a left herpes zoster ophthalmicus not affecting the tip of her nose, that was treated with bacitracin-polymyxin ointment and 0.5% methylcellulose drops. Over the next two months, the left upper lid scarred and retracted and she was hospitalized with a left corneal ulcer, hypopyon and hyphema. Initial treatment included 1% atropine and 3% gentamycin eye drops and oral ampicillin, with the addition three days later of fluorometholone and 10% acetylcysteine drops with an occlusive shield. The hypopyon resolved but the exposed cornea perforated. A plano T soft contact lens was positioned, a saran wrap moisture chamber placed around

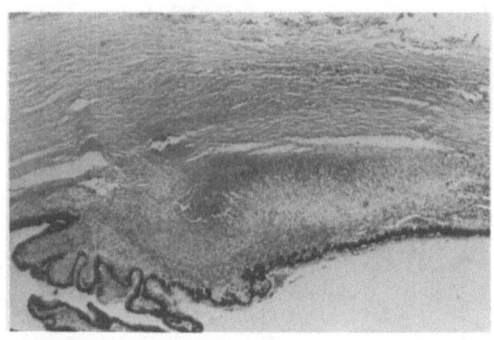

**Fig. 8.** Case 3. Histopathologic section of ciliary body demonstrating a rheumatoid nodule (hematoxylin and eosin, × 10)

the eye, and she was transferred to the University of California, Davis, Medical Center.

Examination of the right eye was normal. There was a thick, black eschar above the left eye and the retracted upper lid was unable to close completely. The tip of her nose was unaffected. Her uncorrected vision was hand motions. Her peripheral cornea was thin but vascularized 360°, probably from her systemic connective tissue disease. The central three-quarters of the cornea was de-epithelialized with necrotic edematous stroma and a central 2 mm diameter perforation. The anterior chamber was flat. Cultures of the corneal ulcer were negative. Immunofluorescent staining of corneal scrapings for herpes simplex and zoster were also negative. Because of her general debility, a left enucleation was performed.

Histopathologic abnormalities of the eye were limited to the anterior segment, where a rheumatoid nodule occupied the ciliary body (Fig. 8). There was no perivasculitis or perineuritis around the long posterior ciliary vessels and nerves or in the posterior pole and no marked inflammatory reaction in the cornea.

## Case 4

An 83 year old white male had medically controlled hypertension, chronic obstructive pulmonary disease, and anemia. In June, 1977, at the age of 80, he developed right herpes zoster ophthalmicus not involving the tip of the nose, treated with oral prednisone and ampicillin and topical gentamycin eye drops. At that

time, his visual acuity was: right eye – 6/20, left eye – 6/60. Two months later, the skin lesions were healed but he had bilateral punctate epithelial keratopathy of suspected viral origin, treated with idoxuridine eye drops every 2 hours over the following 6 weeks. Four months after onset of the herpes zoster, the inferior cornea of the right eye again manifested a punctate epithelial keratopathy presumably caused by nocturnal lagophthalmos, that was treated with artificial tears, and taping the eyelid shut at bedtime. In October, 1978, he developed an infiltrate in the lower one-third of the right cornea unresponsive to fluorometholone eye drops and followed two months later by a spontaneous eight ball hyphema with an intraocular pressure of over 60 mm Hg and corneal blood staining. Oral acetazolamide, topical atropine, and topical corticosteroids controlled the intraocular pressure.

He was referred to the Corneal and External Disease Clinic at the University of California, Davis, Medical Center in May, 1979, with a corneal perforation. At that time, his visual acuity was: right eye – light perception, left eye – 6/120. There was incomplete right eyelid closure nasally, with irregular margins, lash loss, and medial keratinization. At the junction of the lower and middle thirds of the blood-stained cornea was a dense vascularized corneal infiltrate and a perforation plugged with iris. The anterior chamber was flat. In the left eye, a diagnosis of keratoconjunctivitis sicca was made.

After culture, cyanoacrylate adhesive sealed the perforation and a Hydrocurve II soft contact lens applied. Topical neomycin-bacitracin-gramicidin and gentamycin eye drops were instilled. The anterior chamber remained flat, so a penetrating keratoplasty, anterior chamber membranectomy, sector iridectomy, intracapsular lensectomy and anterior vitrectomy were performed. Postoperative treatment included 500 mg acetazolamide sequels, 0.5% timolol, 2% epinephrine, 1% prednisolone acetate, 1% atropine sulfate, and 0.5% chloramphenicol eye drops and artificial tears. The transplant remained clear over the two month follow-up, the intraocular bleeding resolved and the intraocular pressure remained controlled. Candida albicans grew from the original corneal culture and was visible on light microscopy of the host corneal button.

**Table 1.** Factors contributing to corneal perforation in four cases of herpes zoster ophthalmicus

| Case number | Cicatricial reaction of upper eyelid w/corneal exposure | Neurotrophic keratopathy | Keratoconjunctivitis sicca ± connective tissue disease | Systemic Immunosuppression | Topical corticosteroids | Zoster vasculitis | Zoster keratitis | Secondary infection | Tip of nose affected |
|---|---|---|---|---|---|---|---|---|---|
| 1 | + | + | + | − | + | − | − | − | + |
| 2 | + | + | − | + | + | + | + | − | + |
| 3 | + | + | + | + | + | − | − | − | − |
| 4 | + | + | + | − | + | − | − | + | − |

## Discussion

These four cases emphasize the multiple factors that contribute to corneal perforation in herpes zoster ophthalmicus, a danger that exists for years after the initial episode (Tables 1, 2). Each of our patients had at least four of these factors; although only two had involvement of the tip of the nose to suggest involvement of the globe, all had cicatricial retraction of the upper eyelid with corneal exposure, all had neurotrophic keratopathy, and all were given topical glucocorticoids despite a non-healing epithelial defect (Table 1). Both vigorous prophylaxis and meticulous long-term follow-up can help prevent corneal perforation.

### Cicatricial Retraction of Upper Eyelid Causing Corneal Exposure

The vasculitis in herpes zoster causes severe inflammation in the skin of the affected dermatome [13]. In herpes zoster ophthalmicus, the upper eyelid retracts because the raw surfaces of the lid skin adhere to each other, pulling the eyelid up and because the underlying dermis scars and contracts. The lid neither covers the eye nor blinks effectively, and the dry exposed cornea develops erosions aggravated by aberrant eyelashes and by improperly applied eye patches. If inadequately treated, the exposed corneal stroma can melt and perforate. A large tarsorrhaphy performed early in the disease course, fre-

**Table 2.** Factors contributing to corneal perforation in four cases of herpes zoster ophthalmicus

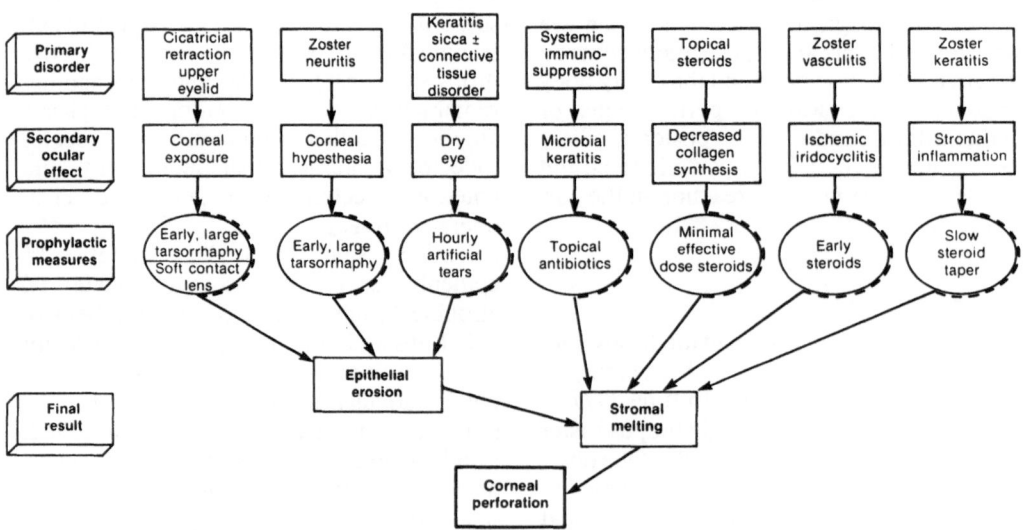

474

quent lubrication, and a thin, high water content soft contact lens protect the cornea and promote healing [10, 13].

Once eyelid retraction occurs, large lateral and medical tarsorrhaphies (Fig. 2), full-thickness skin grafts to the lid (Fig. 4), and disinsertion of the levator palpebrae superioris allow the eyelid to cover the cornea. In spite of these procedures, the cicatrization can progress and expose the cornea again, but the oculoplastic procedures can be repeated. A thin conjunctival flap pulled over the cornea before stromal melting has progressed will also help prevent perforation [13].

### Neurotrophic Keratopathy

Corneal sensory nerves are terminations of the long posterior ciliary nerves, branches of the nasociliary branch of the first division of the trigeminal nerve [15]. The herpes zoster virus causes inflammation, hemorrhage and necrosis of the trigeminal ganglion [16, 17]. The cell nuclei degenerate, and mononuclear cells invade the ganglion. The peripheral nerves are damaged by both the Wallerian degeneration that follows ganglion necrosis and by direct viral invasion [18]. Myelin around large and medium-sized nerve fibers degenerates, lymphocytes and phagocytic mononuclear cells invade the nerve, and the nerves heal with endoneural fibrosis [18].

This damage renders the cornea hypesthetic and a horizontally oval, superficial punctate erosion usually appears in the interpalpebral fissure [9, 11]. This can progress to stromal melting, scarring, and perforation. Corneal anesthesia decreases the blink reflex and reflex tear secretion from the lacrimal gland, and the dry ocular surface retards epithelial healing and promotes stromal melting. The reduction of neurotransmitters also might slow epithelial healing [19].

A large tarsorrhaphy is mandatory at this time, in spite of the patients' complaints about the cosmetic defect.

### Keratoconjunctivitis Sicca With or Without Systemic Connective Tissue Disease

Keratoconjunctivitis sicca may appear alone or as part of a systemic connective tissue disorder. When aqueous tear production is reduced, the lysozymes, beta-lysins and other antimicrobial components of tears are also reduced. The resultant drying of the corneal surface and subsequent abnormal corneal epithelium can cause epithelial erosions and increased susceptibility to increased numbers of pathogenic bacteria present in the ocular flora [20]. These patients have more difficulty epithelializing corneal defects once they occur and have a propensity for corneal stromal melting as part of their connective tissue disorder. To combat surface drying, a lateral tarsorrhaphy (Fig. 2), upper and lower punctal occlusion, occlusive glasses or ocular shields (Fig. 5), and frequent ocular lubrication will reduce tear evaporation, and preserve and supplement what tears are made. Prophylactic topical antibiotics such as chloramphenicol, antibiotics to the affected facial skin, and eyelid hygiene when the skin heals will all decrease the risk of a bacterial keratitis.

The systemic connective tissue disease also contributes directly to the karatolysis in some cases.

### Systemic Immunosuppression Predisposing to Microbial Keratitis

Herpes zoster more frequently affects individuals who are immunosuppressed because of a systemic disease or medication. The estimated incidence of herpes zoster in the general population is 0.2% [21] and in patients with neoplastic disease it is 2.8–9% [22–24]. Conversely, 7.9–20% [25–27] of patients with herpes zoster suffer from an immunosuppressing or debilitating systemic disease like chronic leukemia [25], Hodgkin's disease [28] or carcinoma, or from diseases treated with immunosuppressive agents such as connective tissue disorders or renal transplantation [27]. These disorders predispose not only to herpes zoster but to other microbial infections such as bacterial or fungal keratitis. In addition, the systemic corticosteroids commonly used early in the course of herpes zoster to diminish the vasculitis, skin scarring, and subsequent post-herpetic neuralgia are immunosuppressive [29, 30]. Compared to patients with localized herpes zoster, patients with disseminated herpes zoster have exhibited a late rise in interferon in the vesicles [31] and a delayed development of a virus-specific complement fixing antibody [31, 32], implying that an immune abnormality exists in those individuals in whom the virus disseminates.

Patients with herpes zoster need a complete medical evaluation to rule out an underlying systemic disorder and to assess the safety of using oral corticosteroids. If systemic corticosteroid therapy is initiated, the patient should be hospitalized for four to six days to be observed for virus dissemination [26, 30]. We sometimes use systemic corticosteroids early in the disease in those patients with severe zoster ophthalmicus and ocular involvement but with no underlying immunosuppressing disease. We give prednisone 60 mg daily for a week, 30 mg daily for a week, 15 mg daily for a week, and taper off over the next 7 days [13], watching for dissemination of the virus.

Prophylactic topical antibiotics such as 0.5% chloramphenicol eye drops three times a day reduce the risk of bacterial keratitis [9, 11].

If a bacterial keratitis develops, stromal melting is accelerated by the proteolytic activity of enzymes elaborated by the bacteria and by the invading polymorphonuclear leukocytes. The keratitis must be treated vigorously and promptly.

### Topical Corticosteroids Decreasing Collagen Synthesis and Resistance to Infection

Corticosteroids, judiciously administered, are the cornerstone of therapy in herpes zoster ophthalmicus. Topical corticosteroids are the most effective agents available for suppressing the vasculitis and inflammation of zoster keratouveitis; unfortunately, they decrease host defenses to bacterial and fungal keratitis, decrease stromal keratocyte collagen synthesis [33], and cause a severe rebound keratouveitis if withdrawn too quickly. If there is a corneal epithelial defect, stromal melting accelerates in the presence of topical corticosteroids because destructive processes outstrip reparative ones.

We treat the uveitis with topical cycloplegics, antibiotics and, depending on the severity of the inflammation, topical corticosteroids such as 1% prednisolone acetate eye drops. We taper the corticosteroids gradually over the succeeding months to doses as low as 0.12% prednisolone acetate eye drops once a week before discontinuing them. If there is an epithelial defect and no medical contraindication to systemic steroids, we will give pred-

nisone 60 mg daily, tapering and switching to topical steroids when the epithelium is healed. While the topical corticosteroids are being administered, the potential local complications of the drugs, including stromal melting, secondary infection, or steroid-induced glaucoma, must be remembered.

### Zoster Vasculitis With Iridocyclitis and Corneal Edema

Vasculitis is a major component of the destructive process in herpes zoster. In herpes zoster ophthalmicus, lymphocytes characteristically surround and invade the long posterior ciliary nerves and vessels [17]. An occlusive vasculitis and subsequent ischemic necrosis of the iris and pars plicata of the ciliary body may ensue. The subsequent anterior chamber inflammation and corneal malnutrition can irreversibly damage the cornea, culminating in a bullous keratopathy susceptible to epithelial loss, stromal melting and secondary infection. Kline et al. [34] reported an ischemic conjunctival ulcer in a case of herpes zoster ophthalmicus; this suggests that there may be an ischemic as well as an immune component to the marginal corneal ulcers described by Mondino [35].

We treat the vasculitis, intra- or extraocular, with corticosteroids to reduce inflammation, remaining aware of all the attendant dangers of steroid therapy in an already compromised eye.

### Zoster Keratitis

Herpes zoster keratitis occurs in 35–40% of patients with zoster ophthalmicus [5, 11], and takes different forms at different stages of the disease [11]. In the early stage it may appear as a coarse punctate keratopathy with focal, gray, raised, intraepithelial lesions, sometimes dendritiform [36, 37], that last only a few days and are not exacerbated by topical corticosteroids. Zoster virus can be cultured from the dendrites [36, 37] and virus antigen detected in them [38]. Ten to fourteen days after the onset of the disorder, single or multiple subepithelial focal fluffy infiltrates that consist of fine white granules against a brownish background may appear. Although they resolve spontaneously and more rapidly with corticosteroid therapy, they may recur months later. Histologically, these are areas of edema with a few polymorphonuclear leukocytes [39]. From one to 24 months after the onset, a disciform keratitis may appear either centrally, or peripherally, with its associated corneal edema, concentric immune rings and iritis, characterized histopathologically by the early appearance of polymorphonuclear leukocytes followed by lymphocytes and macrophages [39]. Mondino et al. [35] reported peripheral corneal ulcers in four cases of herpes zoster ophthalmicus and implicated an autoimmune reaction to virus-altered corneal antigen. Rarely, a focal sclerokeratitis appears a few months after the onset of the zoster, sometimes associated with underlying iris atrophy [9, 11].

Each of these types of inflammatory keratitis may appear alone, in sequence, or together either during the skin eruption or months later [9]. In general, these forms of inflammatory keratitis, either singly or in combination, do not produce corneal melting, unless one of the other predisposing factors is present. Treatment of the keratitis is similar to the uveitis: topical cycloplegics, antibiotics, and corticosteroids.

Corneal perforations can be sealed with cyanoacrylate adhesive and a soft contact lens but more frequently require a penetrating keratoplasty (Fig. 6) with sector iridectomy and lensectomy. However, unless the predisposing factors are corrected, perforation may recur in the donor tissue. A lateral tarsorrhaphy (Fig. 2) and possibly upper and lower punctal occlusion at the time of surgery and vigorous ocular lubrication are necessary.

Table 2 summarizes the interactions of the factors predisposing to corneal perforation and possible prophylactic measures. Two patients had involvement of the tip of the nose. Only one (Case 2) had zoster keratitis, a mild punctate keratopathy with involvement of the tip of the nose noted prior to upper eyelid scarring. The other (Case 1) developed an hypopyon ulcer in her exposed, hypesthetic cornea following insertion of a soft contact lens and the use of corticosteroids; no zoster keratitis was documented. However, all four patients had cicatricial lid retraction and exposure of hypesthetic corneas. The corneal epithelium eroded and the subsequent stromal melting was accelerated by topical corticosteroid therapy leading to corneal perforation.

We must not be lulled into a false sense of security by Hutchinson's law; corneas can perforate as a result of herpes zoster ophthalmicus even if there is no nasociliary nerve involvement or zoster keratouveitis.

**Acknowledgment.** Supported in part by a grant from the Medical Research Council of Canada (Dr. Ekins).

# References

1. Hybord A (1873) Du zona ophthalmique et des lesions oculaires qui s'y rattachent. Summarized in New York Medical Journal 17:642 (from Paris-Adrien Delahaye, 1878, p 161)
2. Jeffries BJ (1873) Two cases of herpes zoster ophthalmicus destroying the eye. Trans Am Ophthalmol Soc II:73
3. Calhoun AW (1873) Herpes zoster ophthalmicus. Atlanta Medical and Surgical Journal 11:188
4. Randolph RL (1901) Herpes zoster ophthalmicus resulting in loss of the eye. Arch Ophthalmol 30:414
5. Edgerton AE (1945) Herpes zoster ophthalmicus. Report of cases and review of literature. Arch Ophthalmol 34:40–114
6. Doden W (1960) Zoster ophthalmicus gangraenosus mit Verlust des Augapfels. Klin Monatsbl Augenheilkd 136:230
7. Blodi FC (1968) Ophthalmic zoster in malignant disease. Am J Ophthalmol 65:686
8. Sugar HS (1971) Herpetic keratouveitis: clinical experiences. Ann Ophthalmol 3:335
9. Marsh RJ (1973) Herpes zoster keratitis. Trans Ophthalmol Soc UK 93:181
10. Marsh RJ (1976) Current management of ophthalmic herpes zoster. Trans Ophthalmol Soc UK 96:334
11. Pavan-Langston D (1975) Varicella zoster ophthalmicus. Int Ophthalmol Clin 15:171
12. Duke-Elder S (1965) System of ophthalmology, Vol VIII. Diseases of the Outer Eye. Kimpton, London, p 340
13. Pavan-Langston D (1979) Ocular virus diseases. In: Galasso GJ, Merigan TC, Buchanan RA (eds) Antiviral agents and viral diseases of man. , New York, p 274
14. Achard C (1924) Zona ophthalmique. Paris Med 51:285
15. Wolfe E (1976) Anatomy of the eye and orbit, 7 ed. Saunders, Philadelphia, p 306
16. Head H, Campbell AW (1900) The pathology of herpes zoster and its bearing on sensory location. Brain 23:353

17. Naumann G, Gass JDM, Font RL (1968) Histopathology of herpes zoster ophthalmicus. Am J Ophthalmol 65:533

18. Zacks SI, Langfitt TW, Elliott FA (1964) Herpetic neuritis. A light and electron microscopic study. Neurology 14:744

19. Cavanagh HD, Colley A, Pihlaja DJ (1979) Persistent corneal epithelial defects. Int Ophthalmol Clin 19:197

20. Lemp MA (1979) Diagnosis and treatment of tear deficiencies. In: Wilson LA (ed) External diseases of the eye. Harper and Row, Hagerstown, p 143

21. Vachtenheim J, Grossman J (1963) Herpes zoster and steroid therapy. Br Med J 2:622

22. De Moragas JM, Kierland RR (1957) The outcome of patients with herpes zoster. Arch Dermatol 75:193

23. Wright ER, Winer LH (1961) Herpes zoster and malignancy. Arch Dermatol 84:242

24. Williams HM, Diamond HD, Craver LF (1958) The pathogenesis and management of neurological complications in patients with malignant lymphomas and leukemia. Cancer 11:76

25. Shanbrom E, Miller S, Haar H (1960) Herpes zoster in hematologic neoplasias: some unusual manifestations. Ann Intern Med 53:523

26. Merselis JG, Kay D, Hook EW (1964) Disseminated herpes zoster. A report of 17 cases. Arch Intern Med 113:679

27. Rifkind D (1966) The activation of varicella zoster virus infections by immunosuppressive therapy. J Lab Clin Med 68:463

28. Sokal JE, Firat D (1965) Varicella zoster infection in Hodgkin's disease: Clinical and epidemiological aspects. Am J Med 39:452

29. Elliott FA (1964) Treatment of herpes zoster with high doses of prednisone. Lancet 2:610

30. Sheie HG (1970) Herpes zoster ophthalmicus. Trans Ophthalmol Soc UK 90:899

31. Stevens DA, Merigan TC (1972) Interferon, antibody, and other host factors in herpes zoster. J Clin Invest 51:1170

32. Miller LH, Brunell PA (1970) Zoster, reinfection or activation of latent virus? Observation on the antibody response. Am J Med 49:480

33. Berman M (1978) Regulation of collagenase. Therapeutic considerations. Trans Ophthalmol Soc UK 98:397

34. Kline LB, Jackson WB (1977) Herpes zoster conjunctival ulceration. Can J Ophthalmol 12:66

35. Mondino BJ, Brown SI, Mondzelewski JP (1978) Peripheral corneal ulcers with herpes zoster ophthalmicus. Am J Ophthalmol 86:611

36. Pavan-Langston DM, McCulley JP (1973) Herpes zoster dendritic keratitis. Arch Ophthalmol 89:25

37. Hayashi S (1975) Study of herpes zoster keratitis, demonstration of virus particles in corneal scrapings. Acta Soc Ophthalmol Jpn 79:542

38. Uchida Y, Kameyama K, Kaneko M, Inoue S, Yohda Y, Handa S (1974) Study on herpes zoster keratitis. Acta Soc Ophthalmol Jpn 78:1073

39. Hogan MJ, Zimmerman LE (1962) Ophthalmic pathology. An atlas and text, 2 ed. Saunders, Philadelphia, p 298

# Cytomegalovirus Diseases

Sundmacher, R. (Hrsg.):
Herpetische Augenerkrankungen
© J.F. Bergmann Verlag, München 1981

# Infections With Cytomegalovirus in Adults and the Natural History and Treatment of Cytomegalovirus Retinitis

R.B. Pollard, P.R. Egbert, J.G. Gallagher, T.C. Merigan, Galveston, Stanford

**Key words.** Cytomegalovirus, inclusion retinouveitis in the adult

**Schlüsselwörter.** Cytomegalievirus – Einschluß-Retinouveitis des Erwachsenen

**Summary.** Cytomegalovirus infections occur in the majority of all populations examined and once acquired remain in a latent state throughout the lifespan of the individual infected. Immunosuppressed individuals, particularly transplant recipients have increased severity of primary infections due to this agent and not infrequently reactivate the latent infection. Disseminated infections occur with resultant mortality in patients with underlying diseases, especially bone marrow transplant recipients. Retinitis due to CMV has been reported in over 30 patients and occurs in immunosuppressed patients. Fourteen cases of retinitis were seen at one institution and seven were treated with systemically administered adenine arabinoside. A dosage of 20 mg/kg was associated with improvement in retinitis and a decrease in quantitative shedding of CMV in the urine. Improvement was observed in several cases following lowering of immunosuppression without antiviral therapy. Significant side effects, mainly hematologic and gastrointestinal were observed at the dosages required. Certain patients with progressive retinitis due to CMV may respond to therapy with adenine arabinoside, but require frequent monitoring for side effects before and after such treatments.

**Zusammenfassung.** Zytomegalievirus-(CMV-)Infektionen bei gesunden Erwachsenen lassen sich meist auf ausgedehnte Frischbluttransfusionen zurückführen; sie erfolgen aber auch spontan und gehen dann – soweit sie klinisch manifest sind – mit einem Mononukleose-Syndrom einher. Immunosupprimierte Individuen erleiden allerdings sehr viel ernsthaftere CMV-Infektionen. Insbesondere Patienten, die Nieren- oder Herztransplantate erhalten haben, erkranken mäßig schwer an dieser Infektion, und Empfänger von Knochenmarktransplantaten erkranken ausgesprochen schwer mit einer hohen Mortalität. Bei diesen Transplatempfängern scheinen vorhandene spezifische Antikörper nicht gegen eine Reaktivierung oder gegen eine schwere exogene Infektion zu schützen. CMV-spezifische zellvermittelte Immunitätsreaktionen können aber wahrscheinlich als wesentliches Zeichen für eine wirksame Immunität gegenüber CMV-Infektionen gewertet werden. Bisher sind CMV-Retinitisfälle bei über 30 Erwachsenen mit Immunsuppression beschrieben worden. Das typische ophthalmologische Bild kann ophthalmoskopisch ziemlich eindeutig diagnostiziert werden. Der natürliche Verlauf der Retinitis ist sehr verschieden. Bei der nur begrenzten Fallzahl, die in den einzelnen Zentren beschrieben worden ist, ist es schwierig, sich ein gültiges Bild über den spontanen Verlauf zu machen. Während einer Sechsjahresperiode haben wir bei uns 15 Fälle mit CMV-Chorioretinitis beobachtet. Sie wurden aufgrund ihres typischen ophthalmologischen Erscheinungsbildes diagnostiziert, und die Diagnose wurde durch erhöhte CMV-Antikörper-Titer bei der Mehrzahl der Fälle bestätigt, meist auch durch die zusätzliche CMV-Ausscheidung im Urin. Bei acht Patienten verfolgten wir den Verlauf ohne spezifische Therapie. Zwei Patienten hatten nur sehr geringfügige ophthalmologische Veränderungen, die frühzeitig nach einer Herztransplantation entdeckt wurden. Diese Veränderungen heilten spontan nach Reduzierung der immunsuppressiven Therapie ab. Ein anderer Patient hatte eine rezidivierende und immer wieder exazerbierende Retinitis in Verbindung mit Abstoßungsphasen und entsprechend verstärkter Immunsuppression. Bei mehreren dieser Patienten wurde die Diagnose erst im präterminalen Stadium gestellt. Sie litten bis zu ihrem Tod an einer progressiven Retinitis.

Sieben Patienten behandelten wir mit Adeninarabinosid (ARA-A) in einer Dosierung von 1–20 mg/kg und Tag. Alle diese Patienten hatten trotz einer stark herabgesetzten immunsuppressiven Therapie weiterhin an einer progressiven Chorioretinitis gelitten. Um außer dem klinischen Bild noch ein zusätzliches Kriterium für die Virustatikawirksamkeit zu erhalten, führten wir auch quantitative Virusbestimmungen im Urin durch. Bei vier Patienten, die 20 mg ARA-A/kg Körpergewicht und Tag erhielten, ging die Entzündung zurück und die Retinitis besserte sich mit einem gleichzeitigen signifikanten Abfall der Virusausscheidung im Urin. Die ARA-A-Therapie bei diesen Patienten führte aber zu signifikanten hämatologischen und gastrointestinalen Nebenwirkungen. Die zellvermittelten Immunitätsreaktionen gegenüber CMV wurden bei 10 von 11 darauf untersuchten Patienten wesentlich reduziert gefunden.

## Cytomegalovirus Infections — General

Conditions caused by cytomegalovirus (CMV) were first described via pathologic diagnosis as associated with large inclusion bearing cells in tissue sections [24, 29, 35]. The virus was then isolated by several different investigators independently almost 25 years ago [63, 70, 74]. CMV has been increasingly recognized as a cause of human disease and as a ubiquitous problem in all populations examined throughout the world. Its major impact is in causing congenital infections, wherein at least during primary infection occurring early in pregnancy, intrauterine infection results in the production of a fetus with multiple congenital abnormalities including chorioretinitis. The newborn may also be infected perinatally from women who have virus in the cervix at the time of delivery or from seropositive mothers who transmit via breastmilk. This mode of transmission apparently results in asymptomatic infection of the infant.

The prevalence of antibodies varies in various populations around the world with a majority of infants acquiring virus before one year of life in certain environs. It seems to vary with socioeconomic groups with the lower having a higher incidence of antibody at each age level examined. Infection rates vary with age with approximately 50% having antibody at age 18 and 75 to 100% by age 35–40. Like other herpesviruses, CMV in normal individuals is acquired during an asymptomatic or symptomatic primary infection and then remains in a state of latency throughout the life of the individual, but the virus can be reactivated at any time by sufficient immunosuppression. Several extensive reviews of human CMV infections have been published [34, 47, 75].

### Infections in Normal Adults

The mode of transmission in the majority of cases remains unknown; however, because of the number of individuals infected, the agent must be quite contagious. CMV does not remain viable in the environment on inanimate objects, is relatively labile and probably requires close contact between individuals for transmission to occur. It has been recovered from saliva, urine, and buffy coat of infected individuals and some evidence exists for venereal transmission [14, 37, 39]. Another mode of transmission is via blood products, particularly, fresh whole blood. Persons likely to contract the virus by this mode of transmission include those undergoing massive transfusions following major trauma and those having open heart surgery requiring cardiopulmonary by-pass and large volume blood exchange [38, 60, 76].

The incubation period as has been determined from studies of transfusion acquired disease is apparently quite long, ranging between 6 and 8 weeks in the majority of cases. The primary disease in normal individuals varies in severity with the majority of those infected not experiencing a distinctive syndrome identified as primary CMV infection, but only being detected as seropositive when antibody titers are examined. Clinically recognized disease may last from as little as one week to several weeks to months, and has been frequently reported as the causative agent in cases of fever of unknown etiology in otherwise normal individuals.

The typical pattern is that of a heterophil negative mononucleosis [36]. Patients usually have fever, malaise, mild hepatosplenomegaly, and lymphocytosis with the concomitant appearance of atypical lymphocytes. Lymphadenopathy does occur in some individuals and there are frequently mild abnormalities in liver function tests. No evidence of progression to permanent liver damage has been reported, however, granulomatous hepatitis has been associated with CMV infection [8, 16]. Symptomatic recurrent infection in immunologically normal individuals has not been described, however, seropositive individuals may possibly have recurrent shedding of virus in the urine and certainly in cervical secretions during pregnancy [62].

## Infections in Immunosuppressed Individuals

An increased incidence and severity of infections in many groups of immunosuppressed individuals has been described. These patient groups range from those with rheumatologic diseases receiving cytotoxic therapy [21] to those with underlying malignancies. Organ transplant recipients in particular have been reported to have more severe infections with CMV than noted in any other adult patient population. Whether this increased prevalence is related to the prolonged period of immunosuppression, to the degree of immunosuppression, or to the interaction between the grafted organ and the host immune defenses, or a combination of these has not been clearly established.

Patients with malignancies have increased rates of shedding CMV which approximated 25% in children with leukemia who were cultured repeatedly and in a much smaller percentage of adults with Hodgkins diseases or lymphoma [3, 32]. There have been many reports of severe CMV infections in patients with malignancies, presenting with either pneumonia due to CMV and/or disseminated infection with multiple organ involvement. In general, however, CMV has not been observed to be as severe a problem in this patient population as in transplant recipients.

CMV infections in bone marrow transplant recipients have been the most severe in any patient population thus far described [46, 50, 51]. Approximately 45% of patients experience interstitial pneumonia, about half of which is due to CMV and the mortality in this group approaches 90%. Therefore, at present CMV may be the most important pathogen in bone marrow transplant recipients. The cause of death in such patients has been secondary to the severe interstitial pneumonitis with impairment in oxygenation. Individuals who develop detectable antibody rises early in the course of this illness appear to be at decreased risk for fatal infections, as compared to those who do not develop antibody. If these patients become engrafted successfully and immunosuppression thereby decreases, the risk for significant infection with CMV also decreases

several months post-transplantation. The presence of antibody in the marrow donor appears to influence the risk of subsequent CMV infection in the recipient.

Renal transplant recipients experience a high frequency of CMV infections with the majority of those undergoing primary infection having a syndrome typical of CMV mononucleosis [7, 71]. These symptoms have been self limited for the most part, but there have been individual patients having evidence of CMV pneumonia and disseminated infection resulting in death [68]. Individuals with antibody to CMV prior to transplantation frequently reactivate their latent infection with viral shedding detected. Two separate groups of investigators have reported a significant relationship between the serologic status of the donor kidney and the recipient as to subsequent infection with CMV [6, 33]. Kidneys from seropositive donors which are transplanted into seronegative recipients produce primary infection in recipients significantly more frequently than if seronegative donors are used as a source of kidneys for seronegative recipients. The role of CMV infections in the occurrence of rejection of renal allografts remains controversial. Two recent studies suggested that primary CMV infection and symptomatic recurrent infection were both associated with an increased incidence of rejection of the transplanted organ [40, 53, 77].

CMV infections in cardiac transplant recipients are related to the experience with the virus preceding transplantation [55]. Those patients with antibody prior to transplantation have a high incidence of shedding in throat or urine cultures post-transplant and the majority of these patients have significant increases in antibody titer following transplantation. About half of the patients without antibody pre-transplant undergo primary infection with CMV. The clinical manifestations in this group include fever not traceable to any other cause, leukopenia (<4000 WBC), elevated liver function tests, and atypical lymphocytes in the peripheral blood. Some of these individuals have evidence of disseminated CMV infection resulting in death. Those who lack antibody pretransplant and who do not acquire antibody post-transplant do not shed virus or have any of the symptoms of CMV mononucleosis. Those undergoing primary infection also have an increased incidence of pneumonia due to bacterial organisms or pneumocystis and lung abscess when compared to the group having recurrent or no evidence of infection with CMV [61]. A similar immunosuppressive effect of primary CMV infection has also been reported in mice with increased mortality due to otherwise sublethal challenges with bacterial organisms or Candida [31].

## Diagnosis

Many techniques of measuring antibody to CMV have been reported, and the ability to detect true seronegatives from seropositives appears to be the critical factor. The complement fixation test is performed in most laboratories and when properly standardized should be able to identify the majority of the patients who have no experience with the agent. This has been the case, at least as far as the development of subsequent manifestations of CMV infections in cardiac transplant recipients [55]. Utilizing a titer of < 1:8 as representing significant evidence of prior infection and a fourfold increase in titer or converting from seronegative to seropositive as significant evidence of recent infection identifies persons experiencing recent disease with CMV. More sensitive techniques such as fluorescent antibody staining, indirect hemagglutination and enzyme linked-immunoabsorbent assays, may well replace the CF test in the future.

Virus isolation is performed in diploid tissue culture cells with the urine as the most easily obtained and most likely positive culture material. Most individuals shed the virus for prolonged periods following primary or recurrent infection. The development of typical cytopathogenic effect due to CMV may be noted in 1 to 2 days in the case of congenitally infected infants who are shedding massive quantities of virus or in 1–3 weeks in adults shedding smaller amounts. Virus can be identified by typical changes in the monolayer with slow progression of plaque morphology or by either direct or indirect fluorescent antibody staining. Other tissues such as visceral organs, throat gargles, and buffy coat cultures may also be positive in cases of disseminated infection. Typical inclusion bodies in histologic sections may also enable the diagnosis of CMV disease, but are less frequently present than culturable virus, at least in lung biopsy specimens.

## Cell Mediated Immunity

Immunosuppressed individuals in particular undergo primary infection or reactivation of the latent infection and continue shedding CMV despite the development of significant antibody titers. Lymphocyte transformation responses to CMV antigen are detectable in the majority of normal individuals with antibody to CMV and no history of CMV infection while those undergoing recent primary CMV infection develop elevated lymphocyte transformation responses a few months after acute CMV mononucleosis whether community or transfusion acquired [55]. Cardiac transplant recipients had significant cell mediated immune responses to CMV antigen pre-transplantation but these responses were depressed post-transplantation and remained depressed during the prolonged period of immunosuppression following the transplant. They continued to shed virus during this period, however, in a few individuals studied in the late post-transplant period, the cessation of viral shedding appeared to correlate with a return of significant lymphocyte transformation responses [55].

## Therapeutic Possibilities

The potentials for therapy of CMV infections are limited at present. Human leukocyte interferon depressed the quantity of virus shed in the urine in congenitally infected babies but the dosages required approached toxic levels [2]. In bone marrow transplant recipients interferon therapy may be associated with significant toxicity at low dosages and may potentially interfere with engraftment of the transplanted tissue [30]. Renal transplant recipients had a delay in the onset of shedding following prolonged post-transplantation interferon therapy, however, significant hematologic toxicity was reported [12]. A recently developed compound, acycloguanosine (acyclovir) has potential for the therapy of HSV and VZV infections, however, CMV does not produce the virus specific thymidine kinase detected in cells infected with the other two agents and its usefulness in CMV infections awaits further study [20, 23, 67].

Adenine arabinoside, a purine nucleoside

whose mode of action is to inhibit DNA polymerase has been shown to decrease viral shedding of CMV in several patients populations [13]. This compound inhibits host cell DNA polymerase as well as viral DNA polymerase and this may be responsible for its toxicity, which is manifested by hematologic and gastrointestinal side effects. Adenine arabinoside has recently been shown to decrease mortality in herpes simplex encephalitis, improve some parameters of herpes zoster infections in the immunosuppressed and have some effects on the viral markers of chronic hepatitis B virus infection [56, 78, 79]. It has efficacy against CMV in tissue culture and was felt to be the agent with the greatest potential in the studies of CMV chorioretinitis to be described. Vaccination with live attenuated CMV vaccine remains potentially useful in the control of infections with this agent, but may not protect from reactivation of endogenous infection following immunosuppression [28, 54].

## CMV Chorioretinitis

Chorioretinitis due to CMV was first reported in 1959 when typical inclusion bodies were noted in the retina during a postmortem examination [27]. Since that time over 30 cases of this condition have been reported with all but one occurring in immunosuppressed hosts [1, 4, 5, 10, 11, 15, 18, 19, 25, 26, 41–43, 45, 48, 49, 58, 59, 65, 66, 69, 72, 73, 80]. The retinal lesions are reported to have a very characteristic appearance presenting as an exudative retinitis, which frequently begin perivascularly and becomes hemorrhagic as it progresses. The paucity of vitreous involvement distinguishes this condition from more common forms of retinitis, particularly toxoplasmosis. A possible relationship between dosages of immunosuppressive drugs and progression of the retinitis has emerged from previous reports and remissions of active lesions have followed decreasing dosages in some patients. Retinitis has been progressive in many of the cases with resultant blindness or severe visual loss being reported. Previous trials of therapy with specific transfer factor or adenine arabinoside failed to show any significant beneficial effect [65, 66].

The natural history of CMV retinitis remains to be determined. Many of the previously reported cases have been diagnosed at postmortem with the rate of progression being impossible to determine. Other individuals have had a relentlessly progressive course resulting in blindness. The report of the use of transfer factor concerned a patient with remitting and exacerbating retinitis over several years, finally, resulting in significant visual loss. Fourteen patients were seen at one institution over several years, seven of these received no antiviral therapy and seven were treated with adenine arabinoside [22, 57].

### Methods

The diagnosis of CMV retinitis was made by the typical appearance of retinal lesions and the following criteria. All patients studied before death were shedding CMV in the urine or throat and had elevated CF antibody titers to CMV. The diagnosis was made at postmortem in several cases by the presence of typical inclusions due to CMV in the retina.

Frequent routine follow up of heart transplant recipients enabled the diagnosis of several asymptomatic cases. Eyes were examined frequently and the extent of disease documented by fundus mapping. Cell mediated immunity to CMV was measured with previously reported techniques [55]. Adenine arabinoside was administered intravenously over 12 hrs daily from 5–14 days at dosages ranging from 1–20 mg/kg/day.

### Results and Discussion

Seven patients with CMV chorioretinitis were not treated with antiviral therapy. Four of these were heart transplant recipients, two had undergone renal transplantation, one had non-Hodgkins lymphoma, and one individual had asymptomatic retinitis which was diagnosed at autopsy. Two heart transplant recipients, one with mild visual loss and the other who was asymptomatic, were diagnosed on routine ophthalmologic exam and had spontaneous improvement of their lesions with reductions in immunosuppressive therapy. Another individual who had undergone renal transplantation had improvement in CMV retinitis after removal of the transplanted kidney and withdrawal from immunosuppressive drug therapy.

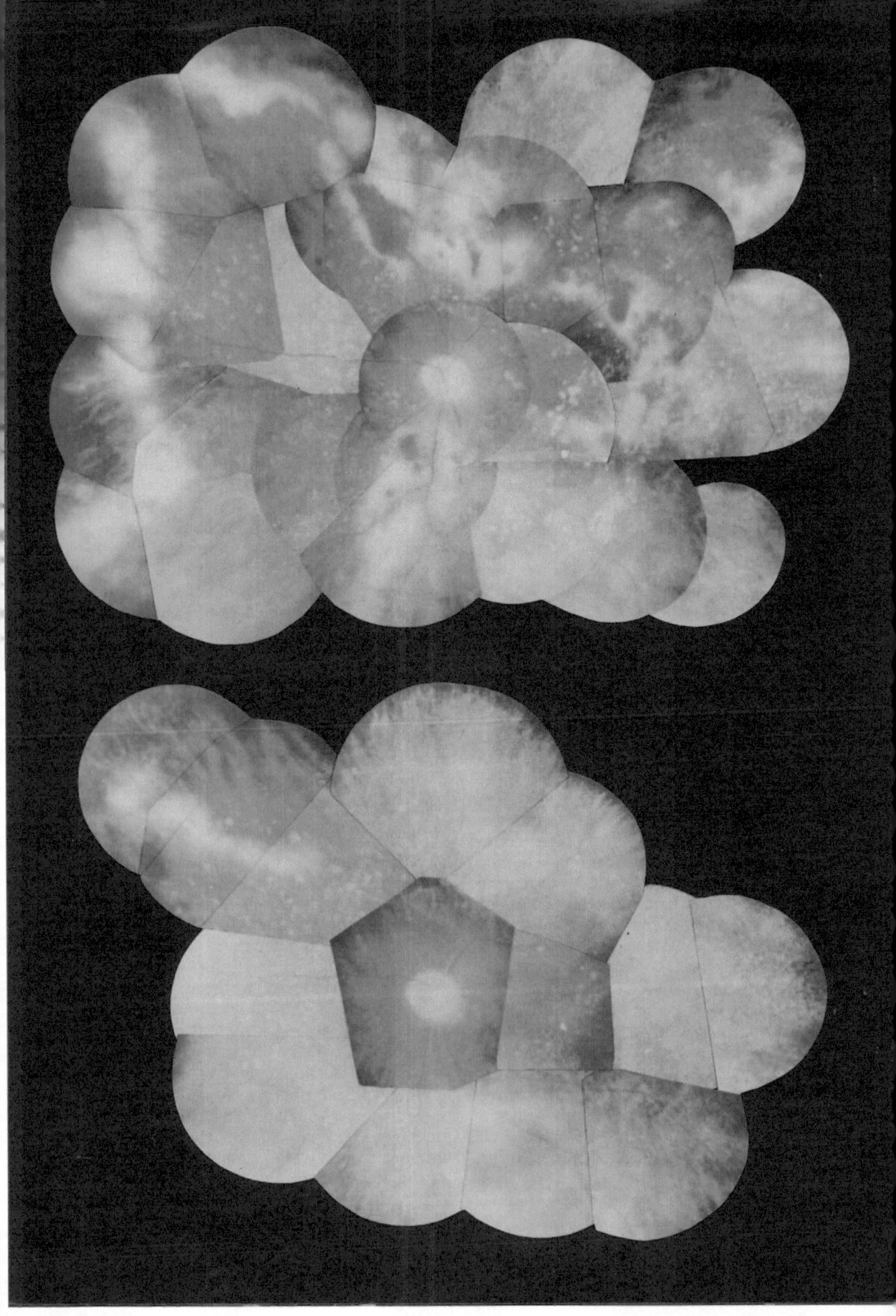

Three other patients had progressive retinitis until they expired and one of these individuals had evidence of disseminated CMV infection at postmortem. The remaining patient presented with a previously unreported manifestation of CMV eye infection. Decreased vision was associated with an observed swelling of the optic nerve thought to be due to lymphoma. However, at postmortem examination, the optic nerve contained multiple inclusions typical of CMV infection.

Quantitative shedding of CMV in the urine proved to be very constant and varied by $\pm$ log $TCID_{50}$ infectious units for many months. The stability of virus shedding facilitated measurement of the effectiveness of antiviral chemotherapy enabling a second parameter other than changes in the retinitis to be monitored. Therapy with adenine arabinoside transiently decreased shedding in the urine in several patients. Shedding was temporarily completely undetectable in two patients and permanently disappeared in one individual. All three noted to have complete depression of urinary CMV received 20 mg/kg/day of adenine arabinoside.

The course of progressive CMV retinitis was apparently improved in several of the treated patients. In one patient, in whom shedding was completely eliminated by the second course of adenine arabinoside, sustained improvement in CMV retinitis was observed. Newly appearing lesions disappeared following therapy and no active retinal lesions reappeared during over a year of followup. Two other patients had significant improvement in CMV retinitis following adenine arabinoside and the improvement appeared to be stable for some time after treatment. Two other patients had definite improvement in retinal lesions following adenine arabinoside courses (Fig. 1, 2), however, retinitis recurred at a later date and was then progressive. One of these two had subsequently progressive disease until death and the other individual had progression of disease in one eye despite improvement in the other.

The side effects due to adenine ara-binoside administration were significant in these patients. Hematologic toxicity was the most troublesome with three of seven having significant depressions of platelet count and in two patients, granulocytopenia occurred during therapy. The white count returned to normal in one of these patients after adenine arabinoside was discontinued. The second patient, however, developed severe depression of white blood cells after the therapy was discontinued and expired with sepsis. Gastrointestinal side effects were observed in four of the seven patients, including two patients who experienced nausea and vomiting and two patients who developed diarrhea. One of the two with diarrhea had received an inadvertant overdosage of adenine ara-binoside, however, the diarrhea was transient, disappearing after therapy was discontinued.

Evaluation of cell mediated immune responses to CMV antigen revealed a specific absence of responsiveness to CMV. Those patients tested prior to cardiac transplantation had detectable reaction to CMV antigen. Another patient who had responded to adenine arabinoside with a significant decrease in the activity of CMV retinitis and elimination of CMV urinary shedding had detectable responsiveness to CMV antigen after treatment was completed. Significant lymphocyte transformation responses were lacking in all other patients tested.

## Ocular Findings

CMV infections with eye involvement in immunosuppressed hosts was characteristically distinct and the diagnosis was supported by changes in antibody titer suggestive of recent infection and by isolation of virus from patient specimens. The early manifestations might possibly lead to other diagnosis considerations, such as choriodal metastasis or cotton wool spots [44]. The later, more extensive lesions may be confused with idiopathic chorioretinitis or when extensive hemorrhage is present, with retinal vein occlusion. Other entities, such as herpes simplex and herpes zoster retinitis appear to be much less frequent in adults, but may be difficult to dis-

Fig. 1. CMV retinitis in the right eye of a 59 y/o renal transplant recipient before and after the first course of therapy with adenine arabinoside. The retinitis involved large areas of the fundus with the typical exudative and hemorrhagic pattern observed with this condition. Improvement began shortly after therapy and resulted in the appearance of 9-7-77

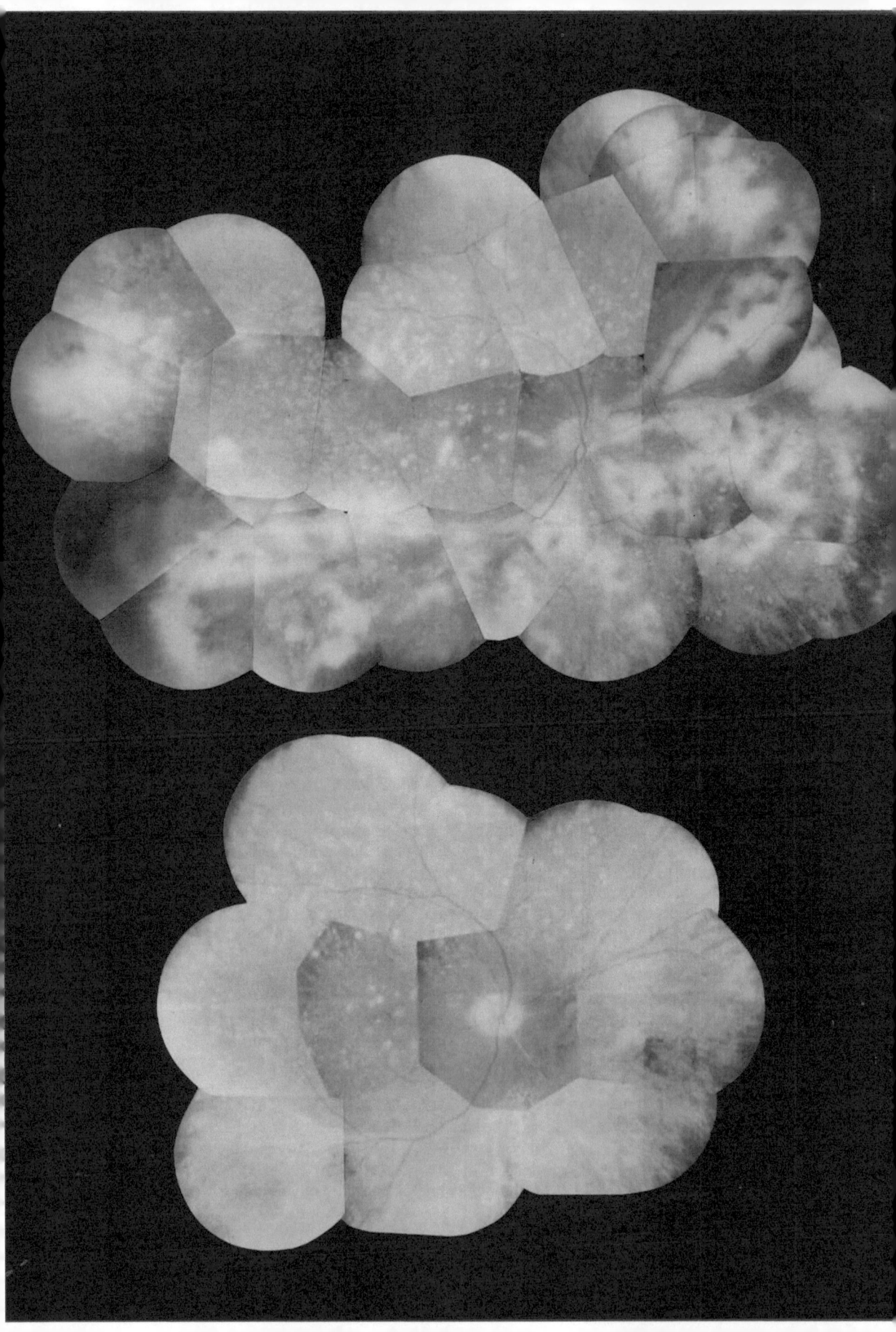

tinguish [17]. Toxoplasmosis presents a special problem when there is less than expected vitreous flare [52]. Only one of the patients in the present study had serologic and clinical evidence of toxoplasmosis.

Extension of the lesions tended to occur around the original site of involvement with a brush fire-like expansion of each focus. Expansion was heralded by faint dots at the edge of the advancing retinitis and a granular appearance of the existing lesion. Later recurrences were mostly observed to occur at sites distant from the original lesions, probably due to the systemic viremic phase of the infection. Progression at sites distant to the original focus occurred in only about 15% of the eyes examined. Therefore, a treatment modality which arrests the progression of the original focus appears indicated as it potentially will prevent continuing visual loss.

Almost a third of the eyes examined had evidence of recurrent disease after healing of the original focus. These recurrences were noted either at the edge of the previous focus or at a distant site. Changes in the immune status of the patient appeared to correlate with the emergence of recurrent disease.

Retinitis was frequently observed to occur peripherally and to spare the macula as has been observed in congenital CMV infection [9]. Although CMV retinitis has been reported to become widespread and be progressive, about half the cases in this series were asymptomatic and lesions resolved spontaneously in one third. Approximately 50% had impairment in central visual acuity especially with macular involvement or in the face of rapidly progressive disease. An absence of satellite lesions and a change of the whitish lesions to grey or transparent scars frequently preceded slowing of progression of the retinitis and was predictive of a phase of healing.

## Conclusion

In this series, as suggested previously, CMV retinitis presented with typical ophthalmologic findings in immunosuppressed hosts. Spontaneous resolution of retinitis was observed in patients in whom significantly decreased dosages of immunosuppressive therapy were possible. Several patients with progressive retinitis, despite the lowest dosages of immunosuppressives possible, had apparent improvement in eye lesions following treatment with adenine arabinoside. Measurements of quantitative virus shedding provided a second parameter of effectiveness during antiviral therapy. The dosages of adenine arabinoside required to influence the course of CMV retinitis were higher than those required in other herpesvirus infections and were associated with significant hematologic and gastrointestinal side effects. Careful monitoring of patients at risk for this infection revealed several cases which resolved spontaneously and may facilitate earlier diagnosis, especially of peripheral retinitis before visual loss has occurred. Careful ophthalmologic followup enabled the accumulation of additional information as to the natural evolution of retinal lesions and the appearance of the lesions which may be predictive of eventual healing.

Acknowledgment. These studies were supported by grant number AI-05629 from the U.S. Public Health Service and by an unrestricted research grant from Research to Prevent Blindness, Inc.

## References

1. Aaberg TM, Cesarez TJ, Rytel MW (1972) Correlation of virology and clinical course of cytomegalovirus retinitis. Am J Ophthalmol 74:407–415
2. Arvin AM, Yeager AS, Merigan TC (1976) Effect of leukocyte interferon on urinary excretion of cytomegalovirus by infants. J Infect Dis 133S:A205–209
3. Arvin AM, Pollard RB, Rasmussen LE, Merigan TC (1980) Cellular and humoral immunity in the pathogenesis of recurrent herpes viral infections in patients with lymphoma. J Clin Invest 65:869–878
4. Ashton N, Cunha-Vaz JG (1966) Cytomegalic inclusion disease in the adult retina. Arqu Port Oftal 18 Suppl 39–50
5. Astle JN, Ellis PP (1974) Ocular complications

Fig. 2. CMV retinitis in the left eye of the same patient as in Fig. 1. with the same interval between photographs. Multiple drusen were noted before the onset of CMV retinitis. This patient relapsed approximately one year later and at postmortem typical inclusions were noted in histologic sections and the drusen also had a typical histologic appearance

in renal transplant patients. Ann Ophthalmol 6:1269-1274

6. Betts RF, Freeman RB, Douglas RG, Talley TE, Rundell B (1975) Transmission of cytomegalovirus infection with renal allograft. Kidney Int 8:385-392

7. Betts RF, Freeman RB, Douglas RG, Talley TE (1977) Clinical manifestations of renal allograft derived primary cytomegalovirus infection. Am J Dis Child 131:759-763

8. Bonkowsky HL, Lee RV, Klatskin G (1975) Acute granulomatous hepatitis: Occurrence in cytomegalovirus mononucleosis. J Am Med Assoc 233:1284-1288

9. Burns RP (1959) Cytomegalic inclusion disease uveitis. Arch Ophthalmol 61:376-387

10. Carson S, Chatterjee SN (1978) Cytomegalovirus retinitis: Two cases occurring after renal transplantation. Ann Ophthalmol 10:275-279

11. Chawla HB, Ford MS, Munro JF, Scorgie RE, Watson AR (1976) Ocular involvement in cytomegalovirus infection in a previously healthy adult. Br Med J 2:281-282

12. Cheesman SH, Rubin RH, Stewart JA, Tolkoff-Rubin NE, Cosimi AB, Cantell K, Gilbert J, Winkle S, Herrin JT, Black PH, Russel PS, Hirsch MS (1979) Controlled clinical trial of prophylactic human leukocyte interferon in renal transplantation. N Engl J Med 300:1345-1349

13. Chien LT, Cannon NJ, Whitley RJ, Diethelm AG, Dismukes WE, Scott CW, Buchanan RA, Alford CA (1974) Effect of adenine arabinoside on cytomegalovirus infections. J Infect Dis 130:32-39

14. Chreitieh JH, McGinniss CG, Muller A (1977) Venereal causes of cytomegalovirus mononucleosis. J Am Med Assoc 238:1644-1645

15. Chumbley LC, Robertson DM, Smith TF, Campbell RJ (1975) Adult cytomegalovirus inclusion retino-uveitis. Am J Ophthalmol 80:807-816

16. Clarke J, Craig RM, Saffro R, Murphy P, Yokoo H (1979) Cytomegalovirus granulomatous hepatitis. Am J Med 66:264-268

17. Cogan DG (1977) Immunosuppression and eye disease. Am J Ophthalmol 83:777-788

18. Coulson AS, Lucas ZJ, Condy M, Cohn R (1974) An epidemic of cytomegalovirus disease in a renal transplant population. West J Med 120:1-3

19. Cox F, Meyer D, Hughes WT (1975) Cytomegalovirus in tears from patients with normal eyes and with acute cytomegalovirus chorioretinitis. Am J Ophthalmol 80:817-824

20. Crumpacker CS, Schnipper LE, Zaia JA, Levin MJ (1979) Growth inhibition by acycloguanosine of herpesviruses isolated from human infections. Antimicrob Agents Chemother 15:642-645

21. Dowling JN, Saslow AR, Armstrong JA, Ho WM (1976) Cytomegalovirus infection in patients receiving immunosuppressive therapy for rheumatologic disorders. J Infect Dis 133:339-408

22. Egbert PR, Pollard RB, Gallagher JG, Merigan TC (1980) Cytomegalovirus retinitis in immunosuppressed hosts. II. Ocular manifestations. Ann Intern Med :

23. Elion GB, Furman PA, Fyfe JA, Miranda P de, Beauchamp L, Schaeffer HJ (1977) Selectivity of action of an antiherpetic agent 9-(2-Hydroxyethoxymethyl) guanine. Proc Natl Acad Sci 74:5716-5720

24. Farber S, Wolbach SB (1932) Intranuclear and cytoplasmic inclusions ("protozoan-like bodies") in salivary glands and other organs of infants. Am J Pathol 8:123-126

25. Fiala M, Payne JE, Berne TV, Moore TC, Henle W, Montgomerie JZ, Chatterjee SN, Guze LB (1975) Epidemiology of cytomegalovirus infection after renal transplantation and immunosuppression. J Infect Dis 132:421-433

26. Fiala M, Chatterjee SN, Carsons S, Poolsawat S, Heiner D, Saxon A, Guze LB (1977) Cytomegalovirus retinitis secondary to chronic viremia in phagocytic leukocytes. Am J Ophthalmol 84:567-573

27. Foester HW (1959) Uveitis symposium. Surv Ophthalmol 4:296

28. Glazer JP, Friedman HM, Grossman RA, Starr SE, Barker LF, Perloff LJ, Huang ES, Plotkin SA (1979) Live cytomegalovirus vaccination of renal transplant candidates. Ann Intern Med 91:676-683

29. Goodpasture EW, Talbot FB (1921) Concerning the nature of "protozoan-like" cells in certain lesions of infancy. Am J Dis Child 21:415-421

30. Greenberg PL, Mosny SA (1977) Cytotoxic effects of interferon in vitro on granulocyte progenitor cells. Cancer Res 37:1794-1799

31. Hamilton JR, Overall JC, Glasgow LA (1976) Synergistic effect on mortality in mice with murine cytomegalovirus and Pseudomonas aeruginosa, Staphylococcus aureus or Candida albicans infections. Infect Immun 14:982-989

32. Hensen D, Siegel SE, Fucillo DA, Matthews E, Levin AS (1972) Cytomegalovirus infections during acute childhood leukemia. J Infect Dis 126:469-481

33. Ho M, Suwansirikul S, Dowling JN, Youngblood LA, Armstrong JA (1975) The transplanted kidney as a source of cytomegalovirus infection. N Engl J Med 293:1109-1112

34. Ho M (1978) Cytomegalovirus infections and diseases. Diseases of the Month, 3-59. Year Book Medical, New York

35. Jesionek A, Kiolemenoglou B (1904) Über einen Befund von protozoenartigen Gebilden in den Organen eines Feten. Münch Med Wochenschr 51:1095–1097

36. Jordan MC, Rousseau WE, Stewart JA, Noble GR, Chin TDY (1973) Spontaneous cytomegalovirus mononucleosis: Clinical and laboratory observations in nine cases. Ann Int Med 79:153–160

37. Jordan MC, Rousseau WE, Noble GR, Stewart JA, Chin TDY (1973) Association of cervical cytomegaloviruses with venereal disease. N Engl J Med 288:932–934

38. Kreel I, Zaroff LI, Cantor JW, Krasna I, Baronofsky ID (1969) Syndrome following total body perfusion. Surg Gynecol Obstet 111:317–321

39. Lang DJ, Kummer JF (1975) Cytomegalovirus in semen: Observations in selected populations. J Infect Dis 132:472–473

40. Light JA, Burke DS (1979) Association of cytomegalovirus infections with increased recipient mortality following transplantation. Transplant Proc 11:79–82

41. Madge GE (1972) Cytomegalovirus infection of the eye in a case of renal homotransplantation. MCV Quarterly 8:251–253

42. Malek GH, Kisken WA (1970) Problems in diagnosis in treatment in renal transplantation. Am J Surg 119:334–336

43. Merritt JC, Callender CD (1978) Adult cytomegalic inclusion retinitis. Ann Ophthalmol 10: 1059–1063

44. Michelson JB, Stephens RF, Shields JA (1979) Clinical conditions mistaken for metastatic cancer to the choroid. Ann Ophthalmol 11: 149–153

45. Murray HW, Knowx DL, Green WR, Susel RM (1977) Cytomegalovirus retinitis in adults: A manifestation of disseminated viral infection. Am J Med 63:574–584

46. Myers JD, Spencer HC, Watts JC, Gregg MB, Stewart JA, Troupin RH, Thomas ED (1975) Cytomegalovirus pneumonia after human marrow transplantation. Ann Intern Med 82: 181–188

47. Nankervis GA, Kumar ML (1978) Diseases produced by cytomegaloviruses. Med Clin North Am 62:1021–1035

48. Naumann G, Hamann KU, Gabrecht M (1974) Zur ophthalmologischen Diagnose der zytomegalie-retinitis. Klin Monatsbl Augenheilkd 164:329–333

49. Nicholson D (1975) Cytomegalovirus infection on the retinal. Intern Ophthalmol Clin 15: 151–162

50. Nieman P, Wasserman PB, Wentworth BB, Kao GF, Lerner KG, Storb R, Buckner LD, Clift RA, Fefer A, Fass L, Glucksberg H,

Thomas ED (1973) Interstitial pneumonia and cytomegalovirus infection as complications of human marrow transplantation. Transplantation 15:478–485

51. Nieman PE, Reeves W, Ray G, Flournay N, Lerner KG, Sale GE, Thomas ED (1977) A prospective analysis of interstitial pneumonia and opportunistic viral infection among recipients of allogeneic bone marrow grafts. J Infect Dis 136:754–767

52. O'Connor GR (1978) Current concepts in ophthalmology: Uveitis in the immunosuppressed host. N Engl J Med 299:130–132

53. Pass RF, Whitley RJ, Diethelm AG, Whelchel JD, Reynolds DW, Alford CA (1979) Outcome of renal transplantation in patients with primary cytomegalovirus infections. Transplant Proc 11:1288–1290

54. Plotkin SA, Farquhar J, Hornberger E (1976) Clinical trials of immunization with the Towne 125 strain of human cytomegalovirus. J Infect Dis 134:470–475

55. Pollard RB, Rand KH, Arvin AM, Merigan TC (1978) Cellmediated immunity to cytomegalovirus infection in normal subjects and cardiac transplant patients. J Infect Dis 137:541–549

56. Pollard RB, Smith JC, Neal EA, Gregory PB, Merigan TC, Robinson WS (1978) Effect of vidarabine on chronic hepatitis B virus infection. J Am Med Assoc 239:1648–1650

57. Pollard RB, Egbert PR, Gallagher JG, Merigan TC (1980) Cytomegalovirus retinitis in immunosuppressed hosts. I. Natural history and effects of treatment with adenine arabinoside. Ann Intern Med 93:655–664

58. Porter R (1972) Acute necrotizing retinitis in a patient receiving immunosuppressive therapy. Br J Ophthalmol 56:555–558

59. Porter R, Crombie AL, Gardner PS, Uldall RP (1972) Incidence of ocular complications in patients undergoing renal transplantation. Br Med J 3:133–136

60. Prince AM, Szmuness W, Millian SJ, David DS (1971) A serologic study of cytomegalovirus infections associated with blood transfusion. N Engl J Med 284:1125–1131

61. Rand KH, Pollard RB, Merigan TC (1978) Increased pulmonary superinfections in cardiac-transplant patients undergoing primary cytomegalovirus infection. N Engl J Med 298: 951–953

62. Reynolds DW, Stagno S, Hosty TS, Tiller M, Alford CA (1973) Maternal CMV excretion and perinatal infection. N Engl J Med 289:1–5

63. Rowe WP, Hartley JW, Waterman S, Turner HC, Huebner RJ (1976) Cytopathogenic agent resembling human salivary gland virus recovered from tissue cultures of human adenoids.

Proc Soc Exp Biol Med 92:418–424

64. Rubin RH, Russell PS, Levin M, Cohen C (1979) Summary of a workshop on cytomegalovirus infections during organ transplantation. J Infect Dis 139:728–734

65. Rytel MW, Aaberg TM, Dee TH, Heim LH (1975) Therapy of cytomegalovirus retinitis with transfer factor. Cell Immun 19:8–21

66. Rytel MW, Kauffman HM (1976) Clinical efficacy of adenine arabinoside in therapy of cytomegalovirus infections in renal allograft recipients. J Infect Dis 133:202–205

67. Schaeffer HJ, Beauchamp L, Miranda P de, Elion GB, Bauer DJ, Collins P (1978) 9-(2-Hydroxyethoxymethyl) guanine activity against viruses of the herpes group. Nature 272:583–585

68. Simmons RL, Matas AJ, Rattazzi LC, Balfour HH, Howard RJ, Najarian JS (1977) Clinical characteristics of the lethal cytomegalovirus infection following renal transplantation. Surgery 82:537–546

69. Smith ME (1964) Retinal involvement in adult cytomegalic inclusion disease. Arch Ophthalmol 72:44–49

70. Smith MG (1956) Propagation in tissue cultures of a cytopathogenic virus from human salivary gland virus (SGV) disease. Proc Soc Exp Biol Med 92:424–430

71. Swansirikul S, Rao N, Dowling JN, Ho M (1977) Primary and secondary cytomegalovirus infection. Arch Intern Med 137:1026–1029

72. Venceia G de, Rhein GMZ, Pratt MV, Kisken W (1971) Cytomegalic inclusion retinitis in an adult. Arch Ophthalmol 86:44–47

73. Wallow L (1970) Nekrotisierende Retinitis bei Schwerer Allgemeiner Krankung. Ber Dtsch Ophthalmol Ges 70:55

74. Weller TH, Macauley JC, Craig JM, Wirth P (1957) Isolation of intranuclear inclusion producing agents from infants with illness resembling cytomegalic inclusion disease. Proc Soc Exp Biol Med 94:4–12

75. Weller TH (1971) The cytomegaloviruses: Ubiquitous agents with protean clinical manifestations. N Engl J Med 285:203–214; 267–274

76. Wheller EQ, Turner JD, Scannell JG (1962) Fever, splenomegaly, and atypical lymphocytes: Syndrome observed after cardiac surgery using pump oxygenator. N Engl J Med 266:454–466

77. Whelchel JD, Pass RF, Diethelm AG, Whitley RJ, Alford CA (1979) Effect of primary and recurrent cytomegalovirus infections upon graft and patient survival after renal transplantation. Transplantation 28:443–446

78. Whitley RJ, Chien LT, Dolin R, Galasso GJ, Alford CA (1976) Adenine arabinoside therapy of herpes zoster in the immunosuppressed. N Engl J Med 294:1193–1199

79. Whitley RJ, Soong S, Dolin R, Galasso GJ, Chien LT, Alford CA (1977) Adenine arabinoside therapy of biopsy-proved herpes simplex encephalitis. N Engl J Med 297:289–294

80. Wyhinny GJ, Apple DJ, Guastella FR, Vygantas CM (1973) Adult cytomegalovirus retinitis. Am J Ophthalmol 76:773–781

## Discussion on the Contribution pp. 481–492

G.O.H. Naumann (Erlangen)
Certainly this is not a rare entity and the clinical ophthalmologist has a rather significant responsibility to diagnose the disease. It has the typical ophthalmoscopical picture of virus retinitis which is indistinguishable between HS or CMV retinitis. We should always think of it in a patient with immunosuppressive or cytostatic therapy suffering from "intraocular inflammation".

O.P. van Bijsterveld (Utrecht)
In one of these patients, who I believe was a non-Hodgkin, there was a swelling of the optic nerve, and cell inclusions in the optic nerve were found on histopathological examination post-mortem. Where, exactly, would one expect such inclusions?

R.B. Pollard (Galveston)
The subretinal layer is where they usually occur to my understanding. It was very much a surprise to find the inclusions in this optic nerve, as it was felt the swelling was due to lymphoma.

R. Sundmacher (Freiburg)
Is it correct that the major difficulty in effectively treating CMV infections results from the fact that cytomegaloviruses do not induce their own thymidine kinase? As most of our currently available antivirals interact in some way or another with virus induced thymidine kinases, you wouldn't really expect that acyclovir or BVDU would be effective against CMV, would you?

R.B. Pollard (Galveston)
No, neither one of those compounds holds much promise for effectiveness against CMV. Adenine arabinoside must be administered in large dosages which are associated with toxicity but its administration in certain cases may be warranted. There are no drugs nearing clinical applications that I am aware of that have exciting effects against CMV. Phosphonoformate may have some activity against CMV, but its tendency to accumulate in bone may affect its usefulness.

T. Ravenscroft (Beckenham)
People may have the impression that acyclovir has

no activity against cytomegalovirus. In fact it does have some activity in vitro even though it lacks thymidine kinase. This is probably due to the slight phosphorylation of acyclovir by host cell enzymes. In the case of the Epstein-Barr Virus which also lacks thymidine kinase, the drug has been shown to have an effect by virtue of the very sensitive DNA polymerase coded by this virus. Several patients with infections caused by these viruses have been treated on an emergency, named patient basis with encouraging results. It is too early to make any claims in these infections.

### R.B. Pollard (Galveston)

It surprises me to hear that you noted some efficacy. At least one patient treated at Stanford with CMV retinitis failed to respond to acyclovir.

### T. Ravenscroft (Beckenham)

We have not used the drug in retinitis yet. An interesting point about the immunocompromised patients who are particularly susceptible is that acyclovir may be given to patients receiving bone marrow grafts without causing loss of graft. This is of significance from the drug toxicity point of view.

### G.O.H. Naumann (Erlangen)

On one occasion we had to treat a desperate patient with bilateral cytomegalic inclusion retinitis. Ara-A had to be discontinued. A very high dosage of systemic interferon was given – without any effect.

### R.B. Pollard (Galveston)

Interferon has been shown to decrease the quantity of CMV shed in urine of congenitally infected babies, but very large dosages which did produce some side effects were required.

No effect on their malformations was noted as the goal was to influence shedding, and if that changed, look for changes in the basic disease process. Only at the highest dosages was a transient decrease in virus in the urine observed.

Sundmacher, R. (Hrsg.):
Herpetische Augenerkrankungen
© J.F. Bergmann Verlag, München 1981

# Histopathological Study of Adult Cytomegalic Inclusion Retino-Uveitis

Y. Masuyama, M. Fukuzaki, Y. Baba, A. Sawada, A. Sumiyoshi, Miyazaki

**Key words.** Cytomegalovirus, inclusion retino-uveitis in the adult

**Schlüsselwörter.** Cytomegalievirus – Einschluß-Retinouveitis des Erwachsenen

**Summary.** Cytomegalic inclusion disease in the adult with ocular involvement has been very rare. About 30 cases have been reported in the world up to date. The case we describe here is the first case with ocular involvement in adult cytomegalic inclusion disease and with ultrastructural confirmation of CMV particles in Japan.

A 29 year old male who suffered from systemic cytomegalic inclusion disease during treatment for Banti's syndrome, had specific retinochoroidal lesions in both eyes. The left eye was removed after death and studied with the light and electron microscope.

Marked retinal degeneration and necrosis with a large number of cytomegalic cells were found. Cytomegalic cells were also found in the epithelium of the iris and in the nonpigmented epithelium of the ciliary body, and were sporadically found in the choroid. In cytomegalic cells a large number of CMV particles of different developmental stages, were clearly demonstrated. Electron-dense round masses were seen in intranuclear inclusion bodies and dense bodies were seen in intracytoplasmic inclusion bodies. No cytomegalic cell was found in occluded retinal vessels.

**Zusammenfassung.** Über Zytomegalovirusinfektionen des Erwachsenen mit Retinitis ist bisher nur in ca. 30 Fällen in der ganzen Welt berichtet worden. Wir präsentieren hier den ersten Fall dieser Art mit elektronenmikroskopischer Bestätigung der Diagnose in Japan.

Bei einem 29jährigen Mann mit systemischer CMV-Erkrankung bei Banti-Syndrom traten beidseits die charakteristischen chorioretinalen Läsionen auf. Das linke Auge konnte nach dem Tod entfernt und mit Licht- und Elektronenmikroskopie untersucht werden.

Wir fanden eine erhebliche retinale Degeneration und Nekrose mit vielen zytomegalen Zellen. Solche Zellen wurden auch im Irisepithel und im nicht-pigmentierten Epithel des Ziliarkörpers gesehen, sehr selten auch einmal in der Chorioidea. In den zytomegalen Zellen ließen sich eindeutig große Mengen von CMV-Partikeln verschiedener Entwicklungsstufen demonstrieren. Elektronendichte runde Massen befanden sich in den intranuklearen Einschlußkörpern und dichte Körperchen in den intrazytoplasmatischen. In verschlossenen Retinagefäßen sahen wir keine zytomegalen Zellen.

## Introduction

Cytomegalic inclusion disease (CID) caused by the infection of cytomegalovirus (CMV) has been usually considered as a disease in the newborn and has rarely involved the eye. Reports on ocular involvement in adult CID have been extremely rare. About 30 cases have been reported in the world [7]. The case we report here is the first case with ocular involvement in adult CID in Japan.

In 1979 we reported the clinical course of a case of a 29-year-old male who suffered from systemic CID with ocular involvement, specific retinochoroidal lesions in both eyes during treatment for Banti's syndrome, and who finally died [7]. In histopathological study after death, marked retinal degeneration and massive necrosis with a large number of cytomegalic cells were found. Cytomegalic cells were sporadically found in the uveal tissue. In cytomegalic cells, a large number of CMV particles were clearly demonstrated under the electron microscope.

In this report we describe localization of CMV particles in ocular tissues and their various kinds of structure, and discuss the similarity between round masses in the nucleus and dense bodies in the cytoplasm.

## Clinical Course

At the first consultation in the Eye Clinic in Miyazaki Medical College Hospital, low-grade fibrinous iridocyclitis and slight vitreous opacity were found in both eyes. In the fundus, the optic disc was of yellow tone. Retinal arterioles and veins were narrowed. White sheath was found everywhere, particularly in the temporal area superior to the optic disc. There were many spots of hemorrhage and yellow-white granular exudation. Four months later, the patient died of pneumonia. At autopsy, CMV infection was found in ocular tissues as well as in the capsule of the pituitary gland, the lungs, the alimentary tract and the adrenal gland.

## Materials for Histopathological Study

Five hours after the death the left eye was removed. Materials for light microscopy were fixed in 10% formalin solution. For electron microscopy the retina and choroid in the superior temporal quadrant from the optic disc,

and the ciliary body and iris connected to them, were excised. The excised materials were fixed with 3% glutaraldehyde, post-fixed with 1% osmic acid solution, embedded in epoxy resins, sectioned by ultramicrotome, Sorvall MT-1, stained with uranium and lead, and observed by electron microscope, JEM-100 B.

## Histopathological Findings

### Retina

Under the light microscope, the retina lost its normal architecture completely, with intense degeneration and massive necrosis seen. A large number of cytomegalic cells which had inclusion bodies in the nucleus and in the cytoplasm, were found. The origin of these cytomegalic cells was uncertain except that some of them apparently originated from retinal pigment epithelial cells. Some retinal arterioles were occluded. No infiltration of these cytomegalic cells into the vitreous beyond the internal limiting membrane was seen (Fig. 1).

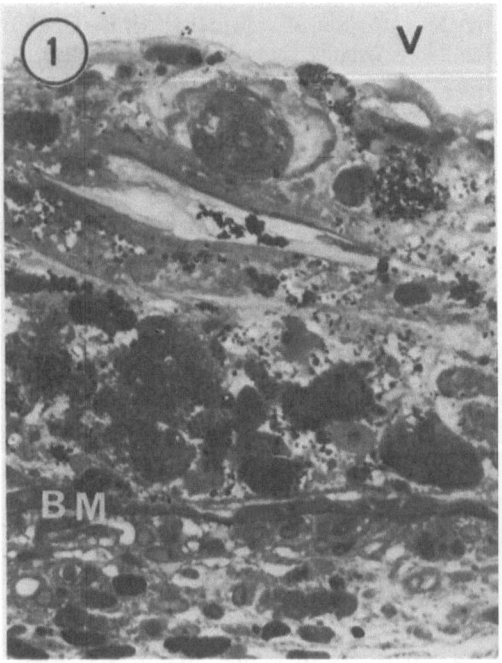
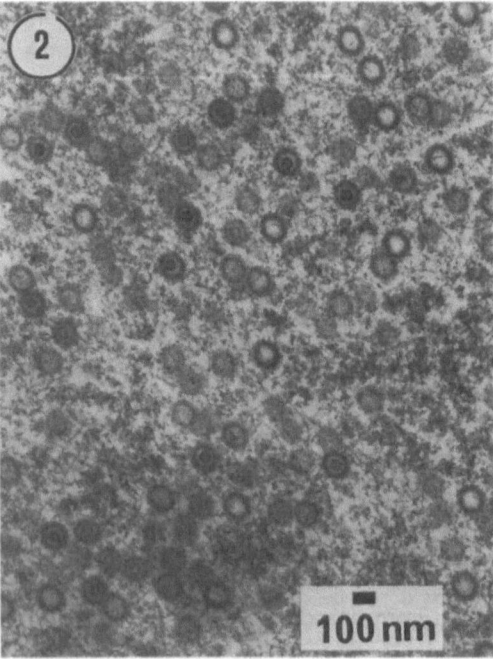

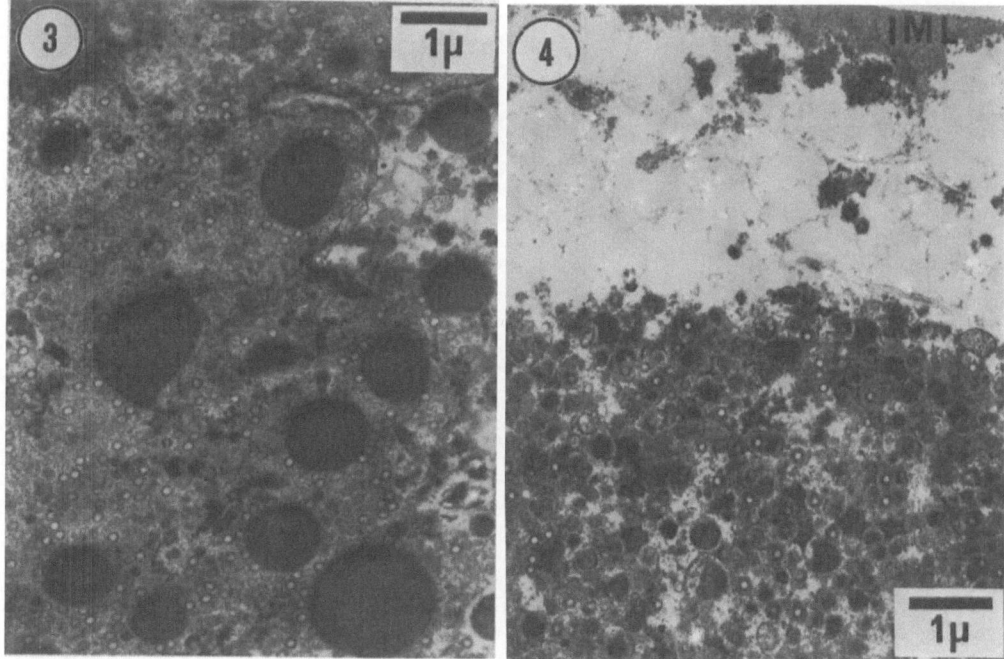

Under the electron microscope, a large number of CMV particles were seen in intranuclear inclusion bodies of infected cells. CMV particles showed different developmental stages: empty capsid, capsid with bar-like structure, and capsid with electron-lucent or electron-dense core (Fig. 2). In some cytomegalic cells, a large number of homogenous electron-dense round masses about 2 to 3 microns in diameter were seen with CMV particles in the nucleus. Sometimes there were round masses larger than 10 microns in diameter. Around these masses, many perichromatin-like granules, the size of which was almost the same as CMV particles, were seen (Fig. 3). In intracytoplasmic inclusion bodies of the cytomegalic cells, enveloped CMV particles in different developmental stages and many dense bodies surrounded by limiting membrane were observed (Fig. 4). Round masses in intranuclear inclusion bodies were apparently similar to dense bodies in intracytoplasmic inclusion bodies. However, the size of round masses was larger than that of dense bodies, although electron-density of round masses was the

same as that of dense bodies or lower (Fig. 3, 4).

In one of occluded retinal arterioles, electron microscopy revealed that endothelial cells of the vessel vanished and the vascular lumen was occluded with proliferating smooth muscle cells of the vascular wall. The basal lamina of the vessel remained (Fig. 5). No CMV particles were found in the lumen of vessels. Small calcified foci were scattered throughout the necrotic retinal tissue.

*Uvea*

Changes in the uveal tissue were generally less than those in the retina. Cytomegalic cells and infiltration of plasma cells were found in places. Cytomegalic cells were in the epithelium of the iris and in the nonpigmented epithelium of the ciliary body (Fig. 6). Cytomegalic cells were sporadically found in the choroid. They had intranuclear inclusion bodies surrounded by a clear halo in paraffin-embedded sections (Fig. 7). In Bruch's membrane no marked changes were found.

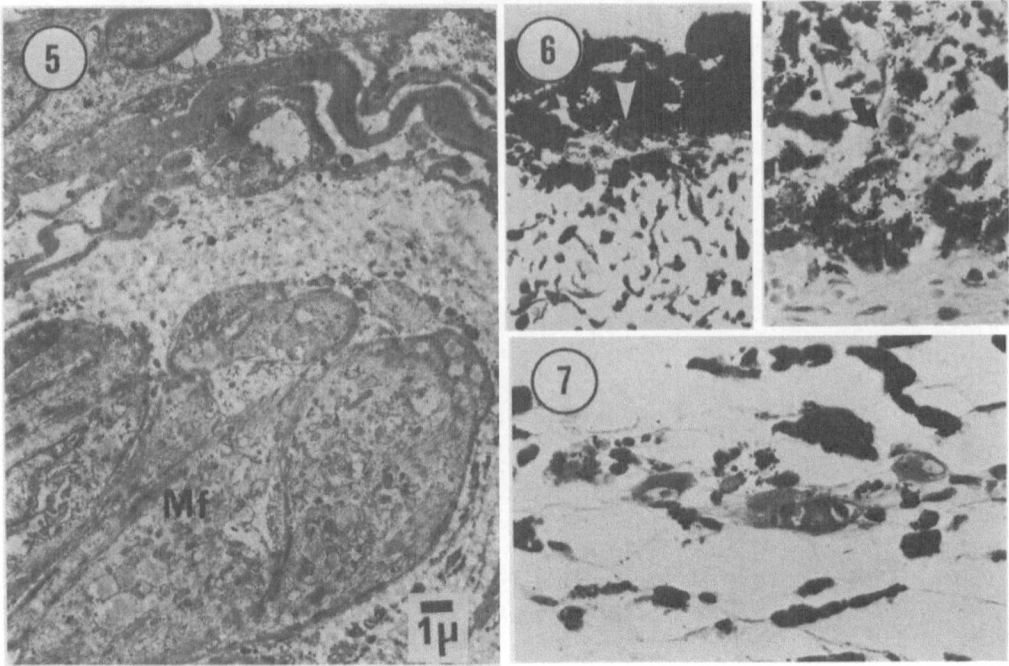

## Discussion

Recently infectious diseases by so-called opportunistic agents such as virus, fungus and Protozoa have increased, due to impairment of the defence mechanism caused by organ transplantation or immunosuppressive therapy. Virus infection, particularly with CMV is said to be the most prevalent [1, 3]. Usually CID occurs in the newborn with weak power of resistance. Ocular involvement in CID of the newborn has been frequently reported. However, ocular involvement in CID of the adult has been very infrequently reported. After Foerster [6], ocular involvements in CID of the adult have been described in only 30 cases. The case we report here is the first case in Japan.

The most characteristic clinical finding of ocular involvement in CID is exudative granular yellow-white spots and marked hemorrhage in the retina. In most cases, inflammatory changes in the anterior segments and in the vitreous were mild. The optic nerve was involved on relatively rare occasions. The

case we report here, has these clinical characteristics.

In histopathological studies, intense degeneration and massive necrosis were seen in the retina with little invasion into the vitreous (Fig. 1). Therefore, the major site of infection in the eye is thought to be the retina. These findings accord with those reported before [2, 3, 4, 5, 13, 14]. The reason why the retina was dominantly involved is possibly due to the affinity of CMV to ectodermal tissues, to which the retina belongs.

CMV produces inclusion bodies in the nucleus and in the cytoplasm. Particularly in the nucleus it produces inclusion bodies of Cowdry A type, which show characteristically so-called "owl eye" appearance with halo in paraffin-embedded sections for light microscopy (Fig. 7). On the other hand, in epoxy resins embedded sections the formation of halo was not seen under the light microscope (Fig. 1). Therefore, halo is considered as an artefact probably produced in the process of embedding [3, 4].

Under the electron microscope, a large

number of CMV particles of different developing stages were seen in intranuclear inclusion bodies (Fig. 2). Lussier et al. [8] divided murine CMV particles into three groups, empty capsid, capsid with electron-lucent core and capsid with electron-dense core, based on their different stages of the development. Besides these three kinds of CMV particles, capsid with bar-like structure and particles similar to perichromatin-like granules described by Smith et al. [12], were found. These two kinds of particles are also considered as those in the process of development. The majority of CMV particles in the cytoplasm were enveloped.

It is one characteristic of CMV infection that round masses are seen in intranuclear inclusion bodies and dense bodies are seen in intraplasmic inclusion bodies. Round masses are very similar to dense bodies except that the size of round masses is 2 to 3 times as large as that of dense bodies. Electron-density of round masses is equal or lower than that of dense bodies. Dense bodies are said to be accumulated structural polypeptides [10]. Smith et al. [12] mentioned that dense bodies appeared in the Golgi complex in the early stage of infection and round masses appeared in the nucleus later. However, there is no evidence that dense bodies and round masses have the same origin.

Retinal necrosis, characteristic of ocular involvement in CID, was said to be caused not by inflammation, but by occlusion of retinal vessels [3]. De Venecia et al. [5] speculated that retinal necrosis was coagulative necrosis resulted from thrombosis caused by CMV infection in endothelial cells, based on the recognition of cytomegalic cells in the endothelium of large retinal veins. In the case described here, histopathological study could not reveal the existence of CMV particles in retinal vessels, which were shown as white sheaths on funduscopy. However, possible concern of CMV particles with occlusion of retinal vessels can not be denied, because cytomegalic cells were found in endothelial cells of vessels in the stomach and other tissues. On the other hand, retinal arterioles occluded with proliferating smooth muscle cells of the vascular wall, were found. The finding is extremely extraordinary, because occlusion of retinal vessels usually results from glial cells, particularly Müller's cells. Yellow-white granular exudation seen in the fundus at the first visit resulted possibly from massive necrosis and calcification in the retina.

Changes in the uveal tissue in adult CID has been very limited [2, 13]. In the present study, cytomegalic cells were distinctly demonstrated in the iris, ciliary body and choroid (Fig. 6, 7). On less involvement of uveal tissue with CMV, Wyhinny et al. [14] said that choroidal involvement might be observed in an infection of longer duration, although the retina was dominantly involved. On the other hand, in experimental cytomegalovirus ophthalmitis Schwartz et al. [11] found that the uvea was dominantly affected and the retina was slightly affected. Therefore, the affinity of CMV to the uvea can not be simply and easily denied.

CMV belongs to herpes virus group. In the fundus of herpes simplex and herpes zoster infection, yellow-white granular spots similar to those in CMV infection are seen. In histopathological studies, severe necrotizing retinopathy were also shown in herpes simplex and herpes zoster infection. As one point of difference, it has been known that herpes simplex and herpes zoster involve the nervous system more frequently than CMV. However, this is nothing but a relative point of differentiation. It is not easy to differentiate these virus infections. Detection of affected cells, isolation of virus, measurement of antibody titers would be useful for the definite diagnosis.

In a histopathological study, specific cytomegalic cells seen under light microscope and dense bodies seen under electron microscope, are characteristic of CMV infection [12]. The case we describe here is fully in agreement with the above-mentioned qualification for CMV infection in ocular tissues.

## References

1. Berger BB, Weinberg RS, Tessler HH, Wyhinny GJ, Vygantas CM (1979) Bilateral cytomegalovirus panuveitis after high-dose corticosteroid therapy. Am J Ophthalmol 88:1020
2. Chumbley LC, Robertson DM, Smith TF, Campbell RJ (1975) Adult cytomegalovirus inclusion retino-uveitis. Am J Ophthalmol 80: 807
3. Cogan DG (1977) Immunosuppression and eye disease. Am J Ophthalmol 83:777
4. Cox F, Meyer D, Hughes WT (1975) Cytomegalovirus in tears from patients with normal

eyes and with acute cytomegalovirus chorioretinitis. Am J Ophthalmol 80:817

5. Venecia G de, Zu Rhein GM, Pratt MV, Kisken W (1971) Cytomegalic inclusion retinitis in an adult. Arch Ophthalmol 86:44
6. Foerster HW (1959) Uveitis symposium. Pathology of granulomatous uveitis. Surv Ophthalmol 4:296
7. Inahara M, Fukuzaki M, Masuyama Y, Kusune E (1979) Ocular involvement in adult systemic cytomegalic inclusion disease. Folia Ophthalmol Jpn 30:1312
8. Lussier G, Berthiaume L, Payment P (1974) Electron microscopy of murine cytomegalovirus: Development of the virus in vivo and in vitro. Arch Ges Virusforsch 46:269
9. Ruebner BH, Hirano T, Slusser R, Osborn J, Medearis jr DN (1966) Cytomegalovirus infection. Viral ultrastructure with particular reference to the relationship of lysosomes to cytoplasmic inclusions. Am J Pathol 48:971
10. Sarov I, Abady I (1975) The morphogenesis of human cytomegalovirus. Isolation and polypeptide characterization of cytomegalovirions and dense bodies. Virology 66:464
11. Schwartz JN, Cashwell F, Hawkins HK, Klintworth GK (1976) Necrotizing retinopathy with herpes zoster ophthalmicus. Arch Pathol Lab Med 100:386
12. Smith JD, Harven E de (1973) Herpes simplex virus and human cytomegalovirus replication in WI-38 cells. 1. Sequence of viral replication. J Virology 12:919
13. Smith ME (1964) Retinal involvement in adult cytomegalic inclusion disease. Arch Ophthalmol 72:44
14. Wyhinny GJ, Apple DJ, Guastella FR, Vygantas CM (1973) Adult cytomegalic inclusion retinitis. Am J Ophthalmol 76:773

## Discussion on the Contribution pp. 495–500

G.O.H. Naumann (Erlangen)

Was there any evidence of the inclusion in the uveal tissue or did you find it only in the epithelial ocular structures? Not in the cells of the iris stroma, not in the cornea, but only in epithelial ocular structures? I think it is important to stress this point, because as clinicians we see the retinal disease and the remarkable sparing of the choroid with the ophthalmoscope. Was it emphasized that you did not find, at least morphologically, the virus in the stroma of the uvea?

Y. Masuyama (Miyazaki)

The cytomegalic cells were seen not only in the neuroepithelial tissues, but also in the uveal tissues. Changes in the uveal tissues were generally less than those in the retina. We found no cytomegalic cells in the cornea or in the iris stroma.

Sundmacher, R. (Hrsg.):
Herpetische Augenerkrankungen
© J.F. Bergmann Verlag, München 1981

# Connatal Monosymptomatic Corneal Endotheliitis by Cytomegalovirus

R. Sundmacher, D. Neumann-Haefelin, A. Mattes, K. Cantell, Freiburg, Helsinki

**Key words.** Cytomegalovirus, endotheliitis, connatal glaucoma, ara-AMP, interferon

**Schlüsselwörter.** Cytomegalievirus, Endotheliitis, konnatales Glaukom, ara-AMP, Interferon

**Summary.** An otherwise healthy male newborn baby was seen post partum with bilaterally cloudy and enlarged corneae, and was first diagnosed to have "congenital glaucoma". The eyes were "white" and the intraocular pressure high. Intraocularly, however, some hyperemia of the iris could be seen. The corneae were swollen without major infiltrates similar to longstanding disciform edema. This led to the presumptive diagnosis of a viral corneal endotheliitis also involving the trabeculum. Virus cultures from urine, conjunctiva and acqeous humour were positive several times for cytomegalovirus. In spite of different therapeutic approaches comprising of adenine-arabinoside-monophosphate and interferon, and in spite of several attempts to lower the pressure by trabeculotomies, the disease could not be brought under control.

**Zusammenfassung.** Ein allgemeinklinisch normal erscheinendes männliches Neugeborenes fiel sofort nach der Geburt durch die vergrößerten und trüben Hornhäute auf. Zunächst dachte man, es handele sich um ein „gewöhnliches" connatales Glaukom. Die Augen waren weitgehend blaß, der intraokulare Druck war hoch. Bei der Narkoseuntersuchung fand sich aber eine deutliche Irishyperämie. Die Hornhäute waren ohne wesentliches Infiltrat geschwollen, wie man dies auch bei einer etwas länger verlaufenden Keratitis disciformis findet. Dies führte zu der Verdachtsdiagnose einer viralen Endotheliitis corneae, die auch auf das Trabekel übergegriffen und so ein Glaukom erzeugt hatte. Viruskulturen aus Urin, von der Bindehaut und aus dem Kammerwasser waren mehrfach positiv und ergaben immer Zytomegalievirus. Trotz verschiedener therapeutischer Versuche, u.a. mit Adeninarabinosid-Monophosphat und Interferon, und trotz mehrfacher Versuche, den intraokularen Druck durch Trabekulotomien zu senken, konnte die Erkrankung nicht unter Kontrolle gebracht werden.

An otherwise healthy male child was born on 30 December 1978, with bilateral corneal clouding and enlarged corneal diameters. A diagnosis of congenital hydrophthalmia was made. Two days later, the eyes were more closely investigated under general anesthesia and it was found that the diagnosis had to be corrected. The corneae were enlarged (re 12.5, le 11.5 mm) and the pressures high (re 27, le 50 mm Hg appl.); but the corneae exhibited gross stromal swelling, without infiltrates, whereas the epithelium was only slightly edematous. This reminded one more of extended disciform edema (see p 203ff) than of pressure-induced edema. Further, the iris vessels were engorged. Thus, a secondary glaucoma due to some intraocular inflammatory process also involving the endothelium seemed likely, although both eyes were mostly white (Fig. 1 was taken a few days later with the child awake and struggling,

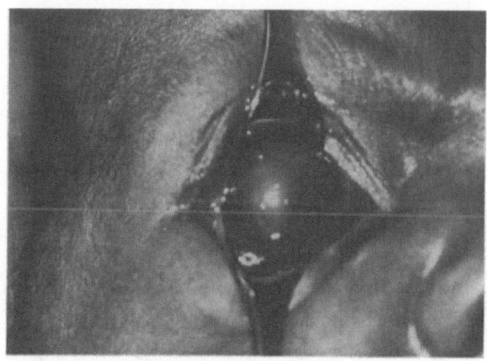

**Fig. 1.** Connatal corneal endotheliitis by cytomegalovirus; appearance 3 weeks after birth with the corneae enlarged, edematous, and moderately cloudy; severe secondary glaucoma

**Table 1.** Course of the disease

| | | 1 | 2 | 3 | 4 | 5 | 6 | 7 | 8 | 9 | 10 | 11 | 12 | 1 | 2 | 3 |
|---|---|---|---|---|---|---|---|---|---|---|---|---|---|---|---|---|
| Corneal Diameter (mm) | RE | 12,5 | | | | 13,0 | 13,5 | | | | = | = | | = | = | |
| | LE | 11,5 | | | | 12,0 | 13,0 | | | | = | = | | = | = | |
| Intraocular Pressure (mm Hg) | RE | 37 | 27 | | 50 | | 47 | | | appr. 50 | | = | | | = | |
| | LE | 50 | 33 | | 43 | | 40 | | | appr. 50 | | = | | | = | |
| CMV Isolated from | | | | | | | | | | | | | | | | |
| Aqueous Humor | RE | + | | | | + | | | | | − | | | | | |
| | LE | + | | | | − | | | | | + | | | | | |
| Conjunctiva | RE | − | | | | | | | | | − | | | | | |
| | LE | + | | | | | | | | | − | | | | | |
| Urine | | ++++++++++ | + | | + | | + | + | + | + | ++++ | + | + | + | + | + (massive) |
| Anti-CMV Serum Antibodies | | | | | | | | | | | | | | | | |
| IgM/IF | | >1:64 | | | | | 1:128 | 1:64 | | | 1:16 | | | | | |
| CBR | | 1:80 | | | | | 1:80 | 1:80 | | | 1:80 | | | | | |
| Systemic Antivirals | | Interferon (1) | | | | | | | | | Interferon (2) Ara-AMP | | | | | |
| Surgery | RE | Trabeculotomie | | | | | Trabeculotomie = | | | | Cyclodialysis | | | | | |
| | LE | | | | Trabeculotomie | | Trabeculotomie = | | | | | | | | | |
| Time Course (Months, 1979/80) | | 1 | 2 | 3 | 4 | 5 | 6 | 7 | 8 | 9 | 10 | 11 | 12 | 1 | 2 | 3 |

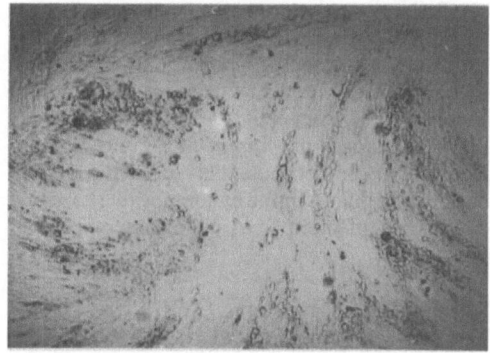

**Fig. 2.** Typical cytopathogenic effects of cytomegalovirus, derived from the acqeous humour, on human foreskin fibroblast cultures

and the conjunctiva red). A trabeculotomie was performed on the left eye under the same anesthesia (see Table 1 for a comprehensive survey of the course of the disease). A few days later, high anti-CMV-IgM serum levels were found in both, mother and child, and the child was checked intensively virologically. CMV could be isolated on many occasions from the urine, the conjunctiva, and also from the acqeous humour of both eyes (Table 1 and Fig. 2). Therefore we believe that this case represents a monosymptomatic congenital secondary glaucoma due to CMV infection. The most probable sites which were infected and led to corneal swelling and secondary glaucoma are the corneal and trabecular endothelium. Corneal involvement and glaucoma together with many other signs of severe general CMV disease have been occasionally reported. Ours seems to be the first observation of a *monosymptomatic*

**Table 2.** Details of first trial with systemic interferon therapy

Human Leucocyte Interferon i.m. for 22 days starting from 26 January 1979.
Dosage: $10^6$ units HLI every 12 hours for 3 days, thereafter $10^6$ units every day (body weight: 3 600–3 800 g)
Local therapy (each eye per day):
2 drops of Scopolamin 0.25%
3 drops of Dexamethasone 0.1%
2 drops of Timolole 0.25%
No side effects were observed; in particular, leucocytes and thrombocytes did not drop
CMV was continuously shed from the urine

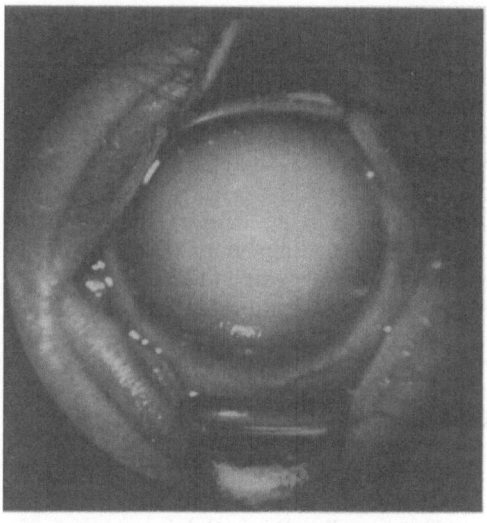

**Fig. 3.** Connatal corneal endotheliitis by cytomegalovirus; appearance 10 months after birth with both corneae already heavily scarred and persistent, therapy-resistant glaucoma

congenital anterior segment CMV disease mimicking congenital hydrophthalmia.

All surgical and medical attempts to lower the intraocular pressure and eradicate lytic CMV infection have been insufficient. Surgical interventions also had no beneficial effect whatsoever. A first interferon regime a few

**Table 3.** Details of second trial with systemic antiviral therapy consisting of interferon and Ara-AMP

Human Leukocyte Interferon i.m. plus Adeninearabinoside-Monophosphate (Ara-AMP) i.v. for 21 days starting from 24 October 1979
Dosage per day: $3 \times 10^6$ units HLI (375 000 units per kg bodyweight), 120 mg Ara-AMP (15 mg per kg bodyweight)

No local therapy

No severe side effects were observed; the leucocytes dropped, however, from 8 600 to 3 600, and the thrombocytes from 317 000 to 96 000 respectively. Also, GPT (65 mU/ml) and GOT (31-mU/ml) rose slightly. All alterations were quickly reversible after cessation of therapy.

CMV was continuously shed from the urine and the impression was that virus excretion some time after therapy was greater than before therapy. No quantitative estimations of CMV excretion, however, were performed

weeks after birth seemed to have had some positive effects, as the left cornea was less dull after than before therapy (Table 2), but this effect was only transient. A second medical attempt with a combination of Adenineara-binoside-Monophosphate and Human Leukocyte Interferon 10 months after birth, both corneae already being scarred (Fig. 3), did not affect CMV shedding, neither from the urine nor from the acqeous (Tables 1 and 3). Further therapeutic attempts have, therefore, as of yet been abandoned.

## Reference

1. Witschel H, Sundmacher R (1980) Virusendotheliitis als Ursache connataler Hornhauttrübungen. Ber Dtsch Ophthalmol Ges 77: 503–507

### Discussion on the Contribution pp. 501–504

O.P. van Bijsterveld (Utrecht)
How would you imagine that the disease spread to the baby in this case? Was it because the mother was immunosuppressed?

R. Sundmacher (Freiburg)
No, the mother was not immunosuppressed; she was apparently healthy and the delivery was normal. She must have acquired, however, asymptomatic cytomegalovirus infection some time before delivery because she had high anti-CMV IgM titers in the serum at the time of delivery.

R.B. Pollard (Galveston)
Classical CMV congenital malformations may occur only in women with primary CMV early in pregnancy. The potential for transmission exists throughout pregnancy, but we don't know for certain what changes develop in those infected at a later date. Another potential for transmission occurs when infants borne by seropositive mothers acquire the infection from genital secretions or breast milk.

R. Sundmacher (Freiburg)
We have been thinking about the first and the last possibilities, but have not found them really convincing. If it had been an infection during embryogenesis, we would expect to find malformations as you said. This was not the case. If it had been an infection in the birth canal, one should not find a well advanced disease immediately after birth. Therefore, the infection must have occurred sometime during the last trimester, and this, of course, is curious. We, too, have not come across any information concerning the infection risk during this time of gravidity and we don't know what kind of diseases may arise. Our case observation may be a first step to broaden our knowledge in this direction.

G.O.H. Naumann (Erlangen)
There is some analogy in cases of buphthalmus that were studied histopathologically where one had a suggestion of rubella disease. Here, apparently only monosymptomatic keratitis and buphthalmus were the complications of transplacental rubella infection. That's a very different virus, of course, but there are some similarities.

Sundmacher, R. (Hrsg.):
Herpetische Augenerkrankungen
© J.F. Bergmann Verlag, München 1981

# Summing-Up

R. Sundmacher, Freiburg

Mr. President, Ladies and Gentlemen,

summing-up the results of this symposium cannot mean mentioning all the facts which were presented, not even all of the most important ones. Rather, let me do it in a more general and subjective way.

When analyzing the causes which lead to any infectious disease, we can identify three of them: 1. the infecting organism, 2. the host with its natural and acquired defense mechanisms, and 3. all kinds of active exogenous factors, namely therapy. The separate topics have been presented roughly in this order, and most of the time, we have been concerned with herpes simplex virus eye diseases.

For about 50 years, we have known that HSV strains behave differently in the rabbit model, and a distinction has been made between dermatotrophic and neurotrophic strains. Also, the hypothesis that different strains are correlated with different courses of disease in patients is not new. This hypothesis, however, has not been unequivocally proven. Although it is very probable that a virus-disease correlation exists, a meaningful in vitro marker for this must still be found. Possibly, studies concentrating on the expression of different surface antigens of HSV and HSV-infected cells offer a better chance than the even more basic DNA-studies in finding such markers. More laboratories should occupy themselves with this topic because positive results will have a strong impact on our understanding of herpes pathophysiology and therapy.

The most important progress in pathophysiology has certainly been the experimental confirmation of neuronal latency. This has led to a better understanding of many things, such as "primary" disciform edema which had been previously difficult to explain. It has taught us that trials for establishing a peripheral prophylaxis of recurrences are aimed at symptoms but not at the root of the problem; and it has enormously focused our interest on the questions: What are the mechanisms which keep the virus in its latent state? What are the failures that allow a virus to escape latency control? How can we get on top of these basic events? The answers must be left open.

It may well be that a certain percentage of human beings is disposed for recurrent HSV disease by some defect in their immunosurveyance system. Some feel that the results of HLA typing – variable as they still are – point in this direction. All hypotheses, however, like defective natural killer cell activity still lack scientific proof. Although a genetic background for herpes diseases must be suspected, it should not a priori be assumed to be a defect in immunology. Other regulatory abnormalities, e.g. on the hormone level, may equally be operative.

From this it seems reasonable to me that one should be reluctant in trying vaccines in humans unless some defect in the immune system of patients has been positively demonstrated. Further, much more basic research with animal models is needed. The results obtained with some of these models are not really disappointing in all respects; the general feeling, however, is that the chances for a successful inhibition of chronic recurrent HSV disease by vaccination are not too good.

Many of our questions thus center on immunology; and here, it is not easy for us to see clinically exploitable progress. We still ponder how we can put together the many puzzle pieces and have not really surpassed the simple, though basic, statement that cellular immune reactions are more decisive in herpes immunology than antibody-mediated ones. I do not of course, say this to blame the immunologists who, without doubt, have the most difficult job of all of us, but it would certainly be useful if even more energy were spent on the development of clinical immunology concomitant with either the models that exist or with those that are being developed. A constant feedback will be instrumental in reaching clinically useful results.

Further, we should not forget that a variety of unspecific cellular and humoral responses are certainly also of importance in the pathophysiology of herpetic disease. We have heard something about this, but not enough.

Turning to therapy, it is almost trivial to state that a clear diagnosis is a prerequisite. A new classification of herpetic eye diseases based on clinico-virologic studies has been offered. Its essential is that, with the exception of so-called metaherpetic diseases all others are viral in nature. There is no hard data for immunologic herpetic disease without associated virus multiplication. Immune reactions are triggered in all viral diseases; their nature and importance, however, vary considerably and need further intensive investigation. That clinical studies may be crucial to our understanding of pathophysiology is, I feel, illustrated by the finding of herpetic endotheliitis in man. This will also help to better understand and eventually modify animal models.

For most herpetic eye diseases, antivirals should be the basic therapy. This therapy is certainly the field in which the most spectacular progress has been made.

There are now four drugs which have shown to be clinically effective against dendritic keratitis in well controlled studies. These are IDU, Ara-A, TFT and ACG – a most interesting newcomer.

Although extremely useful in the beginning of the antiviral era, IDU must now be regarded as the least effective and probably most toxic topical antiherpetic agent. Its role as a reference drug in clinical studies, which is probably due to administrational regulations, should, therefore, be reconsidered. I would favour TFT in this position at the moment because it is the most effective of the three clinically established drugs. Doing this, we would ensure that our prime criterion for acceptance of new drugs in the clinic is efficacy and not lack of side effects which also is important but may be misleading. We have to await whether or not ACG will meet or surpass the therapeutic index of topically applied TFT in the clinic. I was a little bit puzzled by the relatively high incidence of punctate lesions after topical therapy with ACG, but this will certainly be clarified soon. In other respects, however, we can be more optimistic that ACG is a big step forward. Because of its lack of toxicity on host cells it seems to be suitable for systemic application. For the first time in antiviral history, this probably announces decisive progress in the therapy of such complicated diseases as intraocular herpes, zoster and perhaps, herpes simplex encephalitis which is mostly fatal when left untreated.

The biochemical background of antiviral action is becoming clearer and clearer, now that selectivity is, for example, based on the inhibition of one or several virus-coded enzymes. I suspect, however, that our current knowledge is only the beginning of the whole story and that things will become more and more complicated. This does not preclude the hope that, one day, it will be possible to actually design a specific antiviral agent. Up to this remote day however, scientists will still have to rely on the principle of serendipity. Whether other promising antivirals – like BVDU – will be added to the club of the clinically approved has to be awaited, since controlled clinical studies have not as yet been initiated.

There is one aspect of antiviral specificity which seems to be quite important: The more specific the antivirals become, the more we must fear the development of drug resistant viral strains. Whether this theoretical assumption should now lead us to an increased application of combinations of synthetic antivirals will remain a matter of debate. With the presently available data, I would not support this, but rather call for much more intensified clinical research and supervision.

Interferon is a delicate topic for two reasons. First, it has and is being presented to the public as some kind of miracle drug against cancer and all evils of the world. Of course this is not true. Second, the availability of interferon is still limited; not because of difficulties which could not have been overcome but because the big pharmaceutical companies have only recently become seriously interested. It is probably not very wise to stir up the public too much by stressing the excellent results which have been obtained in the therapy of dendritic keratitis

506

with the combination of either debridement of TFT. Rather, we should call for the priority development of mass production of interferons by pharmaceutic companies. It is certainly a rarity that a new mode of therapy has been developed and successfully tested clinically without the pharmaceutical industries being prepared to market the product.

With this we leave medical therapy and turn to surgical therapy which also has greatly improved − maybe less as a consequence of antiviral development and more as a consequence of other achievements like diagnosis and therapy of immune reactions. There has been some debate on how important single factors really are and what therapy and prophylaxis would be necessary, but generally, I think, we are all moving in the same and hopefully the right direction.

I will not make detailed comments to zoster and cytomegalovirus diseases. You have just heard a number of excellent contributions which have offered a lot of exciting news and views. I would suggest, however, that more colleagues engage themselves with the diseases caused by these two herpes viruses. Although they are comparatively rare, the relative threat for vision seems to be higher than in herpes simplex diseases, and this is especially true if therapeutic failures are made in the acute phase of the diseases. There was probably no general agreement on all new views and suggestions; but this is mainly due to the lack of solid knowledge and time will tell what holds true.

Ladies and Gentlemen,

we have come to the end. You have been a really stimulating and cooperative audience and I would like to thank you for this. Also, I am sure you would like to join me in thanking all the technicians and residents of this clinic who, by their silent and effective work, have helped considerably to make this symposium run smoothly and − as I hope − successfully.

Sundmacher, R. (Hrsg.):
Herpetische Augenerkrankungen
© J.F. Bergmann Verlag, München 1981

# Zusammenfassung

R. Sundmacher, Freiburg

Herr Präsident, meine sehr verehrten Damen und Herren,

wenn ich jetzt versuche, ein Resümee der Symposiumsergebnisse zu ziehen, dann kann ich natürlich nicht alle Fakten erwähnen, ja nicht einmal alle wichtigen. Lassen Sie mich deshalb diese Übersicht auf eine mehr allgemeine und natürlich auch subjektive Art geben.

Analysiert man die pathogenetischen Faktoren, die zu einer Infektionskrankheit führen, so stößt man auf drei Gruppen: 1. die infizierenden Keime, 2. die natürlichen und erworbenen Abwehrmechanismen des infizierten Organismus, und 3. verschiedene exogene Faktoren, die einen Einfluß auf das Geschehen nehmen, insbesondere die Therapie. Ungefähr in der Reihenfolge dieser drei Hauptgruppen war auch unser Programm aufgebaut, und entsprechend ihrer größten Häufigkeit haben wir uns die meiste Zeit mit Augenerkrankungen beschäftigt, die durch Herpes simplex-Viren hervorgerufen werden.

Seit ungefähr 50 Jahren weiß man, daß die verschiedenen Herpes simplex-Virusstämme, die man vom Patienten isolieren kann, sich im Kaninchenmodell unterschiedlich verhalten, und man hat z.B zwischen dermatotrophen und neurotrophen Stämmen unterschieden. Auch die Hypothese, daß verschiedene Stamm-Eigenschaften mit verschiedenen Krankheitsverläufen bei Patienten korreliert sind, ist keineswegs neu. Dennoch ist es bis heute nicht zweifelsfrei gelungen, diese Hypothese zu beweisen. Obwohl wir eigentlich alle glauben, daß eine solche Virus-Erkrankungs-Korrelation besteht, kennen wir immer noch kein Kennzeichen dieser Stämme, das man im Labor bestimmen könnte und das uns dann verläßliche Auskunft über die Pathogenität des betreffenden Stammes gibt. Möglicherweise ist es erfolgversprechender, wenn man sich mehr auf die Untersuchung der Virus-codierten Antigene in Herpes simplex-Virus befallenen Zellen konzentriert als wenn man versucht, das Problem sozusagen an der Basis zu lösen, indem man nach korrelierbaren Unterschieden in der DNA-Zusammensetzung der einzelnen Stämme sucht. Es wäre wünschenswert, wenn sich mehr Laboratorien mit diesen Problemen beschäftigten, weil entsprechende Resultate natürlich erhebliche Auswirkungen auf unser Pathophysiologie-Verständnis und unsere Therapie-Vorstellungen haben könnten.

Der wichtigste Fortschritt auf dem Gebiet der Pathophysiologie war sicherlich die experimentelle Bestätigung der schon lange bestehenden neuronalen Latenz-Hypothese. Wir können jetzt viele Dinge, die zuvor vielleicht etwas schwierig zu verstehen waren, besser erklären, z.B. eine sogenannte primäre Keratitis disciformis, der nie eine Keratitis dendritica vorangegangen ist. Wegen der neuronalen Latenz des Herpes simplex-Virus ist es auch völlig klar, daß alle Versuche, eine Rezidivprophylaxe durch periphere Lokaltherapie zu treiben, nur auf Symptome, aber nicht auf die eigentliche Wurzel des Problems gerichtet sein können. Am meisten interessieren uns hierbei die Fragen: Welche Unterdrückungsmechanismen halten das Herpesvirus in seinem latenten Zustand, welche Defekte müssen auftreten, damit das Virus der Latenzkontrolle entweichen kann und wie können wir auf diese grundsätzlichen Mechanismen therapeutischen oder prophylaktischen Einfluß gewinnen? Antworten hierauf sind noch nicht gefunden worden.

Möglicherweise ist ein gewisser Prozentsatz aller Menschen durch einen Defekt im Immunüberwachungssystem zu rezidivierenden Herpes-Infektionen disponiert. Einige Autoren vertreten auf Grund der Ergebnisse der HLA-Typisierungen diese Auffassung, obwohl die Typisierungsergebnisse auffällig unterschiedlich ausfallen. Alle immunogenetischen Hypothesen entbehren bisher aber noch der wissenschaftlichen Bestätigung, so auch die Hypothese, daß ein Defekt in den natürlichen „Killerzellen" hierfür verantwortlich sein könnte. Obwohl eine genetische Disposition für rezidivierende Herpeserkrankungen ziemlich wahrscheinlich ist, bedeutet dies noch keineswegs, daß der Defekt unbedingt immunologischer Art sein muß. Andere Regelstörungen, z.B. auf dem hormonalen Sektor, könnten ebenfalls ursächlich sein.

Wenn dies aber noch derart unklar ist, erscheint es mir nicht ohne weiteres vertretbar und u.U. sogar gefährlich, wenn man ohne positiven Nachweis eines Defektes im Immunsystem von Patienten versucht, diese mit Vakzinen vor Rezidiven zu schützen. Um hierfür eine überzeugende Indikation zu haben, sollten wir über sehr viel mehr Basiswissen anhand von Tiermodellen verfügen. Die Ergebnisse, die mit einigen dieser Tiermodelle bislang erzielt wurden, sind zwar nicht sehr ermutigend, aber auch nicht in jeder Hinsicht enttäuschend. Dennoch kann man wohl sagen, daß allgemein die Erfolgsaussichten für eine erfolgreiche Rezidivprophylaxe der Herpeserkrankungen durch eine Vakzination nicht gut eingeschätzt werden.

Während also unser Denken bei entscheidenden Problemen immer wieder auf die Immunologie zurückkommt, müssen wir leider konstatieren, daß auf diesem Gebiet eigentlich nicht viel klinisch verwertbarer Fortschritt zu erkennen ist. Irgendwie befinden wir uns noch in der Situation eines Kindes, das vor einer Menge Puzzle-Stücken sitzt und diese zusammenfügen will, ohne zu wissen, wie das endgültige Bild aussehen soll. Eigentlich sind wir über die einfache, wenn auch wichtige Feststellung nicht hinausgekommen, daß zelluläre Immunreaktionen in der Herpes-Immunologie offensichtlich wichtiger als Antikörper-vermittelte Reaktionen sind. Dies sage ich natürlich nicht, um den Immunologen wehe zu tun, die zweifellos von uns allen die schwierigste Aufgabe zu lösen haben. Ich sage es in der Hoffnung, daß in Zukunft noch erheblich mehr wissenschaftliche Energie investiert wird, um die *klinische* Immunologie zu entwickeln. Ob und wie schnell man dann zu klinisch nützlichen Ergebnissen kommt, wird ganz entscheidend davon abhängen, in welchem Umfang es gelingt, die klinischen Befunde mit den bestehenden Tiermodellen zu korrelieren, bzw. neue Tiermodelle zu schaffen, die den klinischen Befunden vielleicht besser entsprechen.

Daß diese ständige Rückkoppelung zwischen Klinik und Labor für einen Erfolg unerläßlich ist, ist bisher vielleicht nicht von allen Forschergruppen hinreichend beachtet worden.

Abgesehen von immunologischen Reaktionen gibt es natürlich auch noch eine Vielfalt von unspezifischen zellulären und humoralen Reaktionen auf eine Infektion mit Herpesviren hin. Auch hierüber haben wir ein wenig gehört, sicherlich aber noch nicht genug.

Wenn wir uns jetzt der Therapie zuwenden, so ist es natürlich trivial zu sagen, daß vor der Therapie die Diagnose zu stehen hat. Hierfür wurde eine neue Klassifikation der herpetischen Augenerkrankungen zur Diskussion gestellt, die auf der Grundlage klinisch-virologischer Korrelationsstudien entwickelt wurde. Eine wesentliche Grundlage dieser Klassifikation ist die Auffassung, daß es mit Ausnahme der sogenannten metaherpetischen (= aviralen) Erkrankungen nur virale gibt. Es gibt keinen überzeugenden Beweis für die Existenz immunologischer Herpeserkrankungen ohne gleichzeitige Virusvermehrung. Immunreaktionen sind natürlich bei allen Viruserkrankungen vorhanden; ihr Ausmaß und ihre Bedeutung hingegen sind sehr verschieden und bedürfen weiterer genauerer Untersuchung.

Daß auch klinische Studien neue Anstöße für unser Pathophysiologie-Verständnis geben können, belegt, so meine ich, das Konzept von der herpetischen viralen Endotheliitis (= Keratitis disciformis). Dieses Konzept kann uns nicht nur helfen, die bestehenden Tiermodelle besser zu interpretieren, sondern wird möglicherweise auch dazu führen, daß man diese Modelle entsprechend modifiziert. Wenn die meisten Herpeserkrankungen viraler Natur sind, wie eben ausgeführt, dann sollten natürlich Virostatika zur Basistherapie gehören, und auf diesem Gebiet der Virostatika ist in letzter Zeit zweifelsohne ein immenser Fortschritt erzielt worden.

Bis jetzt sind vier Virustatika in kontrollierten Studien geprüft worden und haben sich bei der Lokaltherapie der Keratitis dendritica als wirksam erwiesen: IDU, Ara-A, TFT und ACG, eine sehr interessante Neuentwicklung.

IDU war zu Beginn der Virustatika-Ära natürlich ein ungeheuer wichtiges Medikament; inzwischen muß man aber feststellen, daß es von allen vieren das am wenigsten wirksame und wahrscheinlich auch das toxischste für die Lokaltherapie ist. Es wäre deshalb sicher auch sinnvoll, wenn man das IDU nicht mehr, wie noch häufig von den Behörden gefordert, als Referenz-Wirkstoff bei der Prüfung neuer Medikamente einsetzt. Hierfür sollte man hingegen das jeweils beste geprüfte Virustatikum nehmen, und dies ist von den drei schon länger bekannten Virustatika im Moment das TFT. Würde so verfahren und nicht immer noch auf IDU als Referenz zurückgegriffen, so wäre auch sichergestellt, daß wir bei der klinischen Prüfung neuer Medikamente unser Hauptaugenmerk auf die verbesserte Wirksamkeit richten und nicht in allererster Linie auf möglichst wenig Nebenwirkungen, was zwar sehr wichtig ist, aber bei der Medikamentenprüfung auch in die Irre führen kann. Ob das neue Mittel ACG den therapeutischen Index lokal angewandten TFT's eindeutig erreichen oder sogar übertreffen wird, bleibt noch abzuwarten. Ein wenig überrascht war ich über die Berichte, daß man nach lokaler ACG-Therapie relativ häufig eine Keratopathia punctata findet. Ob dies mit dem Wirkstoff oder der Salbengrundlage zusammenhängt, wird sich sicher bald klären. In anderer Hinsicht kann das ACG aber wahrscheinlich schon heute als ein großer Fortschritt angesehen werden: seine sehr geringe Toxizität für Wirtszellen macht es für eine systemische Anwendung geeignet. Damit zeichnet sich zum ersten Mal in der Geschichte der Virustatika-Entwicklung ein Zeitpunkt ab, zu dem es wahrscheinlich möglich sein wird, so komplizierte Krankheiten, wie schweren intraokularen Herpes und Zoster, antiviral zu behandeln; und vielleicht ist damit auch ein wichtiges Mittel gegen die Herpes simplex-Encephalitis gefunden, die häufig tödlich endet.

Die biochemischen Grundlagen der Virustatika-Wirkung, die z.B. auf der Hemmung eines oder mehrerer virus-kodierter Enzyme beruhen, sind in letzter Zeit zunehmend besser aufgeklärt worden. Man darf allerdings vermuten, daß unser heutiges Wissen erst einen kleinen Anfang darstellt und daß die Biochemie der Virustatika mit der Zeit nicht einfacher, sondern eher komplizierter werden wird. Dies schließt nicht aus, daß wir vielleicht eines Tages in der Lage sein werden, spezifisch antiviral wirksame Stoffe sozusagen auf dem Reißbrett zu entwickeln. Bis dahin wird aber ganz sicher noch sehr viel Wasser den Rhein herunterfließen und bis zu diesem fernen Tag werden sich die Wissenschaftler weiterhin bei dem Auffinden von Virustatika zu einem guten Teil auf ihren besten Helfer, den Zufall, verlassen müssen.

Ob in absehbarer Zeit noch weitere Virustatika, z. B. BVDU, das Stadium der erfolgreichen klinischen Prüfung absolvieren werden, muß abgewartet werden.

Ein Aspekt der Virustatika-Spezifität verdient noch besondere Beachtung: Je spezifischer die Virustatika werden, desto mehr müssen wir die Entwicklung von Virustatika-resistenten Virusstämmen fürchten. Ob wir auf Grund dieser vorläufig nur hypothetischen Annahme schon jetzt zu einer generellen Kombinations-Therapie mit Virustatika greifen sollten, erscheint mir vorläufig noch zweifelhaft. Auf Grund der wenigen vorliegenden Befunde wäre ich persönlich im Moment noch nicht für eine generelle Kombinationstherapie, vielmehr würde ich eine intensivere klinisch-virologische Forschung und Überwachung auf diesem Gebiet befürworten.

Über Interferon spreche ich aus zwei Gründen eigentlich gar nicht so gern. Zum einen wird es in der Öffentlichkeit häufig als eine Art Wunder-Mittel gegen Krebs und alle möglichen anderen schweren Erkrankungen angepriesen. Dies ist natürlich überhaupt nicht haltbar. Der zweite Grund ist, daß Interferon heute immer noch kaum in größeren Mengen zu bekommen ist; dies nicht deshalb, weil es unmöglich wäre, die Produktionsschwierigkeiten zu lösen, sondern wahrscheinlich in erster Linie, weil sich die großen pharmazeutischen Konzerne erst in allerjüngster Zeit wirklich ernsthaft mit dem Problem der Massenherstellung befassen. Ich würde es vorziehen, die wirklich ausgezeichneten Therapieergebnisse, die wir z.B. bei der Keratitis dendritica mit Interferon + Thermoabrasio bzw. Interferon +

TFT erzielt haben, nicht an die allzu große Glocke zu hängen, solange Interferon nicht allgemein erhältlich ist. Vielmehr sollten wir darauf drängen, daß endlich hinreichende Mengen von Interferon von der pharmazeutischen Industrie produziert werden. Es dürfte schon selten vorkommen, daß ein neues Präparat erfolgreich klinisch getestet wurde, ohne daß die pharmazeutische Industrie vorbereitet ist, es auch zu vermarkten. Meist ist es ja eher umgekehrt.

Damit verlassen wir die medikamentöse Therapie des Herpes und wenden uns der chirurgischen Therapie zu, bei der ebenfalls erhebliche Fortschritte zu verzeichnen sind – vielleicht weniger in der Folge der Virustatika-Entwicklung als vielmehr in der Folge anderer Fortschritte, wie z.B. der Diagnose und Therapie von Immunreaktionen. Wir waren uns nicht ganz einig, wie wichtig die einzelnen postoperativen Störungen eigentlich sind und welche Therapie und Prophylaxe angewandt werden solle; im allgemeinen bestand aber erstaunlich viel Konsens und ich glaube, daß wir uns letztlich alle in dieselbe Richtung bewegen.

Zu den Zoster- und Zytomegalievirus-erkrankungen möchte ich jetzt nicht viel sagen, da Sie gerade eine Reihe ausgezeichneter Beiträge mit interessanten Neuigkeiten und Perspektiven gehört haben. Auch hinsichtlich dieser beiden Erkrankungskreise wäre es sicher wünschenswert, wenn sich mehr Ophthalmologen und Basiswissenschaftler mit ihnen beschäftigten. Obwohl sie seltener sind als die Herpes simplex-Viruserkrankungen, bedrohen sie doch das Sehvermögen in ungleich höherem Maße, und dies ist besonders dann der Fall, wenn in der akuten Erkrankungsphase diagnostische und/oder therapeutische Fehler gemacht werden. Auch bei verschiedenen Aspekten zu diesen Erkrankungen bestand keine generelle Einigkeit; aber dies beruhte im wesentlichen darauf, daß wir noch zu wenig gesichertes Wissen haben.

Meine sehr verehrten Damen und Herren,

damit sind wir am Ende dieses Symposiums. Für Ihre sehr anregende und hilfreiche Teilnahme möchte ich Ihnen ganz herzlich danken, und ich bin mir sicher, daß auch Sie jetzt gern mit mir zusammen all den Helfern und Assistenten dieser Klinik danken möchten, die durch ihre lautlose und effektive Arbeit hinter den Kulissen ganz entscheidend dazu beigetragen haben, daß dieses Symposium so glatt, und wie ich hoffe, auch erfolgreich verlaufen konnte.

Sundmacher, R. (Hrsg.):
Herpetische Augenerkrankungen
© J.F. Bergmann Verlag, München 1981

# Closing Remarks

W. Böke, Kiel, Erster Vorsitzender der Deutschen Ophthalmologischen Gesellschaft

Ladies and Gentlemen,

I would like to apologize for taking your time once more, but I think we should not close the symposium without some closing remarks from the President of the German Ophthalmological Society. On behalf of the Society I would like to thank you again for coming here. We are very pleased that so many experts from all over the world have been able to attend and have stimulated the discussions so much. I am sure that this symposium will be remembered as a highly successful one, at any rate, I was told so by many of the participants. However, only a minor part of the credit goes to the German Ophthalmological Society, although we have welcomed and supported this meeting. The major part of the credit goes to Dr. Sundmacher. Everyone who has arranged and organized a symposium of this magnitude knows about the tremendous amount of work which has to be done in order to prepare and carry it out. I am sure all of the participants truly appreciate what you have done, Dr. Sundmacher, for making this meeting possible. I would like to congratulate you on behalf of both our society and the participants.

I think we should also thank our host, Professor Mackensen, who has not only made the facilities of this hospital available to us, but who has also greatly supported Dr. Sundmacher and his co-workers in arranging this symposium.

Last, but not least, I would like to thank all those who have been working behind the scenes: the secretaries, the projectionists, and all the others who have helped. They have done an excellent job and have contributed quite a lot to the success of this meeting. Well, now we will officially close the symposium on ocular herpetic diseases. I hope you have enjoyed being with us and that you will come again to join the German Ophthalmological Society in the not too distant future. Thank you very much. Good bye. Auf Wiedersehen.

# List of Authors and Discussion Participants

(The page numbers of the contributions are printed semi-bold, those of the discussions in roman type.
Die Seitenzahlen der Beiträge sind halbfett, die der Diskussionen gewöhnlich gesetzt.)

# Index and Key Words

(The page numbers of the contributions are printed in roman type, those of the discussions semi-bold.
Die Seitenzahlen der Beiträge sind gewöhnlich, die der Diskussionen halbfett gesetzt.)

# Verzeichnis der Schlüsselwörter

A. H. Chignell
## Retinal Detachment Surgery
1980. 50 figures. X, 166 pages
Cloth DM 64,–. ISBN 3-540-09475-X

G. Eisner
## Augenchirurgie
Einführung in die operative Technik
Einleitung: P. Niesel
Zeichnungen: P. Schneider
1978. 343 Abbildungen. XII, 184 Seiten
Gebunden DM 132,–. ISBN 3-540-08371-5

S. N. Hassani
## Real Time Ophthalmic Ultrasonography
In collaboration with R. L. Bard
1978. 423 figures. XXI, 214 pages
Cloth DM 76,–. ISBN 3-540-90318-6

## Intraokularer Fremdkörper und Metallose
Internationales Symposium der Deutschen Ophthalmologischen Gesellschaft vom 30. März bis 2. April 1976 in Köln
Herausgeber: H. Neubauer, W. Rüssmann, H. Kilp
1977. 229 Abbildungen, 70 Tabellen. XVI, 470 Seiten
(73 Seiten in Englisch, 17 Seiten in Französisch)
DM 98,–. J. F. Bergmann Verlag, München
ISBN 3-8070-0301-0

## Ionisierende Strahlen in der Augenheilkunde
(Deutsche Ophthalmologische Gesellschaft, Bericht über die 76. Zusammenkunft in Düsseldorf 1978)
Redigiert von W. Jaeger
1979. 539 Abbildungen, 183 Tabellen. XIV, 916 Seiten
DM 208,–. J. F. Bergmann-Verlag, München
ISBN 3-8070-0308-8

## Kunststoffimplantate in der Ophthalmologie
(Deutsche Ophthalmologische Gesellschaft, Bericht über die 75. Zusammenkunft in Heidelberg, 1977)
Redigiert von W. Jaeger
1978. 601 Abbildungen, 111 Tabellen. XIII, 717 Seiten
DM 198,–. J. F. Bergmann-Verlag, München
ISBN 3-8070-0304-5

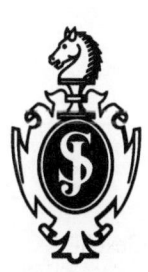

Springer-Verlag
Berlin
Heidelberg
New York

W. Leydhecker

## Manual der Tonographie für die Praxis

1977. 84 Abbildungen, 4 Tabellen, 2 Ausklapptafeln.
VII, 115 Seiten. (Kliniktaschenbücher)
DM 22,80. ISBN 3-540-08093-7

W. Leydhecker

## Die Glaukome in der Praxis

Ein Leitfaden
3., völlig neubearbeitete Auflage. 1979. 64 Abbildungen,
6 Tabellen. XII, 216 Seiten. (Kliniktaschenbücher)
DM 21,–. ISBN 3-540-09184-X

G. O. H. Naumann

## Pathologie des Auges

Unter Mitarbeit von J. D. Apple sowie D. von Domarus,
E. N. Hinzpeter, K. W. Ruprecht, H. E. Völcker und
L. R. Naumann
1980. 546 Abbildungen in 1003 Einzeldarstellungen, davon
115 zweifarbige schematische Skizzen, 1 Farbtafel,
188 differentialdiagnostische Tabellen. XLIX, 994 Seiten
(Spezielle pathologische Anatomie, Band 12)
Gebunden DM 680,–
Subskriptionspreis gültig bei Abnahme des Gesamtwerks
DM 544,–. ISBN 3-540-09209-9

## Plastische Chirurgie der Lider und Chirurgie der Tränenwege

(Deutsche Ophthalmologische Gesellschaft, Bericht über die
77. Zusammenkunft in Heidelberg 1979)
Redigiert von W. Jaeger
1980. 716 Abbildungen, 151 Tabellen. XXXIII, 1049 Seiten
DM 230,–. J. F. Bergmann-Verlag, München
ISBN 3-8070-0321-5

## Therapie in der Augenheilkunde

Herausgeber: H. Pau
Unter Mitarbeit zahlreicher Fachwissenschaftler
1977. 3 Abbildungen, 9 Tabellen. XIX, 279 Seiten
Gebunden DM 68,–. ISBN 3-540-08320-0

## Wundheilung des Auges und ihre Komplikationen

Symposium der Deutschen Ophthalmologischen Gesell-
schaft vom 30. März bis 1. April 1979
Herausgeber: G. O. H. Naumann, B. Gloor
1980. 277 Abbildungen in 377 Teilbildern, 33 Tabellen.
XVII, 468 Seiten. (39 Seiten in Englisch, 3 Seiten in
Französisch)
DM 118,–. J. F. Bergmann-Verlag, München
ISBN 3-8070-0320-7

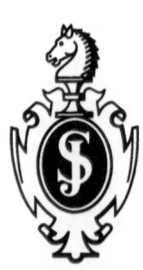

Springer-Verlag
Berlin
Heidelberg
New York